Johannes W. Rohen
Chihiro Yokochi
Elke Lütjen-Drecoll

# Anatomy:
# A Photographic Atlas

Eighth Edition

Coeditions in 20 Languages

Johannes W. Rohen
Chihiro Yokochi
Elke Lütjen-Drecoll

# Anatomy:
# A Photographic Atlas

## Eighth Edition

with 1209 Figures,
1096 in Color,
and 113 Radiographs, CT, and MRI Scans

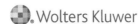

. Wolters Kluwer

Philadelphia · Baltimore · New York · London
Buenos Aires · Hong Kong · Sydney · Tokyo

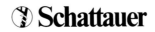

Schattauer

**Prof. Dr. med. Dr. med. h.c. Johannes W. Rohen**
Anatomisches Institut II der Universität Erlangen-Nürnberg
Universitätsstraße 19, 91054 Erlangen, Germany

**Chihiro Yokochi, M.D.**
Professor emeritus, Department of Anatomy
Kanagawa Dental College, Yokosuka, Kanagawa, Japan
Correspondence to:
Prof. Chihiro Yokochi, c/o Igaku-Shoin Ltd., 1-28-23 Hongo,
Bunkyo-ku Tokyo 113-8719, Japan

**Prof. Dr. med. Elke Lütjen-Drecoll**
Anatomisches Institut II der Universität Erlangen-Nürnberg
Universitätsstraße 19, 91054 Erlangen, Germany

8th edition

9  8  7  6  5  4  3  2  1

Printed in Germany

Cataloging-in-Publication Data available on request from publisher.
ISBN: 978-1-4511-9318-3

LWW.com

# Preface to the Eighth Edition

The knowledge of the structure and topography of the various organs of the human body is a prerequisite not only for the education of medical students but also for everyone involved in diagnostic and therapy of human diseases. This knowledge can optimally be gained by dissection of the human body, with an excellent atlas by one's side. Today there exist a number of good anatomic atlases, but most of them contain mainly schematic drawings, which minimally reflect reality. In contrast, the photographs of the actual anatomic specimens have the advantage of conveying the reality of the object with its proportions and spatial dimensions in a more accurate manner.

On the other hand, schematic drawings help us to better understand the photos. Therefore, in this eighth edition, the number of drawings has greatly been increased and old drawings have been replaced by new ones specifically adapted to their accompanying photos.

The didactic purpose of this atlas is not only to help the student understand the topography of the human body. We also hope to provide a way to systematically learn the anatomical structures and functions. Therefore, the chapters of regional anatomy are consequently placed behind a systematic description of the anatomical structures – e.g., before dissecting an extremity, the student can study the systematic anatomy of the involved bones, joints, muscles, nerves, and vessels.

The correlations between clinical images like MRI and CT scans can best be learned if sections of scans can be directly compared with cadaveric anatomical sections of the same region. In this edition, a number of MRI scans have been added that have been taken in a plane of the related anatomical section. In addition, functional MRI scans of the heart and the related anatomical preparations are included, hopefully increasing the importance of the atlas for clinical purposes.

While preparing this new edition, the authors were reminded of how precisely, beautifully, and admirably the human body is constructed. If this book helps the student or physician to appreciate the overwhelming beauty of the anatomical architecture of these tissues and organs, then it greatly fulfills its task. Deep interest and admiration of these anatomical structures may create the "love for the human being," which unhesitatingly becomes the inspiration to pursue the vocation of medicine.

Erlangen, Germany; Spring 2015

**J. W. Rohen**
**C. Yokochi**
**E. Lütjen-Drecoll**

## Acknowledgments

The preparations of the anatomical specimens shown in this atlas were time consuming and required profound knowledge. Therefore, all were prepared by anatomists or surgeons. The majority were prepared by the authors and coworkers either in the Department of Anatomy in Erlangen or in the Department of Anatomy, Kanagawa, Dental College in Tokyo. We would like to express our great gratitude to Prof. S. Nagashima, Prof. K. Okamoto, and Dr. M. Takahashi (all Japan) who worked for extended periods in Germany in the Department of Anatomy in Erlangen, and to Dr. K. Schmidt, Dr. G. Lindner-Funk (both Nuremberg), Dr. M. Rexer (Fürth), R.M. Mc Donnell (Dallas, USA), and Mr. J. Bryant (Erlangen) for dissecting specimens with great skill and knowledge.

We are also greatly indebted to Mr. H. Sommer (SOMSO Co., Coburg, Germany) who kindly provided a number of excellent bone specimens.

All the excellent macro photos of specimens newly included in this eighth edition, most notably those of the skeletal system and of the heart, were contributed by our photographer Mr. M. Gößwein, to whom we express our great gratitude.

Most important for this new eighth edition was the work of our artist Mr. J. Pekarsky. He created many new drawings specifically adapted to the photos in this edition and revised most of the old ones. We express our many thanks to him for his most excellent and time consuming work.

We are greatly indebted to our coworkers from the Department of Radiology, especially Prof. M. Uder and his colleagues (Erlangen) who took the time to perform MRI scans specifically adapted to specimens in our atlas and who added scans to the heart chapter that significantly improved our ability to elucidate the functional aspects of this organ. Also, we extend our thanks to Prof. W. J. Huk and Prof. W. Bautz (both Erlangen), Prof. A. Heuck (Munich), and Dr. Wieners (Berlin) for their excellent MRI and CT scans.

In addition, we express our many thanks to our secretary Mrs. L. Koehler for her untiring and excellent cooperation and to Dr. C. Sims-O'Neil for her careful corrections of the proofs of the new edition.

Finally, we gratefully acknowledge the head of our publisher (Schattauer Verlag, Stuttgart) Mr. D. Bergemann and his coworkers, particularly Mrs. E. Wallstein, who prepared the final layout of the Atlas and worked intensely together with the authors on the new structure of this edition.

# Preface to the First Edition

Today there exist any number of good anatomic atlases. Consequently, the advent of a new work requires justification. We found three main reasons to undertake the publication of such a book.

First of all, most of the previous atlases contain mainly schematic or semischematic drawings, which often reflect reality only in a limited way; the third dimension, i.e., the spatial effect, is lacking. In contrast, the photo of the actual anatomic specimen has the advantage of conveying the reality of the object with its proportions and spatial dimensions in a more exact and realistic manner than the "idealized," colored "nice" drawings of most previous atlases. Furthermore, the photo of the human specimen corresponds to the student's observations and needs in the dissection courses. Thus he has the advantage of immediate orientation by photographic specimens while working with the cadaver.

Secondly, some of the existing atlases are classified by systemic rather than regional aspects. As a result, the student needs several books each supplying the necessary facts for a certain region of the body. The present atlas, however, tries to portray macroscopic anatomy with regard to the regional and stratigraphic aspects of the object itself as realistically as possible. Hence it is an immediate help during the dissection courses in the study of medical and dental anatomy.

Another intention of the authors was to limit the subject to the essential and to offer it didactically in a way that is self-explanatory. To all regions of the body we added schematic drawings of the main tributaries of nerves and vessels, of the course and mechanism of the muscles, of the nomenclature of the various regions, etc. This will enhance the understanding of the details

seen in the photographs. The complicated architecture of the skull bones, for example, was not presented in a descriptive way, but rather through a series of figures revealing the mosaic of bones by adding one bone to another, so that ultimately the composition of skull bones can be more easily understood.

Finally, the authors also considered the present situation in medical education. On one hand there is a universal lack of cadavers in many departments of anatomy, while on the other hand there has been a considerable increase in the number of students almost everywhere. As a consequence, students do not have access to sufficient illustrative material for their anatomic studies. Of course, photos can never replace the immediate observation, but we think the use of a macroscopic photo instead of a painted, mostly idealized picture is more appropriate and is an improvement in anatomic study over drawings alone.

The majority of the specimens depicted in the atlas were prepared by the authors either in the Dept. of Anatomy in Erlangen, Germany, or in the Dept. of Anatomy, Kanagawa Dental College, Yokosuka, Japan. The specimens of the chapter on the neck and those of the spinal cord demonstrating the dorsal branches of the spinal nerves were prepared by Dr. K. Schmidt with great skill and enthusiasm. The specimens of the ligaments of the vertebral column were prepared by Dr. Th. Mokrusch, and a great number of specimens in the chapter of the upper and lower limb was very carefully prepared by Dr. S. Nagashima, Kurume, Japan.

Once again, our warmest thanks go out to all of our coworkers for their unselfish, devoted and highly qualified work.

Erlangen, Germany; Spring 1983

**J. W. Rohen**
**C. Yokochi**

# Contents

## 1 General Anatomy $\qquad$ 1

## 2 Head and Neck $\qquad$ 19

### 2.1 Skull _____ 20

### 2.2 Masticatory Apparatus and Muscles of the Head _____ 53

# 2  Head and Neck

# 3 Trunk    189

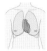

# 4 Thoracic Organs    251

# 5 Abdominal Organs    299

# 6 Retroperitoneal Organs    333

## 7 Upper Limb    380

## 8 Lower Limb    446

## Index _____ 517

# 1 General Anatomy

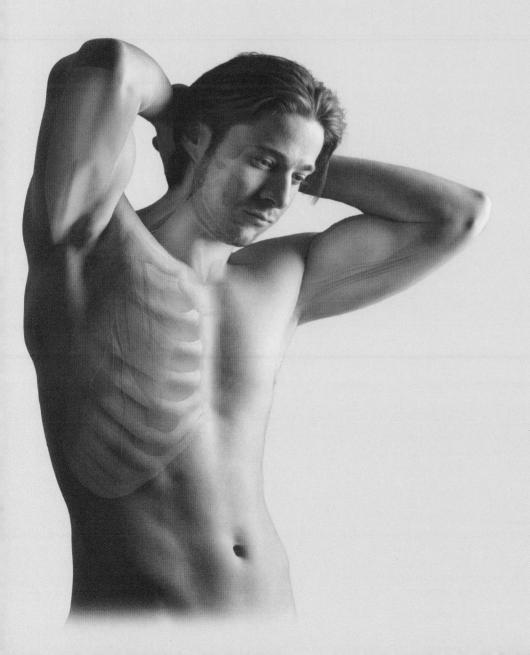

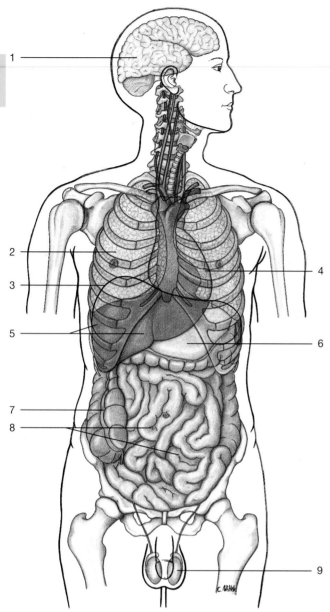

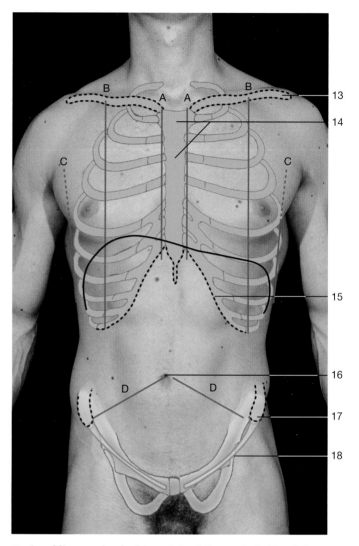

**Position of the inner organs of the human body** (anterior aspect). The main cavities of the body and their contents.

**Regional lines and palpable points at the ventral side of the human body.**

**Regional lines**
A = Parasternal line
B = Midclavicular line
C = Anterior axillary line
D = Umbilical-pelvic line

The bones of the skeletal system are palpable through the skin at different points. This enables physicians to localize the inner organs. On the **ventral side,** the clavicle, sternum, ribs, and intercostal spaces are palpable. Furthermore, the anterior iliac spine and the symphysis can be localized. For better orientation, several **lines of orientation** are used, e.g., the parasternal line, the midclavicular line, the anterior axillary line, the umbilical-pelvic line.

By means of these lines, the heart and the position of the vermiform process can be localized.

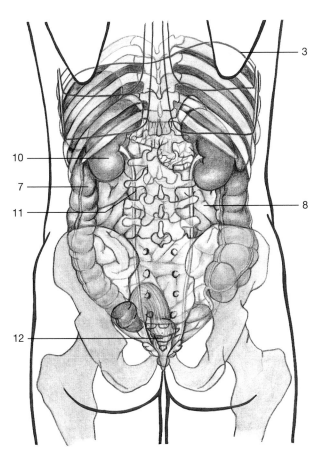

**Position of the inner organs of the human body** (posterior aspect).

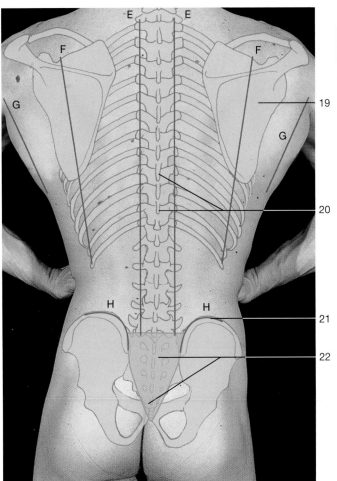

**Regional lines and palpable points at the dorsal side of the human body.**

**Regional lines**
E = Paravertebral line
F = Scapular line
G = Posterior axillary line
H = Iliac crest

1  Brain
2  Lung
3  Diaphragm
4  Heart
5  Liver
6  Stomach
7  Colon
8  Small intestine
9  Testis
10  Kidney
11  Ureter
12  Anal canal
13  Clavicle
14  Manubrium sterni
15  Costal arch
16  Umbilicus
17  Anterior superior iliac spine
18  Inguinal ligament
19  Scapular spine
20  Spinous processes
21  Iliac crest
22  Coccyx and sacrum

At the **dorsal side** of the body, the posterior spines of the vertebral column, the ribs, the scapula, the sacrum, and the iliac crest are palpable. **Lines of orientation** are the paravertebral line, the scapular line, the posterior axillary line, and the iliac crest.

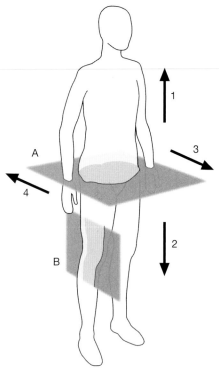

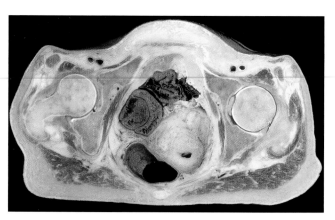

Horizontal section through the pelvic cavity and the hip joints.

**Planes of the body:**
A = Horizontal or axial or transverse plane
B = Sagittal plane (at the level of the knee joint)

**Directions:**
1 = Cranial          3 = Anterior (ventral)
2 = Caudal          4 = Posterior (dorsal)

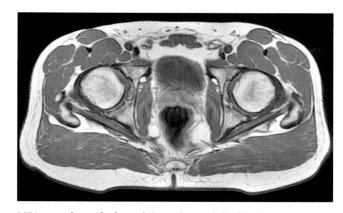

**MRI scan through the pelvic cavity and the hip joints** (horizontal or axial or transverse plane).

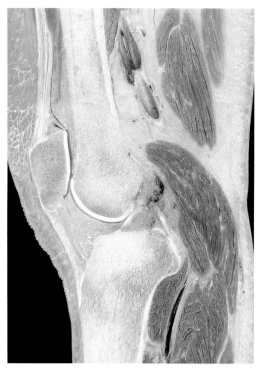

**Sagittal section through the knee joint.**

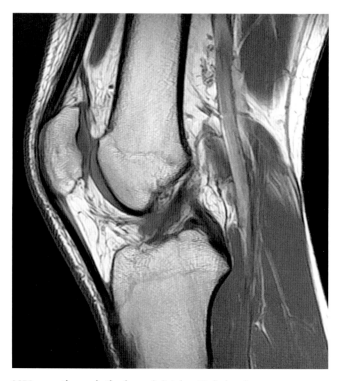

**MRI scan through the knee joint** (sagittal plane).

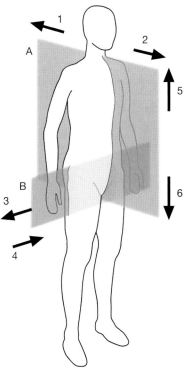

**Planes of the body:**
A = Midsagittal or median plane
B = Frontal or coronal plane (through the pelvic cavity)

**Directions:**
1 = Posterior (dorsal)    4 = Medial
2 = Anterior (ventral)    5 = Cranial
3 = Lateral               6 = Caudal

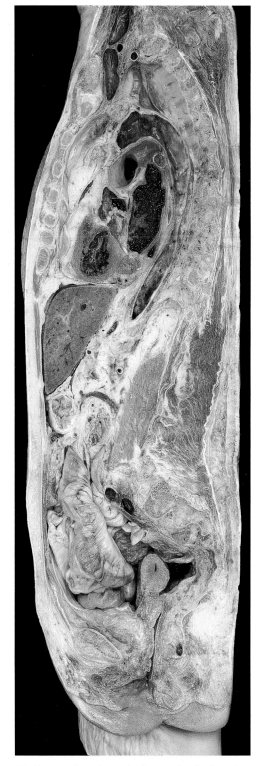

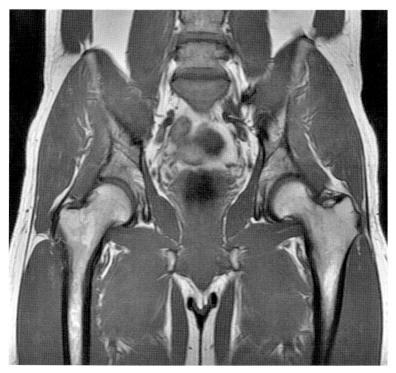

**MRI scan through the pelvic cavity and the hip joints** (frontal or coronal plane).

**Median section through the trunk of a female.**

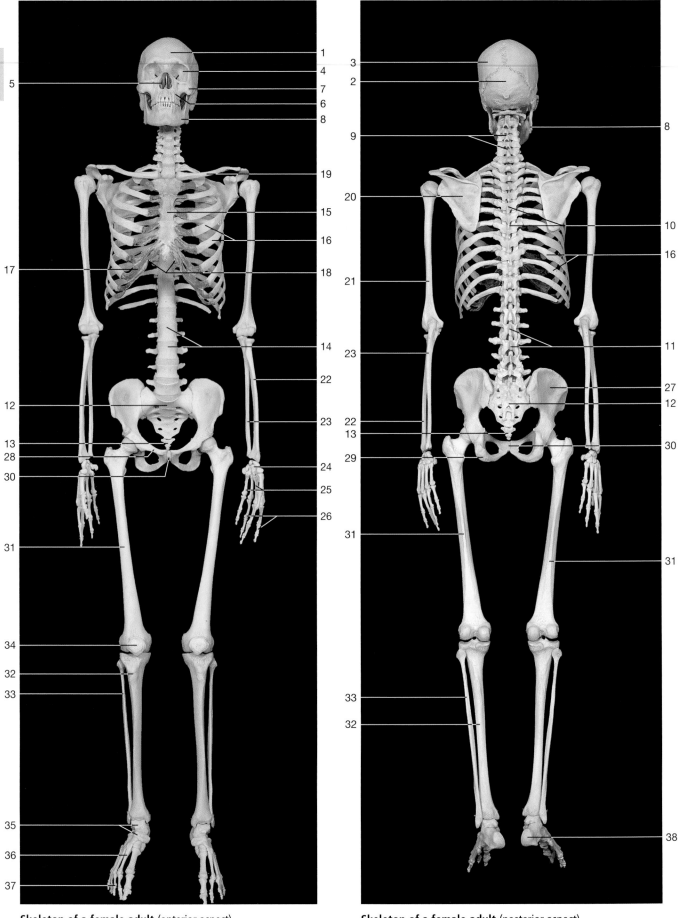

**Skeleton of a female adult** (anterior aspect).

**Skeleton of a female adult** (posterior aspect).

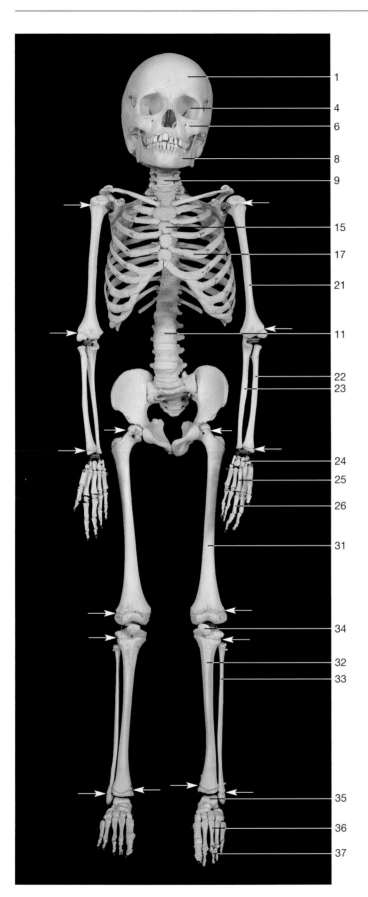

## Axial skeleton
### Head
1 Frontal bone
2 Occipital bone
3 Parietal bone
4 Orbit
5 Nasal cavity
6 Maxilla
7 Zygomatic bone
8 Mandible

### Trunk and thorax
#### Vertebral column
 9 Cervical vertebrae
10 Thoracic vertebrae
11 Lumbar vertebrae
12 Sacrum
13 Coccyx
14 Intervertebral discs
#### Thorax
15 Sternum
16 Ribs
17 Costal cartilage
18 Infrasternal angle

## Appendicular skeleton
### Upper limb and shoulder girdle
19 Clavicle
20 Scapula
21 Humerus
22 Radius
23 Ulna
24 Carpal bones
25 Metacarpal bones
26 Phalanges of the hand

### Lower limb and pelvis
27 Ilium
28 Pubis
29 Ischium
30 Symphysis pubis
31 Femur
32 Tibia
33 Fibula
34 Patella
35 Tarsal bones
36 Metatarsal bones
37 Phalanges of the foot
38 Calcaneus

**Skeleton of a 5-year-old child** (anterior aspect).
The zones of the cartilaginous growth plates are seen (arrows).
In contrast to the adult, the ribs show a predominantly
horizontal position.

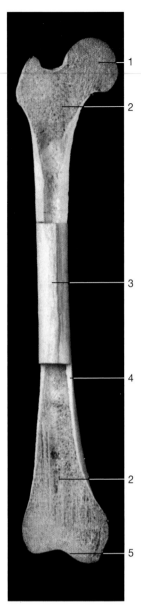

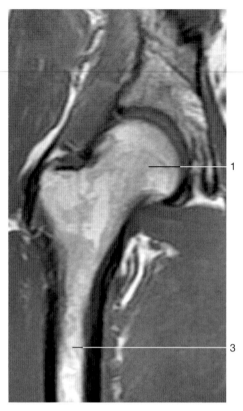

**MRI scan of the right femur and hip joint** (coronal section). (From Heuck et al., MRT-Atlas, 2009.)

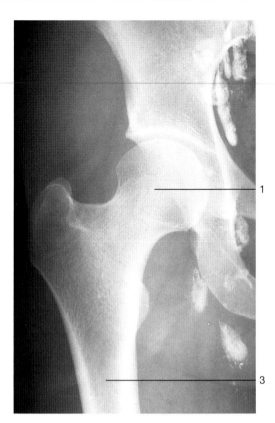

**X-ray of the right femur and hip joint** (a.-p. direction).

◁ **Femur of the adult.** Coronal section of the proximal and distal epiphyses displaying the spongy bone and the medullary cavity.

1   Head of the femur
2   Spongy bone
3   Diaphysis of the femur
4   Compact bone
5   Articular cartilage

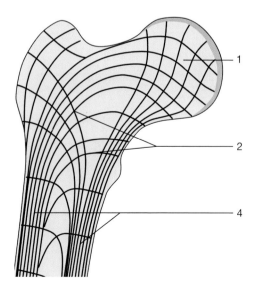

**Three-dimensional representation on the trajectorial lines of the femoral head.**

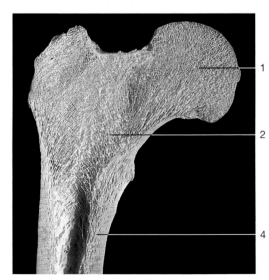

**Coronal section through the proximal end of the adult femur** showing the characteristic structure of the spongy bone.

The **ossification of the bones** of the limbs starts within the ossification centers of the primary cartilagenous bones. Here, the medullary cavity develops. The ossification process of limb bones is not finished at birth.

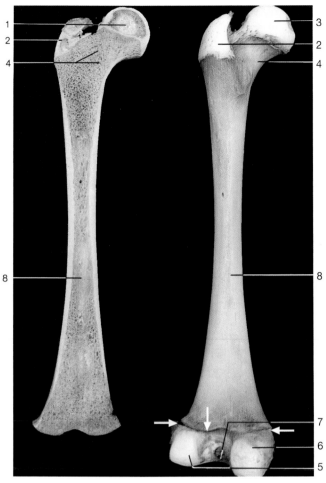

◁ 1  Ossification center
     in the head of the femur
  2  Greater trochanter
  3  Head of the femur
  4  Neck of the femur

  5  Lateral condyle
  6  Medial condyle
  7  Intercondylar notch
  8  Diaphysis

**Ossification of the femur** (left: coronal section, right: posterior aspect of the femur). Arrows: distal epiphysis.

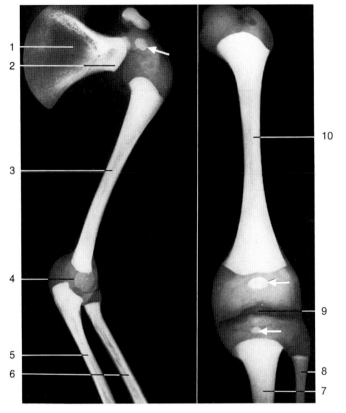

**X-ray of the upper and lower limb of a newborn child** (left: upper limb, right: lower limb). Arrows: ossification centers.

  1  Scapula
  2  Shoulder joint
  3  Humerus
  4  Elbow joint
  5  Ulna

  6  Radius
  7  Tibia
  8  Fibula
  9  Knee joint
 10  Femur

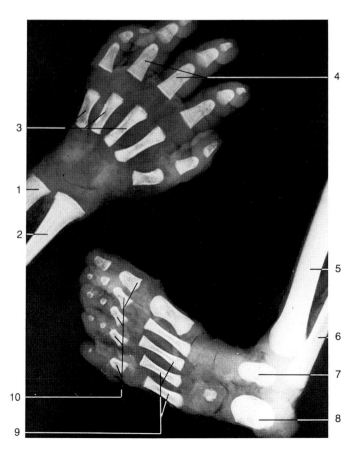

◁ 1  Ulna
  2  Radius
  3  Metacarpal bones
  4  Phalanges
  5  Tibia

  6  Fibula
  7  Talus
  8  Calcaneus
  9  Metatarsal bones
 10  Phalanges

**X-ray of hand and foot of a newborn.**

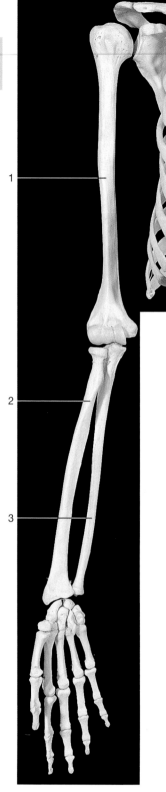

**Skeleton of the arm and shoulder girdle** (anterior aspect).

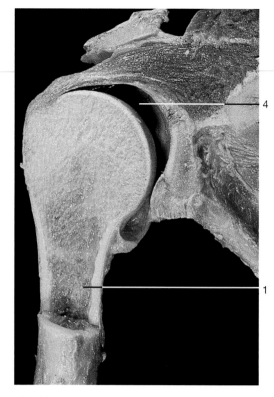

**Shoulder joint** as an example of a multiaxial ball-and-socket joint (coronal section).

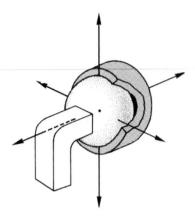

**Ball-and-socket joint** with its different axes. Arrows: axes of movement.

1 Humerus
2 Radius
3 Ulna
4 Articular cavity (shoulder joint)
5 Metacarpophalangeal joint
6 Joints of fingers

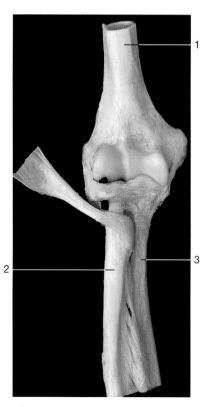

**Elbow joint with ligaments** as an example of a hinge joint (monaxial humero-ulnar joint) in combination with a pivot joint (monaxial radio-ulnar joint), which allows rotation.

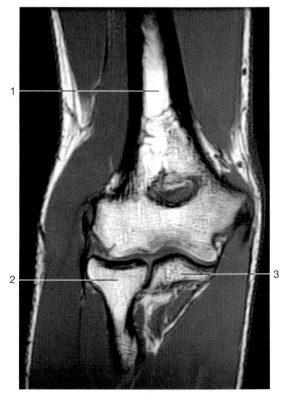

**Coronal section through the elbow joint** (MRI scan). (Courtesy of Prof. Heuck, Munich, Germany.) The possibilities of movement are shown in the schematic drawings on page 11.

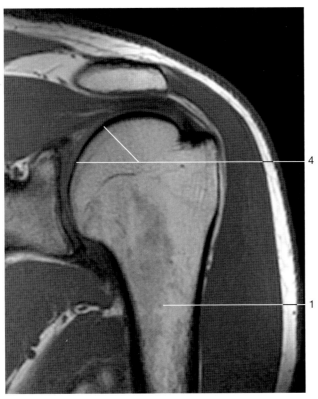

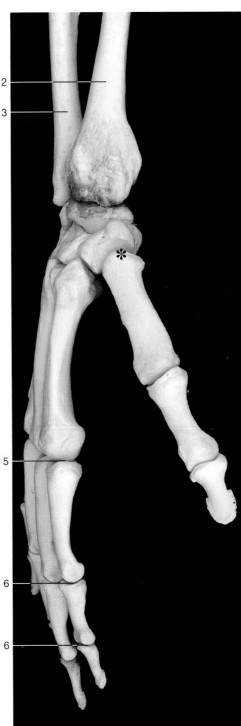

**Coronal section through the shoulder joint** (MRI scan). (From Heuck et al., MRT-Atlas, 2009.)

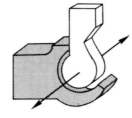

**Hinge joint**
(e.g., humero-ulnar joint). Left: extension, right: flexion. Arrows: axes of movement.

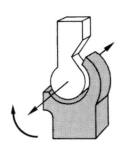

**Pivot joint**
(e.g., radio-ulnar joint).

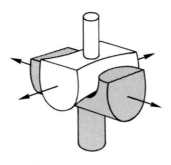

**Saddle joint**
(e.g., carpometacarpal joint of the thumb).

**Skeleton of right wrist and hand** (medial aspect). The metacarpophalangeal joints are biaxial, as is the carpometacarpal joint of the thumb (✳ in the figure). The joints of the fingers, however, are monaxial.

**Joints** exhibit a variety of functions. In general, mobility becomes reduced in the direction from proximal to distal. The hip joint, e.g., is multiaxial; the knee joint is biaxial, and the joints of toes and fingers are monaxial.

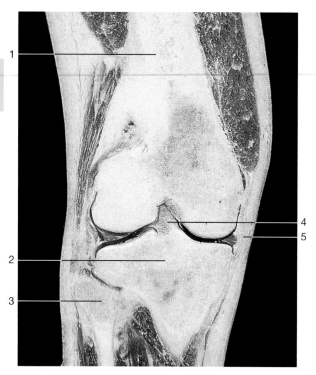

**Coronal section through the knee joint** (anterior aspect of the right joint in extension).

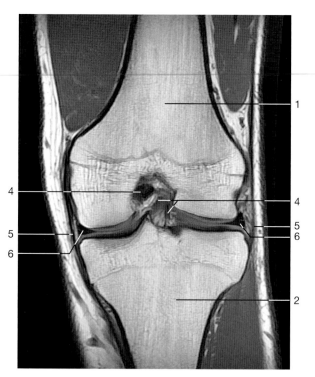

**Coronal section through the knee joint** (MRI scan). (From Heuck et al., MRT-Atlas, 2009.)

1   Femur
2   Tibia
3   Fibula
4   Cruciate ligaments
5   Collateral ligaments
6   Meniscus

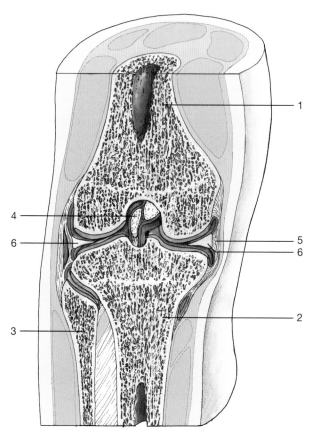

**Joints** are places of articulation allowing movements between bones. Synovial joints are characterized by a joint cavity enclosed by a joint capsule containing synovial fluid, which is produced by the articular capsule. The kind of movements depends not only on form and structure of the articulating bones but also on ligaments incorporated into the articular capsule. In some synovial joints, fibrocartilagenous articular discs develop, when the articulating surfaces of the bones are incongruous.

**Schematic drawing of the knee joint** as an example of a synovial joint, characterized by a joint cavity enclosed by a joint capsule (red) containing synovial fluid. Blue = articular cartilage.

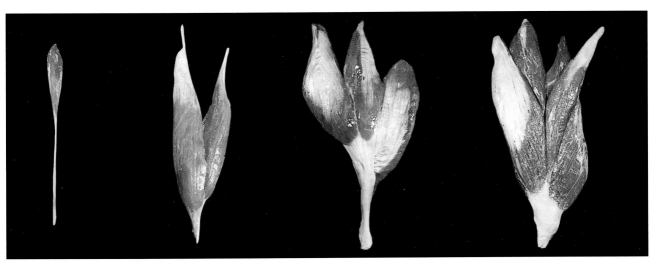

Fusiform
(palmaris longus)

Bicipital
(biceps brachii)

Tricipital (triceps surae,
gastrocnemius, and soleus)

Quadricipital
(quadriceps femoris)

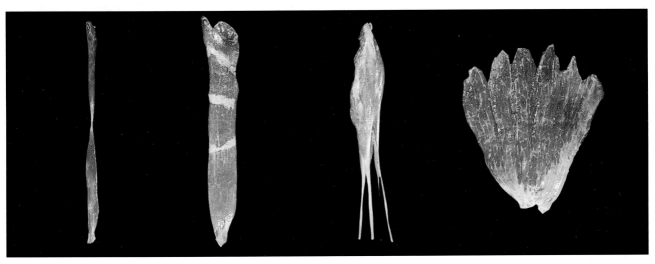

Digastric
(omohyoideus)

Multiventral
(rectus abdominis)

Multicaudal
(flexor digitorum prof.)

Serrated
(serratus anterior)

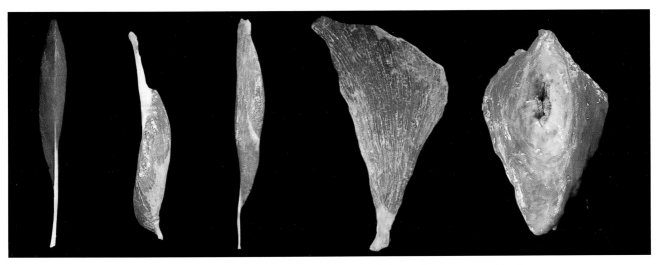

Bipennate
(tibialis anterior)

Unipennate
(semimembranosus)

Semitendinous
(semitendinosus)

Broad, flat muscle
(latissimus dorsi)

Ring-like
(sphincter ani externus)

The human body possesses **a great variety of muscles.** The architecture of the muscles depends on the functional systems in which they are involved, i.e., the kind of movements, the form of the joints with their specific ligaments, etc. The movements themselves vary to a great extent individually.

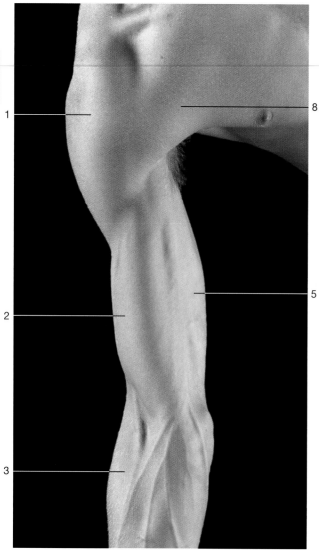

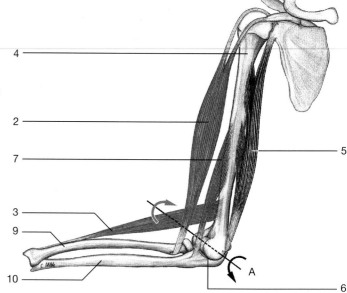

Diagram illustrating the position of the flexor and extensor
muscles of the arm and their effect on the elbow joint.
A: axis of humero-ulnar joint; arrows: direction of movements;
red = flexion; black = extension.

**Ventral aspect of the right arm.** The biceps muscle appears
slightly contracted. In the area of the elbow joint, several
subcutaneous veins can be recognized.

1  Deltoid muscle
2  Biceps brachii muscle
3  Brachioradialis muscle
4  Humerus
5  Triceps brachii muscle
6  Elbow joint
7  Brachialis muscle
8  Pectoralis major muscle
9  Radius
10  Ulna

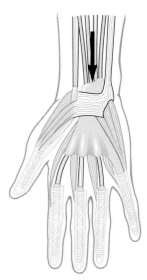

**Synovial sheaths of flexor tendons** (palmar aspect of the right hand).
The flexor retinaculum protects the flexor tendons passing through the
carpal tunnel (arrow).

Joints are moved by muscles. The highly differentiated
movements are coordinated by special groups of muscles
(**synergists**). Their counterparts are called **antagonists**.
Movements can only be carried out harmoniously if the
contraction of the synergists are supported by a corresponding dilatation of the antagonists. This interaction is
controlled by the nervous system. In order to carry out
certain directions of movements, often the tendons of
muscles have to be directed by ligaments. At those places,
the tendons often develop synovial sheaths, e.g., at the
wrist joint or at the fingers.

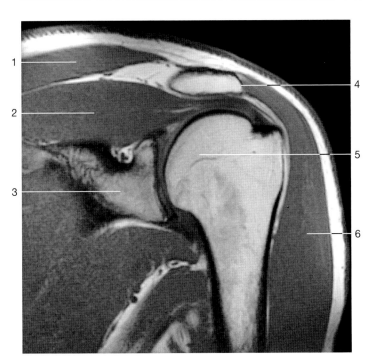

**Frontal section through the shoulder joint** (MRI scan). (From Heuck et al., MRT-Atlas, 2009.)

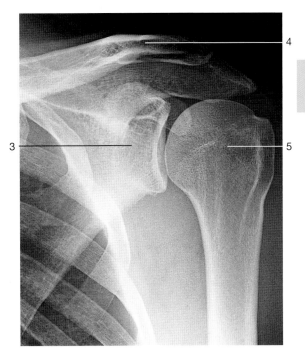

**Frontal section through the shoulder joint** (X-ray, a.-p. direction). (Courtesy of Dr. Holik, Spardorf, Germany.)

1  Trapezius muscle
2  Supraspinatus muscle
3  Scapula
4  Acromion
5  Head of humerus

6  Deltoid muscle
7  Cavity of shoulder joint
8  Articular cartilage
9  Articular cavity
10 Humerus

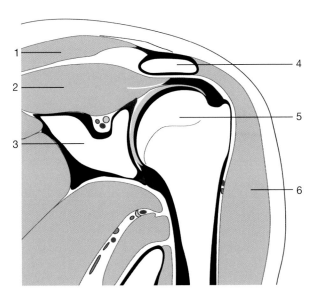

**Frontal section through the shoulder joint** (schematic drawing of the MRI scan above).

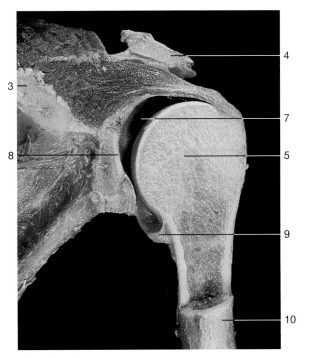

**Frontal section through the shoulder joint** (compare with the two pictures above).

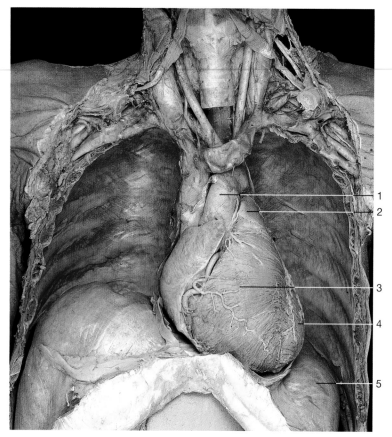

**Heart and related vessels in situ** (anterior aspect). Anterior thoracic wall, pericardium, and epicardium have been removed. The trachea is divided.

1 Aorta
2 Pulmonary artery
3 Right heart

4 Left heart
5 Diaphragm
6 Abdominal aorta

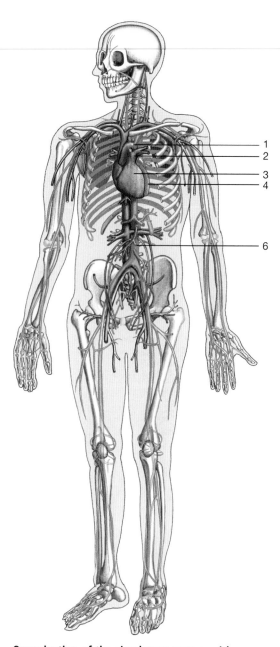

**Organization of the circulatory system with the heart in the center** (anterior aspect).
Red = arteries; blue = veins.

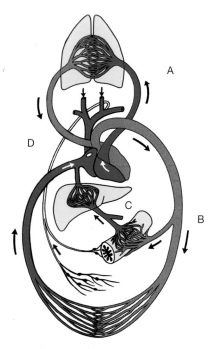

**Organization of the circulatory systems in the human body.**
The center of this system represents the heart.
Red = arteries; blue = veins.

A = Pulmonary circulation    C = Portal circulation
B = Systemic circulation     D = Lymphatic circulation

The center of the circulatory system is the heart, which is situated in the thoracic cavity and in contact with the diaphragm. In the right ventricle, the venous blood is collected and pumped through the pulmonary artery and into the lung where the blood is oxygenated. The veins of the lung transport the blood to the left ventricle, where it is pumped through the aorta and its branches (arteries) in the human body. Arteries and veins mostly run parallel. The venous blood from the intestine reaches the liver via the portal vein.

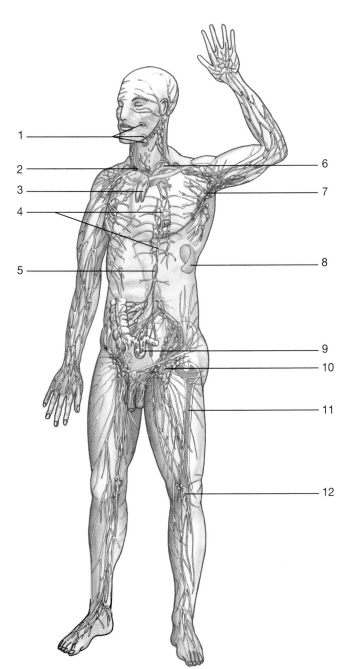

**Organization of the lymphatic system** (anterior aspect). Course of the main lymphatic vessels and location of the most important lymph nodes in the body. Red line = border between the lymphatic vessels draining to the left and right venous angles.

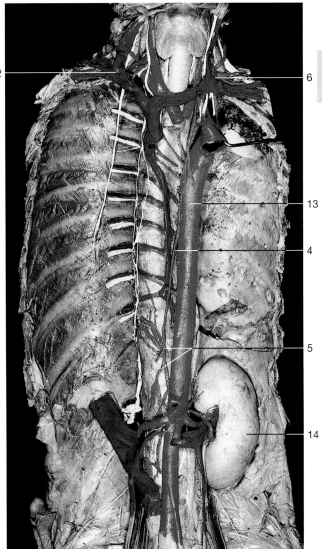

**Major lymph vessels of the trunk** (green). Blue = veins, red = arteries, white = nerves.

| | | | |
|---|---|---|---|
| 1 | Tonsils and submandibular lymph nodes | 8 | Spleen |
| 2 | Right venous angle | 9 | Lymph nodes of the intestinal tract |
| 3 | Remnants of the thymus gland | 10 | Inguinal lymph nodes |
| 4 | Thoracic duct | 11 | Bone marrow |
| 5 | Cisterna chyli | 12 | Lymph nodes of the popliteal fossa |
| 6 | Left venous angle | 13 | Aorta |
| 7 | Axillary lymph nodes | 14 | Left kidney |

Lymphatic vessels originate in the tissue spaces (lymph capillaries) and unite to form larger vessels (lymphatics). These resemble veins but have a much thinner wall, more valves, and are interrupted by lymph nodes at various intervals. Large groups of lymph nodes are located in the inguinal and axillary regions, deep to the mandible and sternocleidomastoid muscle, and within the root of the mesentery of the intestine. The lymphatic vessels of the right half of the head and neck, the right thorax, and the right upper limb drain toward the right venous angle; those of the rest of the body, toward the left venous angle.

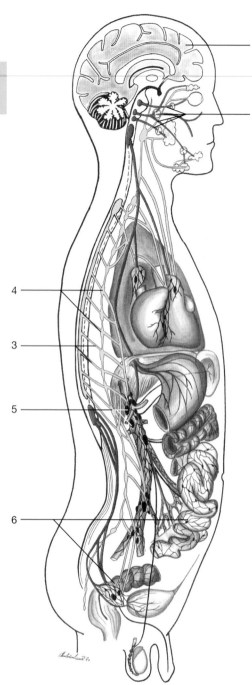

**Posterior part of the trunk.** The **solar plexus** with its connection to the vagus nerve and the sympathetic trunk has been dissected.

**Diagram illustrating the localization of the three functional portions of the nervous system** (brain, spinal cord and autonomic nervous system). Yellow = sympathetic system; red = parasympathetic system.

| | |
|---|---|
| 1  Cerebrum | 6  Nervous plexus |
| 2  Cranial nerves | of the autonomic system |
| 3  Spinal nerves | 7  Aorta |
| 4  Sympathetic trunk | 8  Vagus nerve and esophagus |
| 5  Solar plexus | 9  Bifurcation of trachea |

The nervous system can be divided into three functionally distinct parts:

1. The cranial part, which comprises the great sensory organs and the brain.
2. The spinal cord, which shows a segmental structure and serves predominantly as a reflex organ.
3. The autonomic nervous system, which controls the involuntary functions (subconscious control) of organs and tissues. The autonomic part of the nervous system forms many delicate plexuses near or within the organs.

At certain places these plexuses contain aggregations of nerve cells (prevertebral and intramural ganglia).

The spinal nerves leave the spinal cord at regular intervals. The ventral rami of the spinal nerves form the cervical and brachial plexus, which innervates the upper extremity, and the ventral rami of the lumbar and sacral spinal nerves form the lumbosacral plexus, which innervates the pelvis and genital organs and the lower extremity.

# 2 Head and Neck

# 2.1 Skull

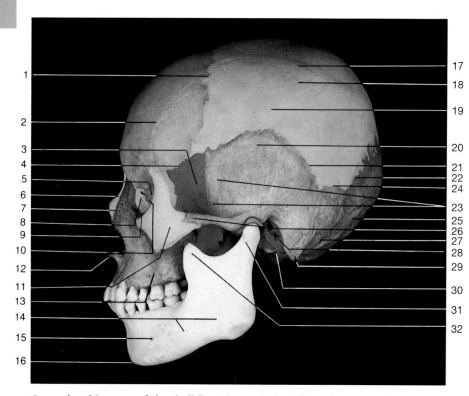

| | |
|---|---|
| 1 | Coronal suture |
| 2 | Frontal bone |
| 3 | Sphenoidal bone |
| 4 | Sphenofrontal suture |
| 5 | Ethmoidal bone |
| 6 | Nasal bone |
| 7 | Nasomaxillary suture |
| 8 | Lacrimal bone |
| 9 | Lacrimomaxillary suture |
| 10 | Ethmoidolacrimal suture |
| 11 | Zygomatic bone |
| 12 | Anterior nasal spine |
| 13 | Maxilla |
| 14 | Mandible |
| 15 | Mental foramen |
| 16 | Mental protuberance |
| 17 | Superior temporal line |
| 18 | Inferior temporal line |
| 19 | Parietal bone |
| 20 | Temporal bone |
| 21 | Squamous suture |
| 22 | Lambdoid suture |
| 23 | Temporal fossa |
| 24 | Parietomastoid suture |
| 25 | Occipital bone |
| 26 | Zygomatic arch |
| 27 | Occipitomastoid suture |
| 28 | External acoustic meatus |
| 29 | Mastoid process |
| 30 | Tympanic portion of temporal bone |
| 31 | Condylar process of mandible |
| 32 | Coronoid process of mandible |

**General architecture of the skull** (lateral aspect). The different bones are indicated in color (compare with the table).

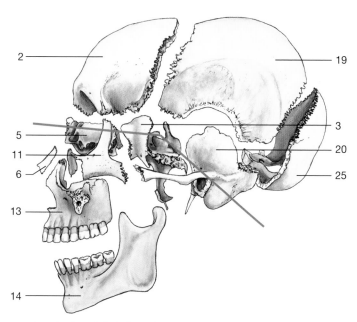

**Disarticulated skull** (lateral aspect). The facial bones are blue colored. Red line = angle of the clivus.

| | | |
|---|---|---|
| 2 | Frontal bone (orange) | Cranial bones |
| 19 | Parietal bone (light yellow) | |
| 3 | Greater wing of sphenoidal bone (red) | |
| 25 | Squama of occipital bone (blue) | |
| 20 | Squama of temporal bone (brown) | |
| 5 | Ethmoidal bone (dark green) | Base of skull |
| 3 | Sphenoidal bone (red) | |
| | Temporal bone excluding squama (brown) | |
| 30 | Tympanic portion of temporal bone (dark brown) | |
| | Occipital bone excluding squama (blue) | |
| 6 | Nasal bone (white) | Facial bones |
| 8 | Lacrimal bone (light yellow) | |
| | Inferior nasal concha | |
| | Vomer | |
| 11 | Zygomatic bone (dark yellow) | |
| | Palatine bone | |
| 13 | Maxilla (violet) | |
| 14 | Mandible (white) | |
| | Malleus ⎫ within petrous portion | Auditory ossicles |
| | Incus ⎬ of temporal bone | |
| | Stapes ⎭ | |
| | Hyoid | |

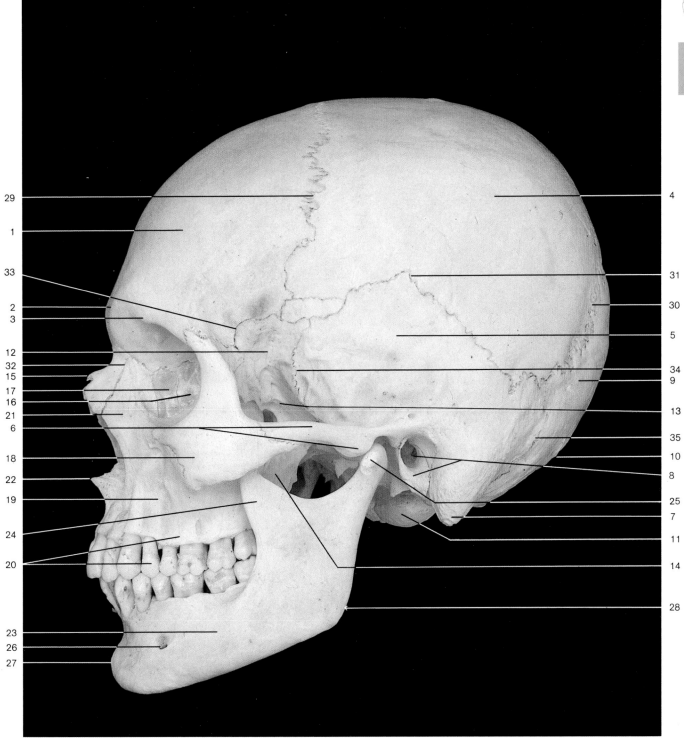

**Lateral aspect of the skull.**

| | | | | | |
|---|---|---|---|---|---|
| 1 | Frontal bone | 12 | Sphenoidal bone (greater wing) | 25 | Condylar process |
| 2 | Glabella | 13 | Infratemporal crest of sphenoid | 26 | Mental foramen |
| 3 | Supraorbital margin | 14 | Pterygoid process (lateral pterygoid plate) | 27 | Mental protuberance |
| 4 | Parietal bone | 15 | Nasal bone | 28 | Angle of the mandible |
| 5 | Temporal bone (squamous part) | 16 | Ethmoidal bone (orbital part) | | |
| 6 | Zygomatic process (articular tubercle) | 17 | Lacrimal bone | | **Sutures** |
| | | 18 | Zygomatic bone | 29 | Coronal suture |
| 7 | Mastoid process | 19 | Maxilla (body) | 30 | Lambdoid suture |
| 8 | Tympanic part (tympanic plate) and external acoustic meatus | 20 | Alveolar process and teeth | 31 | Squamous suture |
| | | 21 | Frontal process | 32 | Nasomaxillary suture |
| 9 | Occipital bone (squamous part) | 22 | Anterior nasal spine | 33 | Frontosphenoid suture |
| 10 | External occipital protuberance | 23 | Mandible (body) | 34 | Sphenosquamosal suture |
| 11 | Occipital condyle | 24 | Coronoid process | 35 | Occipitomastoid suture |

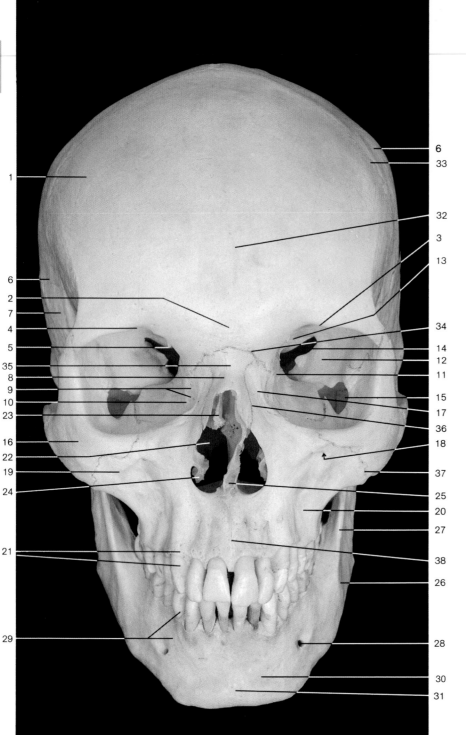

1   Frontal bone
2   Glabella
3   Supra-orbital margin
4   Supra-orbital notch
5   Trochlear spine
6   Parietal bone
7   Temporal bone
8   Nasal bone

**Orbit**
9   Lacrimal bone
10  Posterior lacrimal crest
11  Ethmoidal bone

**Sphenoidal bone**
12  Greater wing of sphenoidal bone
13  Lesser wing of sphenoidal bone
14  Superior orbital fissure
15  Inferior orbital fissure
16  Zygomatic bone

**Maxilla**
17  Frontal process
18  Infra-orbital foramen
19  Zygomatic process
20  Body of maxilla
21  Alveolar process with teeth

**Nasal cavity**
22  Anterior nasal aperture
23  Middle nasal concha
24  Inferior nasal concha
25  Nasal septum, vomer

**Mandible**
26  Body of mandible
27  Ramus of mandible
28  Mental foramen
29  Alveolar part with teeth
30  Base of mandible
31  Mental protuberance

**Sutures**
32  Frontal suture
33  Coronal suture
34  Frontonasal suture
35  Internasal suture
36  Nasomaxillary suture
37  Zygomaticomaxillary suture
38  Intermaxillary suture

**Anterior aspect of the skull.**

The skull comprises a mosaic of numerous complicated bones that form the cranial cavity protecting the brain **(neurocranium)** and several cavities such as the nasal and oral cavities in the facial region. The neurocranium consists of large bony plates that develop directly from the surrounding sheets of connective tissue **(desmocranium).**

The bones of the skull base are formed out of cartilaginous tissue **(chondrocranium),** which ossifies secondarily. The **visceral skeleton,** which in fish gives rise to the gills, has in higher vertebrates been transformed into the bones of the masticatory and auditory apparatus (maxilla, mandible, auditory ossicles, and hyoid bone).

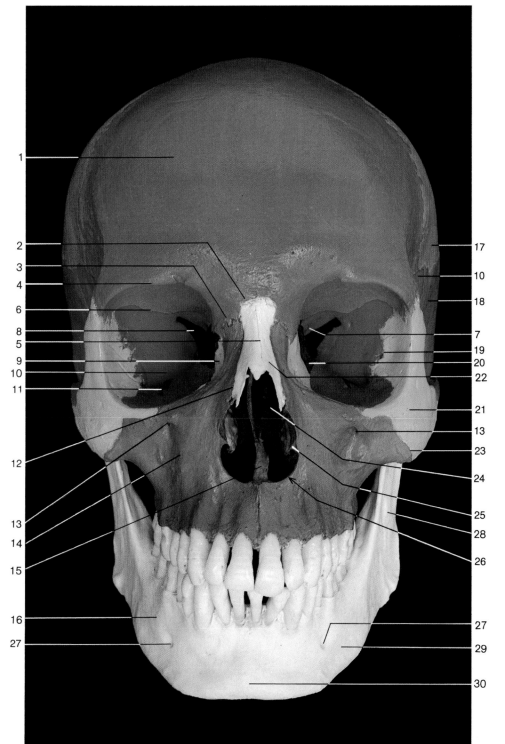

1  Frontal bone
2  Frontonasal suture
3  Frontomaxillary suture
4  Supra-orbital margin
5  Internasal suture
6  Sphenofrontal suture
7  Optic canal in lesser wing
   of sphenoidal bone
8  Superior orbital fissure
9  Lacrimal bone
10  Sphenoidal bone (greater wing)
11  Inferior orbital fissure
12  Nasomaxillary suture
13  Infra-orbital foramen
14  Maxilla
15  Vomer
16  Body of mandible
17  Parietal bone
18  Temporal bone
19  Sphenozygomatic suture
20  Ethmoidal bone
21  Zygomatic bone
22  Nasal bone
23  Zygomaticomaxillary suture
24  Middle nasal concha
25  Inferior nasal concha
26  Anterior nasal aperture
27  Mental foramen
28  Ramus of mandible
29  Base of mandible
30  Mental protuberance

**Bones**

| | | |
|---|---|---|
| Brown | = | frontal bone |
| Light green | = | parietal bone |
| Dark brown | = | temporal bone |
| Red | = | sphenoidal bone |
| Yellow | = | zygomatic bone |
| Dark green | = | ethmoidal bone |
| Yellow | = | lacrimal bone |
| Orange | = | vomer |
| Violet | = | maxilla |
| White | = | nasal bone |
| White | = | mandible |

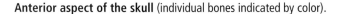

**Anterior aspect of the skull** (individual bones indicated by color).

The following series of figures are arranged so that the mosaic-like pattern of the skull becomes understandable. It starts with the bones of the **skull base** (sphenoidal and occipital bones) to which the other bones are added step by step. The facial skeleton is built up by the ethmoidal bone to which the palatine bone and maxilla are attached laterally; the small nasal and lacrimal bones fill the remaining spaces. Cartilages remain only in the external part of the nose.

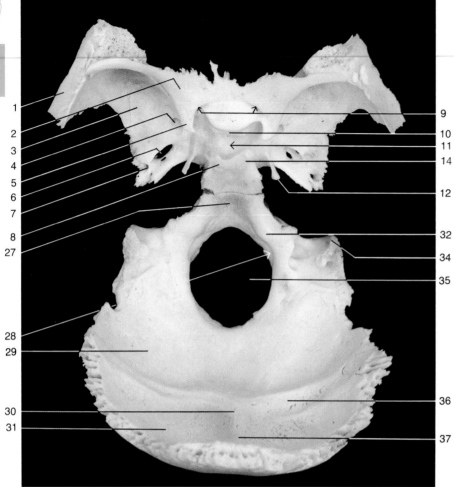

**Sphenoidal and occipital bones** (from above).

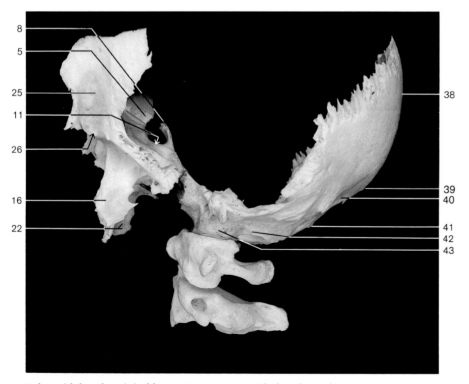

**Sphenoidal and occipital bones** in connection with the atlas and axis
(first and second cervical vertebrae) (left lateral view).

**Sphenoidal bone**
1   Greater wing
2   Lesser wing
3   Cerebral or superior surface of greater wing
4   Foramen rotundum
5   Anterior clinoid process
6   Foramen ovale
7   Foramen spinosum
8   Dorsum sellae
9   Optic canal
10  Chiasmatic groove (sulcus chiasmatis)
11  Hypophysial fossa (sella turcica)
12  Lingula
13  Opening of sphenoidal sinus
14  Posterior clinoid process
15  Pterygoid canal
16  Lateral pterygoid plate of pterygoid process
17  Pterygoid notch
18  Pterygoid hamulus
19  Orbital surface of greater wing
20  Sphenoidal crest
21  Sphenoidal rostrum
22  Medial pterygoid plate
23  Superior orbital fissure
24  Spine of sphenoid
25  Temporal surface of greater wing
26  Infratemporal crest

**Occipital bone**
27  Clivus with basilar part of occipital bone
28  Hypoglossal canal
29  Fossa for cerebellar hemisphere
30  Internal occipital protuberance
31  Fossa for cerebral hemisphere
32  Jugular tubercle
33  Condylar canal
34  Jugular process
35  Foramen magnum
36  Groove for transverse sinus
37  Groove for superior sagittal sinus
38  Squamous part of the occipital bone
39  External occipital protuberance
40  Superior nuchal line
41  Inferior nuchal line
42  Condylar fossa
43  Condyle
44  Pharyngeal tubercle
45  External occipital crest

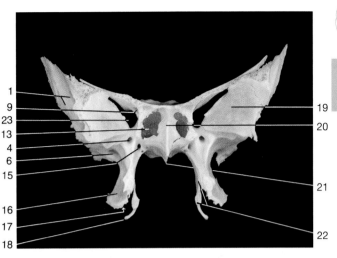

**Sphenoidal bone** (anterior aspect).

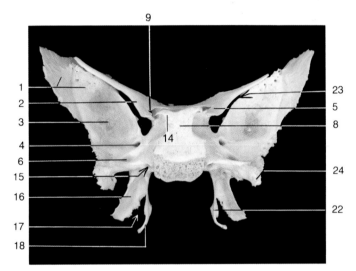

**Sphenoidal bone** (posterior aspect).

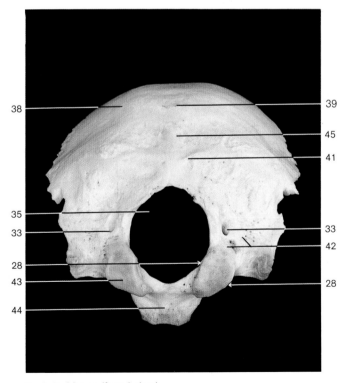

**Occipital bone** (from below).

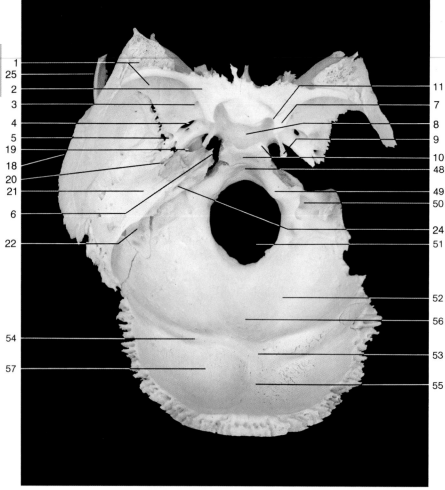

**Sphenoidal bone**
1   Greater wing
2   Lesser wing
3   Foramen rotundum
4   Foramen ovale
5   Foramen spinosum
6   Foramen lacerum
7   Anterior clinoid process
8   Hypophysial fossa (sella turcica)
9   Lingula
10  Dorsum sellae and
    posterior clinoid process
11  Optic canal
12  Sphenoidal rostrum
13  Medial pterygoid plate
14  Lateral pterygoid plate
15  Pterygoid hamulus
16  Infratemporal crest
17  Body of the sphenoidal bone

**Sphenoidal, occipital, and left temporal bones** (from above). Internal aspect of the base of the skull. The left temporal bone has been added to the preceding figure.

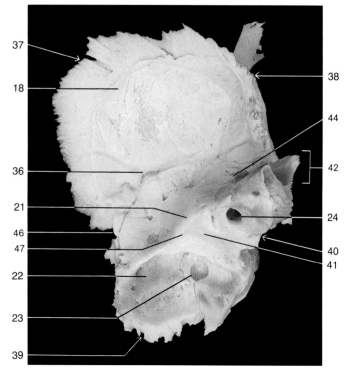

**Left temporal bone** (medial aspect).

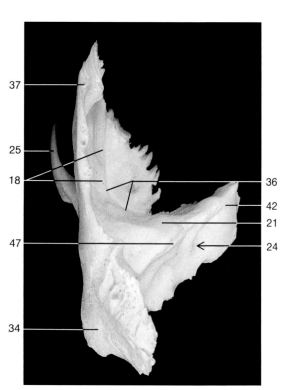

**Left temporal bone** (from above).

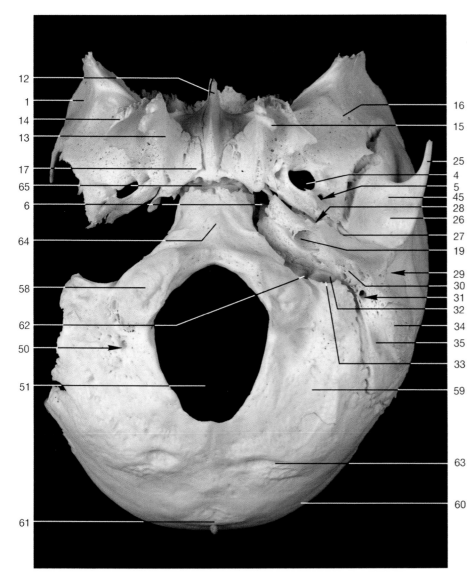

**Temporal bone**
18 Squamous part
19 Carotid canal
20 Hiatus of facial canal
   (for the greater petrosal nerve)
21 Arcuate eminence
22 Groove for the sigmoid sinus
23 Mastoid foramen
24 Internal acoustic meatus
25 Zygomatic process
26 Mandibular fossa
27 Petrotympanic fissure
28 Canalis musculotubarius
   (bony part of auditory tube)
29 External acoustic meatus
30 Styloid process (remnant only)
31 Stylomastoid foramen
32 Mastoid canaliculus
33 Jugular fossa
34 Mastoid process
35 Mastoid notch
36 Groove for middle meningeal vessels
37 Parietal margin
38 Sphenoidal margin
39 Occipital margin
40 Cochlear canaliculus
41 Aqueduct of the vestibule
42 Apex of the petrous part
43 Tympanic part
44 Trigeminal impression
45 Articular tubercle
46 Parietal notch
47 Groove for the superior petrosal sinus

**Occipital bone**
48 Clivus
49 Jugular tubercle
50 Condylar canal
51 Foramen magnum
52 Lower part
   of squamous occipital bone
   (cerebellar fossa)
53 Internal occipital protuberance
54 Groove for the transverse sinus
55 Groove for the superior sagittal sinus
56 Internal occipital crest
57 Upper part
   of squamous occipital bone
   (cerebral fossa)
58 Condyle
59 Nuchal plane
60 Superior nuchal line
61 External occipital protuberance
62 Jugular foramen
63 Inferior nuchal line
64 Pharyngeal tubercle
65 Spheno-occipital synchondrosis

**Sphenoidal, occipital, and left temporal bones.** Base of the skull (external aspect).

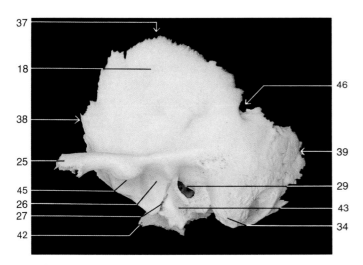

**Left temporal bone** (lateral aspect).

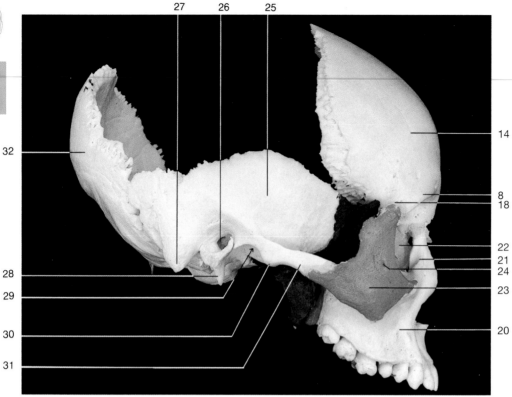

**Part of a disarticulated skull** (right lateral aspect). The frontal bone and the maxilla are connected with the temporal bone by the zygomatic bone (orange). Sphenoidal bone (black), palatine bone (red), lacrimal bone (yellow).

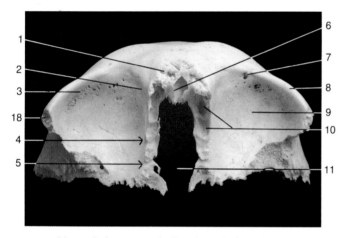

**Frontal bone** (inferior aspect). The ethmoidal foveolae cover the ethmoidal cavities of the ethmoidal bone.

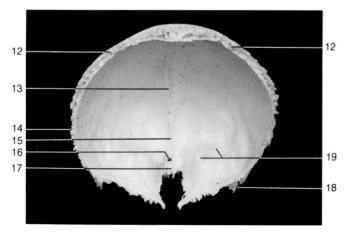

**Frontal bone** (posterior aspect).

**Frontal bone**
1 Nasal margin
2 Trochlear fossa
3 Fossa for lacrimal gland
4 Anterior ethmoidal foramen
5 Posterior ethmoidal foramen
6 Nasal spine
7 Supra-orbital notch
8 Supra-orbital margin
9 Orbital plate
10 Roofs of the ethmoidal air cells
11 Ethmoidal notch
12 Parietal margin
13 Groove for superior sagittal sinus
14 Squamous part of frontal bone
15 Frontal crest
16 Foramen cecum
17 Nasal spine
18 Zygomatic process of frontal bone
19 Juga cerebralia

**Facial bones**
20 Maxilla
21 Frontal process of maxilla
22 Lacrimal bone (yellow)
23 Zygomatic bone (orange)
24 Zygomaticofacial foramen

**Temporal bone**
25 Squamous part of temporal bone
26 External acoustic meatus
27 Mastoid process
28 Styloid process
29 Mandibular fossa
30 Articular tubercle
31 Zygomatic process

**Occipital bone**
32 Squamous part of occipital bone

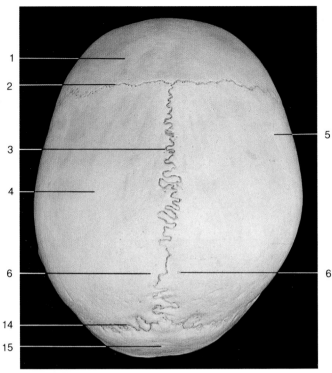

**Calvaria** (superior aspect).

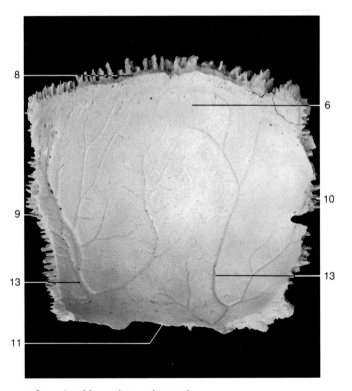

**Calvaria** (posterior aspect).

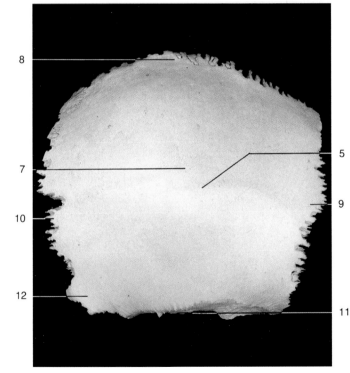

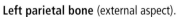

**Left parietal bone** (external aspect).

**Left parietal bone** (internal aspect).

| | | | |
|---|---|---|---|
| 1 | Frontal bone | 8 | Sagittal margin |
| 2 | Coronal suture | 9 | Occipital margin |
| 3 | Sagittal suture | 10 | Frontal margin |
| 4 | Parietal bone | 11 | Squamous margin |
| 5 | Superior temporal line | 12 | Sphenoidal angle |
| 6 | Parietal foramen | 13 | Groove for middle meningeal artery |
| 7 | Parietal tuber or eminence | 14 | Lambdoid suture |

| | |
|---|---|
| 15 | Occipital bone |
| 16 | External occipital protuberance |
| 17 | Inferior nuchal line |
| 18 | Occipitomastoid suture |
| 19 | Temporal bone |
| 20 | Mastoid process |
| 21 | Mastoid notch |

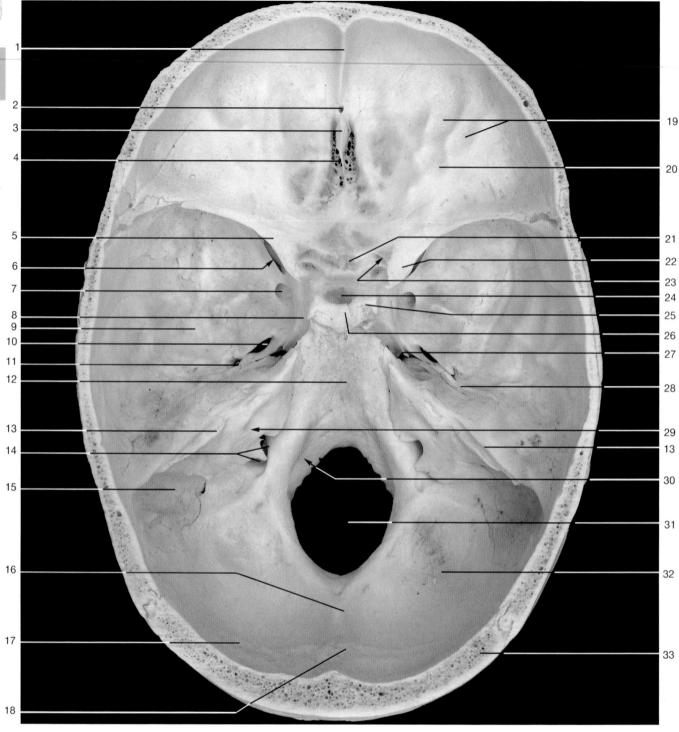

**Base of the skull,** calvaria removed (internal aspect).

| | | |
|---|---|---|
| 1  Frontal crest | 12  Clivus | 23  Optic canal |
| 2  Foramen cecum | 13  Groove for superior petrosal sinus | 24  Sella turcica (hypophysial fossa) |
| 3  Crista galli | 14  Jugular foramen | 25  Posterior clinoid process |
| 4  Cribriform plate of ethmoidal bone | 15  Groove for sigmoid sinus | 26  Dorsum sellae |
| 5  Lesser wing of sphenoidal bone | 16  Internal occipital crest | 27  Foramen lacerum |
| 6  Superior orbital fissure | 17  Groove for transverse sinus | 28  Groove for greater petrosal nerve |
| 7  Foramen rotundum | 18  Internal occipital protuberance | 29  Internal acoustic meatus |
| 8  Carotid sulcus | 19  Digitate impressions | 30  Hypoglossal canal |
| 9  Middle cranial fossa | 20  Anterior cranial fossa | 31  Foramen magnum |
| 10  Foramen ovale | 21  Chiasmatic sulcus | 32  Posterior cranial fossa |
| 11  Foramen spinosum | 22  Anterior clinoid process | 33  Diploe |

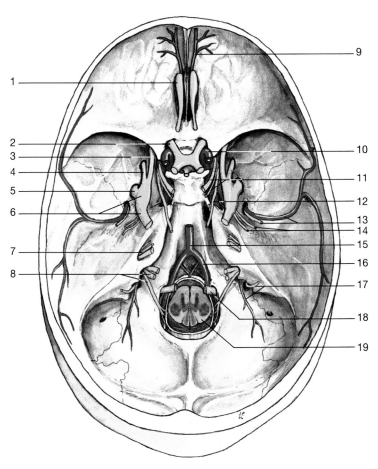

1 Olfactory bulb
2 Optic nerve (n. II)
3 Ophthalmic nerve (n. V₁)
4 Maxillary nerve (n. V₂)
5 Mandibular nerve (n. V₃)
6 Trigeminal nerve (n. V)
  with trigeminal ganglion
7 Facial nerve (n. VII) and
  vestibulocochlear nerve (n. VIII)
8 Glossopharyngeal nerve (n. IX),
  vagus nerve (n. X) and
  accessory nerve (n. XI)
9 Anterior meningeal artery
10 Internal carotid artery
11 Oculomotor nerve (n. III) and
   trochlear nerve (n. IV)
12 Abducent nerve (n. VI)
13 Middle meningeal artery and
   meningeal branch of mandibular
   nerve
14 Greater and lesser petrosal nerves
15 Basilar artery
16 Vertebral artery
17 Posterior meningeal artery and
   recurrent meningeal nerve
18 Hypoglossal nerve (n. XII)
19 Medulla oblongata

**Base of the skull** with cranial nerves and meningeal arteries
(internal aspect).

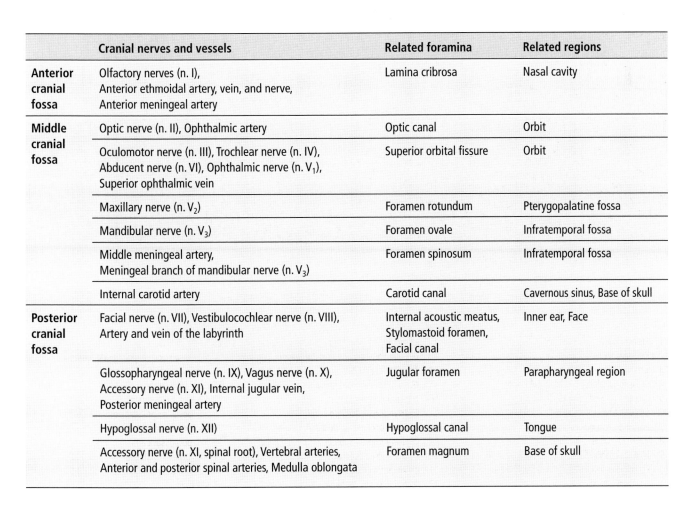

|  | Cranial nerves and vessels | Related foramina | Related regions |
|---|---|---|---|
| **Anterior cranial fossa** | Olfactory nerves (n. I), Anterior ethmoidal artery, vein, and nerve, Anterior meningeal artery | Lamina cribrosa | Nasal cavity |
| **Middle cranial fossa** | Optic nerve (n. II), Ophthalmic artery | Optic canal | Orbit |
| | Oculomotor nerve (n. III), Trochlear nerve (n. IV), Abducent nerve (n. VI), Ophthalmic nerve (n. V₁), Superior ophthalmic vein | Superior orbital fissure | Orbit |
| | Maxillary nerve (n. V₂) | Foramen rotundum | Pterygopalatine fossa |
| | Mandibular nerve (n. V₃) | Foramen ovale | Infratemporal fossa |
| | Middle meningeal artery, Meningeal branch of mandibular nerve (n. V₃) | Foramen spinosum | Infratemporal fossa |
| | Internal carotid artery | Carotid canal | Cavernous sinus, Base of skull |
| **Posterior cranial fossa** | Facial nerve (n. VII), Vestibulocochlear nerve (n. VIII), Artery and vein of the labyrinth | Internal acoustic meatus, Stylomastoid foramen, Facial canal | Inner ear, Face |
| | Glossopharyngeal nerve (n. IX), Vagus nerve (n. X), Accessory nerve (n. XI), Internal jugular vein, Posterior meningeal artery | Jugular foramen | Parapharyngeal region |
| | Hypoglossal nerve (n. XII) | Hypoglossal canal | Tongue |
| | Accessory nerve (n. XI, spinal root), Vertebral arteries, Anterior and posterior spinal arteries, Medulla oblongata | Foramen magnum | Base of skull |

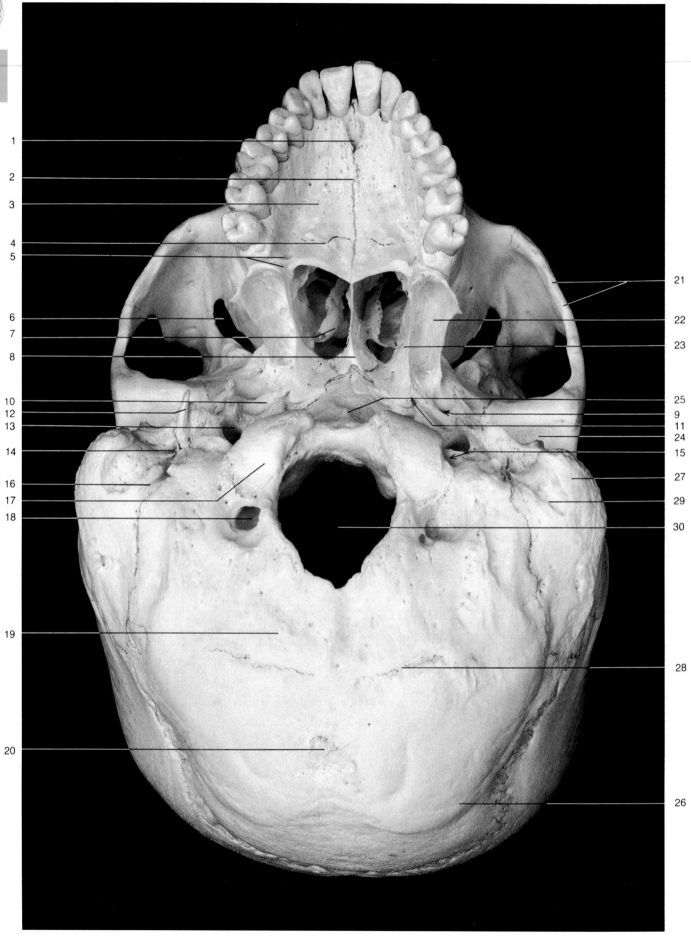

**Base of the skull** (inferior aspect).

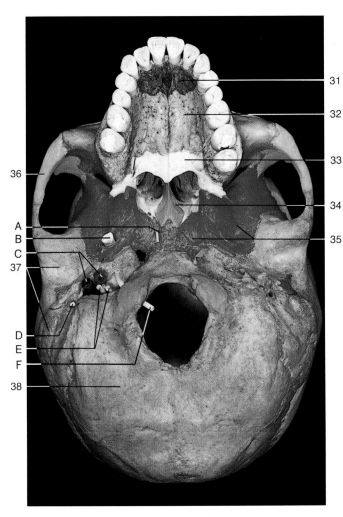

**Base of the skull** (from below). The individual bones are indicated by different colors.

A = **Pterygoid canal**
B = **Foramen ovale**
C = Internal carotid artery within **carotid canal** and internal jugular vein within the venous part of jugular foramen
D = **Stylomastoid foramen** (facial nerve)
E = **Jugular foramen** (glossopharyngeal, vagus and accessory nerves)
F = **Hypoglossal canal** (hypoglossal nerve)

1  Incisive canal
2  Median palatine suture
3  Palatine process of maxilla
4  Palatomaxillary suture
5  Greater and lesser palatine foramina
6  Inferior orbital fissure
7  Middle concha (process of ethmoidal bone)
8  Vomer
9  Foramen ovale
10 Groove for auditory tube
11 Pterygoid canal
12 Styloid process
13 Carotid canal
14 Stylomastoid foramen
15 Jugular foramen
16 Groove for occipital artery
17 Occipital condyle
18 Condylar canal
19 Nuchal plane
20 External occipital protuberance
21 Zygomatic arch
22 Lateral pterygoid plate
23 Medial pterygoid plate
24 Mandibular fossa
25 Pharyngeal tubercle
26 Superior nuchal line
27 Mastoid process
28 Inferior nuchal line
29 Mastoid notch
30 Foramen magnum
31 Incisive bone or premaxilla (dark violet)
32 Maxilla (violet)
33 Palatine bone (white)
34 Vomer (orange)
35 Sphenoidal bone (red)
36 Zygomatic bone (yellow)
37 Temporal bone (brown)
38 Occipital bone (blue)
39 Palatine process of maxilla
40 Vomer
41 Sphenoidal bone
42 Petrous part of temporal bone
43 Basilar part ⎫
44 Lateral part  ⎬ of occipital bone
45 Squamous part ⎭
46 Mandible
47 Zygomatic arch
48 Choana
49 Pterygoid process of sphenoidal bone
50 Carotid canal
51 External acoustic meatus (tympanic anulus)
52 Sphenoidal fontanelle
53 Parietal bone
54 Mastoid fontanelle

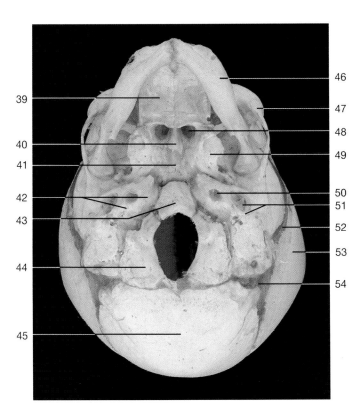

**Skull of the newborn** (inferior aspect).

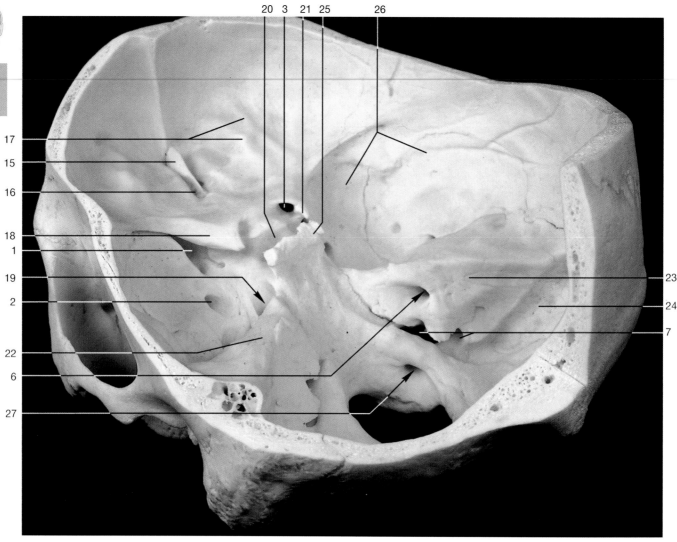

20  3  21  25      26

17
15
16
18
1
19
2
22
6
27

23
24
7

**Base of the skull** (internal aspect, oblique-lateral view from left side).

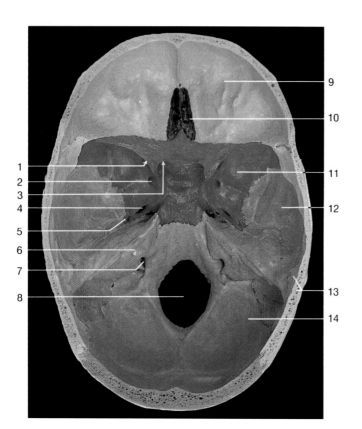

9
10

1
2
3
4
5
6
7
8

11
12

13
14

**Base of the skull** (internal aspect, superior view).
The individual bones are indicated by different colors.

**Canals, fissures, and foramina of the base of the skull**
1   Superior orbital fissure
2   Foramen rotundum
3   Optic canal
4   Foramen ovale
5   Foramen spinosum
6   Internal acoustic meatus
7   Jugular foramen
8   Foramen magnum

**Bones**
9   Frontal bone (orange)
10  Ethmoidal bone (dark green)
11  Sphenoidal bone (red)
12  Temporal bone (brown)
13  Parietal bone (yellow)
14  Occipital bone (blue)

**Details of bones**
15  Crista galli
16  Cribriform plate

17  Digitate impressions (frontal bone)
18  Lesser wing of sphenoidal bone
19  Foramen lacerum
20  Hypophysial fossa (sella turcica)
21  Anterior clinoid process
22  Trigeminal impression
23  Petrous part of temporal bone
24  Groove for sigmoid sinus
25  Dorsum sellae (posterior clinoid process)
26  Greater wing of sphenoidal bone, groove for middle meningeal artery
27  Hypoglossal canal

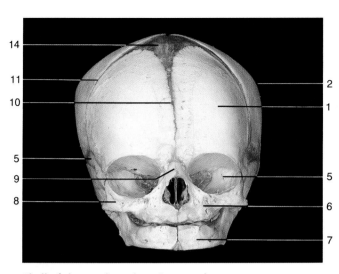

**Skull of the newborn** (anterior aspect).

**Cranial skeleton**
1  Frontal tuber or eminence
2  Parietal tuber or eminence
3  Occipital tuber or eminence
4  Squamous part of temporal bone
5  Greater wing of sphenoidal bone

**Facial skeleton**
6  Maxilla
7  Mandible
8  Zygomatic bone
9  Nasal bone

**Sutures and fontanelles**
10  Frontal suture
11  Coronal suture
12  Sagittal suture
13  Lambdoid suture
14  Anterior fontanelle
15  Posterior fontanelle
16  Sphenoidal (anterolateral) fontanelle
17  Mastoid (posterolateral) fontanelle

**Base of the skull**
18  Frontal bone
19  Ethmoidal bone
20  Sphenoidal bone
21  Hypophysial fossa (sella turcica)
22  Dorsum sellae
23  Temporal bone
24  Mastoid (posterolateral) fontanelle
25  Occipital bone

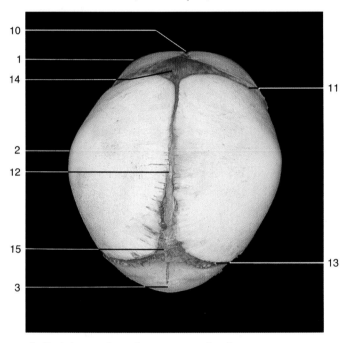

**Skull of the newborn** (superior aspect). Calvaria.

In the newborn, the facial skeleton, in contrast to the cranial skeleton, appears relatively small. There are no teeth presenting. The bones of the cranium are separated by wide fontanelles.

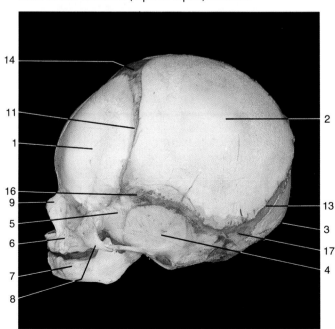

**Skull of the newborn** (lateral aspect).

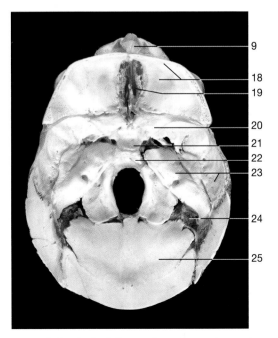

**Base of the skull of the newborn** (internal aspect).

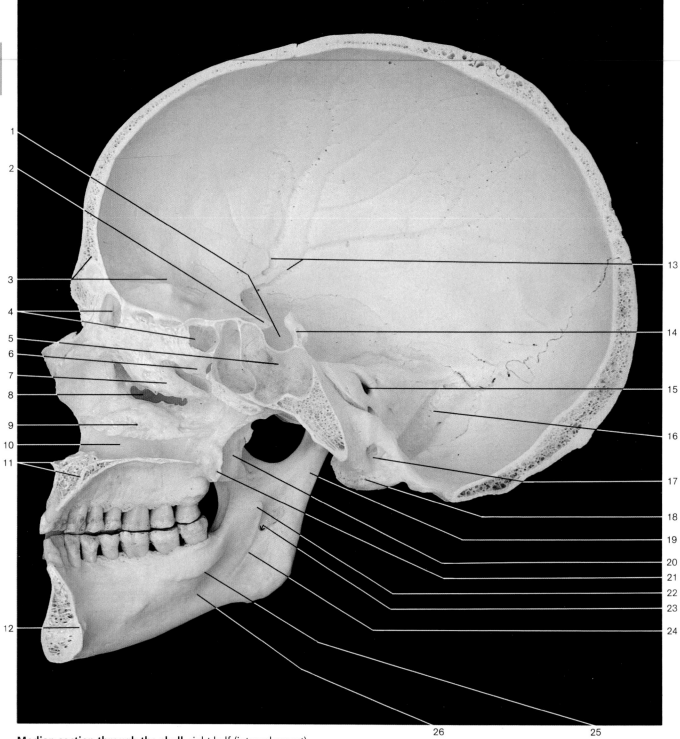

**Median section through the skull,** right half (internal aspect).

1 Hypophysial fossa (sella turcica)
2 Anterior clinoid process
3 Frontal bone
4 Ethmoidal air cells
5 Sphenoidal sinus
6 Superior concha
7 Middle concha
8 Maxillary hiatus
9 Inferior concha
10 Inferior meatus
11 Anterior nasal spine and maxilla
12 Mental spine or genial tubercle
13 Groove for middle meningeal artery

14 Dorsum sellae
15 Internal acoustic meatus
16 Groove for sigmoid sinus
17 Hypoglossal canal
18 Occipital condyle
19 Condylar process
20 Lateral pterygoid plate ⎫
21 Medial pterygoid plate ⎬ of pterygoid process
⎭
22 Lingula of mandible
23 Mandibular foramen
24 Mylohyoid groove
25 Mylohyoid line
26 Submandibular fovea

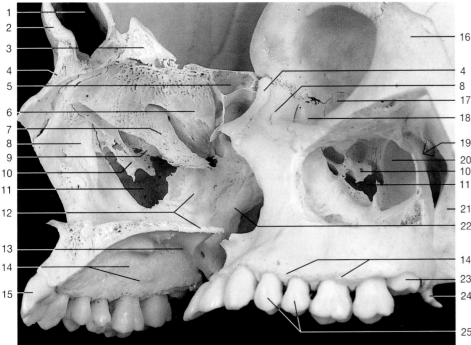

1 Frontal sinus
2 Frontal bone
3 Crista galli
4 Nasal bone
5 Sphenoidal sinus
6 Superior concha ⎫ of ethmoidal
7 Middle concha  ⎭ bone
8 Frontal process
  of maxilla
9 Ethmoidal bulla
10 Uncinate process
11 Maxillary hiatus
12 Palatine bone
13 Greater palatine foramen
14 Alveolar process of maxilla
15 Central incisor
16 Zygomatic bone
17 Ethmoidal bone
18 Lacrimal bone
19 Pterygopalatine fossa
20 Maxillary sinus
21 Lateral pterygoid plate
22 Medial pterygoid plate
23 Third molar tooth
24 Pterygoid hamulus
25 Two premolar teeth

**Facial part of the skull (viscerocranium),** divided in two halves (lateral and medial aspect). Right inferior concha has been removed to show the maxillary hiatus. Left maxillary sinus opened.

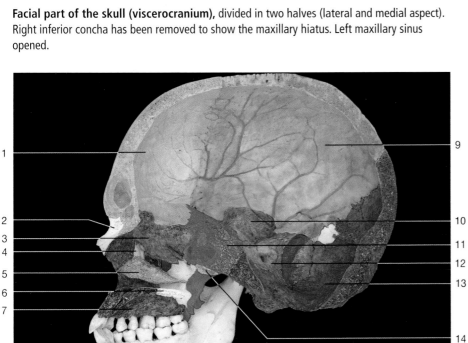

**Bones** (indicated by colors)
1 Frontal bone (yellow)
2 Nasal bone (white)
3 Ethmoidal bone (dark green)
4 Lacrimal bone (yellow)
5 Inferior nasal concha (pink)
6 Palatine bone (white)
7 Maxilla (violet)
8 Mandible (white)
9 Parietal bone (light green)
10 Temporal bone (brown)
11 Sphenoidal bone (red)
12 Petrous part of temporal bone
   (brown)
13 Occipital bone (blue)
14 Ala of vomer (light brown)

**Median section through the skull.** The nasal septum has been removed. The individual bones are indicated by different colors.

Because of the upright posture that the human developed in the course of evolution, the cranial cavity greatly increased in size, whereas the facial skeleton decreased. As a result, the base of the skull developed an angulation of about 120° between the clivus and the cribriform plate (see drawing on page 20). The hypophysial fossa containing the pituitary gland lies at the angle formed between these two planes.

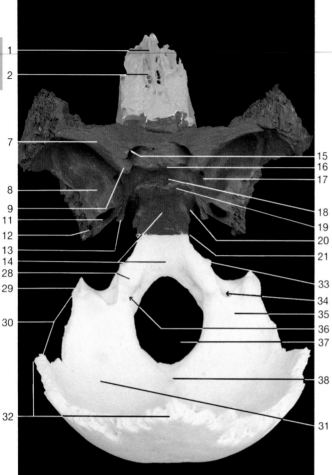

**Ethmoidal bone**
1 Crista galli
2 Cribriform plate
3 Ethmoidal air cells
4 Middle concha
5 Perpendicular plate (part of nasal septum)
6 Orbital plate

**Sphenoidal bone**
7 Lesser wing
8 Greater wing
9 Anterior clinoid process
10 Posterior clinoid process
11 Foramen ovale
12 Foramen spinosum
13 Lingula of the sphenoidal bone
14 Clivus
15 Optic canal
16 Tuberculum sellae
17 Foramen rotundum (right side)
18 Hypophysial fossa (sella turcica)
19 Dorsum sellae
20 Carotid sulcus
21 Spheno-occipital synchondrosis
22 Lateral pterygoid plate
23 Greater wing of sphenoidal bone (orbital surface)
24 Greater wing of sphenoidal bone (maxillary surface)
25 Foramen rotundum (left side)
26 Superior orbital fissure
27 Infratemporal crest of the greater wing

**Part of a disarticulated base of the skull.**
Ethmoidal, sphenoidal, and occipital bones (from above).
Green = sphenoidal bone; yellow = ethmoidal bone.

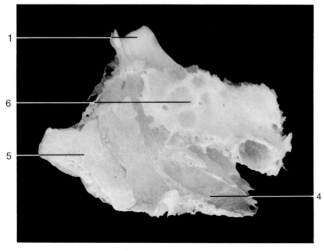

**Ethmoidal bone** (lateral aspect), posterior portion to the right.

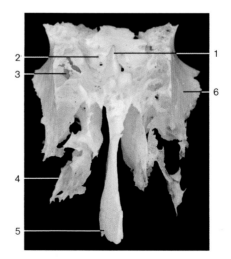

**Ethmoidal bone** (anterior aspect).

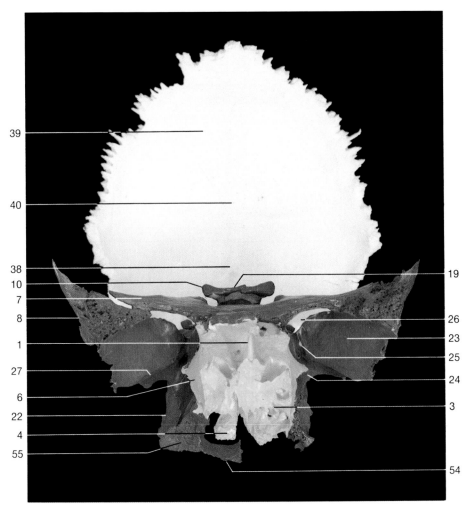

**Occipital bone**
28  Jugular tubercle
29  Jugular process
30  Mastoid margin
31  Posterior cranial fossa
32  Lambdoid margin
33  Intrajugular process
34  Condylar canal
35  Lateral part of occipital bone
36  Hypoglossal canal
37  Foramen magnum
38  Internal occipital crest
39  Squamous part of occipital bone
40  Internal occipital protuberance

**Maxilla**
41  Orbital surface
42  Infra-orbital groove
43  Maxillary tuberosity with foramina
44  Frontal process
45  Nasolacrimal groove
46  Infra-orbital margin
47  Anterior nasal spine
48  Zygomatic process
49  Alveolar process

**Palatine bone**
50  Orbital process
51  Sphenopalatine notch
52  Sphenoidal process
53  Perpendicular plate
54  Horizontal plate
55  Pyramidal process

**Part of a disarticulated base of the skull** (anterior aspect). Green = sphenoidal bone; yellow = ethmoidal bone; red = palatine bone.

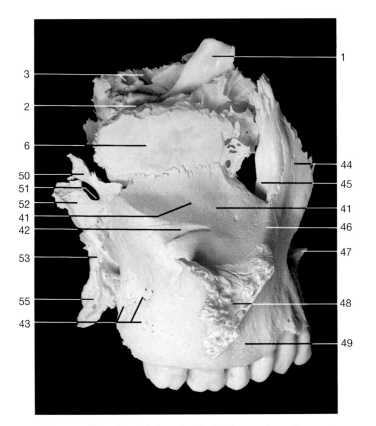

**Right maxilla, ethmoidal, and palatine bones** (lateral aspect).

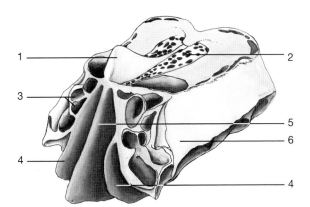

**Ethmoidal bone** (oblique-anterior aspect).

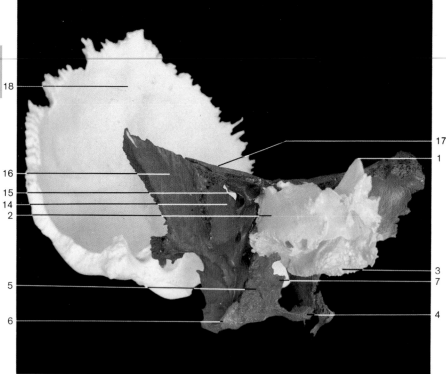

**Ethmoidal bone**
1  Crista galli
2  Orbital plate
3  Middle concha

**Palatine bone**
4  Horizontal plate of palatine bone
5  Greater palatine canal
6  Pyramidal process
7  Maxillary process
8  Orbital process
9  Sphenopalatine notch
10  Perpendicular plate of palatine bone
11  Conchal crest
12  Nasal crest
13  Sphenoidal process

**Sphenoidal bone**
14  Greater wing
15  Superior orbital fissure
16  Greater wing (orbital surface)
17  Lesser wing

**Occipital bone**
18  Squamous part of occipital bone

**Maxilla**
19  Maxillary tuberosity
20  Frontal process
21  Orbital surface
22  Infra-orbital margin
23  Infra-orbital groove
24  Zygomatic process
25  Alveolar process

**Part of a disarticulated base of the skull,** similar to the preceding figures, but with palatine bone. Green = sphenoidal bone; yellow = ethmoidal bone; red = palatine bone.

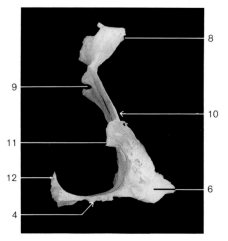

**Left palatine bone** (medial aspect, posterior aspect to the left).

**Left palatine bone** (anterior aspect).

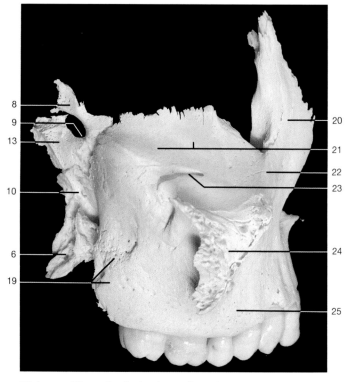

**Right maxilla and palatine bone** (lateral aspect).

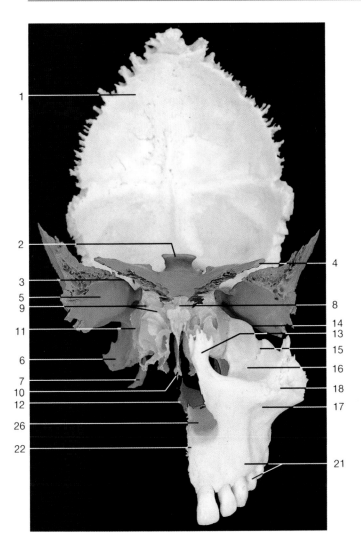

**Occipital bone**
1   Squamous part

**Sphenoidal bone**
2   Dorsum sellae
3   Superior orbital fissure
4   Lesser wing
5   Greater wing (orbital surface)
6   Lateral pterygoid plate
7   Medial pterygoid plate

**Ethmoidal bone**
8   Crista galli
9   Ethmoidal air cells
10  Perpendicular plate
11  Orbital plate

**Palatine bone**
12  Horizontal plate (nasal crest)

**Maxilla**
13  Frontal process
14  Inferior orbital fissure
15  Infra-orbital groove
16  Orbital surface
17  Infra-orbital foramen
18  Zygomatic process
19  Anterior lacrimal crest
20  Canine fossa
21  Alveolar process with teeth
22  Anterior nasal spine
23  Juga alveolaria (elevations formed by roots of teeth)
24  Lacrimal groove
25  Maxillary tuberosity with alveolar foramina
26  Palatine process of maxilla

**Part of a disarticulated base of the skull** (anterior aspect).
The left **maxilla** is added to the preceding specimen.

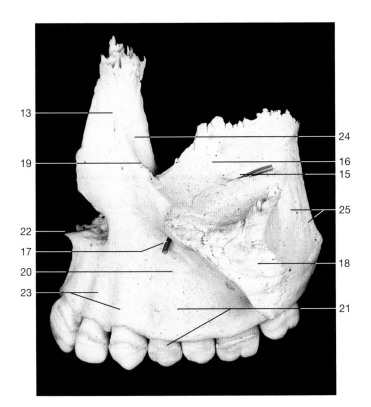

**Left maxilla** (lateral aspect). Probe = infra-orbital canal.

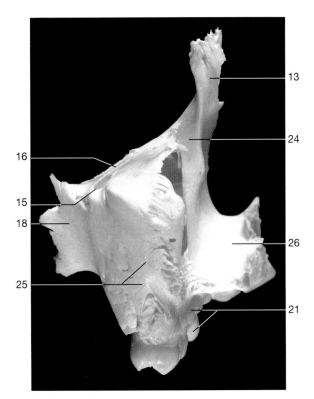

**Left maxilla** (posterior aspect).

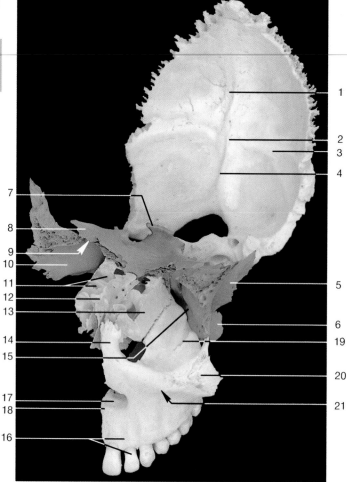

**Part of a disarticulated base of the skull.** The mosaic of the facial bones [sphenoidal bone (green), ethmoidal bone (yellow), and palatine bone (red)] is seen from the antero-lateral aspect.

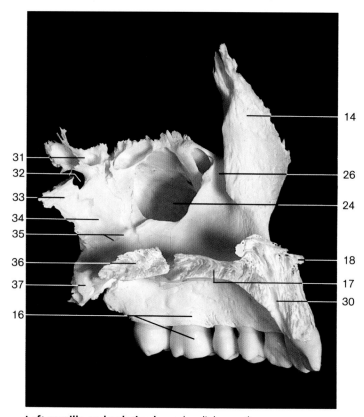

**Left maxilla and palatine bone** (medial aspect).

**Occipital bone**
1   Groove for superior sagittal sinus
2   Internal occipital protuberance
3   Groove for transverse sinus
4   Internal occipital crest

**Sphenoidal bone**
5   Greater wing (temporal surface)
6   Lateral pterygoid plate
7   Dorsum sellae
8   Lesser wing
9   Superior orbital fissure
10  Greater wing (orbital surface)

**Ethmoidal bone**
11  Ethmoidal air cells
12  Crista galli
13  Orbital plate

**Maxilla**
14  Frontal process
15  Inferior orbital fissure
16  Alveolar process with teeth
17  Palatine process
18  Anterior nasal spine
19  Infra-orbital groove
20  Zygomatic process
21  Location of infra-orbital foramen
22  Middle nasal meatus
23  Inferior nasal meatus
24  Maxillary hiatus
     (leading to maxillary sinus)
25  Third molar
26  Lacrimal groove
27  Conchal crest
28  Body of maxilla (nasal surface)
29  Nasal crest
30  Incisive canal

**Palatine bone**
31  Orbital process
32  Sphenopalatine notch
33  Sphenoidal process
34  Perpendicular plate
35  Conchal crest
36  Horizontal plate
37  Pyramidal process

**Frontal bone**
38  Squamous part
39  Supra-orbital foramen
40  Frontal notch
41  Frontal spine

**Inferior nasal concha**
42  Inferior nasal concha
     with maxillary process

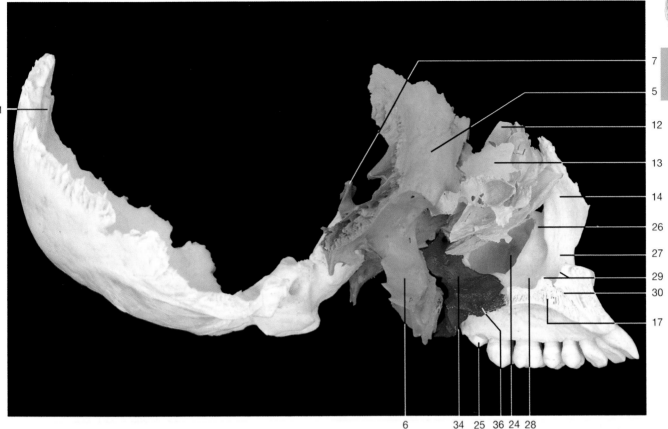

**Part of a disarticulated base of the skull** (medial aspect). Green = sphenoidal bone; yellow = ethmoidal bone; red = palatine bone; natural colored = left maxilla.

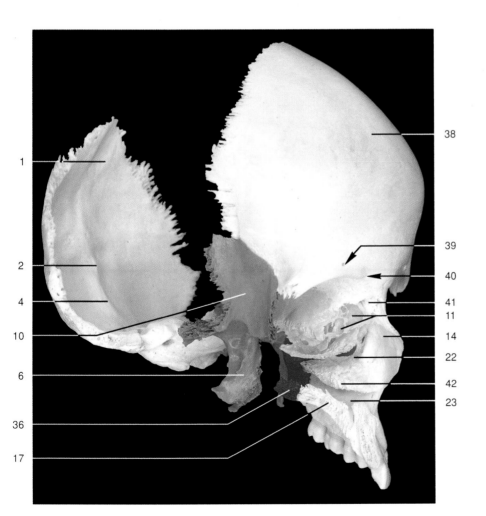

**Part of a disarticulated base of the skull** (oblique-lateral aspect). The same specimen as shown above but with frontal bone.

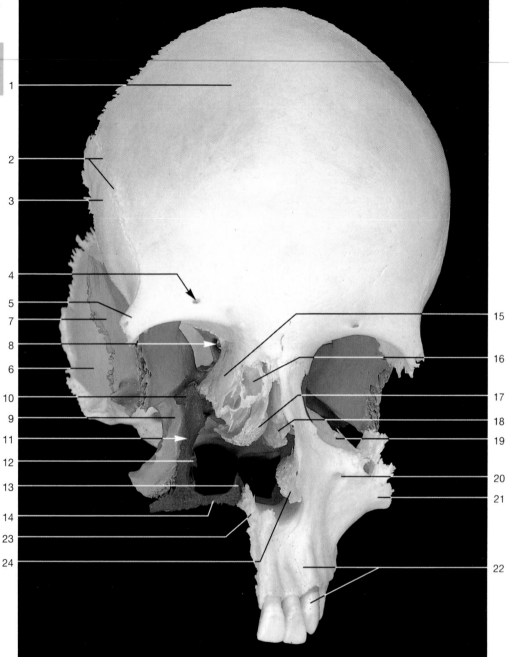

**Part of a disarticulated skull** showing the connection of the palatine bone (red) and the maxilla with ethmoidal bone (yellow) and sphenoidal bone (green) (anterior aspect).

**Frontal bone**
1 Squamous part
2 Inferior temporal line
3 Temporal surface
4 Supra-orbital foramen
5 Zygomatic process

**Occipital bone**
6 Squamous part

**Sphenoidal bone**
7 Greater wing (temporal surface)
8 Optic canal within the lesser wing
9 Lateral pterygoid plate

**Palatine bone**
10 Orbital process
11 Perpendicular plate
12 Conchal crest
13 Nasal crest
14 Horizontal plate

**Ethmoidal bone**
15 Orbital plate
16 Ethmoidal air cell
17 Middle concha
18 Perpendicular plate
(part of bony nasal septum)

**Maxilla**
19 Infra-orbital groove
20 Infra-orbital foramen
21 Zygomatic process
22 Alveolar process with teeth
23 Palatine process

**Left inferior nasal concha**
24 Anterior part
of inferior concha

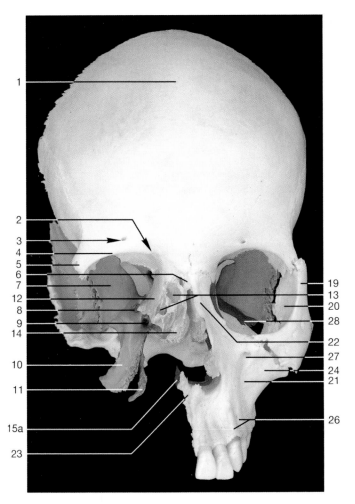

**Frontal bone**
1 Squamous part
2 Frontal notch
3 Supra-orbital foramen
4 Supra-orbital margin
5 Zygomatic process
6 Frontal spine

**Sphenoidal bone**
7 Greater wing (orbital surface)
8 Foramen rotundum
9 Pterygoid or Vidian canal
10 Lateral pterygoid plate
11 Medial pterygoid plate

**Ethmoidal bone**
12 Orbital plate
13 Ethmoidal air cells
14 Middle concha

**Palatine bone**
15 Horizontal plate
15a Nasal crest
16 Pyramidal process
17 Lesser palatine foramen
18 Greater palatine foramen

**Zygomatic bone**
19 Frontal process
20 Orbital surface

**Maxilla**
21 Canine fossa
22 Frontal process
23 Palatine process
24 Zygomatic process
25 Alveolar process and teeth
26 Juga alveolaria
27 Infra-orbital foramen
28 Infra-orbital groove
29 Anterior nasal aperture
30 Anterior nasal spine

**Incisive bone**
31 Central incisor and incisive bone or premaxilla
32 Incisive fossa

**Vomer**
33 Ala of the vomer

**Sutures and choanae**
34 Median palatine suture
35 Transverse palatine suture
36 Choanae

**Part of a disarticulated skull** showing the connection of the maxilla with the frontal and zygomatic bones (anterior aspect).
Yellow = ethmoidal bone; red = palatine bone; green = sphenoidal bone.

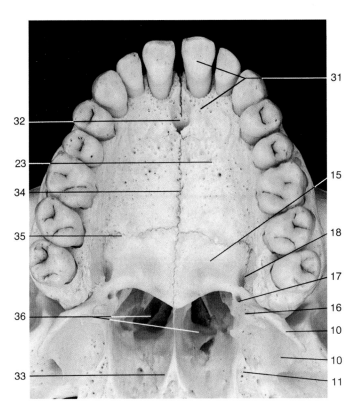

**Bony palate and teeth of the maxillae** (from below).

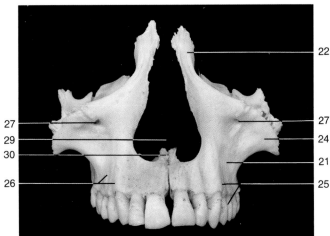

**Anterior view of both maxillae** forming the anterior bony aperture of the nose.

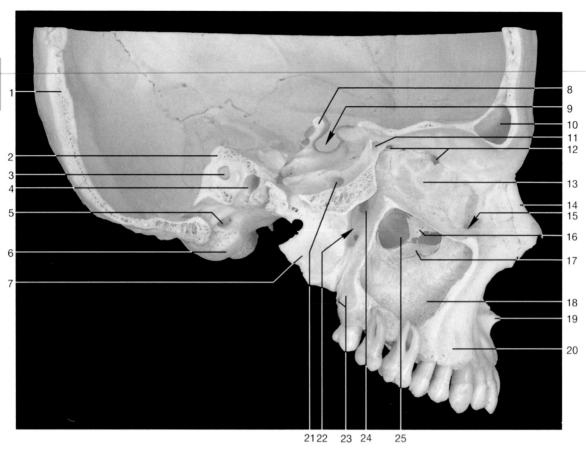

**Pterygopalatine fossa, maxillary sinus, and orbit.** Paramedian section through the skull (right side, lateral aspect). Frontal and maxillary sinuses are opened.

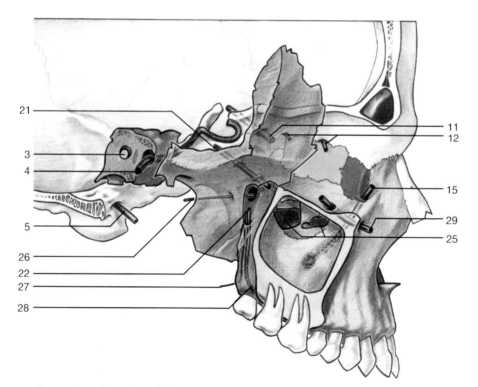

**Illustration of canals and foramina connected with the right orbit and pterygopalatine fossa** (compare with the figure above). The greater wing of sphenoidal bone (green) is shown as being transparent. Brown = temporal bone; yellow = ethmoidal bone; red = lacrimal bone; light red = inferior nasal concha; violet = maxilla; red = palatine bone.

1  Occipital bone
2  Temporal bone (petrous part)
3  Internal acoustic meatus
4  Carotid canal
5  Hypoglossal canal
6  Occipital condyle
7  Lateral plate of pterygoid process
8  Dorsum of sella turcica
9  Sella turcica
10 Frontal sinus
11 Optic canal
12 Posterior and anterior
   ethmoidal foramina
13 Orbital plate of ethmoidal bone
14 Nasal bone
15 Nasolacrimal canal
16 Uncinate process
17 Inferior nasal concha
   (maxillary process)
18 Maxillary sinus
19 Anterior nasal spine
20 Alveolar process of maxilla
21 Foramen rotundum
22 Pterygopalatine fossa
23 Tuberosity of maxilla
   with alveolar foramina
24 Sphenopalatine foramen
25 Maxillary hiatus
26 Pterygoid or Vidian canal
27 Lesser palatine canal
28 Greater palatine canal
29 Infra-orbital canal

1    Occipital bone
2    Temporal bone
3    Frontal bone
4    Nasal spine of frontal bone
5    Zygomatic bone
6    Maxilla
7    Frontal process of maxilla
8    Ethmoidal bone
9    Orbital plate of ethmoidal bone
10   Perpendicular plate of ethmoidal bone
11   Site of lacrimal bone
12   Lacrimal groove of lacrimal bone
13   Posterior lacrimal crest
14   Fossa for lacrimal sac
15   Lacrimal hamulus
16   Nasolacrimal canal
17   Site of nasal bone
18   Nasal foramina of nasal bone
19   Anterior nasal spine of maxilla
20   Vomer
21   Greater wing of sphenoidal bone
22   Anterior and posterior ethmoidal foramina
23   Optic canal
24   Superior orbital fissure
25   Inferior orbital fissure
26   Infra-orbital groove
27   Infra-orbital foramen

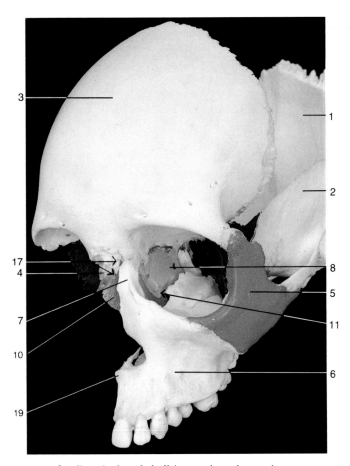

**Part of a disarticulated skull** (antero-lateral aspect).
Orange = zygomatic bone; yellow = ethmoidal bone;
dark green = sphenoidal bone. The arrows indicate the locations
of the lacrimal bone (11) and the nasal bone (17).

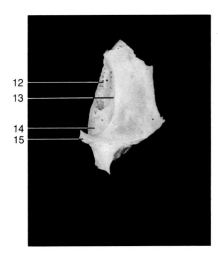

**Left lacrimal bone** (anterior aspect).

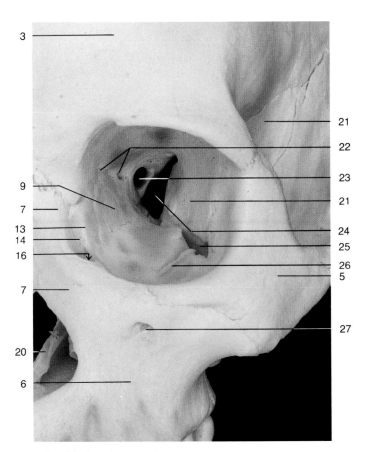

**Left orbit** (anterior aspect).

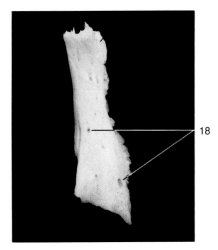

**Left nasal bone** (anterior aspect).

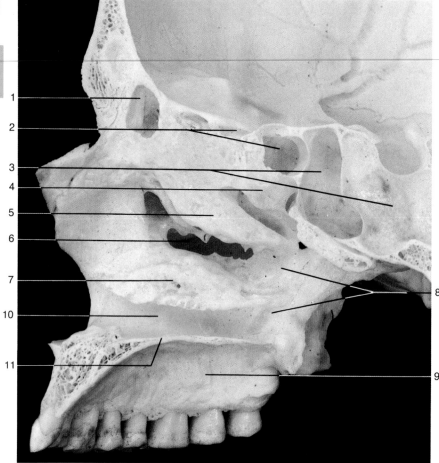

1    Frontal sinus
2    Ethmoidal air cells
3    Sphenoidal sinus
4    Superior nasal concha
5    Middle nasal concha
6    Maxillary hiatus
7    Inferior nasal concha
8    Palatine bone
9    Maxilla
10   Inferior meatus
11   Palatine process of the maxilla

▷

**To page 49:**

| | | |
|---|---|---|
| Blue | = | Occipital bone |
| Light green | = | Parietal bone |
| Yellow | = | Frontal bone |
| Dark brown | = | Temporal bone |
| Red | = | Sphenoidal bone |
| Dark green | = | Ethmoidal bone |
| Light blue | = | Nasal bone |
| Pink | = | Inferior concha |
| Orange | = | Vomer |
| Violet | = | Maxilla |
| White | = | Palatine bone |
| White | = | Mandible |

**Lateral wall of the nasal cavity.** Median section through the skull.

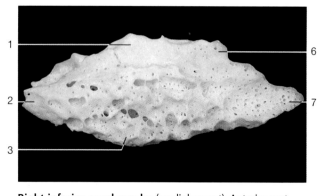

**Right inferior nasal concha** (medial aspect). Anterior part to the left.

**Inferior concha and vomer**
1    Ethmoidal process
2    Anterior part of concha
3    Inferior border
4    Ala of vomer
5    Posterior border of nasal septum
6    Lacrimal process
7    Posterior part of concha
8    Maxillary process

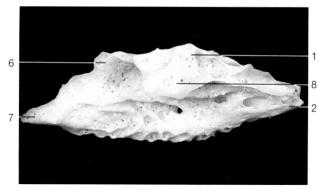

**Right inferior nasal concha** (lateral aspect). Anterior part to the right.

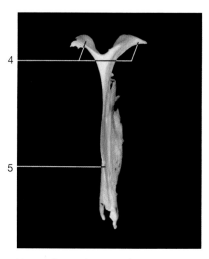

**Vomer** (posterior aspect).

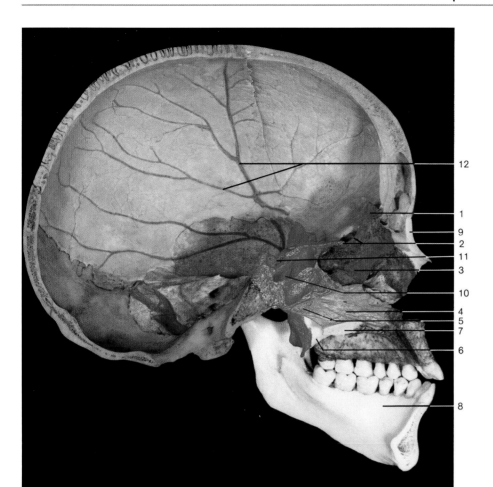

1 Crista galli
2 Cribriform plate
  of ethmoidal bone
3 Perpendicular plate
  of ethmoidal bone
4 Vomer
5 Ala of the vomer
6 Palatine bone
  (perpendicular process)
7 Palatine bone (horizontal plate)
8 Mandible
9 Nasal bone
10 Sphenoidal sinus
11 Hypophysial fossa (sella turcica)
12 Grooves for the middle
   meningeal artery

**Cartilages of the nose**
13 Lateral nasal cartilage
14 Greater alar cartilage
15 Lesser alar cartilages
16 Septal cartilage
17 Location of nasal bone

**Paramedian sagittal section through the skull including the nasal septum.**

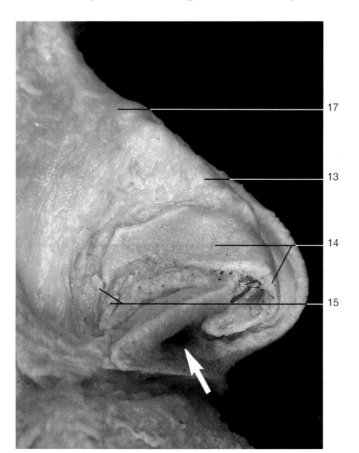

**Cartilages of the nose** (right anterior aspect). Arrow: nostril, framed by nasal wing.

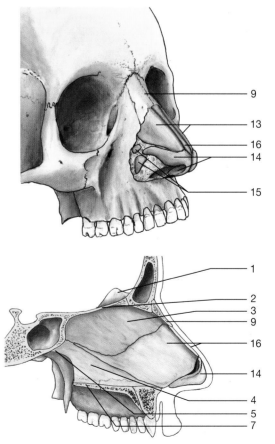

**Shape of the cartilages of the nose.**

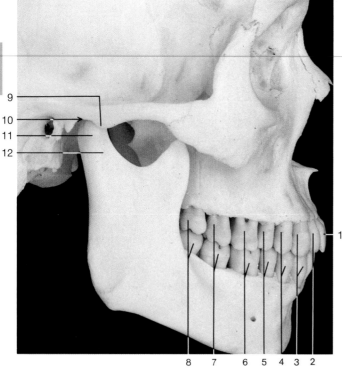

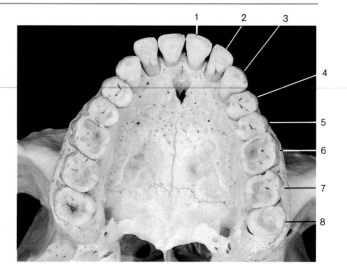

**Upper teeth of the adult** (inferior aspect).

**Normal position of the teeth.** Dentition in centric occlusion (lateral aspect).

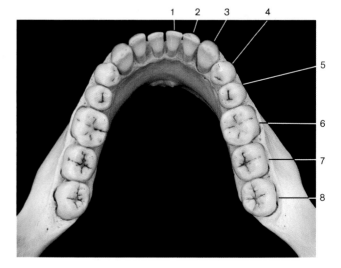

**Lower teeth of the adult** (superior aspect).

1   Central incisor
2   Lateral incisor
3   Canines
4   First premolars or bicuspids
5   Second premolars or bicuspids
6   First molars
7   Second molars
8   Third molars
9   Articular tubercle
10  Mandibular fossa
11  Head of mandible
12  Condylar process
13  Hard palate and palatine glands
14  Oral cavity
15  Upper molar
16  Oral vestibule
17  Lower molar
18  Platysma muscle
19  Mandible
20  Maxillary sinus
21  Superior longitudinal muscle of tongue
22  Transverse muscle of tongue
23  Buccinator muscle
24  Inferior longitudinal muscle of tongue
25  Sublingual gland
26  Genioglossus muscle

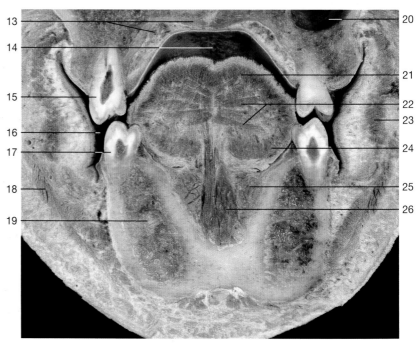

**Coronal section through the oral cavity** (anterior aspect).

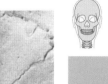

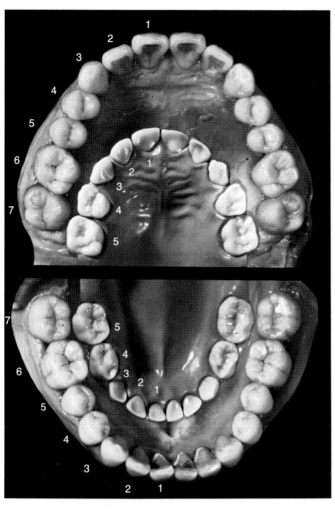

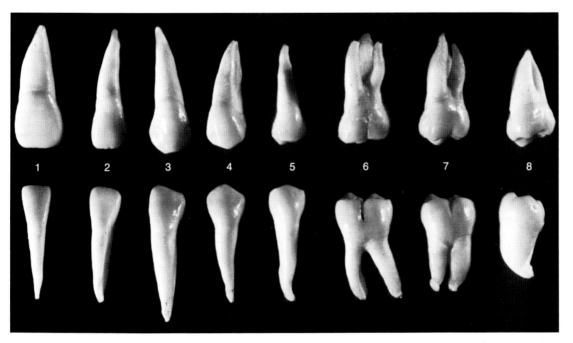

**Deciduous teeth in a child's skull.** The developing crowns of the permanent teeth are displayed in their crypts in the maxilla and mandible.

1    Permanent incisors
2    Permanent cuspid (canine)
3    Premolars
4    First permanent molar
5    Second permanent molar
6    Mental foramen

**Comparison of the deciduous and permanent teeth.**
Notice that the breadth of the alveolar arch of the child's mandible and maxilla holding the deciduous teeth is nearly the same as the comparable portion in the jaws of the adult. Note the emergence of the third molars. The numbers of the teeth correspond to the numbers in the figure below.

**Isolated teeth of the alveolar part of the maxilla** (top row) and the mandible (lower row), labial surface of the teeth.

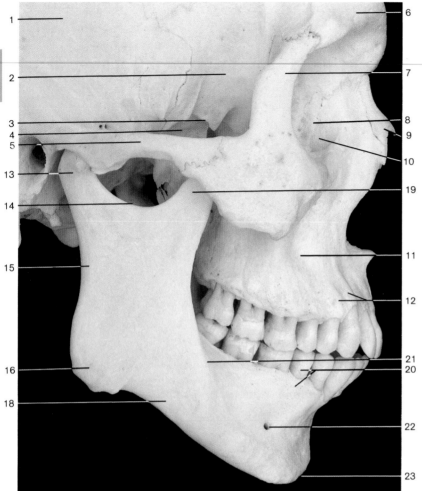

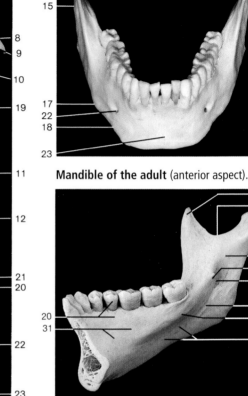

**Mandible of the adult** (anterior aspect).

**Lateral aspect of the facial bones.** Mandible and teeth in the position of occlusion. Upper and lower jaw occluded.

**Right half of the mandible** (medial aspect).

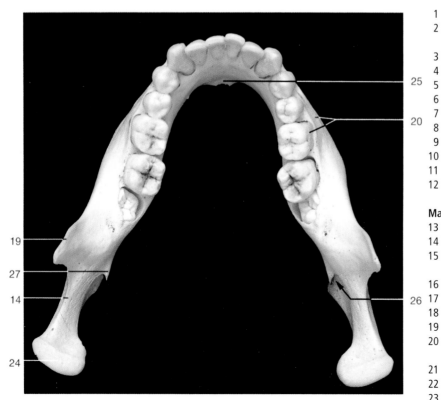

**Mandible of the adult** (superior aspect).

1 Temporal bone
2 Temporal fossa
   (greater wing of sphenoidal bone)
3 Infratemporal crest
4 Infratemporal fossa
5 Zygomatic arch
6 Frontal bone
7 Zygomatic bone (frontal process)
8 Lacrimal bone
9 Nasal bone
10 Lacrimal groove
11 Maxilla (canine fossa)
12 Alveolar process of maxilla

**Mandible**

13 Condylar process
14 Mandibular notch
15 Ramus of the
   mandible
16 Masseteric tuberosity
17 Angle of the mandible
18 Body of the mandible
19 Coronoid process
20 Alveolar process
   including teeth
21 Oblique line
22 Mental foramen
23 Mental protuberance
24 Head of the mandible

25 Genial tubercle
   or mental spine
26 Mandibular foramen
   (entrance to
   mandibular canal)
27 Lingula
28 Mylohyoid sulcus
29 Mylohyoid line
30 Submandibular
   fossa
31 Sublingual fossa

# 2.2 Masticatory Apparatus and Muscles of the Head

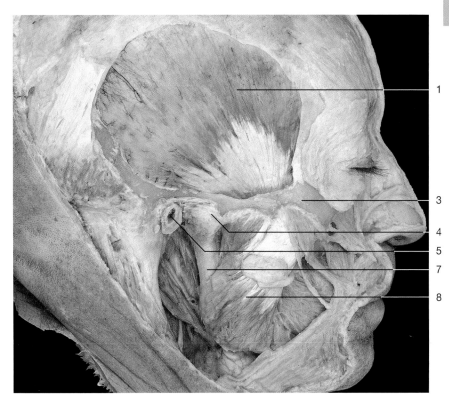

**Muscles of mastication and facial muscles** (lateral aspect). The auricle has been removed.

1 Temporal muscle
2 Frontal bone
3 Zygomatic arch
4 Temporomandibular joint
5 External acoustic meatus
6 Maxilla
7 Mandible
8 Masseter muscle

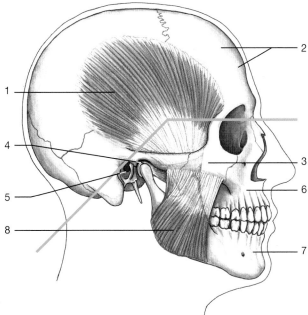

**Temporomandibular joint and muscles of mastication** (lateral aspect).
The base of the skull is bent (gray line).

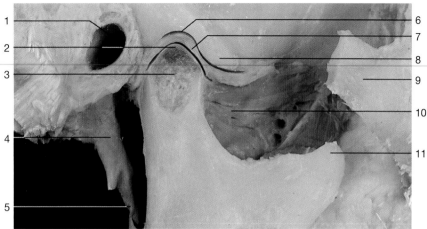

1 External acoustic meatus
2 Articular cartilage of condylar process
3 Condylar process of mandible
4 Styloid process
5 Stylomandibular ligament
6 Mandibular fossa
7 Articular disc
8 Articular tubercle
9 Zygomatic bone
10 Lateral pterygoid muscle
11 Coronoid process of mandible
12 Posterior belly of digastric muscle
13 Masseter muscle
14 Temporal muscle
15 Medial pterygoid muscle
16 Parotid duct
17 Buccinator muscle
18 Mandible
19 Mandibular foramen

**Temporomandibular joint** (sagittal section).

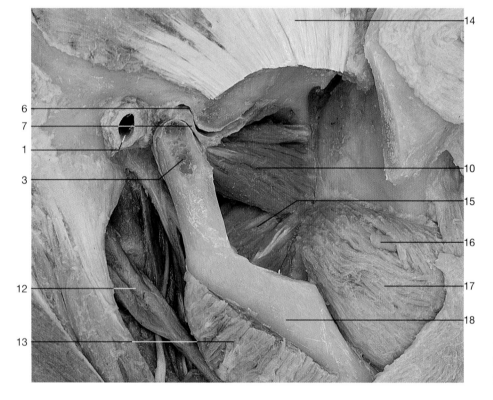

**Temporomandibular joint.**
Dissection of the articular disc and the related muscles (lateral aspect).

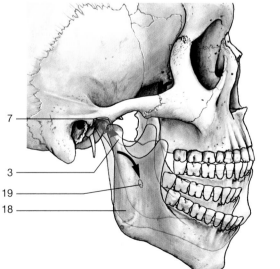
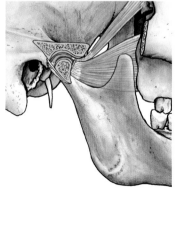
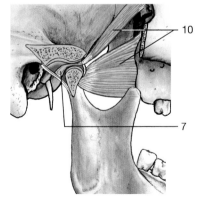

**Movements of the temporomandibular joint and the related lateral pterygoid muscles.**

1   Groove for sigmoid sinus
2   Mandibular nerve
3   Lateral pterygoid muscle
4   Styloid process
5   Sphenomandibular ligament
6   Stylomandibular ligament
7   Mylohyoid groove
8   Ethmoidal air cells
9   Ethmoidal bulla
10  Hiatus semilunaris
11  Middle meatus
12  Inferior nasal concha
13  Limen nasi
14  Vestibule with hairs
15  Inferior meatus
16  Hard palate
17  Soft palate
18  Vestibule of oral cavity
19  Lower lip
20  Mandible
21  Zygomatic arch
22  External acoustic meatus
23  Articular capsule
24  Lateral ligament
25  Mandibular notch
26  Zygomatic bone
27  Coronoid process
28  Maxilla
29  Mastoid process
30  Mandibular foramen

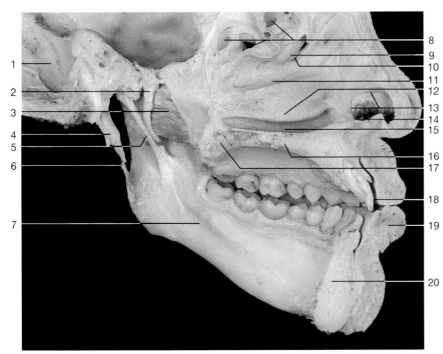

**Ligaments of temporomandibular joint.** Left half of the head (medial aspect).

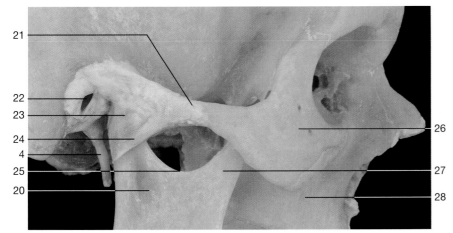

**Temporomandibular joint with ligaments** (lateral aspect).

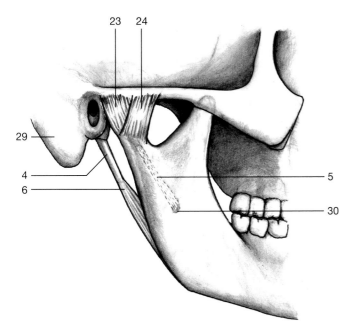

**Ligaments of temporomandibular joint** (lateral aspect).

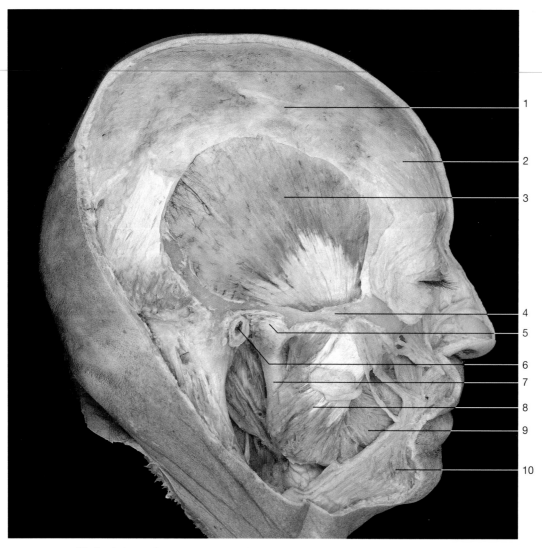

**Temporomandibular joint and masticatory muscles.** The masseter and temporal muscles are shown.

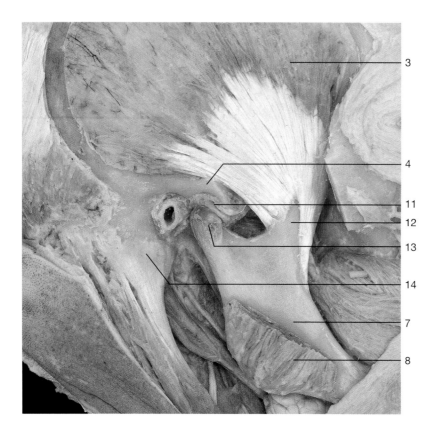

1  Galea aponeurotica
2  Frontal belly of occipitofrontalis muscle
3  Temporal muscle
4  Zygomatic arch
5  Temporomandibular joint
6  External acoustic meatus
7  Mandible
8  Masseter muscle
9  Buccinator muscle
10 Platysma muscle
11 Articular disc of temporomandibular joint
12 Coronoid process of mandible
13 Condylar process of mandible
14 Mastoid process

**Temporal muscle** with insertion at the mandible and the temporomandibular joint. Zygomatic arch and masseter muscle have been partly removed.

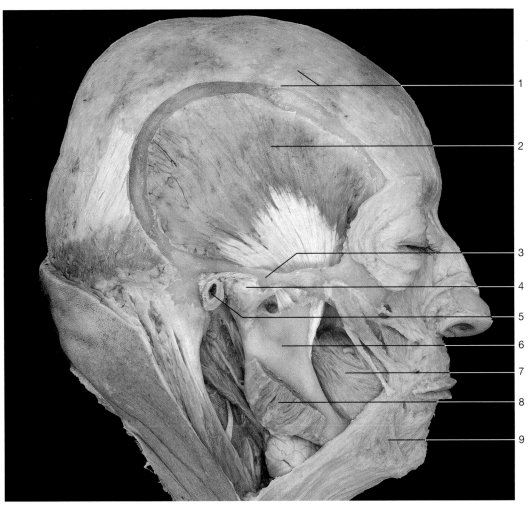

**Temporomandibular joint and masticatory muscles.** The masseter muscle has been partly removed.

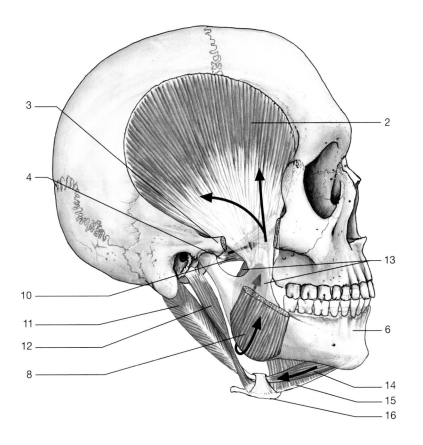

1  Galea aponeurotica
2  Temporal muscle
3  Zygomatic arch
4  Temporomandibular joint
5  External acoustic meatus
6  Mandible
7  Buccinator muscle
8  Masseter muscle (cut)
9  Platysma muscle
10 Lateral pterygoid muscle
11 Posterior belly of digastric muscle
12 Stylohyoid muscle
13 Medial pterygoid muscle
14 Anterior belly of digastric muscle
15 Mylohyoid muscle
16 Hyoid bone

**Effect of the masticatory muscles on the temporomandibular joint** (arrows).

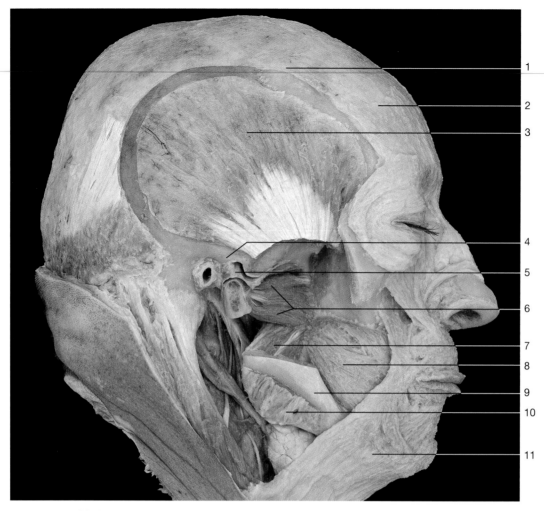

**Temporomandibular joint and masticatory muscles.** The zygomatic arch and part of the mandible have been removed to reveal the medial and lateral pterygoid muscles.

| | | | |
|---|---|---|---|
| 1 | Galea aponeurotica | 7 | Medial pterygoid muscle |
| 2 | Frontal belly of occipitofrontalis muscle | 8 | Buccinator muscle |
| 3 | Temporal muscle | 9 | Mandible |
| 4 | Zygomatic arch | 10 | Masseter muscle |
| 5 | Articular disc of temporomandibular joint | 11 | Platysma muscle |
| 6 | Lateral pterygoid muscle | | |

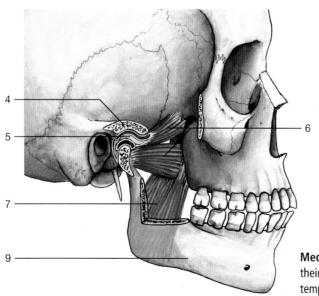

**Medial and lateral pterygoid muscles** and their connections with the articular disc of the temporomandibular joint.

1 Lateral pterygoid muscles
2 Medial pterygoid muscle
3 Temporomandibular joint
4 External acoustic meatus
5 Mandible
6 Nasal septum
7 Facial muscle
8 Cerebellum

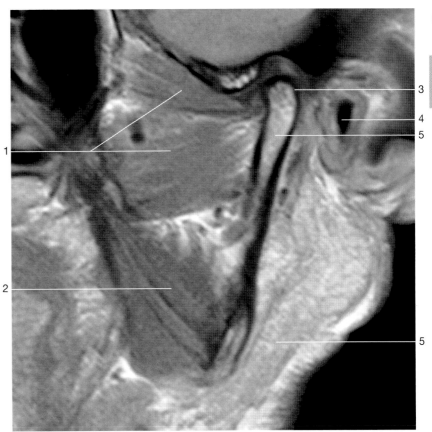

**Temporomandibular joint and masticatory muscles,** sagittal section (MRI scan).
(Prof. Uder, Dept. of Radiology, Univ. Erlangen-Nuremberg, Germany.)

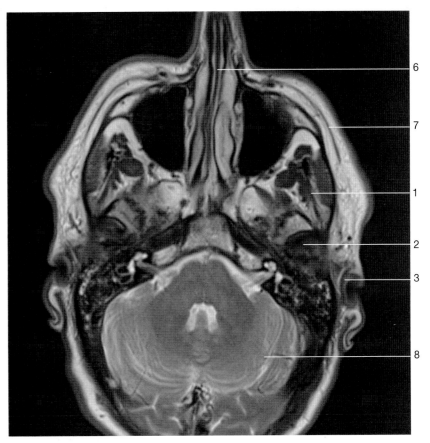

**Temporomandibular joint and masticatory muscles,** axial section (MRI scan).
(Prof. Uder, Dept. of Radiology, Univ. Erlangen-Nuremberg, Germany.)

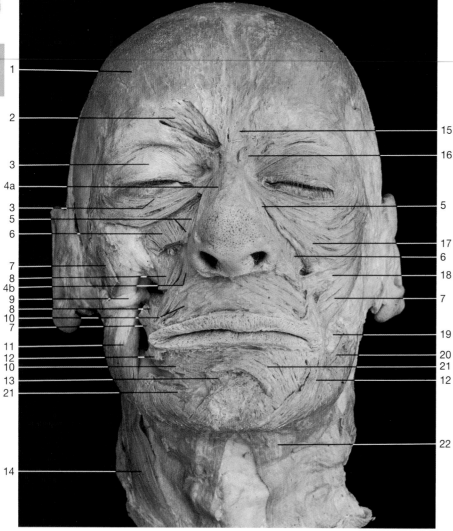

1  Frontal belly of occipitofrontalis muscle
2  Corrugator supercilii muscle
3  Palpebral part of orbicularis oculi muscle
4a Transverse part of nasalis muscle
4b Alar part of nasalis muscle
5  Levator labii superioris alaeque
   nasi muscle
6  Levator labii superioris muscle
7  Zygomaticus major muscle
8  Levator anguli oris muscle
9  Parotid duct
10 Orbicularis oris muscle
11 Masseter muscle
12 Depressor anguli oris muscle
13 Mentalis muscle
14 Sternocleidomastoid muscle
15 Procerus muscle
16 Depressor supercilii muscle
17 Orbital part of orbicularis oculi muscle
18 Zygomaticus minor muscle
19 Buccinator muscle
20 Risorius muscle
21 Depressor labii inferioris muscle
22 Platysma muscle
23 Galea aponeurotica
24 Temporoparietalis muscle
25 Occipital belly of occipitofrontalis muscle
26 Parotid gland with fascia
27 Temporal fascia
28 Orbicularis oculi muscle
29 Parotid duct and masseter muscle

**Facial muscles** (anterior aspect). Left side: superficial layer, right side: deeper layer.

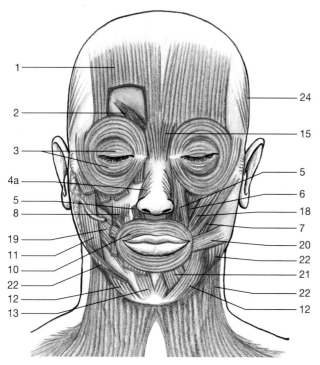

**Facial muscles** (anterior aspect).
Left side: superficial layer, right side: deeper layer.

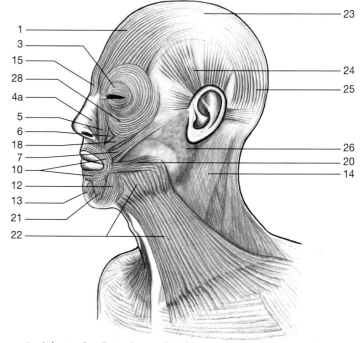

**Facial muscles** (lateral aspect). Sphincter-like muscles surround the orifices of the head. Radially arranged muscles work as their antagonists.

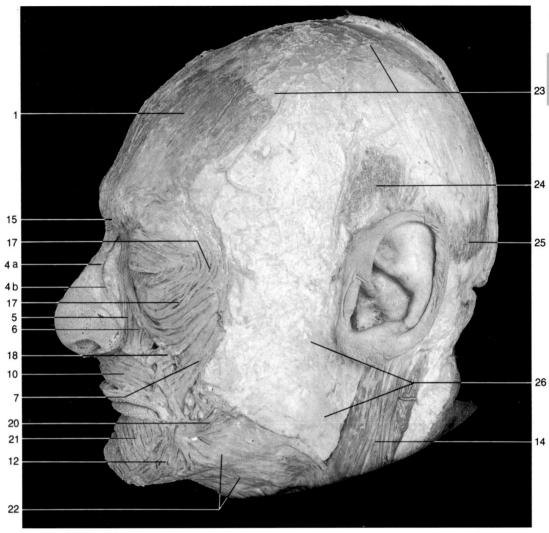

**Facial muscles** (lateral aspect).

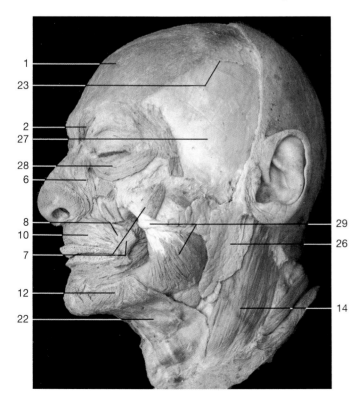

**Facial muscles and parotid gland** (lateral aspect).

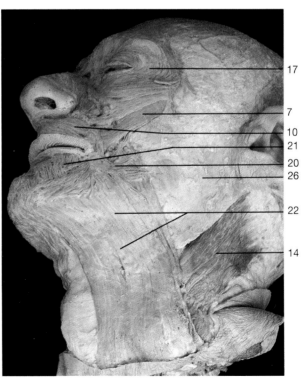

**Platysma muscle** (oblique-lateral aspect). Superficial lamina of cervical fascia partly removed.

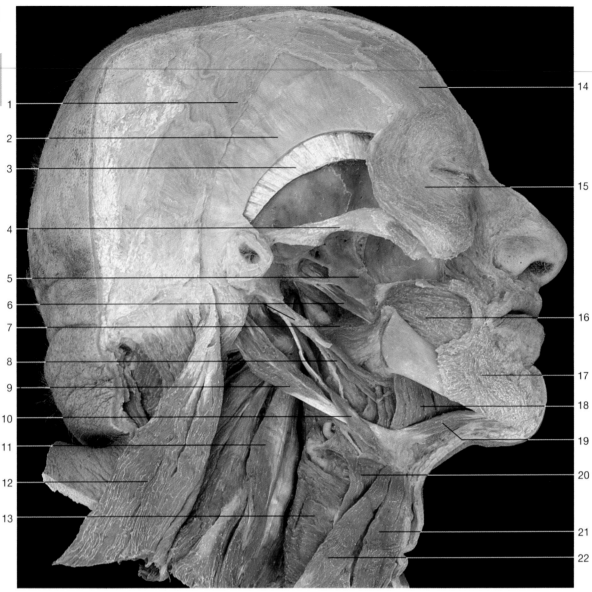

**Supra- and infrahyoid muscles and pharynx** (lateral aspect). Ramus of mandible, pterygoid muscles, and insertion of temporal muscle removed.

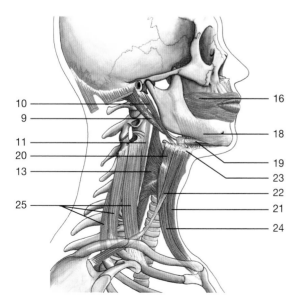

**Supra- and infrahyoid muscles** (lateral aspect).

1 Galea aponeurotica
2 Temporal fascia
3 Tendon of temporal muscle
4 Zygomatic arch
5 Lateral pterygoid plate
6 Tensor veli palatini muscle (styloid process)
7 Superior constrictor muscle of pharynx
8 Styloglossus muscle
9 Posterior belly of digastric muscle
10 Stylohyoid muscle
11 Longus capitis muscle
12 Sternocleidomastoid muscle (reflected)
13 Inferior constrictor of pharynx
14 Frontal belly of occipitofrontalis muscle
15 Orbital part of orbicularis oculi muscle
16 Buccinator muscle
17 Depressor anguli oris muscle
18 Mylohyoid muscle
19 Anterior belly of digastric muscle
20 Thyrohyoid muscle
21 Sternohyoid muscle
22 Omohyoid muscle
23 Hyoid bone
24 Sternothyroid muscle
25 Scalene muscles

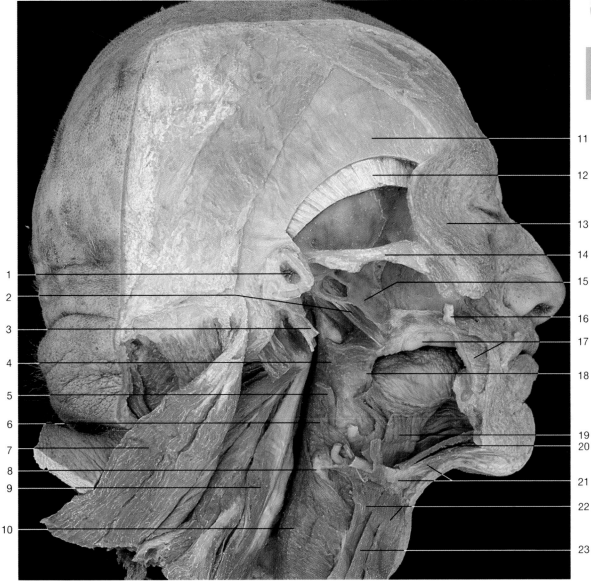

**Supra- and infrahyoid muscles and pharynx** (lateral aspect). Buccinator muscle removed; oral cavity opened.

1   External acoustic meatus
2   Tensor veli palatini muscle
3   Styloid process
4   Superior constrictor muscle of pharynx
5   Stylopharyngeus muscle (divided)
6   Middle constrictor muscle of pharynx
7   Sternocleidomastoid muscle
8   Greater horn of hyoid bone
9   Longus capitis muscle
10  Inferior constrictor muscle of pharynx
11  Temporal fascia
12  Tendon of temporal muscle
13  Orbicularis oculi muscle
14  Zygomatic arch
15  Lateral pterygoid plate
16  Parotid duct
17  Gingiva of upper jaw (without teeth) and
     buccinator muscle (divided)
18  Pterygomandibular raphe
19  Hyoglossus muscle
20  Mylohyoid muscle
21  Anterior belly of digastric muscle (hyoid bone)
22  Sternohyoid and thyrohyoid muscles
23  Omohyoid muscle

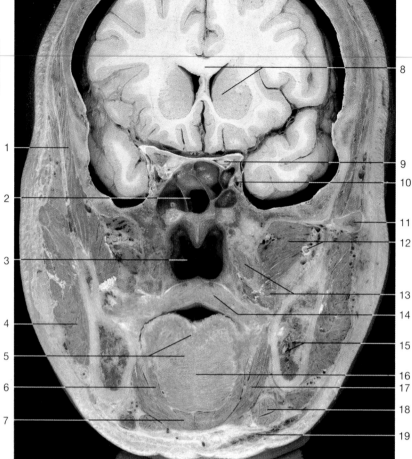

1  Temporal muscle
2  Sphenoidal sinus
3  Nasopharynx
4  Masseter muscle
5  Superior longitudinal, transverse and vertical muscles of tongue
6  Hyoglossus muscle
7  Geniohyoid muscle
8  Corpus callosum (caudate nucleus)
9  Optic nerve
10  Cavernous sinus
11  Zygomatic arch
12  Cross section of lateral pterygoid muscle and maxillary artery
13  Section of medial pterygoid muscle
14  Soft palate
15  Mandible and inferior alveolar nerve
16  Septum of the tongue
17  Mylohyoid muscle
18  Submandibular gland
19  Platysma muscle
20  Foramen magnum, vertebral artery and spinal cord
21  Internal carotid artery
22  Head of mandible
23  Styloid process
24  Inferior alveolar nerve
25  Lingual nerve and chorda tympani nerve
26  Medial pterygoid muscle
27  Uvula
28  Anterior belly of digastric muscle (cut)
29  Condyle of occipital bone
30  Mastoid process
31  Lateral pterygoid muscle
32  Auditory tube and levator veli palatini muscle
33  Tensor veli palatini muscle

**Coronal section through cranial, nasal, and oral cavities** at the level of sphenoidal sinus.

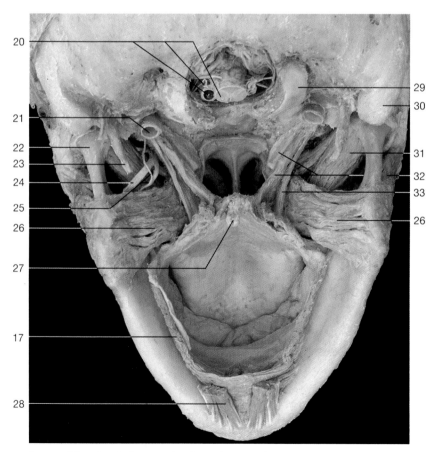

**Pterygoid and palatine muscles** (posterior aspect).

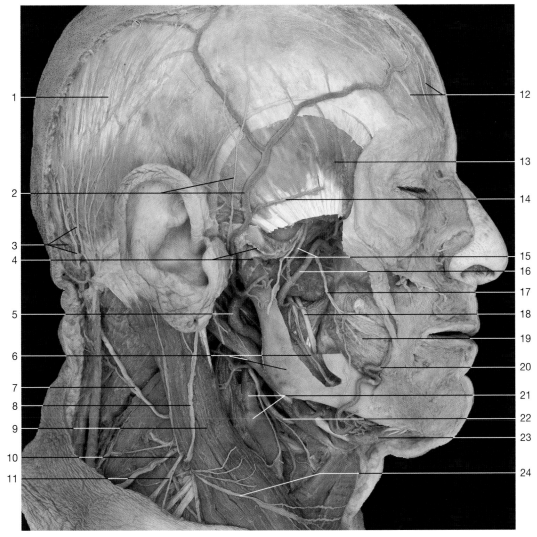

1 Galea aponeurotica
2 Superficial temporal artery and auriculo-temporal nerve
3 Occipital artery and greater occipital nerve (C₂)
4 Temporomandibular joint (opened)
5 External carotid artery
6 Mandible and inferior mandibular artery and nerve
7 Accessory nerve (var.)
8 Great auricular nerve
9 Sternocleidomastoi-deus muscle
10 Punctum nervosum
11 Supraclavicular nerves
12 Supra-orbital nerves
13 Temporal muscle
14 Transverse facial artery
15 Masseteric nerve and deep temporal branch of maxillary artery
16 Maxillary artery
17 Buccal nerve
18 Lingual nerve
19 Buccinator muscle
20 Facial artery
21 External carotid artery and sinus caroticus
22 Hypoglossal nerve
23 Digastric muscle
24 Transverse cervical nerves

**Dissection of maxillary artery** (lateral aspect). The ramus mandibulae has been partly removed and the canalis mandibulae has been opened.

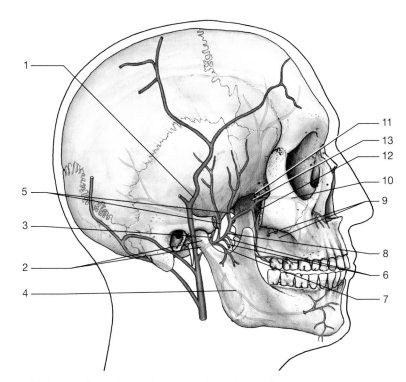

1 Superficial temporal artery

**Branches of the first part**
2 Deep auricular artery and anterior tympanic artery
3 Middle meningeal artery
4 Inferior alveolar artery

**Branches of the second part**
5 Deep temporal branches
6 Pterygoid branches
7 Masseteric artery
8 Buccal artery

**Branches of the third part**
9 Posterior superior alveolar artery
10 Infra-orbital artery
11 Sphenopalatine artery and branches to the nasal cavity
12 Descending palatine artery
13 Artery of the pterygoid canal

**Main branches of maxillary artery** (lateral aspect).

# 2.3 Brain and Regions of the Head

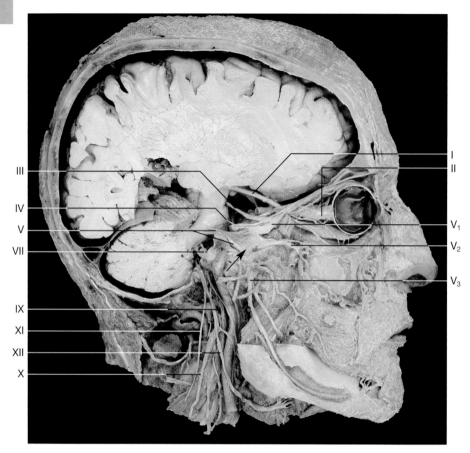

**Cranial nerves**

|       |   |                          |
|-------|---|--------------------------|
| I     | = | Olfactory nerves         |
| II    | = | Optic nerve              |
| III   | = | Oculomotor nerve         |
| IV    | = | Trochlear nerve          |
| V     | = | Trigeminal nerve         |
| $V_1$ | = | Ophthalmic nerve         |
| $V_2$ | = | Maxillary nerve          |
| $V_3$ | = | Mandibular nerve         |
| VI    | = | Abducent nerve           |
| VII   | = | Facial nerve             |
| VIII  | = | Vestibulocochlear nerve  |
| IX    | = | Glossopharyngeal nerve   |
| X     | = | Vagus nerve              |
| XI    | = | Accessory nerve          |
| XII   | = | Hypoglossal nerve        |

**Dissection of the cranial nerves** (indicated by I–XII) (lateral aspect). Brain, brain stem, and cerebellum have been partly removed. Arrow: trigeminal ganglion.

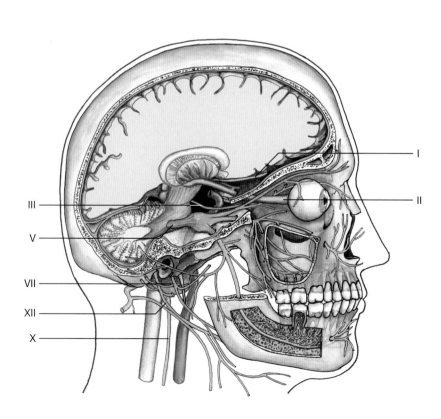

**Schematic drawing of the cranial nerves** (indicated by I–XII) (lateral aspect).

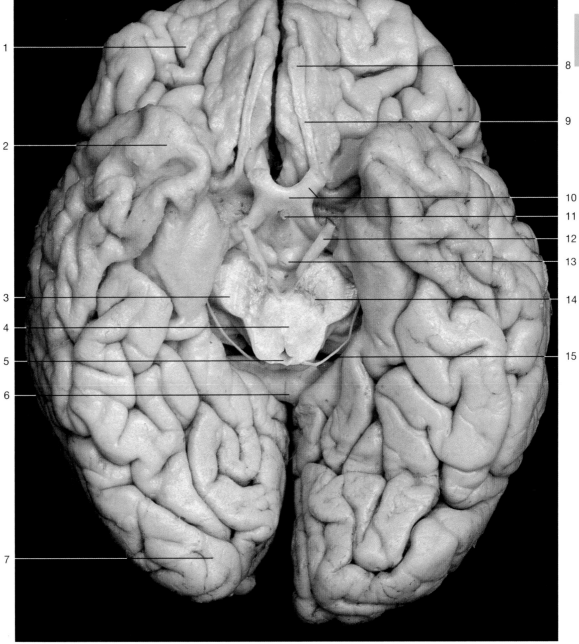

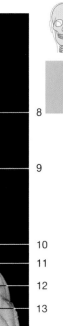

**Brain with cranial nerves** (inferior aspect). Midbrain divided.

| | | | |
|---|---|---|---|
| 1 | Frontal lobe | 9 | Olfactory tract |
| 2 | Temporal lobe | 10 | Optic nerve and optic chiasma |
| 3 | Pedunculus cerebri | 11 | Infundibulum |
| 4 | Midbrain (divided) | 12 | Oculomotor nerve (n. III) |
| 5 | Cerebral aqueduct | 13 | Mamillary body |
| 6 | Splenium of corpus callosum | 14 | Substantia nigra |
| 7 | Occipital lobe | 15 | Trochlear nerve (n. IV) |
| 8 | Olfactory bulb | | |

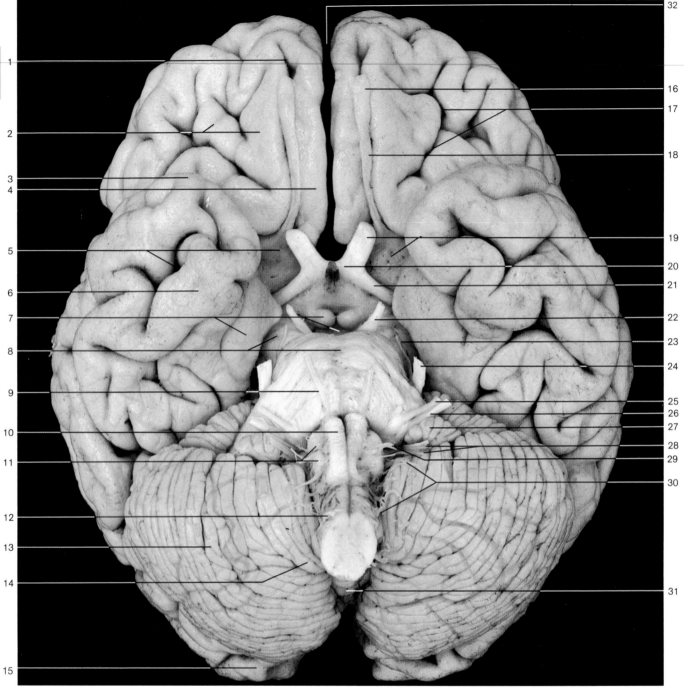

**Brain with cranial nerves** (inferior aspect). Meninges removed.

1  Olfactory sulcus (termination)
2  Orbital gyri
3  Temporal lobe
4  Straight gyrus
5  Olfactory trigone and inferior temporal sulcus
6  Medial occipitotemporal gyrus
7  Parahippocampal gyrus, mamillary body, and interpeduncular fossa
8  Pons and cerebral peduncle
9  Abducent nerve (n. VI)
10  Pyramid
11  Inferior olive

12  Cervical spinal nerves
13  Cerebellum
14  Tonsil of cerebellum
15  Occipital lobe (posterior pole)
16  Olfactory bulb
17  Orbital sulci of frontal lobe
18  Olfactory tract
19  Optic nerve (n. II) and anterior perforated substance
20  Optic chiasma
21  Optic tract
22  Oculomotor nerve (n. III)

23  Trochlear nerve (n. IV)
24  Trigeminal nerve (n. V)
25  Facial nerve (n. VII)
26  Vestibulocochlear nerve (n. VIII)
27  Flocculus of cerebellum
28  Glossopharyngeal nerve (n. IX) and vagus nerve (n. X)
29  Hypoglossal nerve (n. XII)
30  Accessory nerve (n. XI)
31  Vermis of cerebellum
32  Longitudinal fissure

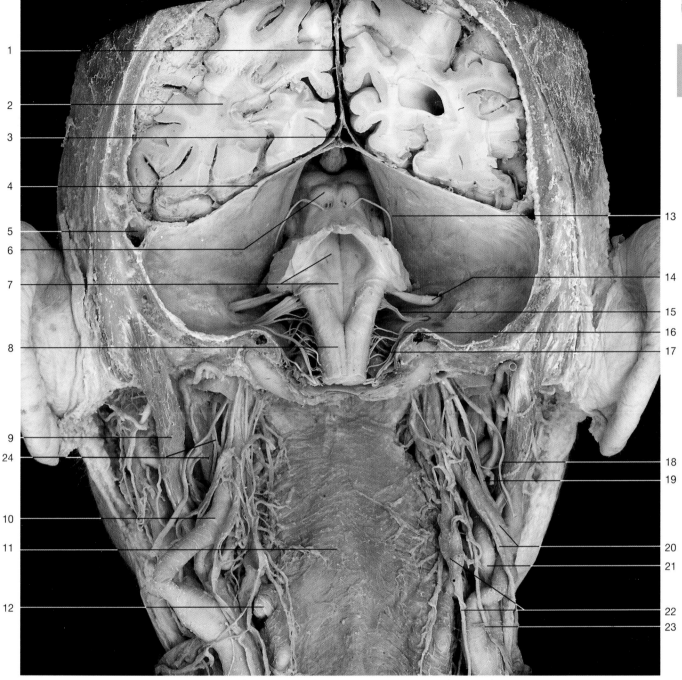

**Brain stem and pharynx with cranial nerves** (posterior aspect). **Dissection of trochlear (n. IV), facial (n. VII), vestibulocochlear (n. VIII), glossopharyngeal (n. IX), vagus (n. X), accessory (n. XI), and hypoglossal (n. XII) nerves.** The cranial cavity has been opened and the cerebellum removed.

| | | |
|---|---|---|
| 1 Falx cerebri | 11 Pharynx (middle constrictor muscle) | 19 Hypoglossal nerve (n. XII) |
| 2 Occipital lobe | 12 Hyoid bone (greater horn) | 20 Vagus nerve (n. X) and internal carotid artery |
| 3 Straight sinus | 13 Trochlear nerve (n. IV) | 21 External carotid artery |
| 4 Cerebellar tentorium | 14 Facial nerve (n. VII) and | 22 Sympathetic trunk and superior cervical ganglion |
| 5 Transverse sinus | vestibulocochlear nerve (n. VIII) | 23 Ansa cervicalis (superior root |
| 6 Inferior colliculus of midbrain | 15 Glossopharyngeal nerve (n. IX) | of hypoglossal nerve) |
| 7 Rhomboid fossa | and vagus nerve (n. X) | 24 Glossopharyngeal nerve (n. IX) and |
| 8 Medulla oblongata | 16 Accessory nerve (intracranial portion) (n. XI) | stylopharyngeus muscle |
| 9 Posterior belly of digastric muscle | 17 Hypoglossal nerve (intracranial portion) (n. XII) | |
| 10 Internal carotid artery | 18 Accessory nerve (n. XI) | |

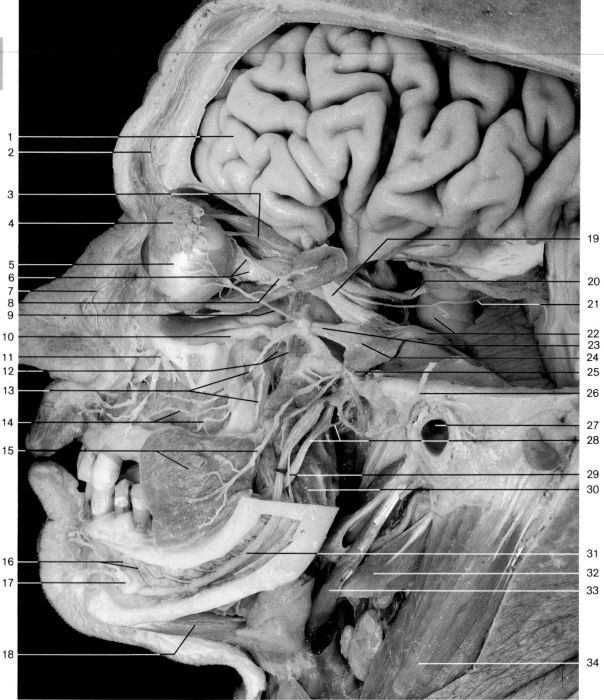

**Dissection of the trigeminal nerve (n. V) in its entirety.** Lateral wall of cranial cavity, lateral wall of orbit, zygomatic arch, and ramus of the mandible have been removed and the mandibular canal opened.

| | |
|---|---|
| 1 | Frontal lobe of cerebrum |
| 2 | Supra-orbital nerve |
| 3 | Lacrimal nerve |
| 4 | Lacrimal gland |
| 5 | Eyeball |
| 6 | Optic nerve and short ciliary nerves |
| 7 | External nasal branch of anterior ethmoidal nerve |
| 8 | Ciliary ganglion |
| 9 | Zygomatic nerve |
| 10 | Infra-orbital nerve |
| 11 | Infra-orbital foramen and terminal branches of infra-orbital nerve |
| 12 | Pterygopalatine ganglion and pterygopalatine nerves |
| 13 | Posterior superior alveolar nerves |
| 14 | Superior dental plexus |
| 15 | Buccinator muscle and buccal nerve |
| 16 | Inferior dental plexus |
| 17 | Mental foramen and mental nerve |
| 18 | Anterior belly of digastric muscle |
| 19 | Ophthalmic nerve (n. V$_1$) |
| 20 | Oculomotor nerve (n. III) |
| 21 | Trochlear nerve (n. IV) |
| 22 | Trigeminal nerve (n. V) and pons |
| 23 | Maxillary nerve (n. V$_2$) |
| 24 | Trigeminal ganglion |
| 25 | Mandibular nerve (n. V$_3$) |
| 26 | Auriculotemporal nerve |
| 27 | External acoustic meatus (divided) |
| 28 | Lingual nerve and chorda tympani |
| 29 | Mylohyoid nerve |
| 30 | Medial pterygoid muscle |
| 31 | Inferior alveolar nerve |
| 32 | Posterior belly of digastric muscle |
| 33 | Stylohyoid muscle |
| 34 | Sternocleidomastoid muscle |

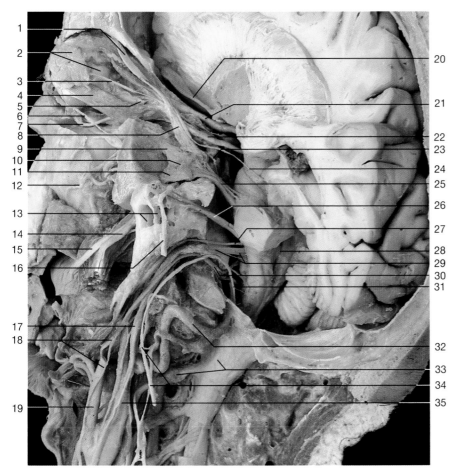

1   Frontal nerve
2   Lacrimal gland and eyeball
3   Lacrimal nerve
4   Lateral rectus muscle
5   Ciliary ganglion lateral to optic nerve
6   Zygomatic nerve
7   Inferior branch of oculomotor nerve
8   Ophthalmic nerve (n. V$_1$)
9   Maxillary nerve (n. V$_2$)
10  Trigeminal ganglion
11  Mandibular nerve (n. V$_3$)
12  Posterior superior alveolar nerves
13  Tympanic cavity, external acoustic meatus, and tympanic membrane
14  Inferior alveolar nerve
15  Lingual nerve
16  Facial nerve (n. VII)
17  Vagus nerve (n. X)
18  Hypoglossal nerve (n. XII) and superior root of ansa cervicalis
19  External carotid artery
20  Olfactory tract (n. I)
21  Optic nerve (n. II) (intracranial part)
22  Oculomotor nerve (n. III)
23  Abducent nerve (n. VI)
24  Trochlear nerve (n. IV)
25  Trigeminal nerve (n. V)
26  Vestibulocochlear nerve (n. VIII) and facial nerve (n. VII)
27  Glossopharyngeal nerve (n. IX) (leaving brain stem)
28  Rhomboid fossa
29  Vagus nerve (n. X) (leaving brain stem)
30  Hypoglossal nerve (n. XII) (leaving medulla oblongata)
31  Accessory nerve (n. XI) (ascending from foramen magnum)
32  Vertebral artery
33  Spinal ganglion and dura mater of spinal cord
34  Accessory nerve (n. XI)
35  Internal carotid artery
36  Lateral and medial branch of supra-orbital nerve
37  Infratrochlear nerve
38  Infra-orbital nerve
39  Pterygopalatine ganglion and pterygopalatine nerves
40  Middle superior alveolar nerves (entering superior dental plexus)
41  Buccal nerve
42  Mental nerve and mental foramen
43  Auriculotemporal nerve
44  Otic ganglion
45  Chorda tympani
46  Mylohyoid nerve
47  Submandibular gland
48  Hyoid bone

**Cranial nerves in connection with the brain stem.** Left side (lateral superior aspect). Left half of brain and head partly removed. Notice the location of the trigeminal ganglion.

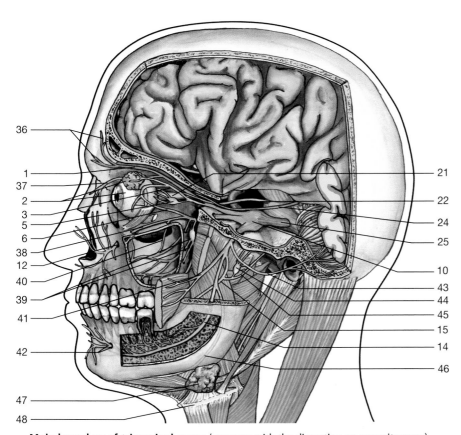

**Main branches of trigeminal nerve** (compare with the dissection on opposite page).

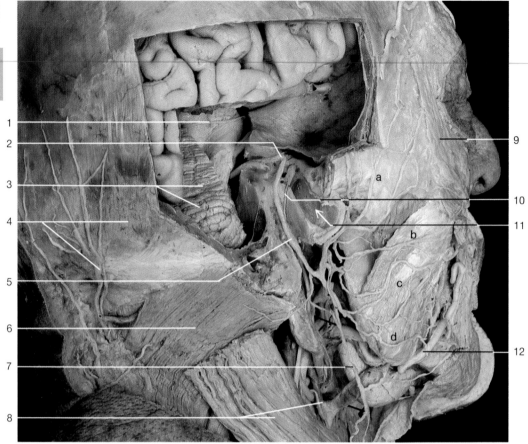

**Dissection of the facial nerve (n. VII) in its entirety.** Cranial cavity fenestrated, temporal lobe partly removed. Facial canal and tympanic cavity opened, posterior wall of external acoustic meatus removed.
**Branches of the facial nerve:** a = temporal branch; b = zygomatic branches; c = buccal branches; d = marginal mandibular branch.

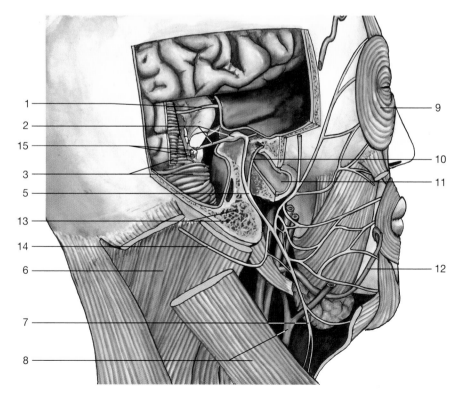

**Facial nerve** (compare with the dissection above).

1   Trochlear nerve (n. IV)
2   Facial nerve (n. VII) with geniculate ganglion
3   Cerebellum (right hemisphere)
4   Occipital belly of occipitofrontalis muscle
    and greater occipital nerve
5   Facial nerve (n. VII) at stylomastoid foramen
6   Splenius capitis muscle
7   Cervical branch of facial nerve (n. VII)
8   Sternocleidomastoid muscle and
    retromandibular vein
9   Orbicularis oculi muscle
10  Chorda tympani
11  External acoustic meatus
12  Facial artery
13  Mastoid air cells
14  Posterior auricular nerve
15  Nucleus and genu of facial nerve

**Cranial nerves in connection with
the brain stem** (oblique-lateral aspect).
Lateral portion of the skull, brain, neck
and facial structures, lateral wall of orbit
and oral cavity have been removed. The
tympanic cavity has been opened.
The mandible has been divided and
the muscles of mastication have been
removed.

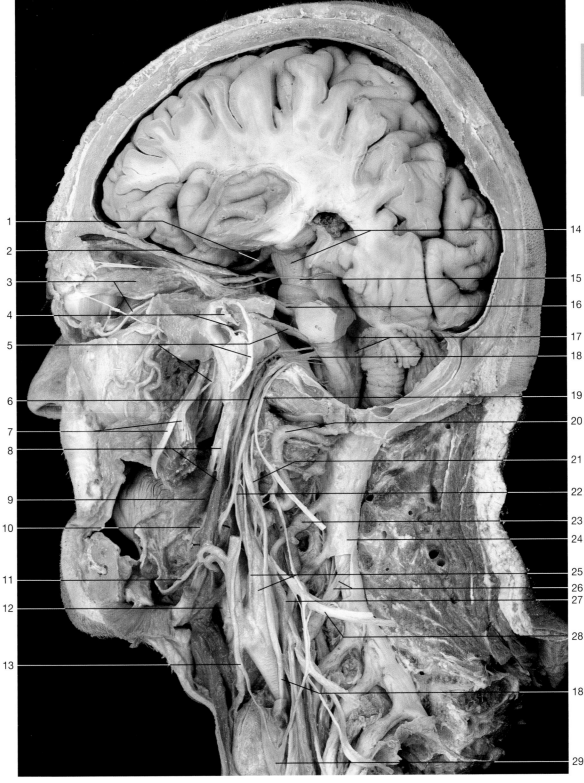

| | | |
|---|---|---|
| 1 Optic tract | 11 Lingual branch of hypoglossal nerve | 22 Hypoglossal nerve (n. XII) |
| 2 Oculomotor nerve (n. III) | 12 External carotid artery | 23 Spinal ganglion with dural sheath |
| 3 Lateral rectus muscle and inferior branch of oculomotor nerve | 13 Superior root of ansa cervicalis (branch of hypoglossal nerve, derived from $C_1$) | 24 Dura mater of spinal cord |
| 4 Malleus and chorda tympani | 14 Lateral ventricle with choroid plexus and cerebral peduncle | 25 Internal carotid artery and carotid sinus branch of glossopharyngeal nerve |
| 5 Chorda tympani, facial nerve (n. VII), and vestibulocochlear nerve (n. VIII) | 15 Trochlear nerve (n. IV) | 26 Dorsal roots of spinal nerve |
| 6 Glossopharyngeal nerve (n. XI) | 16 Trigeminal nerve (n. V) | 27 Sympathetic trunk |
| 7 Lingual nerve and inferior alveolar nerve | 17 Fourth ventricle and rhomboid fossa | 28 Branch of cervical plexus (ventral primary ramus of third cervical spinal nerve) |
| 8 Styloid process and stylohyoid muscle | 18 Vagus nerve (n. X) | |
| 9 Styloglossus muscle | 19 Accessory nerve (n. XI) | 29 Ansa cervicalis |
| 10 Lingual branches of glossopharyngeal nerve | 20 Vertebral artery | |
| | 21 Superior cervical ganglion | |

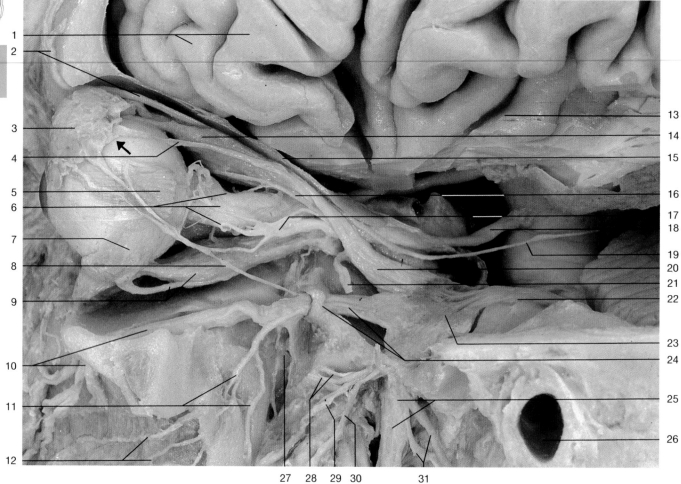

**Cranial nerves of the orbit and pterygopalatine fossa** (left orbit, lateral aspect). **Dissection of optic (n. II), oculomotor (n. III), trochlear (n. IV), ophthalmic (n. V$_1$), and abducent (n. VI) nerves.** Note the zygomaticolacrimal anastomosis (arrow).

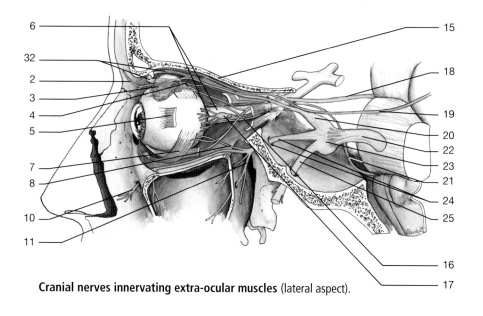

**Cranial nerves innervating extra-ocular muscles** (lateral aspect).

| | | |
|---|---|---|
| 1  Frontal lobe | 6  Optic nerve (n. II) and short ciliary nerves | 10  Infra-orbital nerve |
| 2  Supra-orbital nerve | 7  Inferior oblique muscle | 11  Posterior superior alveolar nerves |
| 3  Lacrimal gland | 8  Zygomatic nerve | 12  Branches of superior alveolar plexus |
| 4  Lacrimal nerve | 9  Inferior branch of oculomotor nerve (n. III) and | adjacent to mucous membrane |
| 5  Lateral rectus muscle (divided) | inferior rectus muscle | of maxillary sinus |

13  Central sulcus of insula
14  Superior rectus muscle
15  Periorbita (roof of orbit)
16  Nasociliary nerve
17  Ciliary ganglion
18  Oculomotor nerve (n. III)
19  Trochlear nerve (n. IV)
20  Ophthalmic nerve (n. V$_1$)
21  Abducent nerve (n. VI) (divided)
22  Trigeminal nerve (n. V)
23  Trigeminal ganglion
24  Maxillary nerve (n. V$_2$) and
     foramen rotundum
25  Mandibular nerve (n. V$_3$)
26  External acoustic meatus
27  Pterygopalatine nerves
28  Deep temporal nerves
29  Buccal nerve
30  Masseteric nerve
31  Auriculotemporal nerve
32  Trochlea and superior oblique muscle

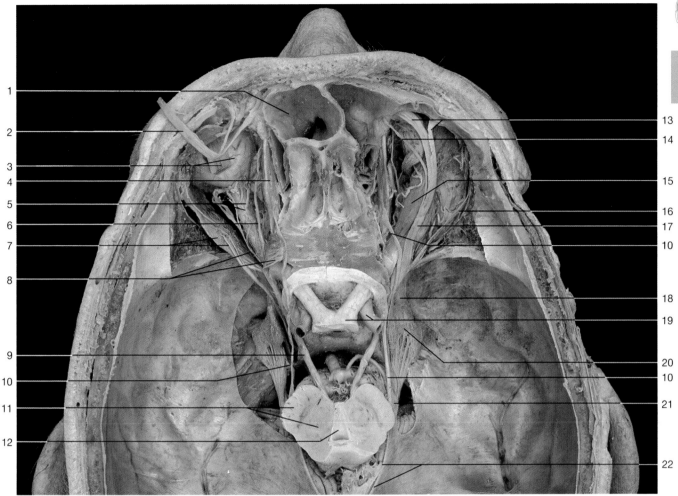

**Cranial nerves of the orbit** (superior aspect). Right side: superficial layer, left side: middle layer of the orbit. Superior rectus muscle and frontal nerve divided and reflected. Tentorium and dura mater partly removed.

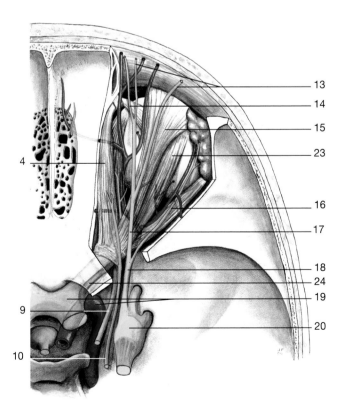

**Cranial nerves within the orbit** (superior aspect).

1    Frontal sinus (enlarged)
2    Frontal nerve (divided and reflected)
3    Superior rectus muscle (divided) and eyeball
4    Superior oblique muscle
5    Short ciliary nerves and optic nerve (n. II)
6    Nasociliary nerve
7    Abducent nerve (n. VI) and
     lateral rectus muscle
8    Ciliary ganglion and superior rectus muscle
     (reflected)
9    Oculomotor nerve (n. III)
10   Trochlear nerve (n. IV)
11   Crus cerebri and midbrain
12   Inferior wall of the third ventricle
     connected with cerebral aqueduct
13   Lateral and medial branches of supra-orbital
     nerve
14   Supratrochlear nerve
15   Superior levator palpebrae muscle
16   Lacrimal nerve
17   Frontal nerve
18   Ophthalmic nerve (n. V₁)
19   Optic chiasma and internal carotid artery
20   Trigeminal ganglion
21   Trigeminal nerve (n. V)
22   Tentorial notch
23   Superior rectus muscle
24   Ophthalmic artery

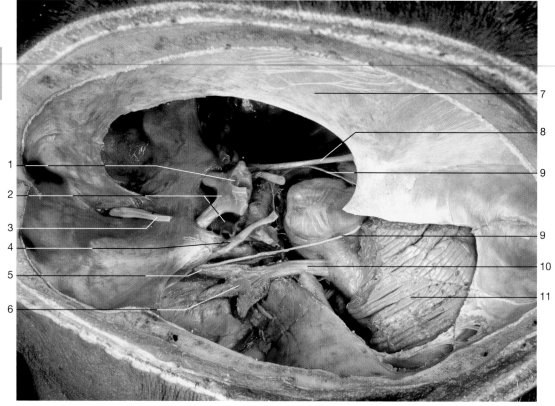

**Base of the skull with cranial nerves.** The brain stem was divided and the tentorium fenestrated. Both hemispheres were removed.

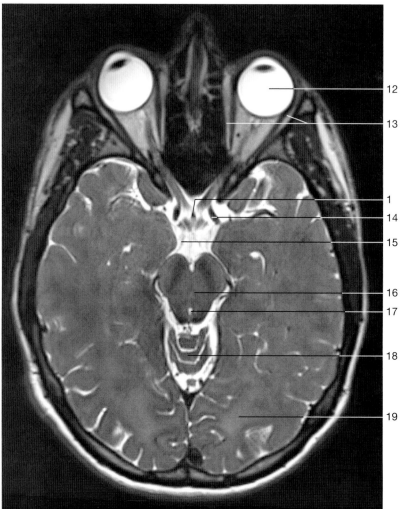

1  Infundibulum
2  Optic chiasma and internal carotid artery
3  Olfactory tract
4  Oculomotor nerve (n. III)
5  Ophthalmic nerve (n. V₁)
6  Trigeminal ganglion
7  Falx cerebri
8  Tentorial notch
9  Trochlear nerve (n. IV)
10  Trigeminal nerve (n. V)
11  Cerebellum
12  Eyeball
13  Medial and lateral rectus muscles
14  Internal carotid artery
15  Oculomotor nerve (n. III)
16  Midbrain
17  Cerebral aqueduct
18  Vermis of cerebellum
19  Occipital lobe of the cerebrum

**Axial section through the head** at the level of the sella turcica demonstrating cranial nerves (MRI scan). (Dept. of Neurosurgery, Univ. Erlangen-Nuremberg, Germany.)

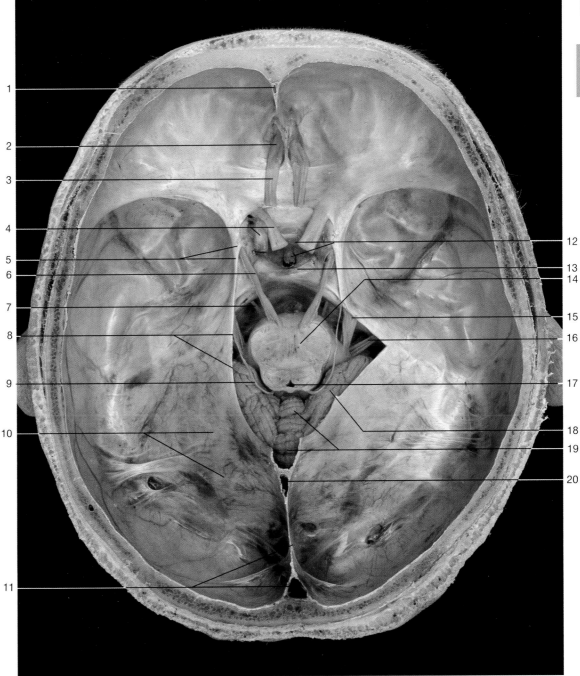

**Base of the skull with cranial nerves** (internal aspect). Both cerebral hemispheres and upper part of the brain stem have been removed. Incision on the right cerebellar tentorium to display the cranial nerves of the infratentorial space.

1   Superior sagittal sinus with falx cerebri
2   Olfactory bulb
3   Olfactory tract
4   Optic nerve and internal carotid artery
5   Anterior clinoid process and
    anterior attachment of cerebellar tentorium
6   Oculomotor nerve (n. III)
7   Abducent nerve (n. VI)
8   Tentorial notch (incisura tentorii)
9   Trochlear nerve (n. IV)
10  Cerebellar tentorium
11  Falx cerebri and confluence of sinuses

12  Hypophysial fossa, infundibulum, and
    diaphragma sellae
13  Dorsum sellae
14  Midbrain (divided)
15  Trigeminal nerve (n. V)
16  Facial nerve (n. VII), nervus intermedius, and
    vestibulocochlear nerve (n. VIII)
17  Cerebral aqueduct
18  Right hemisphere of cerebellum
19  Vermis of cerebellum
20  Straight sinus

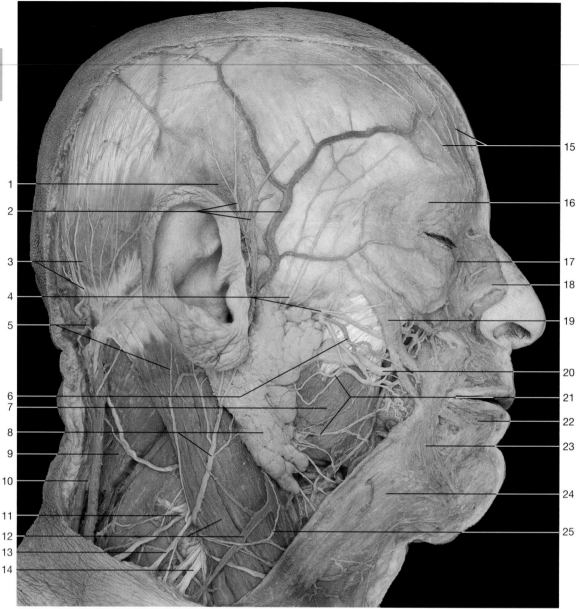

**Superficial dissection of lateral region of the face.** Peripheral distribution of facial nerve (n. VII).

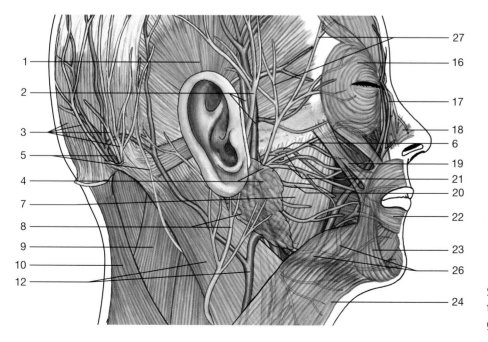

**Superficial region of the face.** Note the facial plexus within the parotid gland (lateral aspect).

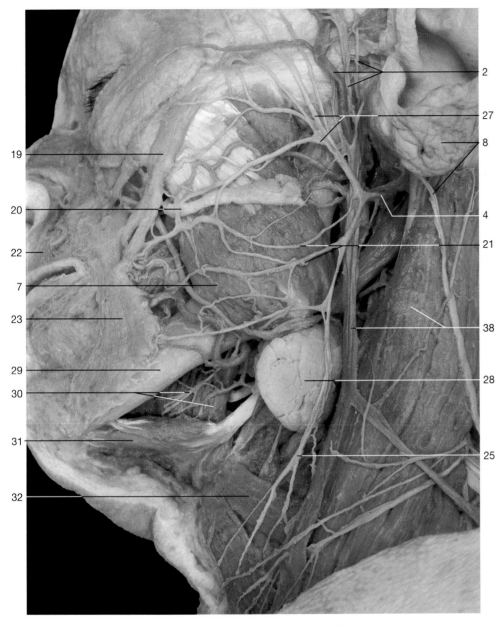

**Deep dissection of facial nerve. Retromandibular and submandibular regions** (lateral aspect). The parotid gland has been removed.

1   Temporoparietalis muscle
2   Superficial temporal artery and vein, and auriculotemporal nerve
3   Occipital belly of occipitofrontalis muscle and greater occipital nerve (C₂)
4   Facial nerve (n. VII)
5   Lesser occipital nerve and occipital artery
6   Transverse facial artery
7   Masseter muscle
8   Parotid gland and great auricular nerve
9   Splenius capitis muscle
10  Trapezius muscle
11  Punctum nervosum, point of distribution of cutaneous nerves of cervical plexus
12  Sternocleidomastoid muscle and external jugular vein
13  Supraclavicular nerves
14  Brachial plexus
15  Supra-orbital nerves
16  Orbicularis oculi muscle
17  Angular artery (terminal branch of facial artery)
18  Nasalis muscle
19  Zygomaticus major muscle
20  Parotid duct
21  Zygomatic and buccal branches of facial nerve
22  Orbicularis oris muscle
23  Depressor anguli oris muscle
24  Platysma muscle
25  Cervical branch of facial nerve (anastomosing with transverse cervical nerve of cervical plexus)
26  Facial artery and vein
27  Temporal branches of facial nerve
28  Submandibular gland
29  Mandible
30  Mylohyoideus muscle and nerve
31  Anterior belly of digastric muscle
32  Omohyoid muscle
33  Greater petrosal nerve
34  Geniculate ganglion
35  Chorda tympani
36  Posterior auricular nerve
37  Stylomastoid foramen
38  Sternocleidomastoid muscle and retromandibular vein

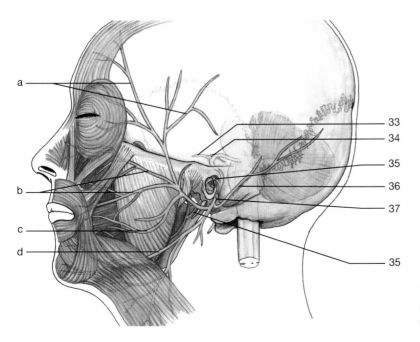

**Main branches of facial nerve** (lateral aspect).
a = temporal branches; b = zygomatic branches;
c = buccal branches; d = marginal mandibular branch.

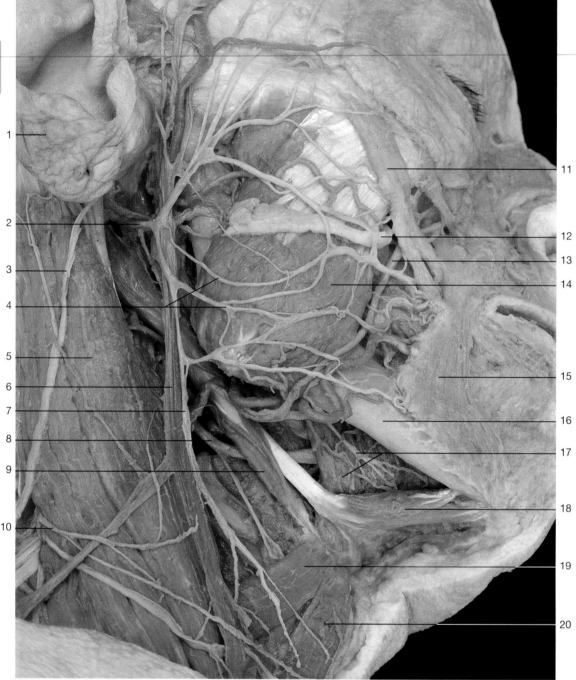

**Deep dissection of facial nerve. Retromandibular and submandibular regions** (lateral aspect).
The parotid gland and the submandibular gland have been removed. The parotid plexus (4) is formed by anastomosis of the temporal, zygomatic, buccal, marginal mandibular, and cervical branches of the facial nerve, arising in the parotid gland.

| | | | | |
|---|---|---|---|---|
| 1 | Parotid gland | 8 | Hypoglossal nerve (n. XII) | 15 Depressor anguli oris muscle |
| 2 | Facial nerve (n. VII) | 9 | Stylohyoid muscle | 16 Mandible |
| 3 | Great auricular nerve | 10 | Transverse cervical nerve | 17 Mylohyoid muscle and nerve |
| 4 | Parotid plexus | 11 | Zygomaticus major muscle | 18 Anterior belly of digastric muscle |
| 5 | Sternocleidomastoid muscle | 12 | Parotid duct | 19 Omohyoid muscle |
| 6 | Retromandibular vein | 13 | Facial artery | 20 Sternohyoid muscle |
| 7 | Cervical branch of facial nerve | 14 | Masseter muscle | |

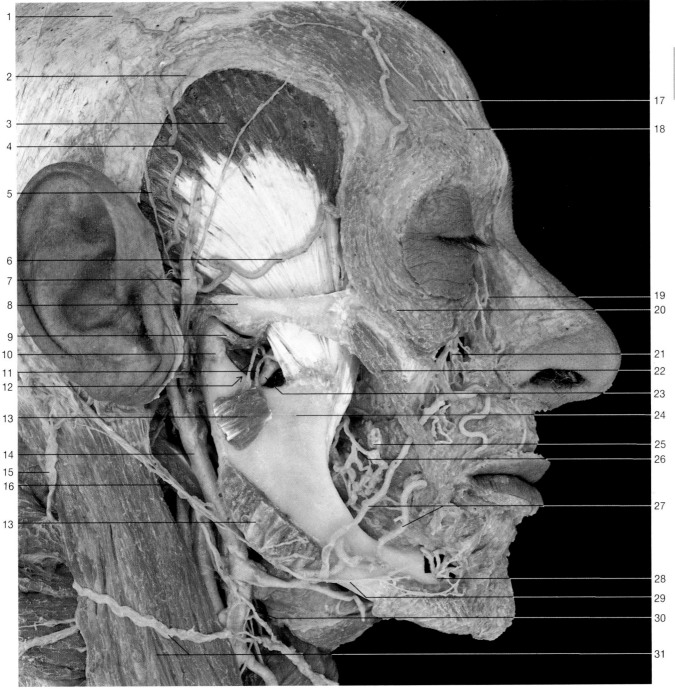

**Superficial dissection of lateral region of the face.** Masseter muscle and temporal fascia have been partly removed to display the masseteric artery and nerve.

1   Galea aponeurotica
2   Temporal fascia
3   Temporal muscle
4   Parietal branch
    of superficial temporal artery
5   Auriculotemporal nerve
6   Frontal branch
    of superficial temporal artery
7   Superficial temporal vein
8   Zygomatic arch
9   Articular disc
    of temporomandibular joint

10   Head of mandible
11   Masseteric artery and nerve
12   Mandibular notch
13   Masseter muscle (divided)
14   External carotid artery
15   Great auricular nerve
16   Facial nerve (reflected)
17   Frontal belly of occipitofrontalis muscle
18   Medial branch of supra-orbital nerve
19   Angular artery
20   Orbicularis oculi muscle
21   Infra-orbital nerve

22   Zygomaticus major muscle
23   Maxillary artery
24   Coronoid process
25   Parotid duct (divided)
26   Buccal nerve
27   Facial artery and vein
28   Mental nerve
29   Mandibular branch of facial nerve
30   Cervical branch of facial nerve
31   Transverse cervical nerve
     (communicating branch with facial nerve)
     and sternocleidomastoid muscle

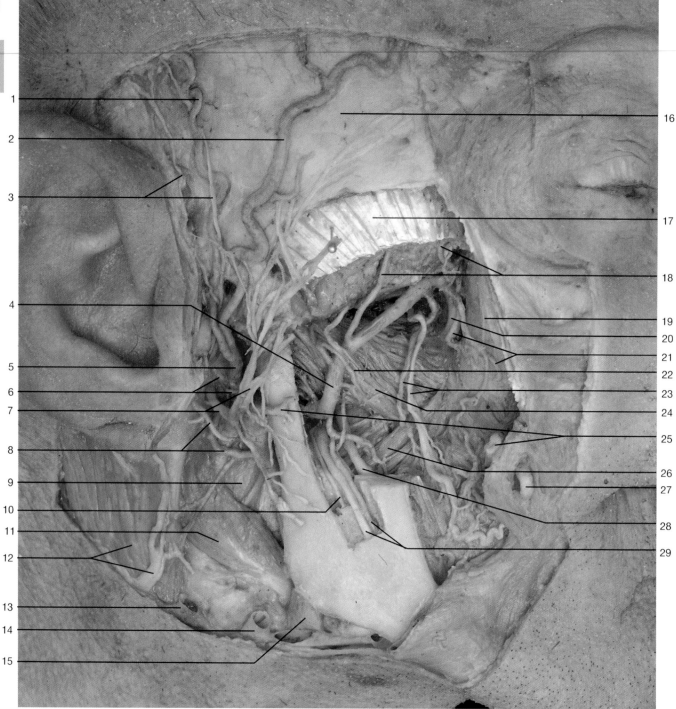

**Deep dissection of facial and retromandibular regions.** The coronoid process together with the insertions of temporal muscle have been removed to display the maxillary artery. The upper part of the mandibular canal has been opened.

| | | |
|---|---|---|
| 1 Parietal branch of superficial temporal artery | 9 Internal jugular vein | 21 Posterior superior alveolar arteries |
| 2 Frontal branch of superficial temporal artery | 10 Mylohyoid nerve | 22 Masseteric artery and nerve |
| 3 Auriculotemporal nerve | 11 Posterior belly of digastric muscle | 23 Buccal nerve and artery |
| 4 Maxillary artery | 12 Great auricular nerve and sternocleidomastoid muscle | 24 Lateral pterygoid |
| 5 Superficial temporal artery | 13 External jugular vein | 25 Transverse facial artery and parotid duct (divided) |
| 6 Communicating branches between facial and auriculotemporal nerves | 14 Retromandibular vein | 26 Medial pterygoid muscle |
| 7 Facial nerve | 15 Submandibular gland | 27 Facial artery |
| 8 Posterior auricular artery and anterior auricular branch of superficial temporal artery | 16 Temporal fascia | 28 Lingual nerve |
| | 17 Temporal tendon | 29 Inferior alveolar artery and nerve (mandibular canal opened) |
| | 18 Deep temporal arteries | |
| | 19 Posterior superior alveolar nerve | |
| | 20 Sphenopalatine artery | |

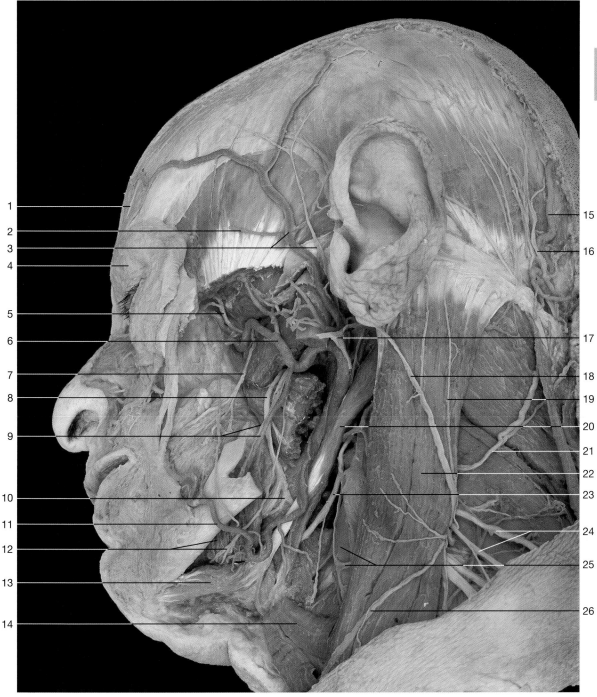

**Dissection of peripharyngeal and retromandibular regions.** The mandible has been partly removed (oblique-lateral aspect).

1  Supra-orbital nerve (medial branch)
2  Temporal muscle
3  Superficial temporal artery and auriculotemporal nerve
4  Orbicularis oculi muscle
5  Anterior deep temporal artery
6  Maxillary artery
7  Buccal nerve
8  Lingual nerve
9  Inferior alveolar nerve and artery
10  Submandibular ganglion
11  Facial artery
12  Mylohyoid muscle and nerve
13  Anterior belly of digastric muscle
14  Omohyoid muscle
15  Occipital artery
16  Greater occipital nerve (C₂)
17  Facial nerve (cut) (n. VII)
18  Great auricular nerve
19  Lesser occipital nerve
20  Posterior belly of digastric muscle
21  Accessory nerve (Var.)
22  Sternocleidomastoid muscle
23  Hypoglossus nerve (n. XII)
24  Supraclavicular nerves (lateral and intermedial branches)
25  Internal jugular vein and ansa cervicalis
26  Anterior supraclavicular nerve

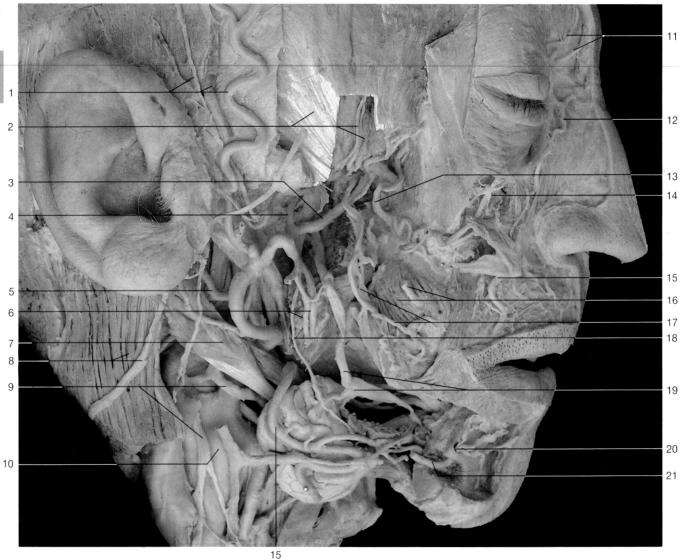

**Deep dissection of facial and retromandibular regions.** The mandible and pterygoid muscles have been removed, the temporal muscle was fenestrated.

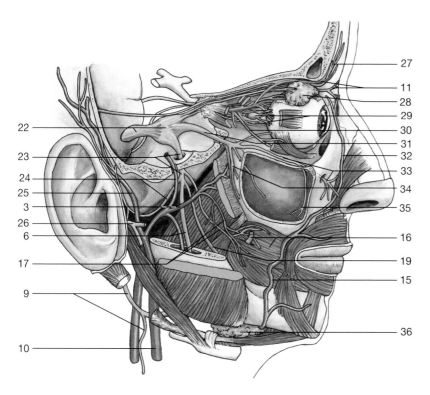

**Deep region of the face with arteries and nerves,** particularly dissection of maxillary artery and trigeminal nerve.

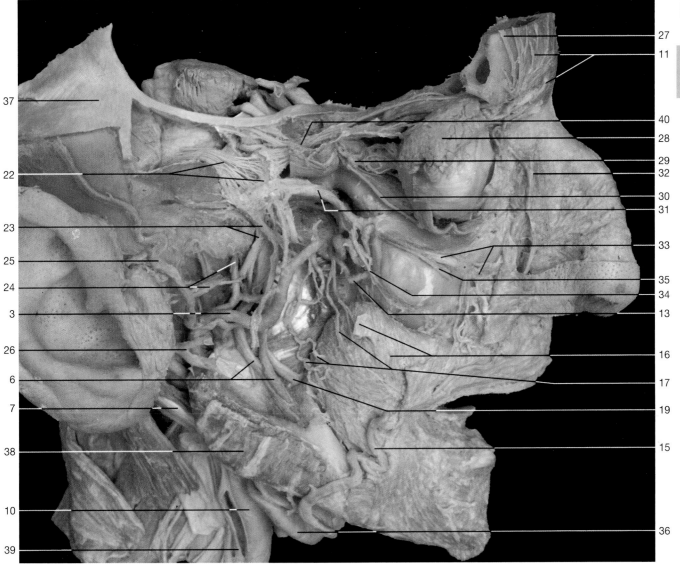

**Dissection of para- and retropharyngeal regions.** The mandible and the lateral wall of the orbit have been removed. The main branches of the trigeminal nerve and its ganglion are displayed.

1 Superficial temporal artery and vein and auriculotemporal nerve
2 Tendon of temporal muscle, deep temporal nerves and artery
3 Maxillary artery
4 Middle meningeal artery
5 Occipital artery
6 Inferior alveolar artery and nerve
7 Posterior belly of digastric muscle
8 Great auricular nerve and sternocleidomastoid muscle
9 Hypoglossal nerve and superior root of ansa cervicalis
10 External carotid artery
11 Supratrochlear nerve and medial branch of supra-orbital artery

12 Angular artery
13 Posterior superior alveolar artery
14 Infra-orbital nerve
15 Facial artery
16 Parotid duct (divided) and buccinator muscle
17 Buccal artery and nerve
18 Mylohyoid nerve
19 Lingual nerve and submandibular ganglion
20 Mental nerve and foramen
21 Inferior alveolar nerve
22 Trigeminal nerve and ganglion
23 Mandibular nerve (n. V₃)
24 Auriculotemporal nerve and middle meningeal artery

25 Superficial temporal artery
26 Facial nerve
27 Lateral branch of supra-orbital nerve
28 Lacrimal gland
29 Ciliary ganglion and short ciliary nerves
30 Inferior branch of oculomotor nerve
31 Maxillary nerve (n. V₂)
32 Angular artery
33 Infra-orbital nerve
34 Posterior superior alveolar nerve
35 Anterior superior alveolar nerve
36 Submandibular gland
37 Cerebellar tentorium
38 Masseter muscle
39 Superior root of ansa cervicalis
40 Ophthalmic nerve (n. V₁)

# 2.4 Brain and Sensory Organs

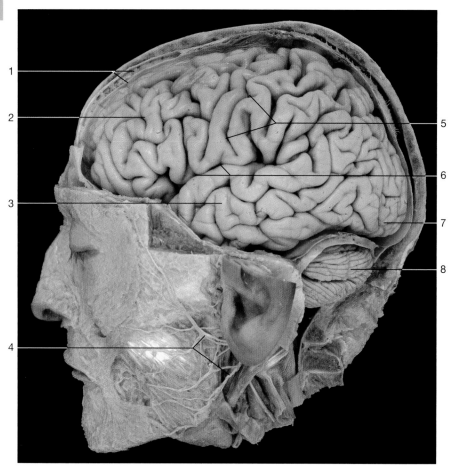

| | |
|---|---|
| 1 | Vertex of the skull and dura mater |
| 2 | Frontal lobe |
| 3 | Temporal lobe |
| 4 | Facial nerve (n. VII) |
| 5 | Central sulcus |
| 6 | Lateral sulcus |
| 7 | Occipital lobe |
| 8 | Cerebellum |
| 9 | Frontal sinus |
| 10 | Eye and optic nerve (n. II) |
| 11 | Nasal cavity |
| 12 | Oral cavity |
| 13 | Tongue |
| 14 | Brain stem |
| 15 | Base of skull |
| 16 | Spinal cord |
| 17 | Vertebral column |

**Dissection of the head to show the brain with pia mater and arachnoid in situ** (lateral aspect).

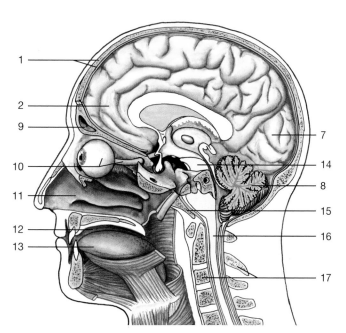

**Sagittal section through the head with brain and sensory organs.** The eye with the optic nerve is located within the orbit; the labyrinth organ, within the petrous bone.

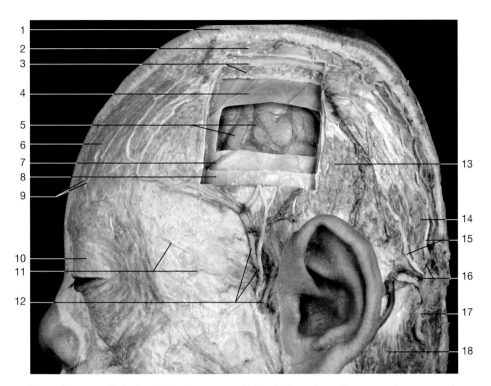

1   Skin
2   Galea aponeurotica
3   Skull diploe
4   Dura mater
5   Arachnoid and pia mater
    with cerebral vessels
6   Frontal belly
    of occipitofrontalis muscle
7   Branch of middle meningeal artery
8   Pericranium (periosteum)
9   Lateral and medial branches
    of supra-orbital nerve
10  Orbicularis oculi muscle
11  Zygomatico-orbital artery
12  Auriculotemporal nerve and
    superficial temporal artery and vein
13  Superior auricular muscle
14  Occipital belly
    of occipitofrontalis muscle
15  Occipital nerve
16  Occipital artery and vein
17  Greater occipital nerve
18  Sternocleidomastoid muscle
19  Frontal lobe
20  Chiasmatic cistern
21  Interpeduncular cistern
22  Arachnoid granulations
23  Subarachnoid space
24  Superior sagittal sinus
25  Inferior sagittal sinus
26  Corpus callosum
27  Straight sinus
28  Confluence of sinuses
29  Cerebellum
30  Cerebellomedullar cistern
31  Cerebral cortex

**Lateral aspect of the head. Scalp, vertex of the skull, and meninges** are demonstrated by a series of window-like openings.

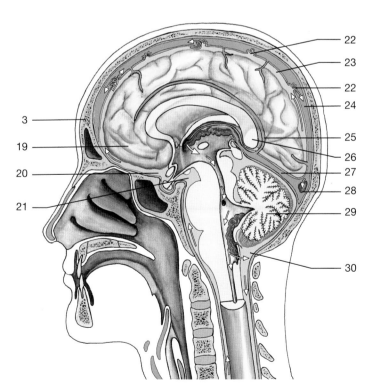

**Subarachnoid cisterns of the brain** (midsagittal section).
Green = cisterns; blue = dural sinus and ventricles;
red = choroid plexus of third and fourth ventricles;
arrows: flow of cerebrospinal fluid.

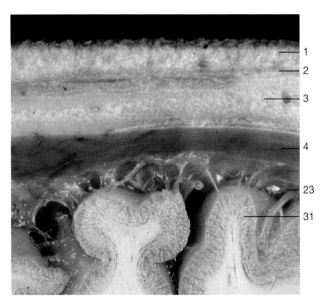

**Cross section of the scalp and the meninges.**
The subarachnoid space (23) is shown.

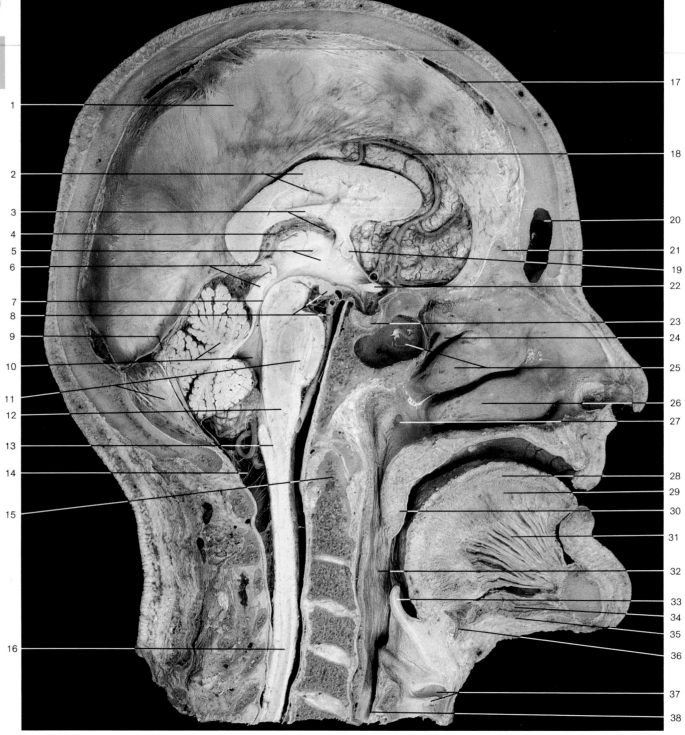

**Median sagittal section through the head and neck.**

1   Falx cerebri
2   Corpus callosum and septum pellucidum
3   Interventricular foramen and fornix
4   Choroid plexus of third ventricle and
     internal cerebral vein
5   Third ventricle and interthalamic adhesion
6   Pineal body and colliculi of the midbrain
7   Cerebral aqueduct
8   Mamillary body and basilar artery
9   Straight sinus
10  Fourth ventricle and cerebellum
11  Pons and falx cerebelli
12  Medulla oblongata
13  Central canal

14  Cerebellomedullary cistern
15  Dens of the axis (odontoid process)
16  Spinal cord
17  Superior sagittal sinus
18  Anterior cerebral artery
19  Anterior commissure
20  Frontal sinus
21  Crista galli
22  Optic chiasma
23  Pituitary gland (hypophysis)
24  Superior nasal concha
25  Middle nasal concha and
     sphenoid sinus
26  Inferior nasal concha

27  Pharyngeal opening of auditory tube
28  Superior longitudinal muscle of tongue
29  Vertical muscle of the tongue
30  Uvula
31  Genioglossus muscle
32  Pharynx
33  Epiglottis
34  Geniohyoid muscle
35  Mylohyoid muscle
36  Hyoid bone
37  Vocal fold and sinus of larynx
38  Esophagus

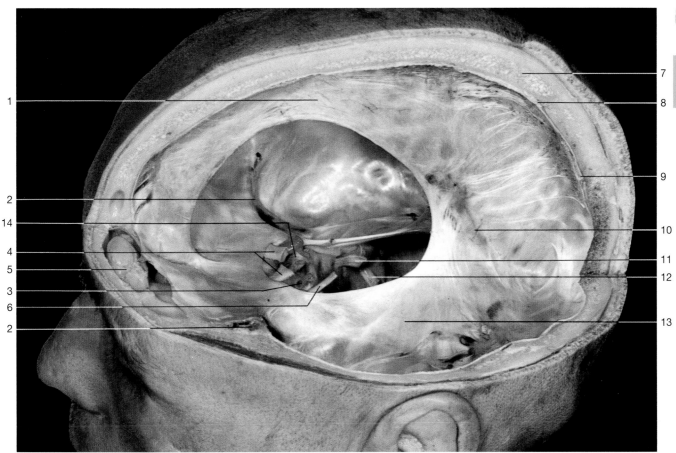

**Dura mater and venous sinuses of the dura mater.** The brain has been removed (oblique-lateral aspect).

1  Falx cerebri
2  Position of middle meningeal
   artery and vein
3  Internal carotid artery
4  Optic nerve (n. II)
5  Frontal sinus
6  Oculomotor nerve (n. III)
7  Diploe
8  Dura mater
9  Superior sagittal sinus
10  Straight sinus
11  Trigeminal nerve (n. V)
12  Facial and vestibulocochlear nerve
   (n. VII and n. VIII)
13  Cerebellar tentorium
14  Pituitary gland (hypophysis)
15  Inferior sagittal sinus
16  Sigmoid sinus
17  Confluence of sinuses
18  Inferior petrosal sinus
19  Transverse sinus
20  Superior petrosal sinus
21  Cavernous and intercavernous sinuses
22  Sphenoparietal sinus

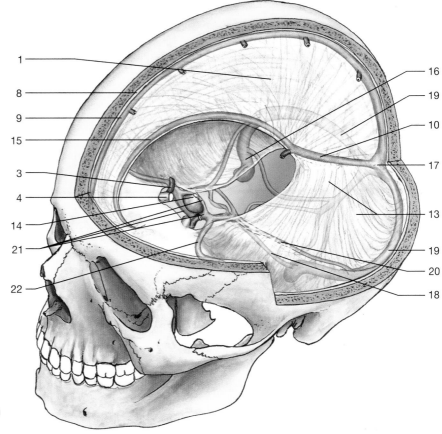

**Dura mater and venous sinuses of the dura mater** (left lateral aspect).

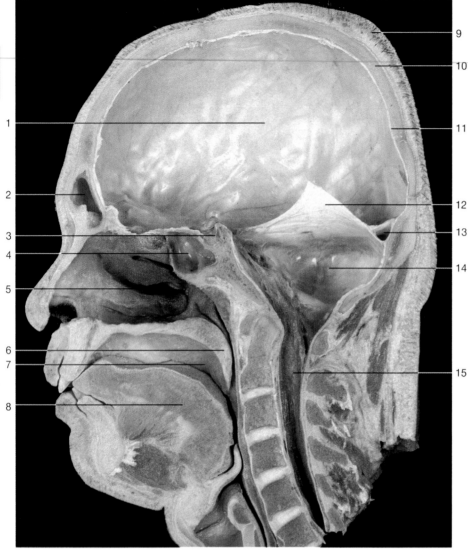

1 Cranial cavity with dura mater (right cerebral hemisphere has been removed)
2 Frontal sinus
3 Hypophysial fossa with pituitary gland
4 Sphenoidal sinus
5 Nasal cavity
6 Soft palate (uvula)
7 Oral cavity
8 Tongue
9 Skin
10 Calvaria
11 Dura mater
12 Cerebellar tentorium
13 Confluence of sinuses
14 Infratentorial space (cerebellum and part of the brain stem have been removed)
15 Vertebral canal
16 Frontal branch of middle meningeal artery and veins
17 Middle meningeal artery
18 Diploe
19 Parietal branch of middle meningeal artery and vein
20 Occipital pole of left hemisphere covered with dura mater

**Median section through the head. Demonstration of dura mater covering the cranial cavity.** Brain and spinal cord are removed (right half of the head, as seen from medial).

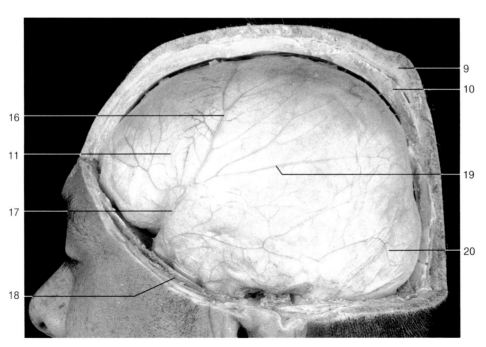

**Dissection of dura mater and meningeal vessels.** Left half of calvaria removed.

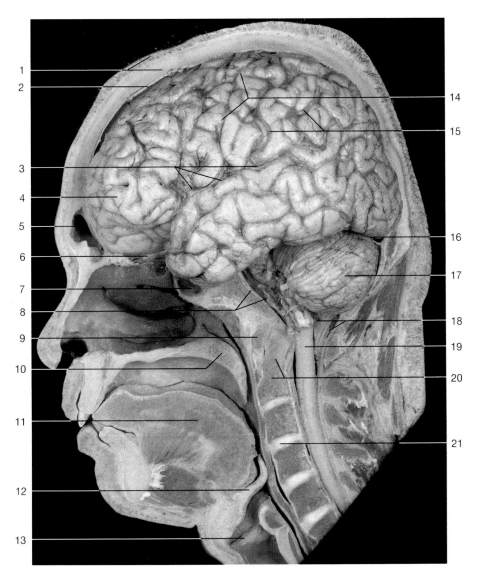

1 Calvaria and
   skin of the scalp
2 Dura mater (divided)
3 Position of lateral sulcus
4 Frontal lobe covered by
   arachnoid and pia mater
5 Frontal sinus
6 Olfactory bulb
7 Sphenoidal sinus
8 Dura mater on clivus and
   basilar artery
9 Atlas (anterior arch, divided)
10 Soft palate
11 Tongue
12 Epiglottis
13 Vocal fold
14 Position of central sulcus
15 Superior cerebral veins
16 Tentorium (divided)
17 Cerebellum
18 Cerebellomedullary cistern
19 Position of foramen magnum
   and spinal cord
20 Dens of axis
21 Intervertebral disc

**Dissection of the brain with pia mater and arachnoid in situ.** The head is cut in half except for the brain, which is shown in its entirety.

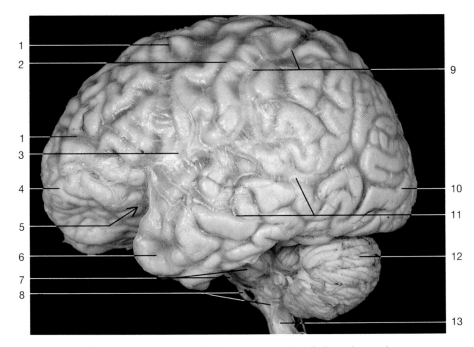

1 Superior cerebral veins
2 Position of central sulcus
3 Position of lateral sulcus and
   cistern of lateral cerebral fossa
4 Frontal pole
5 Lateral sulcus (arrow)
6 Temporal pole
7 Pons and basilar artery
8 Vertebral arteries
9 Superior anastomotic vein
10 Occipital pole
11 Inferior cerebral veins
12 Hemisphere of cerebellum
13 Medulla oblongata

**Brain with pia mater and arachnoid.** Frontal pole to the left (lateral aspect).

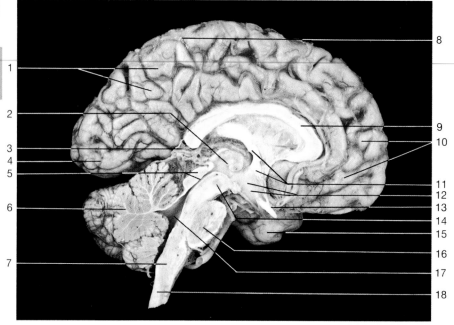

1. Parietal lobe
2. Thalamus, third ventricle, and intermediate mass
3. Great cerebral vein
4. Occipital lobe
5. Colliculi of the midbrain and cerebral aqueduct
6. Cerebellum
7. Medulla oblongata
8. Central sulcus
9. Corpus callosum
10. Frontal lobe
11. Fornix and anterior commissure
12. Hypothalamus
13. Optic chiasma
14. Midbrain
15. Temporal lobe
16. Pons
17. Fourth ventricle
18. Spinal cord
19. Cerebellomedullar cistern
20. Olfactory bulb
21. Hypophysial fossa (sella turcica) with pituitary gland
22. Sphenoid sinus
23. Basilar artery
24. Ligaments to the dens of axis
25. Tongue

**Median section through brain and brain stem.** Frontal pole to the right.

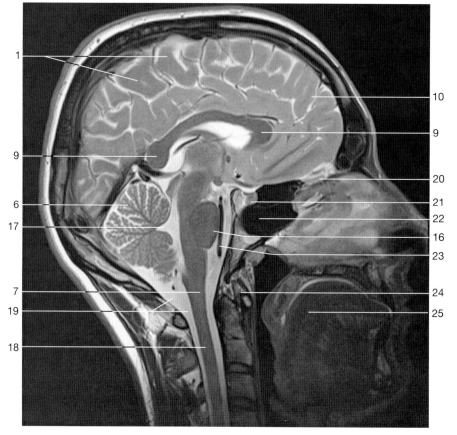

**Median section through the head** (MRI scan). (Prof. Uder, Dept. of Radiology, Univ. Erlangen-Nuremberg, Germany.)

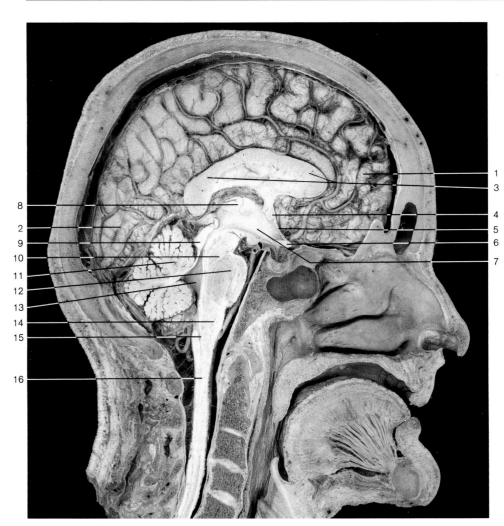

1   Frontal lobe of cerebrum
2   Occipital lobe of cerebrum
3   Corpus callosum
4   Anterior commissure
5   Lamina terminalis
6   Optic chiasma
7   Hypothalamus
8   Thalamus and
    third ventricle
9   Colliculi of the midbrain
10  Midbrain (inferior portion)
11  Cerebellum
12  Pons
13  Fourth ventricle
14  Medulla oblongata
15  Central canal
16  Spinal cord

**Median section through the head.** Regions of the brain. Falx cerebri removed.

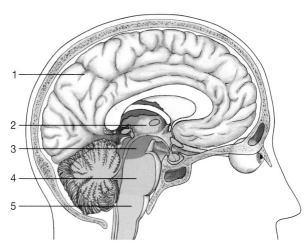

**Median section through the head with colored high-lighting of the brain divisions.**

1   Telencephalon (yellow) with lateral ventricles
2   Diencephalon (orange) with third ventricle, optic nerve, and retina
3   Mesencephalon (blue) with cerebral aqueduct
4   Metencephalon (green) with fourth ventricle
5   Myelencephalon (yellow-green)

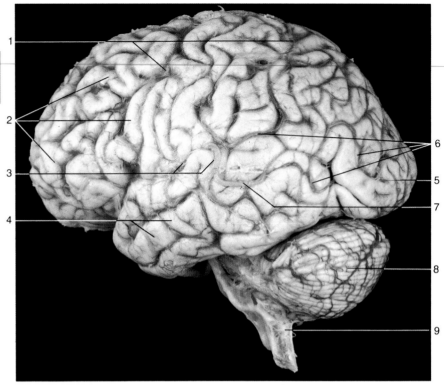

1   Superior cerebral veins and
    parietal lobe
2   Frontal lobe
3   Superficial middle cerebral vein and
    cistern of lateral cerebral fossa
4   Temporal lobe
5   Occipital lobe
6   Inferior cerebral veins and
    transverse occipital sulcus
7   Inferior anastomotic vein
8   Cerebellum
9   Medulla oblongata

**Brain with pia mater and arachnoid** (lateral aspect). **Cerebral veins** (bluish). In the lateral sulcus the cistern of the lateral fossa is recognizable. Frontal lobe to the left.

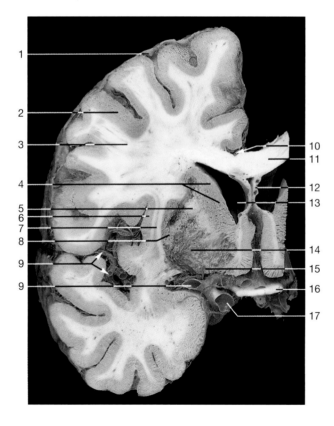

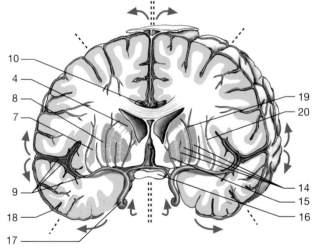

**Arteries of the brain** (coronal section). Areas supplied by cortical and central arteries. Dotted lines indicate boundaries of arterial supply areas. Arrows: direction of blood flow.

◁ **Coronal section through the right hemisphere,** showing arachnoid, pia mater, and the arterial blood supply (anterior aspect).

1   Arachnoid
2   Cortex
3   Frontal lobe (white matter)
4   Caudate nucleus
5   Internal capsule
6   Insular lobe
7   Claustrum
8   Putamen
9   Middle cerebral arteries
10  Anterior cerebral artery
11  Corpus callosum
12  Septum pellucidum
13  Lateral ventricle
14  Globus pallidus and
    pallidostriate artery
15  Thalamic artery
16  Optic chiasma
17  Internal carotid artery
18  Posterior cerebral artery
19  Posterior striate branch
20  Insular artery

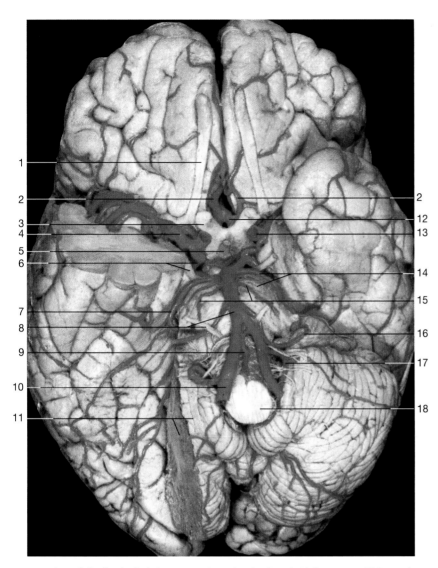

1   Olfactory tract
2   Anterior cerebral artery
3   Optic nerve (n. II)
4   Middle cerebral artery
5   Infundibulum
6   Oculomotor nerve (n. III) and
    posterior communicating artery
7   Posterior cerebral artery
8   Basilar artery and
    abducent nerve (n. VI)
9   Anterior spinal artery
10  Vertebral artery
11  Cerebellum
12  Anterior communicating artery
13  Internal carotid artery
14  Superior cerebellar artery
    and pons
15  Labyrinthine arteries
16  Inferior anterior cerebellar artery
17  Inferior posterior cerebellar artery
18  Medulla oblongata
19  Supratrochlear artery
20  Anterior ciliary arteries
21  Lacrimal artery
22  Posterior ciliary arteries
23  Ophthalmic artery
    with central retinal artery
24  Trigeminal nerve (n. V)
25  Facial nerve (n. VII) and
    vestibulocochlear nerve (n. VIII)
26  Glossopharyngeal nerve (n. IX),
    vagus nerve (n. X), and
    accessory nerve (n. XI)
27  Olfactory bulb
28  Posterior spinal artery

**Arteries of the brain** (inferior aspect, frontal pole above). Right temporal lobe and cerebellum partly removed.

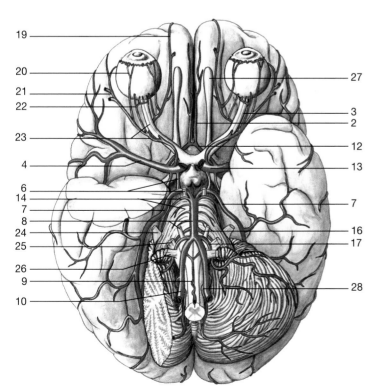

**Arteries of the brain** (inferior aspect). Right temporal lobe and cerebellum partly removed. Note the arterial circle of Willis around the infundibulum.

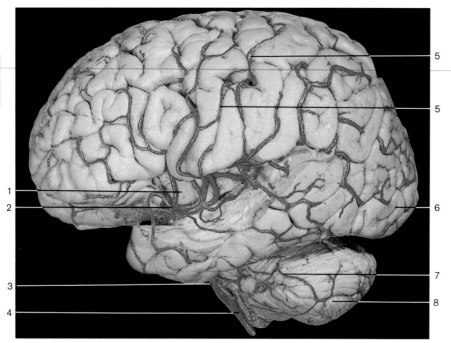

1   Insula
2   Middle cerebral artery with two branches:
    a Parietal branches    b Temporal branches
3   Basilar artery
4   Vertebral artery
5   Central sulcus
6   Occipital lobe
7   Superior cerebellar artery
8   Cerebellum
9   Anterior cerebral artery
10  Ethmoidal arteries
11  Ophthalmic artery
12  Internal carotid artery
13  Posterior communicating artery
14  Posterior cerebral artery
15  Anterior inferior cerebellar artery
16  Posterior inferior cerebellar artery

**Arteries of the brain** (lateral aspect of the left hemisphere). The upper part of the temporal lobe has been removed to display the insula and cerebral arteries (injected with red resin).

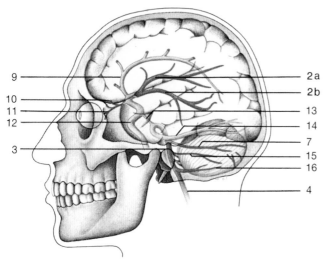

◁ **Arteries of the brain** (lateral aspect).

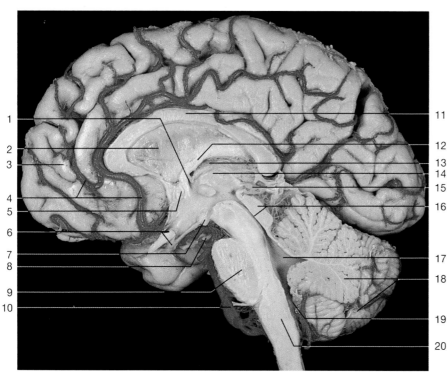

1   Interventricular foramen
2   Septum pellucidum
3   Frontal lobe
4   Anterior cerebral artery
5   Anterior commissure
6   Optic chiasma and infundibulum
7   Mamillary body
8   Oculomotor nerve (n. III)
9   Pons
10  Basilar artery
11  Corpus callosum
12  Fornix
13  Choroid plexus
14  Third ventricle
15  Pineal body
16  Tectum and cerebral aqueduct
17  Fourth ventricle
18  Cerebellum (arbor vitae, vermis)
19  Median aperture of Magendie
20  Medulla oblongata

**Median section through the brain and brain stem.** Cerebral arteries injected with red resin.

1   Skull diploe
2   Middle cerebral artery
3   Internal carotid artery
4   Anterior cerebral artery
5   Nasal cavity
6   Arterial circle of Willis
7   Vertebral artery
8   Common carotid artery
9   Subclavian artery
10  Posterior communicating artery
11  Posterior cerebral artery
12  Basilar artery
13  Aortic arch

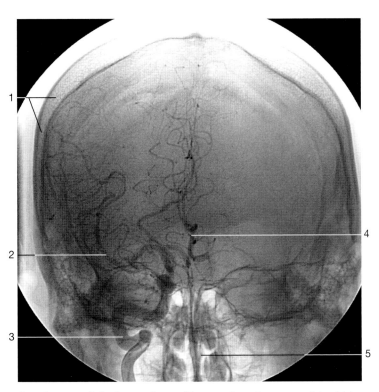

**Arteriogram of the internal carotid artery** (anterior aspect, right side). (Dr. Wieners, Dept. of Radiology, Univ. Berlin, Germany.)

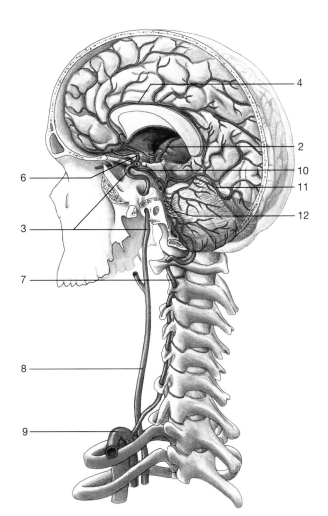

**Arteries of the brain.** Left hemisphere and brain stem have been removed. Note the arterial circle of Willis around the sella turcica.

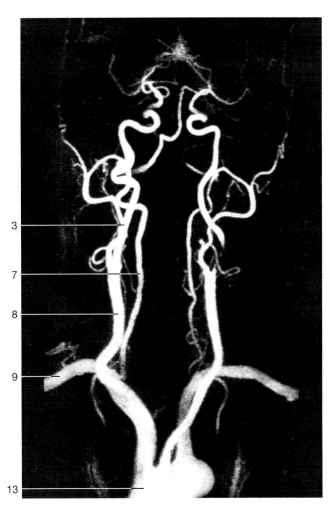

**Main arteries for brain supply** (anterior aspect; MRI angiograph). (Prof. Bautz, Univ. Erlangen-Nuremberg, Germany.)

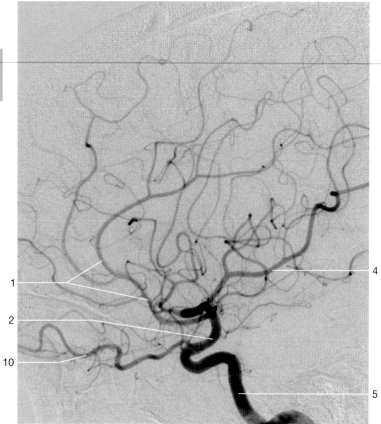

1 Anterior cerebral artery
2 Loop of the internal carotid artery
3 Middle cerebral artery
4 Posterior cerebral artery
5 Internal carotid artery
6 Superior cerebellar artery
7 Anterior inferior cerebellar artery
8 Posterior inferior cerebellar artery
9 Vertebral artery
10 Ophthalmic artery

**Arteriogram of the internal carotid artery** (lateral aspect).
(Prof. Huck, Dept. of Neuroradiology, Univ. Erlangen-Nuremberg, Germany.)

**Arteries of the brain** (lateral aspect). The areas supplied by the main arteries are indicated by different colors.

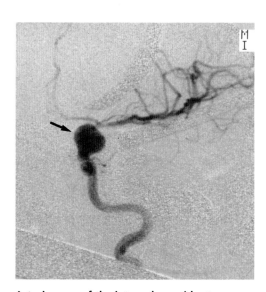

**Arteriogram of the internal carotid artery.**
Arrow: aneurysm located in the region of the sella turcica.

**Areas of blood supply of the brain**
(cerebellum = light blue).
A = Anterior cerebral artery (upper and medial parts of the cortex) (orange)
B = Middle cerebral artery (lateral areas of the frontal, parietal, and temporal lobes) (white)
C = Posterior cerebral artery (occipital lobe and inferior parts of the temporal lobe) (blue)

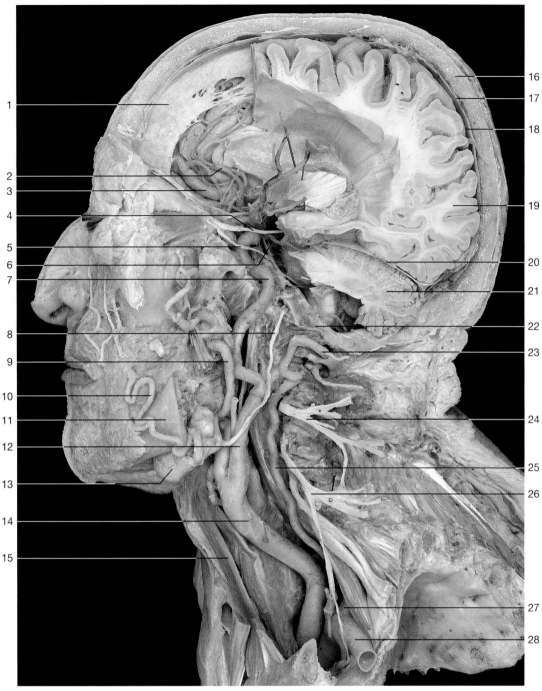

**Dissection of the arteries of the brain and head** (lateral aspect). Superficial layers of facial region and left hemisphere and cerebellum partly removed.

| | | | |
|---|---|---|---|
| 1 | Falx cerebri | 16 | Calvaria |
| 2 | Anterior cerebral artery | 17 | Dura mater |
| 3 | Frontal lobe | 18 | Subarachnoidal space |
| 4 | Oculomotor nerve (n. III) | 19 | Occipital lobe |
| 5 | Abducent nerve (n. VI) | 20 | Tentorium of cerebellum |
| 6 | Posterior cerebral artery | 21 | Cerebellum |
| 7 | Internal carotid artery, entering sinus cavernosus | 22 | Base of skull |
| | | 23 | Vertebral artery (on the posterior arch of the atlas) |
| 8 | Hypoglossus nerve (n. XII) | | |
| 9 | Maxillary artery | 24 | Cervical plexus |
| 10 | Facial artery | 25 | Vertebral artery (removed from the cervical vertebrae) |
| 11 | Mandible | | |
| 12 | External carotid artery | 26 | Brachial plexus |
| 13 | Submandibular gland | 27 | Vertebral artery (branching from the subclavian artery) |
| 14 | Common carotid artery | | |
| 15 | Sternohyoid muscle | 28 | Subclavian artery |

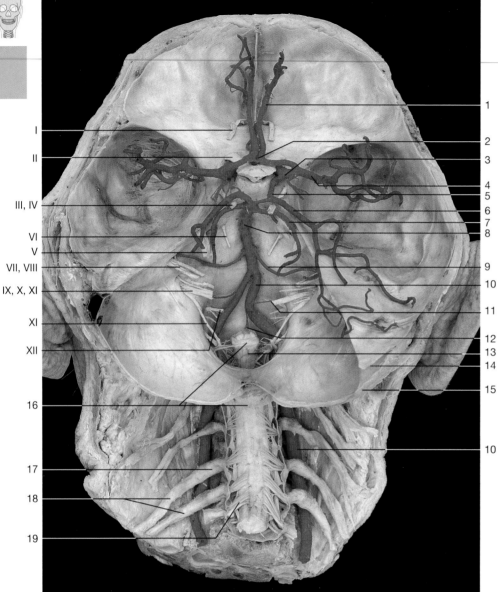

1 Anterior cerebral artery
2 Anterior communicating artery
3 Internal carotid artery
4 Medial cerebral artery
5 Posterior communicating artery
6 Posterior cerebral artery
7 Superior cerebellar artery
8 Basilar artery
9 Anterior inferior cerebellar artery
   with artery of the labyrinth
10 Vertebral artery
11 Posterior inferior cerebellar
   artery
12 Anterior spinal artery
13 Pia mater of spinal cord
14 Cerebellar tentorium
15 Dura mater of the cranial cavity
16 Spinal cord
17 Spinal ganglion
18 Spinal nerves (C₃, C₄)
19 Posterior root filaments
   (fila radicularia post.)
20 Ophthalmic artery
   (within the orbit)
21 Internal carotid artery
   (within carotid canal)

I    =  Olfactory tract
II   =  Optic nerve
III  =  Oculomotor nerve
IV   =  Trochlear nerve
V    =  Trigeminal nerve
VI   =  Abducent nerve
VII  =  Facial nerve
VIII =  Vestibulocochlear nerve
IX   =  Glossopharyngeal nerve
X    =  Vagus nerve
XI   =  Accessory nerve
XII  =  Hypoglossus nerve

**Dissection of the arterial circle of Willis at the base of the skull** (superior aspect).
Calvaria and brain have been removed. Red = arteries; yellow = cranial nerves (n. I–n. XII).

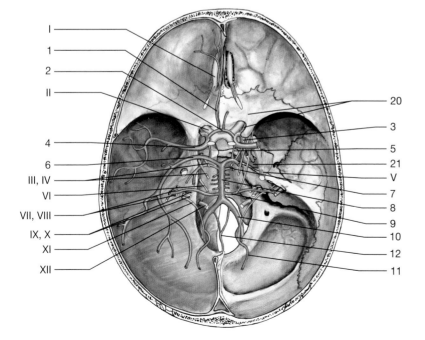

**Arterial circle of Willis at the base of the skull** (superior aspect). Red = arteries; yellow = cranial nerves (n. I–n. XII).

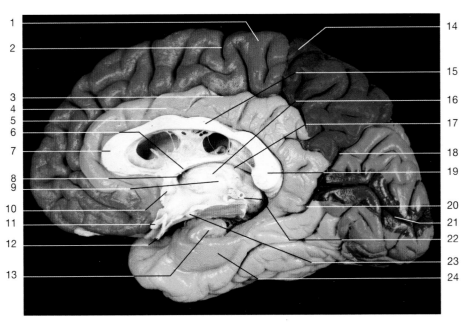

1  Precentral gyrus
2  Precentral sulcus
3  Cingulate sulcus
4  Cingulate gyrus
5  Sulcus of corpus callosum
6  Fornix
7  Genu of corpus callosum
8  Interventricular foramen
9  Intermediate mass
10  Anterior commissure
11  Optic chiasma
12  Infundibulum
13  Uncus hippocampi
14  Postcentral gyrus
15  Body of corpus callosum
16  Third ventricle and thalamus
17  Stria medullaris
18  Parieto-occipital sulcus
19  Splenium of corpus callosum
20  Communication of calcarine and parieto-occipital sulcus
21  Calcarine sulcus
22  Pineal body
23  Mamillary body
24  Parahippocampal gyrus
25  Olfactory bulb
26  Olfactory tract
27  Gyrus rectus
28  Optic nerve
29  Infundibulum and optic chiasma
30  Optic tract
31  Oculomotor nerve
32  Pedunculus cerebri
33  Red nucleus
34  Cerebral aqueduct
35  Corpus callosum
36  Longitudinal fissure
37  Orbital gyri
38  Lateral root of olfactory tract
39  Medial root of olfactory tract
40  Olfactory tubercle and anterior perforated substance
41  Tuber cinereum
42  Interpeduncular fossa
43  Substantia nigra
44  Colliculi of the midbrain
45  Lateral occipitotemporal gyrus
46  Medial occipitotemporal gyrus

**Brain, right hemisphere** (medial aspect). Midbrain divided, cerebellum and inferior part of brain stem removed. Frontal pole to the left.

| | | | | | |
|---|---|---|---|---|---|
| Red | = | Frontal lobe | Dark blue | = | Postcentral lobe |
| Blue | = | Parietal lobe | Dark green | = | Calcarine sulcus |
| Green | = | Occipital lobe | Dark yellow | = | Limbic cortex (cingulate and parahippocampal gyri) |
| Yellow | = | Temporal lobe | | | |
| Dark red | = | Precentral lobe | | | |

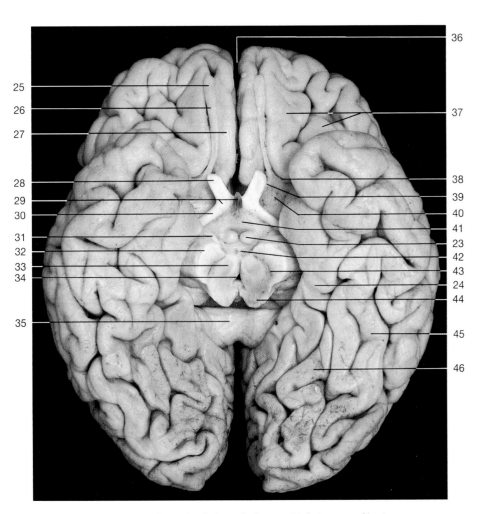

**Brain** (inferior aspect). Midbrain divided, cerebellum and inferior part of brain stem removed. Frontal pole at the top.

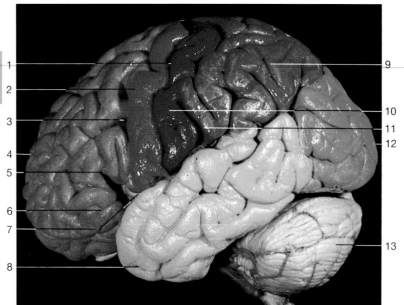

1  Central sulcus
2  Precentral gyrus
3  Precentral sulcus
4  Frontal lobe
5  Anterior ascending ramus of lateral sulcus
6  Anterior horizontal ramus of lateral sulcus
7  Lateral sulcus
8  Temporal lobe
9  Parietal lobe
10  Postcentral gyrus
11  Postcentral sulcus
12  Occipital lobe
13  Cerebellum
14  Superior frontal sulcus
15  Middle frontal gyrus
16  Lunate sulcus
17  Longitudinal fissure
18  Arachnoid granulations

**Brain, left hemisphere** (lateral aspect). Frontal pole to the left.

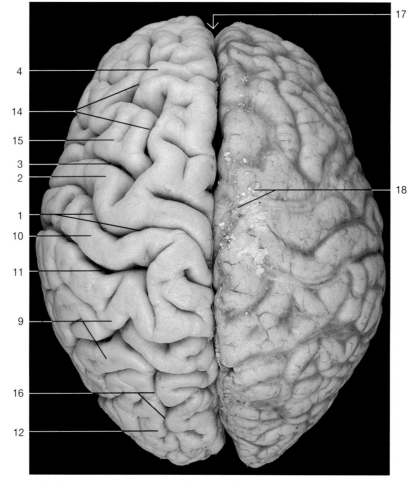

Pink      = Frontal lobe
Blue      = Parietal lobe
Green     = Occipital lobe
Yellow    = Temporal lobe
Dark red  = Precentral gyrus
Dark blue = Postcentral gyrus

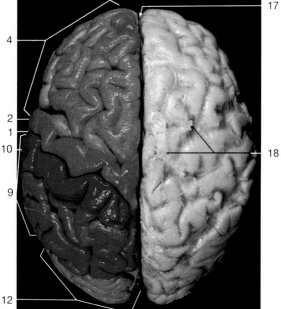

**Brain** (superior aspect). Right hemisphere with arachnoid and pia mater.

**Brain** (superior aspect). Lobes of the left hemisphere indicated by color; right hemisphere is covered with arachnoid and pia mater.

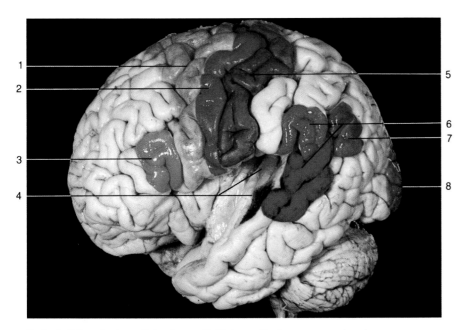

1  Premotor area
2  Somatomotor area
3  Motor speech area of Broca
4  Acoustic area
   (red: high tone, dark green: low tone)
5  Somatosensory area
6  Sensory speech area of Wernicke
7  Reading comprehension area
8  Visuosensory area

**Brain, left hemisphere** (lateral aspect). **Main cortical areas** are colored.
The lateral sulcus has been opened to display the insula and the inner surface of the temporal lobe.

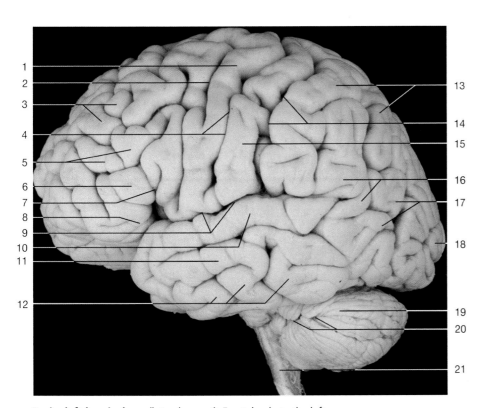

1  Precentral gyrus
2  Precentral sulcus
3  Superior frontal gyrus
4  Central sulcus
5  Middle frontal gyrus
6  Inferior frontal gyrus
7  Ascending ramus ⎫
8  Horizontal ramus ⎬ of lateral sulcus
9  Posterior ramus ⎭
10  Superior temporal gyrus
11  Middle temporal gyrus
12  Inferior temporal gyrus
13  Parietal lobe
14  Postcentral sulcus
15  Postcentral gyrus
16  Supramarginal gyrus
17  Angular gyrus
18  Occipital lobe
19  Cerebellum
20  Horizontal fissure of cerebellum
21  Medulla oblongata

**Brain, left hemisphere** (lateral aspect). Frontal pole to the left.

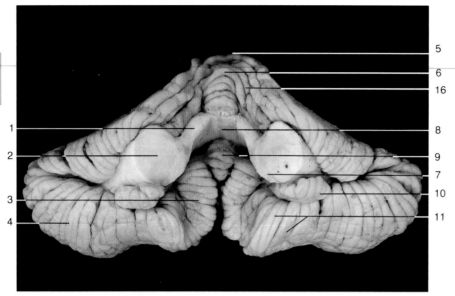

| | |
|---|---|
| 1 | Superior cerebellar peduncle |
| 2 | Middle cerebellar peduncle |
| 3 | Cerebellar tonsil |
| 4 | Inferior semilunar lobule |
| 5 | Vermis |
| 6 | Central lobule of vermis |
| 7 | Inferior cerebellar peduncle |
| 8 | Superior medullary velum |
| 9 | Nodule of vermis |
| 10 | Flocculus of cerebellum |
| 11 | Biventral lobule |
| 12 | Left cerebellar hemisphere |
| 13 | Inferior semilunar lobule |
| 14 | Biventral lobule |
| 15 | Vermis of cerebellum |
| 16 | Tuber of vermis |
| 17 | Pyramid of vermis |
| 18 | Uvula of vermis |
| 19 | Tonsil of cerebellum |
| 20 | Flocculus of cerebellum |
| 21 | Right cerebellar hemisphere |
| 22 | Vermis (central lobule) |
| 23 | Cerebellar lingula |
| 24 | Ala of central lobule |
| 25 | Superior cerebellar peduncle |
| 26 | Fastigium |
| 27 | Fourth ventricle |
| 28 | Middle cerebellar peduncle |
| 29 | Nodule of vermis |
| 30 | Flocculus of cerebellum |
| 31 | Cerebellar tonsil |
| 32 | Culmen of vermis |
| 33 | Declive of vermis |
| 34 | Tuber of vermis |
| 35 | Inferior semilunar lobule |
| 36 | Pyramid of vermis (cut) |
| 37 | Uvula of vermis |

**Cerebellum** (infero-anterior aspect). The cerebellar peduncles have been severed.

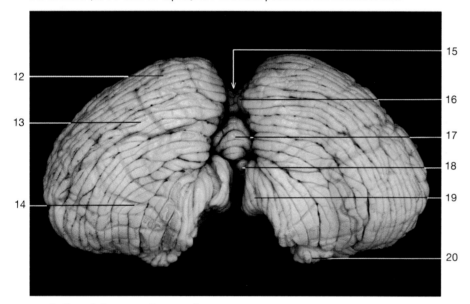

**Cerebellum** (infero-posterior aspect).

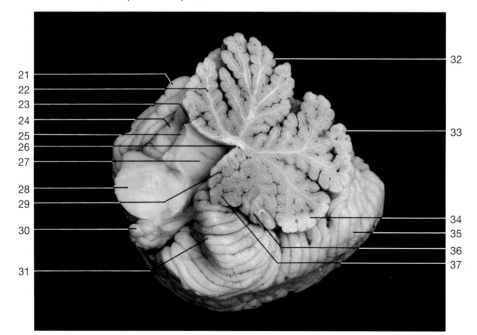

**Median section through the cerebellum.** Right cerebellar hemisphere and right half of vermis.

1  Olfactory bulb
2  Olfactory tract
3  Lateral olfactory stria
4  Anterior perforated substance
5  Infundibulum (divided)
6  Mamillary body
7  Substantia nigra
8  Cerebral peduncle (cut)
9  Red nucleus
10 Decussation of superior cerebellar peduncle
11 Cerebellar hemisphere
12 Medial olfactory stria
13 Optic nerve
14 Optic chiasma
15 Optic tract
16 Posterior perforated substance
17 Interpeduncular fossa
18 Superior cerebellar peduncle and cerebellorubral tract
19 Dentate nucleus
20 Vermis of cerebellum
21 Cingulate gyrus
22 Corpus callosum
23 Stria terminalis
24 Septum pellucidum
25 Columna fornicis
26 Cerebral peduncle at midbrain level
27 Pons
28 Inferior olive
29 Medulla oblongata with lateral pyramidal tract
30 Occipital lobe
31 Calcarine sulcus
32 Thalamus
33 Inferior colliculus with brachium
34 Medial lemniscus
35 Superior cerebellar peduncle
36 Inferior cerebellar peduncle
37 Middle cerebellar peduncle
38 Cerebellar hemisphere

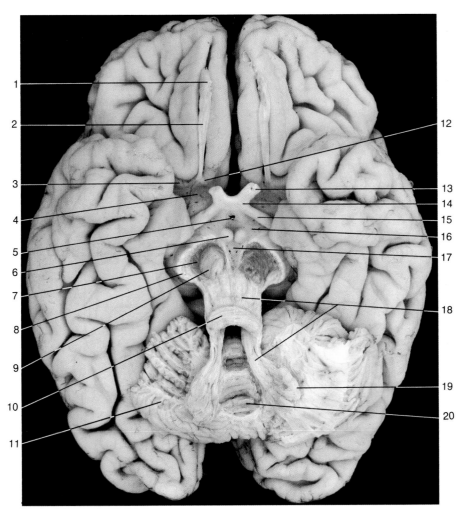

**Brain and cerebellum** (inferior aspect). Parts of the cerebellum have been removed to display the dentate nucleus and the main pathway to the midbrain (cerebellorubral tract).

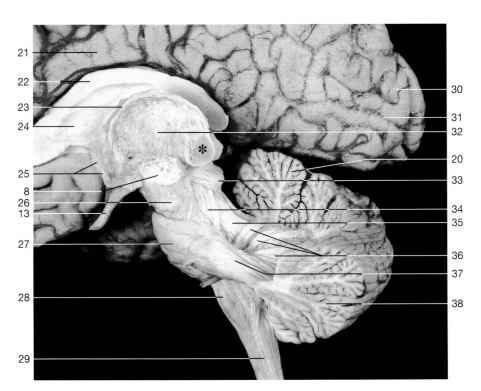

**Dissection of the cerebellar peduncles and their connection with midbrain and diencephalon.** A small part of pulvinar thalami (✳) has been cut to show inferior brachium.

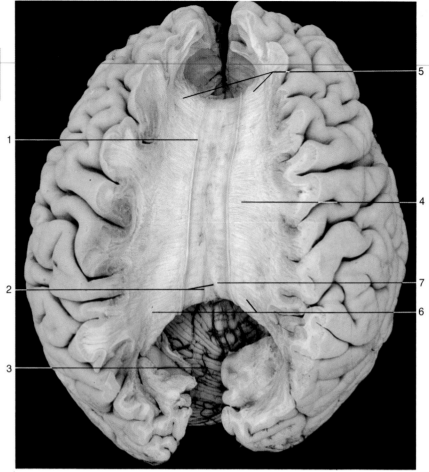

1  Lateral longitudinal stria
   of indusium griseum
2  Medial longitudinal stria
   of indusium griseum
3  Cerebellum
4  Radiating fibers of the corpus callosum
5  Forceps minor of corpus callosum
6  Forceps major of corpus callosum
7  Splenium of corpus callosum

**Dissection of the brain I.** The fiber system of the corpus callosum has been displayed by removing the cortex lying above it. Frontal pole at the top.

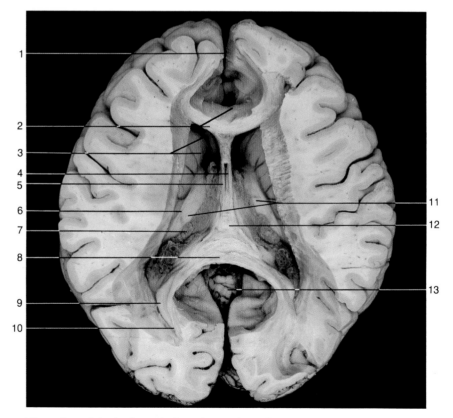

1  Longitudinal cerebral fissure
2  Genu of corpus callosum
3  Head of caudate nucleus and
   anterior horn of lateral ventricle
4  Cavum of septum pellucidum
5  Septum pellucidum
6  Stria terminalis
7  Choroid plexus of lateral ventricle
8  Splenium of corpus callosum
9  Calcar avis
10 Posterior horn of lateral ventricle
11 Thalamus (lamina affixa)
12 Commissure of fornix
13 Vermis of cerebellum

**Dissection of the brain II.** The lateral ventricles and subcortical nuclei of the brain are dissected. The corpus callosum has been partly removed. Frontal pole at the top.

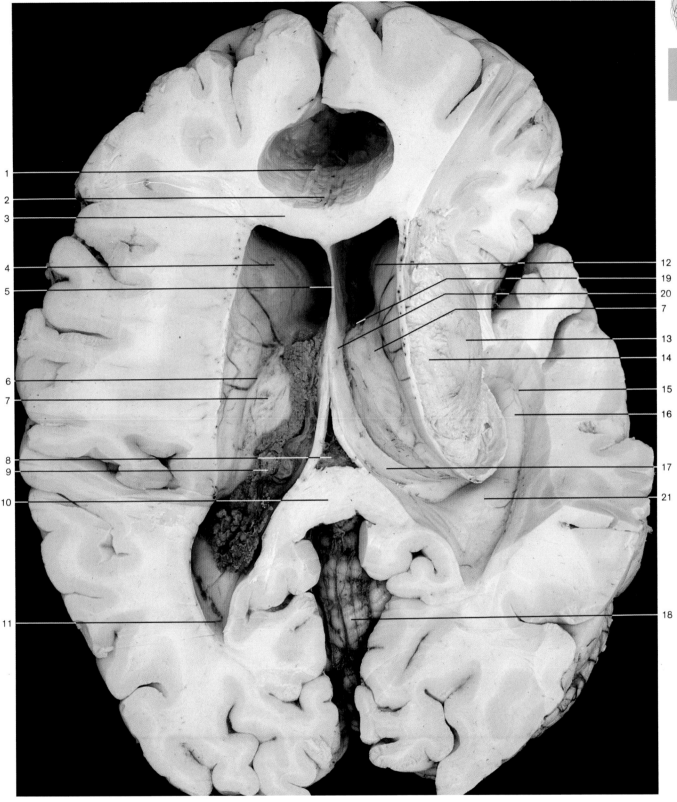

**Dissection of the brain III** (superior aspect of lateral ventricle and subcortical nuclei of the brain). Corpus callosum partly removed. At right, the entire lateral ventricle has been opened, the insula with claustrum and the extreme and external capsules have been removed, exposing the lentiform nucleus and the internal capsule.

| | | |
|---|---|---|
| 1 Lateral longitudinal stria | 9 Choroid plexus of lateral ventricle | 16 Pes hippocampi |
| 2 Medial longitudinal stria | 10 Splenium of corpus callosum | 17 Crus of fornix |
| 3 Genu of corpus callosum | 11 Posterior horn of lateral ventricle | 18 Vermis of cerebellum with arachnoid and |
| 4 Head of caudate nucleus | 12 Anterior horn of lateral ventricle | pia mater |
| 5 Septum pellucidum | (head of caudate nucleus) | 19 Interventricular foramen |
| 6 Stria terminalis | 13 Putamen of lentiform nucleus | 20 Right column of fornix |
| 7 Thalamus (lamina affixa) | 14 Internal capsule | 21 Collateral eminence |
| 8 Choroid plexus of third ventricle | 15 Inferior horn of lateral ventricle | |

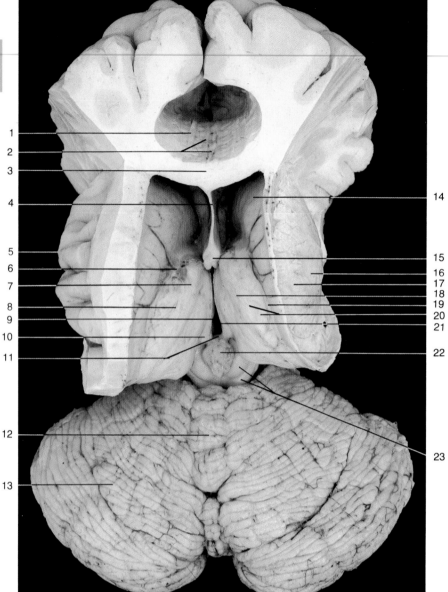

| | |
|---|---|
| 1 | Lateral longitudinal stria |
| 2 | Medial longitudinal stria |
| 3 | Corpus callosum |
| 4 | Septum pellucidum |
| 5 | Insular gyri |
| 6 | Thalamostriate vein |
| 7 | Anterior tubercle of thalamus |
| 8 | Thalamus |
| 9 | Stria medullaris of thalamus |
| 10 | Habenular trigone |
| 11 | Habenular commissure |
| 12 | Vermis of cerebellum |
| 13 | Left hemisphere of cerebellum |
| 14 | Head of caudate nucleus |
| 15 | Columns of fornix |
| 16 | Putamen of lentiform nucleus |
| 17 | Internal capsule |
| 18 | Taenia of choroid plexus |
| 19 | Stria terminalis and thalamostriate vein |
| 20 | Lamina affixa |
| 21 | Third ventricle |
| 22 | Pineal body |
| 23 | Superior and inferior colliculus of midbrain |

**Dissection of the brain IVa.** Temporal lobe, fornix, and the posterior corpus callosum have been removed (this part of the specimen is depicted below). Frontal pole at the top (superior aspect).

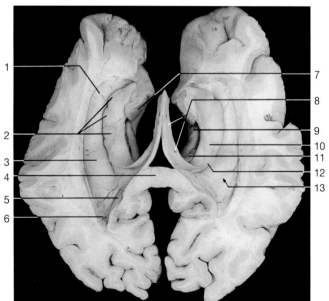

| | |
|---|---|
| 1 | Inferior horn of lateral ventricle |
| 2 | Hippocampal digitations |
| 3 | Collateral eminence |
| 4 | Splenium of corpus callosum |
| 5 | Calcar avis |
| 6 | Posterior horn of lateral ventricle |
| 7 | Uncus of parahippocampal gyrus |
| 8 | Body and crus of fornix |
| 9 | Parahippocampal gyrus |
| 10 | Pes hippocampi |
| 11 | Dentate gyrus |
| 12 | Hippocampal fimbria |
| 13 | Lateral ventricle |

**Dissection of the brain IVb.** Depicted is the portion of the brain removed from the specimen above: temporal lobe and limbic system. Columns of fornix are cut (superior aspect).

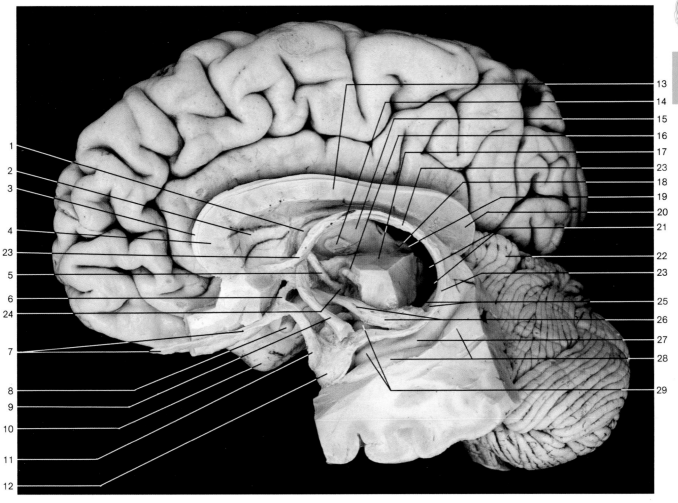

**Dissection of the limbic system** (left side, lateral aspect). Corpus callosum has been cut in the median plane. The left thalamus and the left hemisphere have been partly removed.

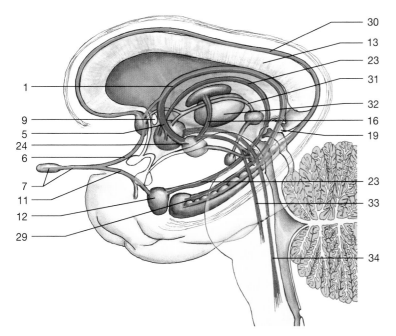

**Main pathways of limbic and olfactory system.** Blue = afferent pathways; red = efferent pathways.

| | | | |
|---|---|---|---|
| 1 | Body of fornix | 21 | Colliculi of midbrain |
| 2 | Septum pellucidum | 22 | Vermis of cerebellum |
| 3 | Lateral longitudinal stria | 23 | Stria terminalis |
| 4 | Genu of corpus callosum | 24 | Mamillary body |
| 5 | Column of fornix | 25 | Fimbria of hippocampus and pes hippocampi |
| 6 | Medial olfactory stria | | |
| 7 | Olfactory bulb and olfactory tract | 26 | Left optic tract and lateral geniculate body |
| 8 | Optic nerve | 27 | Lateral ventricle and parahippocampal gyrus |
| 9 | Anterior commissure (left half) | | |
| 10 | Right temporal lobe | 28 | Collateral eminence |
| 11 | Lateral olfactory stria | 29 | Hippocampal digitations |
| 12 | Amygdala | 30 | Supracallosal gyrus (longitudinal stria) |
| 13 | Body of corpus callosum | | |
| 14 | Interthalamic adhesion | 31 | Stria medullaris of thalamus |
| 15 | Third ventricle and right thalamus | | |
| 16 | Mamillothalamic fasciculus | 32 | Dorsomedial nucleus of thalamus |
| 17 | Part of the thalamus | | |
| 18 | Habenular commissure | 33 | Mamillotegmental fasciculus |
| 19 | Pineal body | | |
| 20 | Splenium of corpus callosum | 34 | Dorsal longitudinal fasciculus (Schütz) |

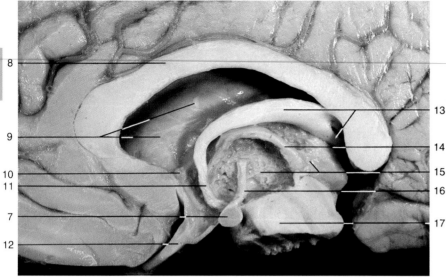

| | |
|---|---|
| 1 | Paraventricular nucleus ⎫ |
| 2 | Pre-optic nucleus ⎪ |
| 3 | Ventromedial nucleus ⎪ Hypothalamic |
| 4 | Supra-optic nucleus ⎬ nuclei |
| 5 | Posterior nucleus ⎪ |
| 6 | Dorsomedial nucleus ⎭ |
| 7 | Mamillary body |
| 8 | Corpus callosum |
| 9 | Lateral ventricle (showing caudate nucleus) |
| 10 | Anterior commissure |
| 11 | Column of fornix |
| 12 | Optic chiasma |
| 13 | Crus of fornix |
| 14 | Stria medullaris of thalamus |
| 15 | Thalamus and interthalamic adhesion |
| 16 | Mamillothalamic fasciculus of Vicq d'Azyr |
| 17 | Cerebral peduncle |
| 18 | Pineal body |
| 19 | Tectum of midbrain |

**Median section through the diencephalon.** Medial part of the thalamus and septum pellucidum have been removed to show the fornix and mamillothalamic fasciculus.

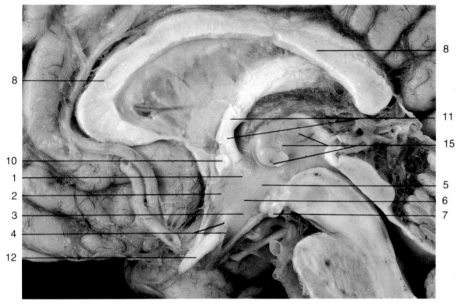

**Median section through diencephalon and midbrain. Location of the hypothalamic nuclei.**

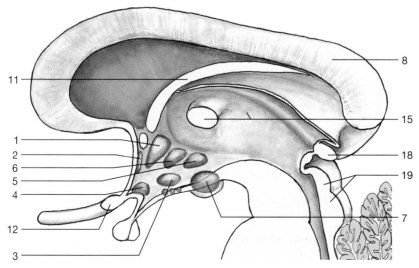

**Location of the main hypothalamic nuclei.**

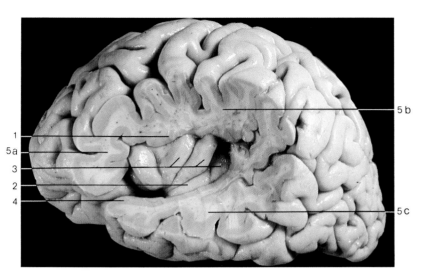

**Insula (Reili),** left hemisphere. The opercula of the frontal, parietal, and temporal lobes have been removed to display the insular gyri.

1   Circular sulcus of insula
2   Long gyrus of insula
3   Short gyri of insula
4   Limen insulae
5   Opercula (cut)
    a   Frontal operculum
    b   Frontoparietal operculum
    c   Temporal operculum
6   Corona radiata
7   Lentiform nucleus
8   Anterior commissure
9   Olfactory tract
10  Cerebral arcuate fibers
11  Optic radiation
12  Cerebral peduncle
13  Trigeminal nerve (n. V)
14  Flocculus of cerebellum
15  Pyramidal tract
16  Decussation of pyramidal tract
17  Internal capsule
18  Optic tract
19  Optic nerve (n. II)
20  Infundibulum
21  Temporal lobe (right side)
22  Mamillary bodies
23  Oculomotor nerve (n. III)
24  Transverse fibers of pons

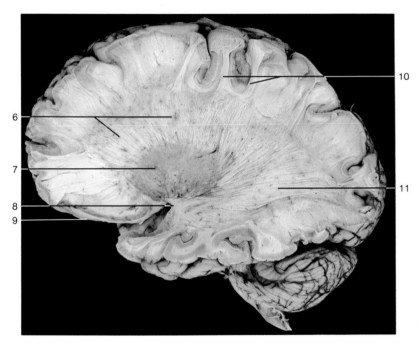

**Corona radiata,** left hemisphere. Frontal pole to the left.

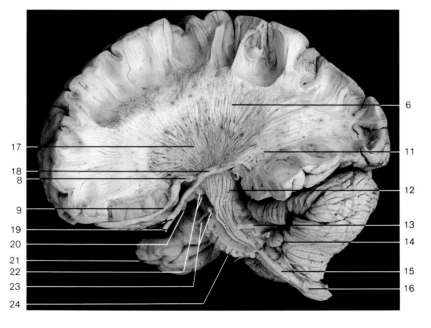

◁  **Corona radiata and internal capsule,** left hemisphere. Lentiform nucleus removed. Frontal pole to the left.

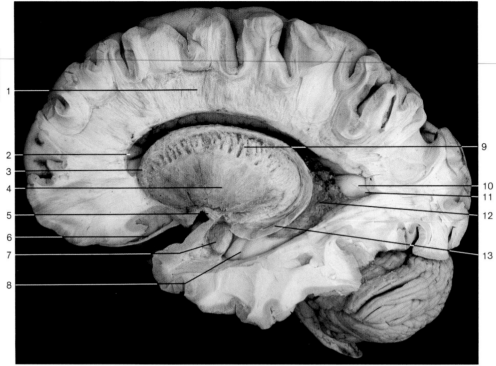

1    Corona radiata
2    Anterior horn
     of lateral ventricle
3    Head of caudate nucleus
4    Putamen
5    Anterior commissure
6    Olfactory tract
7    Amygdala
8    Hippocampal digitations
9    Internal capsule
10   Calcar avis
11   Posterior horn
     of lateral ventricle
12   Choroid plexus
     of lateral ventricle
13   Caudal extremity
     of caudate nucleus
14   Pulvinar of thalamus
15   Mamillary body
16   Optic tract
17   Anterior commissure
18   Fornix
19   Longitudinal stria
20   Dentate gyrus
21   Hippocampal fimbria
22   Pes hippocampi

**Dissection of the subcortical nuclei and internal capsule,** left hemisphere (lateral aspect). The lateral ventricle has been opened, and the insular gyri and claustrum have been removed, revealing the lentiform nucleus and the internal capsule. Frontal pole to the left.

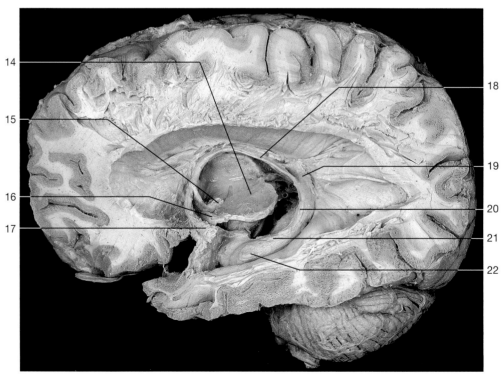

**Dissection of the limbic system and fornix,** left hemisphere (lateral aspect). Frontal pole to the left.

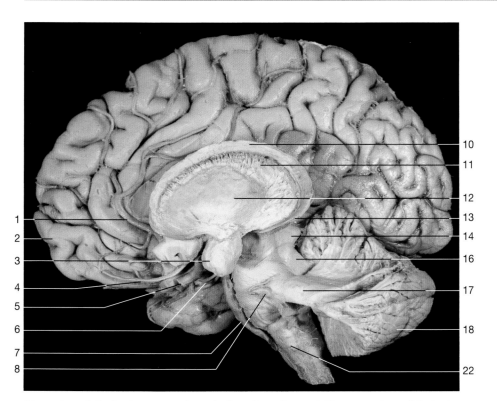

1  Anterior cerebral artery
2  Frontal lobe
3  Amygdala (amygdaloid body)
4  Olfactory tract
5  Internal carotid artery
6  Oculomotor nerve (n. III)
7  Basilar artery
8  Trigeminal nerve (n. V)
9  Hypoglossal nerve (n. XII)
10  Caudate nucleus
11  Internal capsule
12  Lentiform nucleus
13  Caudal extremity
     of caudate nucleus
14  Inferior colliculus of midbrain
15  Trochlear nerve (n. IV)
16  Superior cerebellar peduncle
17  Middle cerebellar peduncle
18  Cerebellum
19  Facial nerve (n. VII) and
     vestibulocochlear nerve (n. VIII)
20  Abducent nerve (n. VI)
21  Glossopharyngeal nerve (n. IX),
     vagus nerve (n. X), and
     accessory nerve (n. XI)
22  Inferior olive

**Dissection of the brain stem and cerebellum** (lateral aspect). The connections of the brain stem with the cerebellum are dissected. The amygdala of the left hemisphere is shown. The corpus callosum has been partly removed. Frontal pole to the left.

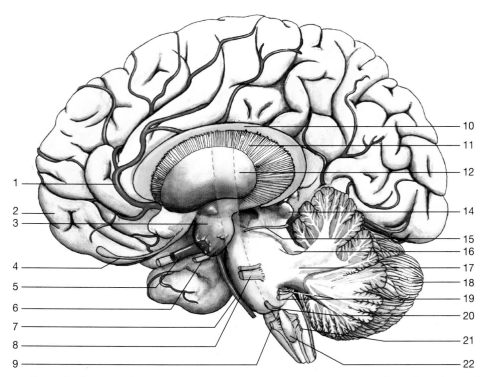

**Schematic drawing of the dissected brain stem and cerebellum** shown above (lateral aspect). The course of the pyramidal tracts is indicated in red. Yellow = cranial nerves.

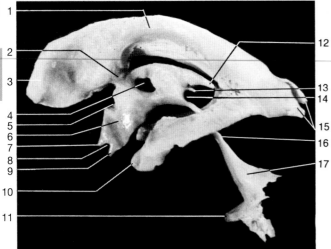

**Cast of ventricular cavities of the brain** (lateral aspect). Frontal pole to the left.

1   Central part of the lateral ventricle
2   Interventricular foramen of Monro
3   Anterior horn of the lateral ventricle
4   Site of interthalamic adhesion
5   Notch for anterior commissure
6   Third ventricle
7   Optic recess
8   Notch for optic chiasma
9   Infundibular recess
10  Inferior horn of lateral ventricle
    with indentation of amygdaloid body
11  Lateral recess and lateral aperture of Luschka
12  Suprapineal recess
13  Pineal recess
14  Notch for posterior commissure
15  Posterior horn of lateral ventricle
16  Cerebral aqueduct
17  Fourth ventricle
18  Median aperture of Magendie

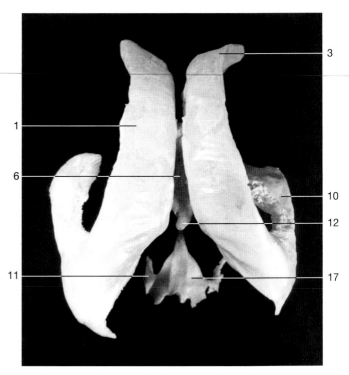

**Cast of ventricular cavities of the brain** (superior aspect). Frontal pole at the top.

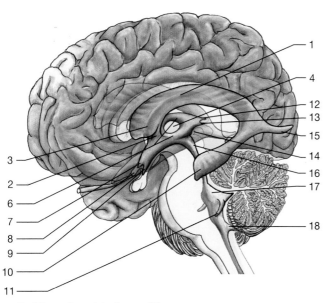

**Position of ventricular cavities.**

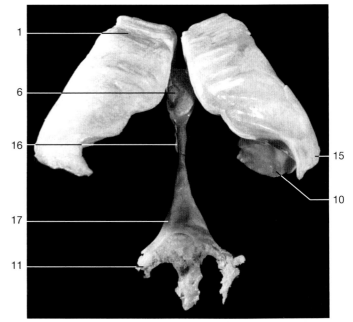

**Cast of ventricular cavities of the brain and cerebral aqueduct** (posterior aspect). Posterior horns of the lateral ventricles (15) are shown. Fourth ventricle (17) from below.

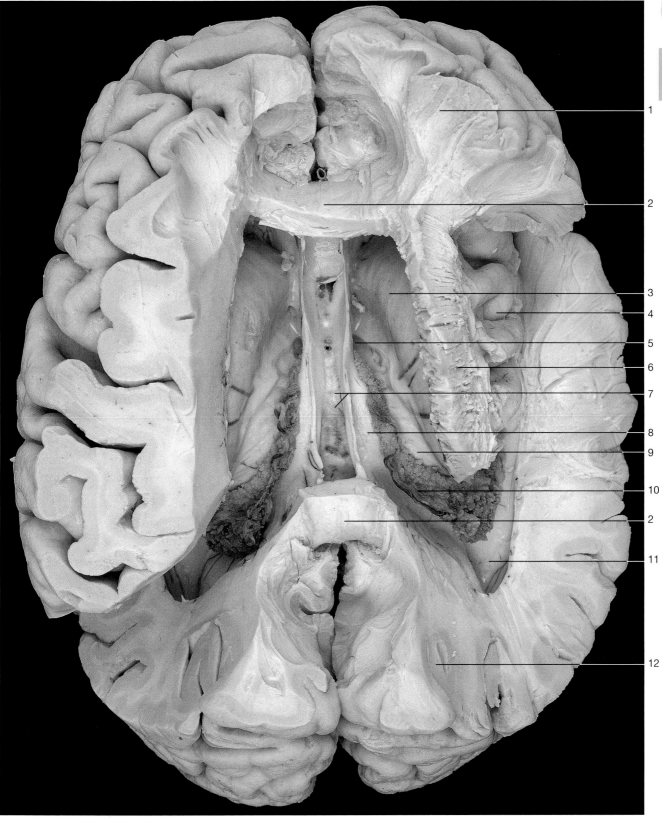

**Dissection of the brain** (superior aspect of the lateral ventricle and of the subcortical nuclei of the brain). Corpus callosum partly removed. Fornix and choroid plexus of the left lateral ventricle are shown.

| | |
|---|---|
| 1 Frontal lobe of brain | 7 Choroid plexus of third ventricle |
| 2 Corpus callosum | 8 Body of fornix |
| 3 Caudate nucleus (head) | 9 Thalamus |
| 4 Insular cortex | 10 Choroid plexus |
| 5 Interventricular foramen | 11 Lateral ventricle (occipital horn) |
| 6 Internal capsule | 12 Occipital lobe of brain |

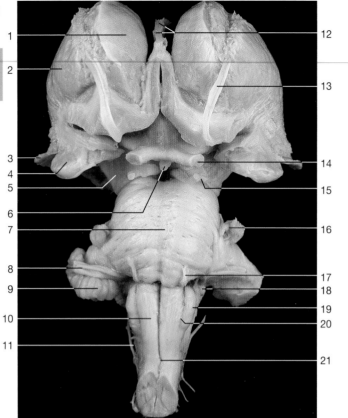

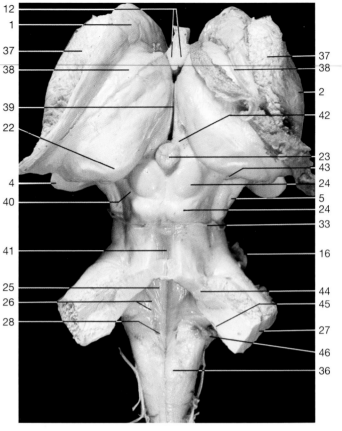

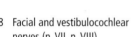

**Brain stem** (anterior aspect). Cerebrum removed.

**Brain stem** (posterior aspect). Cerebellum removed.

1   Caudate nucleus
2   Lentiform nucleus
3   Caudal extremity of caudate nucleus
4   Amygdaloid body
5   Cerebral peduncle
6   Infundibulum
7   Pons

8   Facial and vestibulocochlear nerves (n. VII, n. VIII)
9   Cerebellar flocculus
10  Medulla oblongata
11  Accessory nerve (n. XI)
12  Fornix and column of fornix
13  Olfactory tract
14  Optic nerve (n. II)

15  Oculomotor nerve (n. III)
16  Trigeminal nerve (n. V)
17  Abducent nerve (n. VI)
18  Glossopharyngeal and vagus nerves (n. IX, n. X)
19  Inferior olive
20  Hypoglossal nerve (n. XII)
21  Decussation of the pyramids
22  Thalamus
23  Epiphysis
24  Tectum of midbrain (superior and inferior colliculus)
25  Motor nucleus of trigeminal nerve (n. V)
26  Facial nucleus (n. VII)
27  Middle cerebellar peduncle
28  Visceral nucleus of glossopharyngeal and vagus nerves (n. IX and n. X), salivatory nucleus
29  Vestibular nucleus (n. VIII)
30  Ambiguus nucleus (n. IX, n. X, n. XI)
31  Spinal nucleus of accessory nerve (n. XI)
32  Motor nucleus of oculomotor nerve (n. III)
33  Trochlear nucleus and nerve (n. IV)
34  Sensory nucleus of trigeminal nerve (n. V)
35  Abducent nucleus (n. VI)
36  Hypoglossal nucleus (n. XII)
37  Internal capsule
38  Lamina affixa
39  Third ventricle
40  Brachium of inferior colliculus
41  Superior medullary velum
42  Habenular trigone
43  Medial geniculate body
44  Superior cerebellar peduncle
45  Inferior cerebellar peduncle
46  Choroid plexus of fourth ventricle

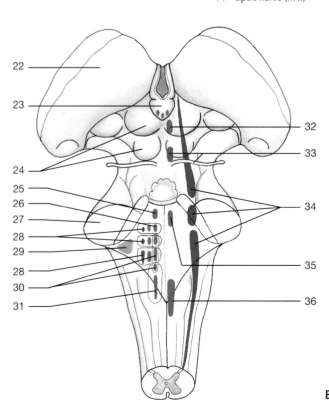

**Brain stem** (posterior aspect). Location of cranial nerve nuclei.

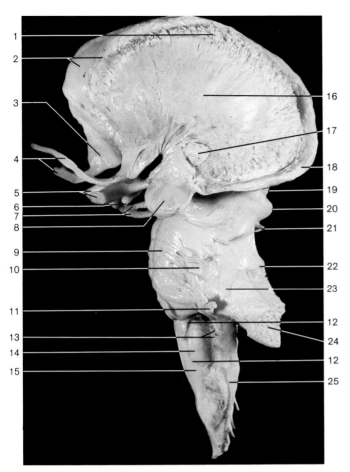

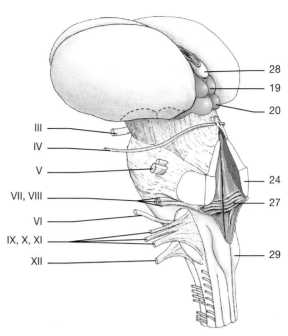

**Brain stem** (lateral aspect). Note the location of the cranial nerves. III–XII = cranial nerves.

**Brain stem** (left lateral aspect). Cerebellar peduncles have been severed, cerebellum and cerebral cortex have been removed.

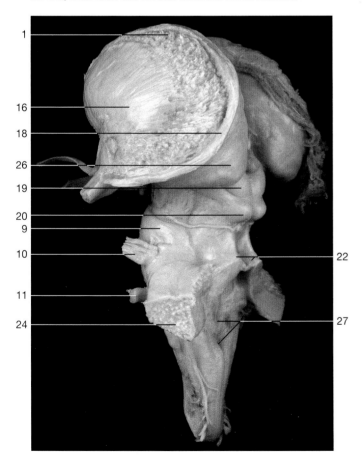

**Brain stem** (dorso-lateral aspect). Cerebellum removed.

1 Internal capsule
2 Head of the caudate nucleus
3 Olfactory trigone
4 Olfactory tracts
5 Optic nerves (n. II)
6 Infundibulum
7 Oculomotor nerve (n. III)
8 Amygdaloid body
9 Pons
10 Trigeminal nerve (n. V)
11 Facial and vestibulocochlear nerves (n. VII, n. VIII)
12 Hypoglossal nerve (n. XII)
13 Glossopharyngeal and vagus nerves (n. IX, n. X)
14 Inferior olive
15 Medulla oblongata
16 Lentiform nucleus
17 Anterior commissure
18 Tail of caudate nucleus
19 Superior colliculus
20 Inferior colliculus
21 Trochlear nerve (n. IV)
22 Superior cerebellar peduncle
23 Inferior cerebellar peduncle
24 Middle cerebellar peduncle
25 Accessory nerve (n. XI)
26 Pulvinar of thalamus
27 Striae medullares and rhomboid fossa
28 Pineal body
29 Clava

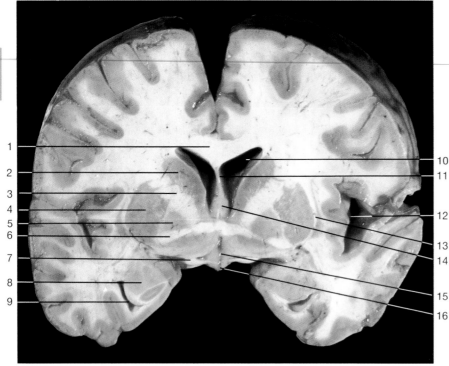

**Coronal section through the brain** at the level of the anterior commissure. Section 1.

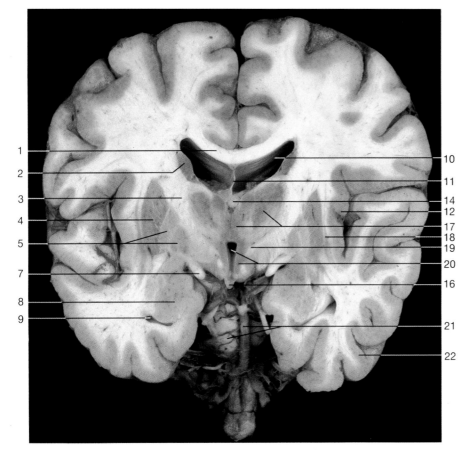

**Coronal section through the brain** at the level of the third ventricle and the interthalamic adhesion. Section 2.

1  Corpus callosum
2  Head of caudate nucleus
3  Internal capsule
4  Putamen
5  Globus pallidus
6  Anterior commissure
7  Optic tract
8  Amygdaloid body
9  Inferior horn of lateral ventricle
10  Lateral ventricle
11  Septum pellucidum
12  Lobus insularis (insula)
13  External capsule
14  Column of fornix
15  Optic recess
16  Infundibulum
17  Thalamus
18  Claustrum
19  Lenticular ansa
20  Third ventricle and hypothalamus
21  Basilar artery and pons
22  Cortex of temporal lobe
23  Inferior colliculus
24  Superior colliculus
25  Cerebral aqueduct
26  Red nucleus
27  Substantia nigra
28  Cerebral peduncle
29  Trochlear nerve (n. IV)
30  Gray matter
31  Nucleus of oculomotor nerve
32  Fibers of oculomotor nerve (n. III)
33  Vermis of cerebellum
34  Fourth ventricle
35  Reticular formation
36  Pons and transverse pontine fibers
37  Emboliform nucleus
38  Dentate nucleus
39  Middle cerebellar peduncle
40  Choroid plexus
41  Hypoglossal nucleus at rhomboid fossa
42  Medial longitudinal fasciculus
43  Trigeminal nerve (n. V.)
44  Inferior olivary nucleus
45  Corticospinal fibers and arcuate fibers
46  Fourth ventricle with choroid plexus
47  Vestibular nuclei
48  Nucleus and tractus solitarius
49  Inferior cerebellar peduncle (restiform body)
50  Reticular formation
51  Medial lemniscus
52  Cuneate nucleus of Burdach
53  Central canal
54  Pyramidal tract
55  Flocculus of cerebellum
56  Cerebellar hemisphere with pia mater
57  "Arbor vitae" of cerebellum
58  Nucleus gracilis of Goll
59  Lateral recess of choroid plexus of fourth ventricle
60  Posterior inferior cerebellar artery
61  Choroid plexus of lateral ventricle

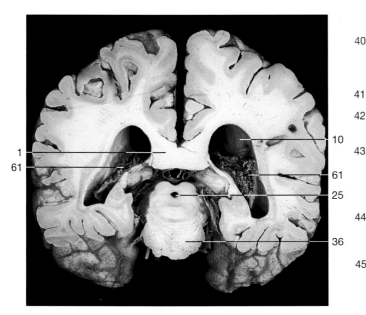

**Coronal section through the brain** at the level of the inferior colliculus (posterior aspect). Section 3.

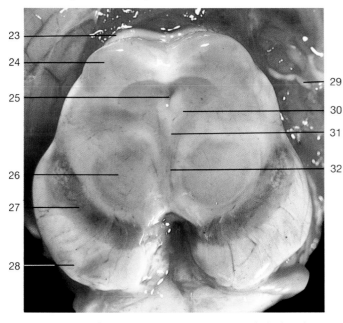

**Cross section through the midbrain** (mesencephalon) at the level of the superior colliculus (superior aspect). Section 4.

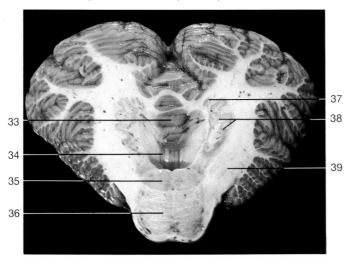

**Cross section through the rhombencephalon** at the level of the pons (inferior aspect). Section 5.

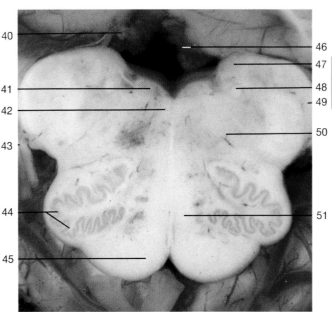

**Cross section through the rhombencephalon** at the level of the olive (inferior aspect). Section 6.

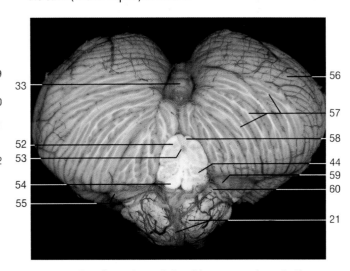

**Cross section through medulla oblongata and cerebellum** (inferior aspect). Section 7.

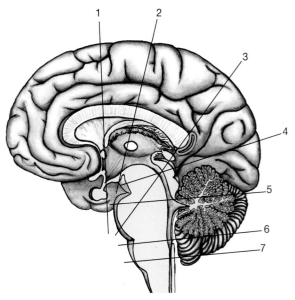

**Right half of the brain.** Levels of the sections are indicated.

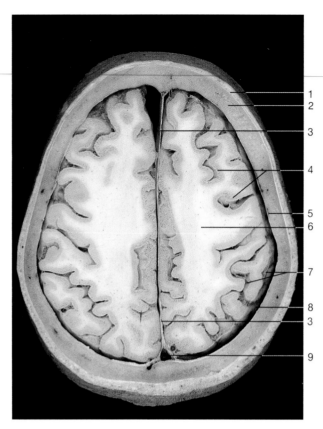

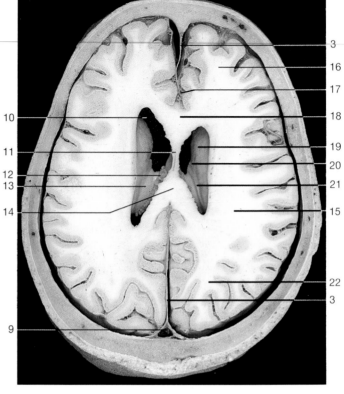

**Horizontal section through the head and brain.**
Section 1.

**Horizontal section through the head and brain.**
Section 2.

| | | | |
|---|---|---|---|
| 1 | Skin of scalp | 7 | Arachnoid and pia mater with vessles |
| 2 | Calvaria (diploe of the skull) | 8 | Subdural space (slightly expanded due to shrinkage of the brain) |
| 3 | Falx cerebri | 9 | Superior sagittal sinus |
| 4 | Gray matter of brain (cortex) | 10 | Anterior horn of lateral ventricle |
| 5 | Dura mater | | |
| 6 | White matter of brain | | |

| | | | |
|---|---|---|---|
| 11 | Septum pellucidum | 17 | Anterior cerebral artery |
| 12 | Choroid plexus | 18 | Genu of corpus callosum |
| 13 | Thalamus | 19 | Caudate nucleus |
| 14 | Splenium of corpus callosum | 20 | Central part of lateral ventricle |
| 15 | Parietal lobe | 21 | Stria terminalis |
| 16 | Frontal lobe | 22 | Occipital lobe |

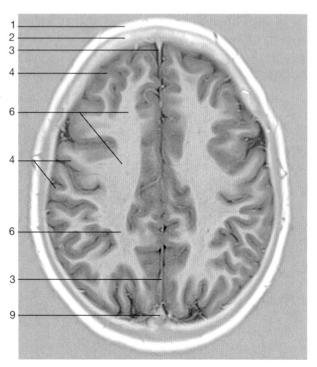

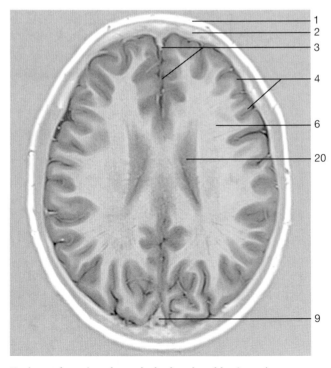

**Horizontal section through the head and brain** at the level of section 1 (MRI scan). (Prof. Uder, Dept. of Radiology, Univ. Erlangen-Nuremberg, Germany.)

**Horizontal section through the head and brain** at the level of section 2 (MRI scan). (Prof. Uder, Dept. of Radiology, Univ. Erlangen-Nuremberg, Germany.)

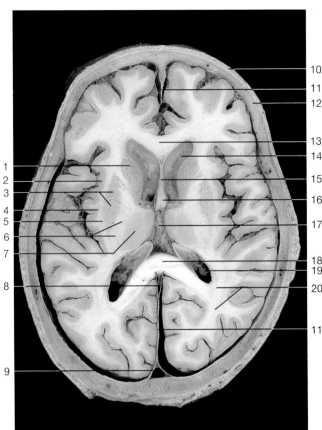

1   Caudate nucleus
2   Lobus insularis (insula)
3   Putamen
4   Claustrum
5   External capsule
6   Internal capsule
7   Thalamus
8   Inferior sagittal sinus
9   Superior sagittal sinus
10  Skin of scalp
11  Falx cerebri
12  Calvaria (diploe of the skull)
13  Genu of corpus callosum
14  Anterior horn of lateral ventricle
15  Septum pellucidum
16  Column of fornix
17  Choroid plexus of third ventricle
18  Splenium of corpus callosum
19  Entrance to inferior horn of lateral ventricle
    with choroid plexus
20  Optic radiation
21  Third ventricle

**Horizontal section through the head and brain** at the level
of third ventricle of internal capsule and neighboring nuclei.
Section 3.

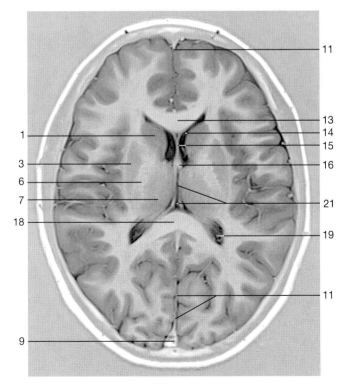

**Horizontal section through the head and brain** at the
level of section 3 (MRI scan). (Prof. Uder, Dept. of Radiology,
Univ. Erlangen-Nuremberg, Germany.)

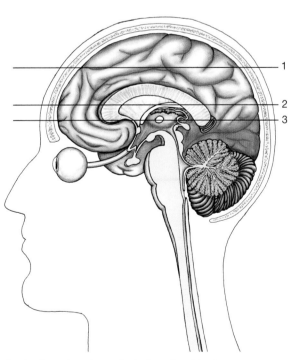

**Sagittal section through the head and brain.**
Levels of the sections are indicated.

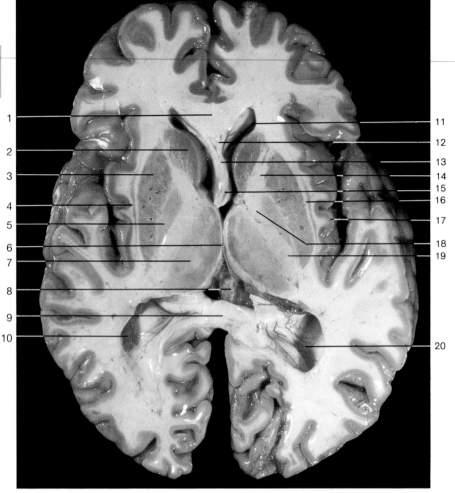

1    Genu of corpus callosum
2    Head of caudate nucleus
3    Putamen
4    Claustrum
5    Globus pallidus
6    Third ventricle
7    Thalamus
8    Pineal body
9    Splenium of corpus callosum
10   Choroid plexus
     of the lateral ventricle
11   Anterior horn of lateral ventricle
12   Cavity of septum pellucidum
13   Septum pellucidum
14   Anterior limb of internal capsule
15   Column of fornix
16   External capsule
17   Lobus insularis (insula)
18   Genu of internal capsule
19   Posterior limb of internal capsule
20   Posterior horn of lateral ventricle
21   Anterior commissure
22   Optic radiation
23   Falx cerebri
24   Maxillary sinus
25   Position of auditory tube
26   Tympanic cavity
27   External acoustic meatus
28   Medulla oblongata
29   Fourth ventricle
30   Cerebellum (left hemisphere)
31   Temporomandibular joint
32   Tympanic membrane
33   Base of cochlea
34   Mastoid air cells
35   Sigmoid sinus
36   Vermis of cerebellum
37   Intermediate mass

**Horizontal section through the brain,** showing the subcortical nuclei and internal capsule. Section 1.

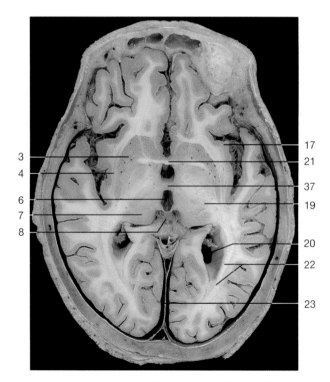

**Horizontal section through the head and brain.** Section 2.

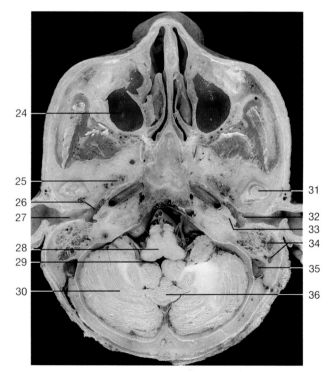

**Horizontal section through the head and brain.** Section 4.

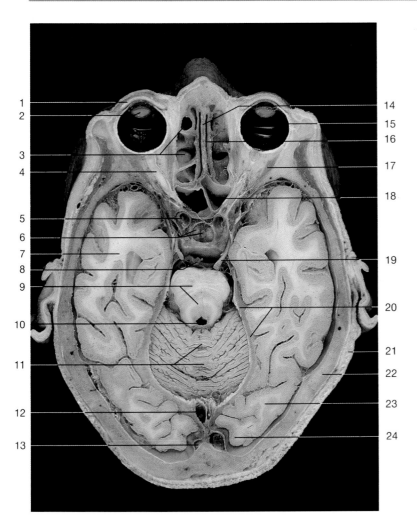

1   Upper lid (tarsal plate)
2   Lens
3   Ethmoidal sinus
4   Optic nerve (n. II)
5   Internal carotid artery
6   Infundibulum and pituitary gland
7   Temporal lobe
8   Basilar artery
9   Pons (cross section of brain stem)
10  Cerebral aqueduct (beginning of fourth ventricle)
11  Vermis of cerebellum
12  Straight sinus
13  Transverse sinus
14  Nasal septum
15  Eyeball (sclera)
16  Nasal cavity
17  Lateral rectus muscle
18  Sphenoidal sinus
19  Oculomotor nerve (n. III)
20  Cerebellar tentorium
21  Skin of scalp
22  Calvaria (diploe of the skull)
23  Occipital lobe
24  Striate cortex (visual cortex)

**Horizontal section through the head and brain.** Section 3.

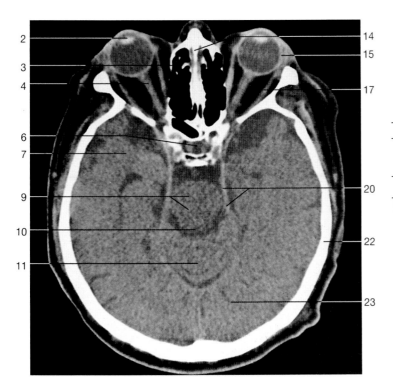

**Horizontal section through the head and brain** at the level of section 3 (CT scan).

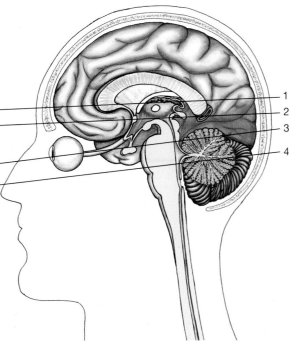

**Sagittal section through the head and brain.**
Levels of the sections are indicated.

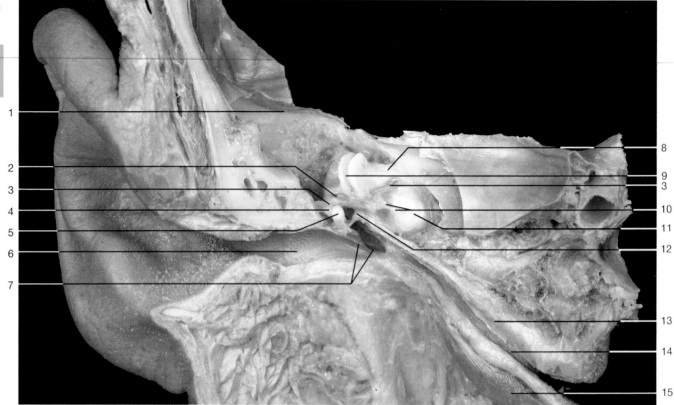

**Longitudinal section through the right outer, middle, and inner ear** (anterior aspect). The cochlea and semicircular canals have been further dissected.

1 Roof of tympanic cavity
2 Lateral osseous semicircular canal
3 Facial nerve
4 Incus
5 Malleus
6 External acoustic meatus
7 Tympanic cavity and tympanic membrane
8 Vestibulocochlear nerve
9 Anterior osseous semicircular canal
10 Geniculate ganglion and greater petrosal nerve
11 Cochlea
12 Stapes
13 Tensor tympani muscle
14 Auditory tube
15 Levator veli palatini muscle

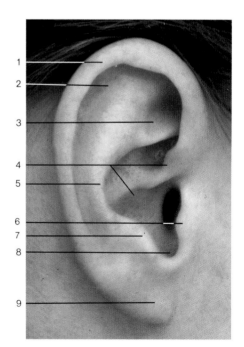

◁
1 Helix
2 Scaphoid fossa
3 Triangular fossa
4 Concha
5 Antihelix
6 Tragus
7 Antitragus
8 Intertragic notch
9 Lobule

**Right auricle** (lateral aspect).

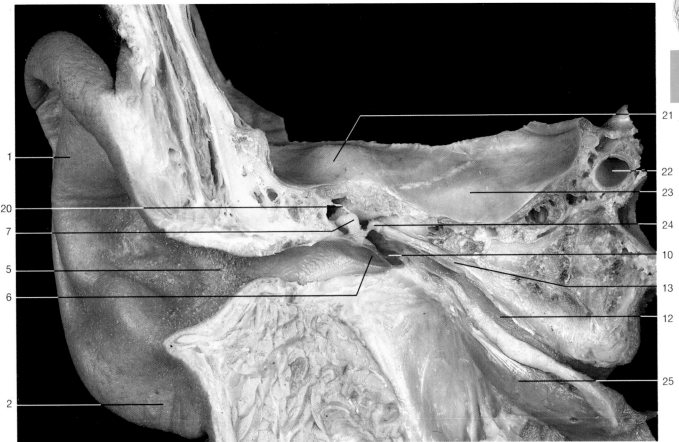

**Longitudinal section through the right outer, middle, and inner ear** (anterior aspect).

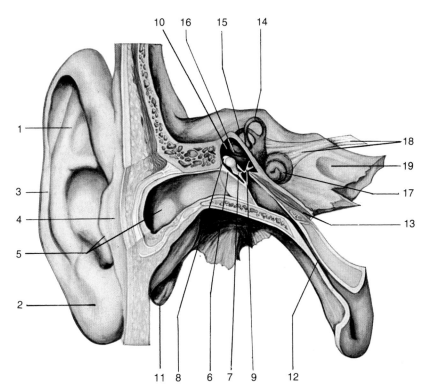

**Right auditory and vestibular apparatus** (anterior aspect).

**Outer ear**
1  Auricle
2  Lobule of auricle
3  Helix
4  Tragus
5  External acoustic meatus

**Middle ear**
6  Tympanic membrane
7  Malleus
8  Incus
9  Stapes
10  Tympanic cavity
11  Mastoid process
12  Auditory tube
13  Tensor tympani muscle

**Inner ear**
14  Anterior semicircular duct
15  Posterior semicircular duct
16  Lateral semicircular duct
17  Cochlea
18  Vestibulocochlear nerve (n. VIII)
19  Petrous part of the temporal bone

**Additional structures**
20  Superior ligament of malleus
21  Arcuate eminence
22  Internal carotid artery
23  Anterior surface of pyramid
    with dura mater
24  Stapes
25  Levator veli palatini muscle

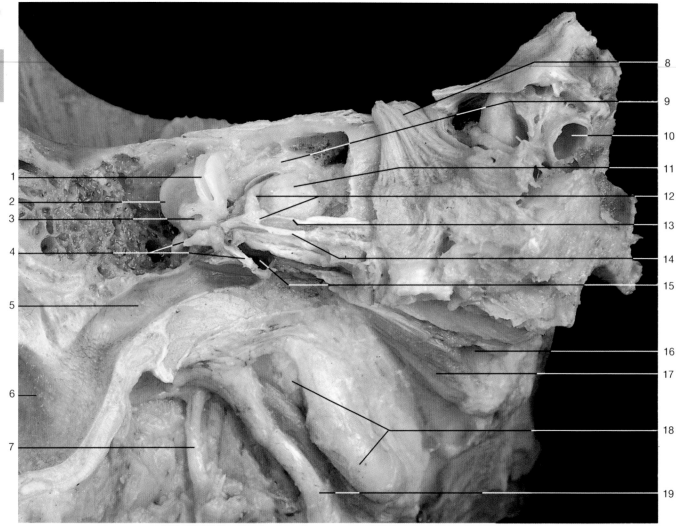

**Longitudinal section through the outer, middle, and inner ear** (anterior aspect). Deeper dissection to display facial nerve and lesser and greater petrosal nerves.

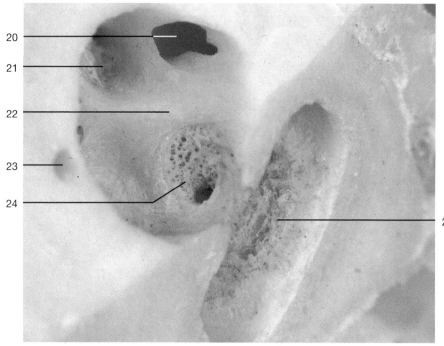

**Internal acoustic meatus,** left side. The bone was partly removed to show the bottom of the meatus.

1 Anterior osseous semicircular canal (opened)
2 Posterior osseous semicircular canal
3 Lateral osseous semicircular canal (opened)
4 Facial nerve and chorda tympani
5 External acoustic meatus
6 Auricle
7 Facial nerve
8 Trigeminal nerve
9 Bony base of internal acoustic meatus
10 Internal carotid artery within cavernous sinus
11 Cochlea
12 Facial nerve with geniculate ganglion
13 Greater petrosal nerve
14 Lesser petrosal nerve
15 Tympanic cavity
16 Auditory tube
17 Levator veli palatini muscle
18 Internal carotid artery and internal jugular vein
19 Styloid process
20 Area of facial nerve
21 Superior vestibular area
22 Transverse crest
23 Foramen singulare
24 Foraminous spiral tract (outlet of cochlear part of vestibulocochlear nerve)
25 Base of cochlea

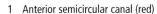

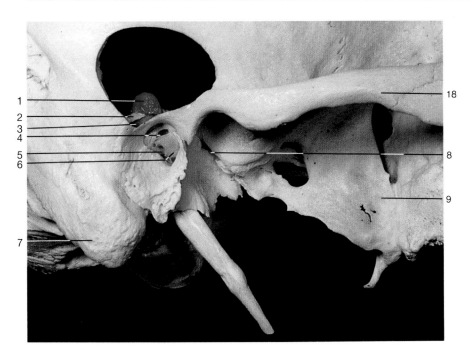

1   Anterior semicircular canal (red)
2   Posterior semicircular canal
    (yellow)
3   Lateral or horizontal semicircular canal
    (green)
4   Fenestra vestibuli
5   Fenestra cochleae
6   Tympanic cavity
7   Mastoid process
8   Petrotympanic fissure
    (red probe: chorda tympani)
9   Lateral pterygoid plate
10  Mastoid air cells
11  Facial canal (blue)
12  Foramen ovale
13  Carotid canal (red)
14  Tympanic ring
15  Petromastoid part of temporal bone
16  Squamous part of temporal bone
17  Squamomastoid suture
18  Zygomatic process
    of temporal bone
19  Incisure of tympanic ring
20  Promontory
21  Apex of cochlea (cupula)
22  Spiral canal of cochlea
    at base of cochlea
23  Epitympanic recess
24  Auditory ossicles and
    tympanic cavity
25  Hypotympanic recess
26  Canaliculus chordae tympani
    (green probe)
27  Mastoid process
28  Canaliculus for stapedius nerve (red)
29  Cochlea
30  Canaliculus mastoideus (red probe)

**Right temporal bone** (lateral aspect). Petrosquamous portion has been partly removed to display the semicircular canals.

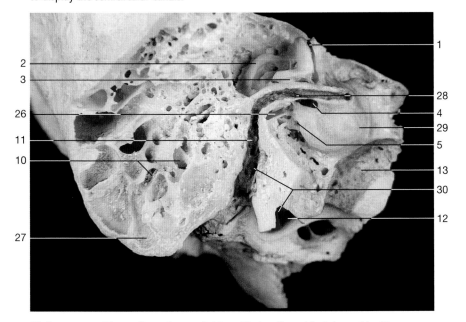

**Right temporal bone** (lateral aspect). Mastoid air cells and facial canal had been opened. The three semicircular canals were dissected.

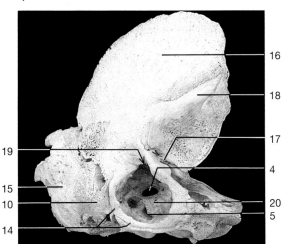

**Right temporal bone of the newborn** (lateral aspect).

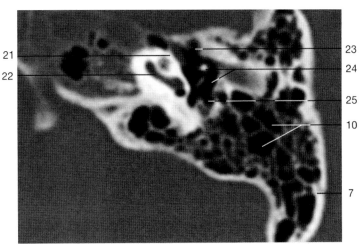

**Frontal section through the petrous part of temporal bone** (CT scan).

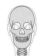

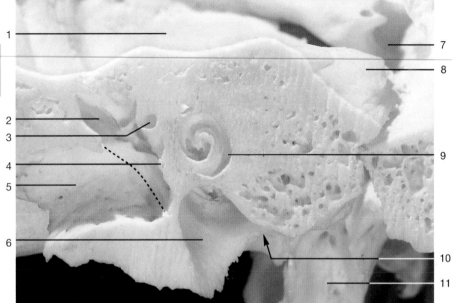

**Frontal section through the petrous part of the left temporal bone** at the level of the cochlea (posterior aspect). The position of the tympanic membrane is indicated by a dotted line.

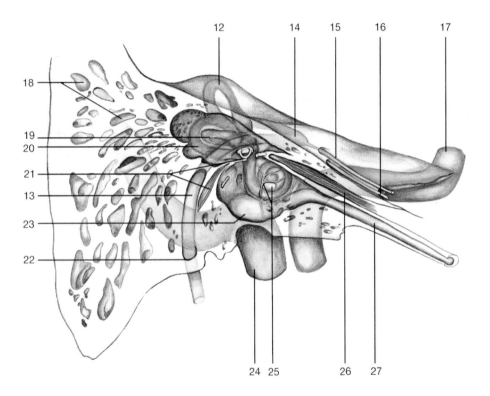

**Medial wall of the tympanic cavity** and its relation to neighboring structures of the inner ear, facial nerve, and blood vessels. Frontal section through the right temporal bone (anterior aspect).

| | | |
|---|---|---|
| 1 Anterior surface of the pyramid | 10 Carotid canal | 20 Posterior semicircular duct |
| 2 Mastoid antrum | 11 Pterygoid process | 21 Stapes with stapedius muscle |
| 3 Lateral semicircular canal | 12 Anterior semicircular duct | 22 Stylomastoid foramen |
| 4 Cochleariform process | 13 Facial nerve | 23 Inferior recess of tympanic cavity |
| 5 External acoustic meatus | 14 Geniculate ganglion | (hypotympanon) |
| 6 Jugular fossa | 15 Greater petrosal nerve | 24 Internal jugular vein |
| 7 Foramen lacerum | 16 Lesser petrosal nerve | 25 Promontory with tympanic plexus |
| 8 Apex of petrous part | 17 Internal carotid artery | (position of cochlea) |
| 9 Position of cochlea | 18 Mastoid air cells | 26 Tensor muscle of tympanum |
| (modiolus with crista spiralis ossea) | 19 Lateral semicircular duct | 27 Auditory tube |

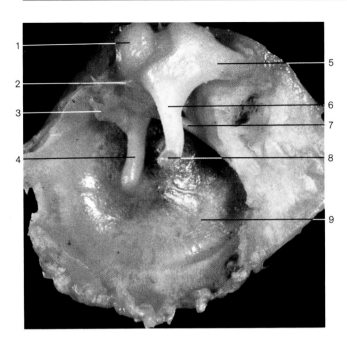

1  Head of malleus
2  Anterior ligament of malleus
3  Tendon of tensor tympani muscle
4  Handle of malleus
5  Short crus of incus
6  Long crus of incus
7  Chorda tympani
8  Lenticular process
9  Tympanic membrane

**Tympanic membrane with malleus and incus** (internal aspect, right side).

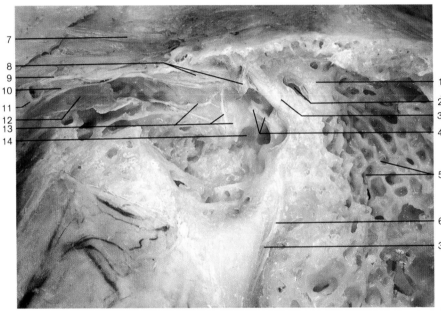

1  Tympanic antrum
2  Lateral semicircular canal (opened)
3  Facial canal
4  Stapes with tendon of stapedius
5  Mastoid air cells
6  Chorda tympani (intracranial part)
7  Greater petrosal nerve
8  Tensor tympani muscle
   (processus cochleariformis)
9  Lesser petrosal nerve
10 Anterior tympanic artery
11 Middle meningeal artery
12 Auditory tube
13 Promontory with tympanic plexus
14 Fenestra cochleae

**Tympanic cavity, medial wall** (left side). External acoustic meatus and lateral wall of tympanic cavity together with incus. Malleus and tympanic membrane have been removed; mastoid air cells are opened.

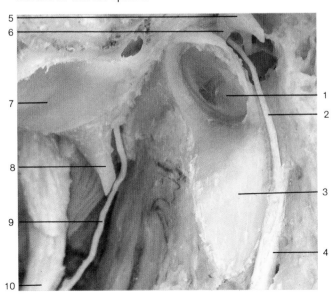

1  Tympanic membrane
2  Chorda tympani (intracranial part)
3  Floor of the external acoustic meatus
4  Facial nerve and facial canal
5  Incus
6  Head of malleus
7  Mandibular fossa
8  Spine of sphenoid
9  Chorda tympani (extracranial part)
10 Styloid process

**Tympanic membrane** (lateral aspect, left side). External acoustic meatus and facial canal have been opened to expose the chorda tympani (magn. ~1.5×).

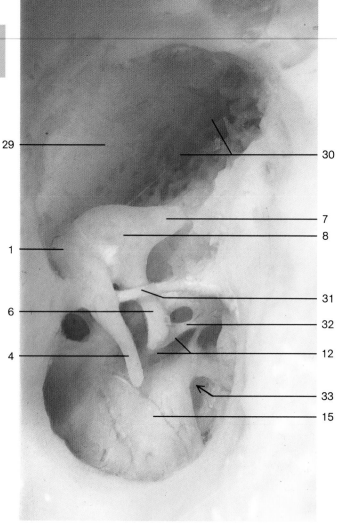

29
30
7
8
1
31
6
32
4
12
33
15

**Tympanic cavity with malleus, incus, and stapes** (lateral aspect, left side). Tympanic membrane removed, mastoid antrum opened.

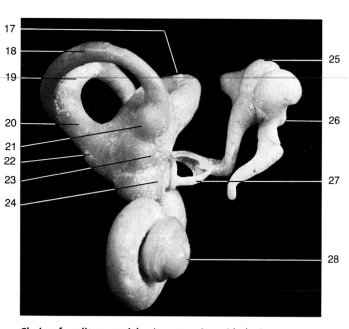

17
18
19
20
21
22
23
24
25
26
27
28

**Chain of auditory ossicles** in connection with the inner ear (antero-lateral aspect, left side).

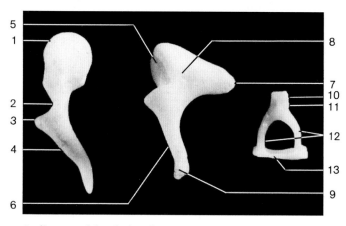

5
1
2
3
4
6
8
7
10
11
12
13
9

**Auditory ossicles** (isolated).

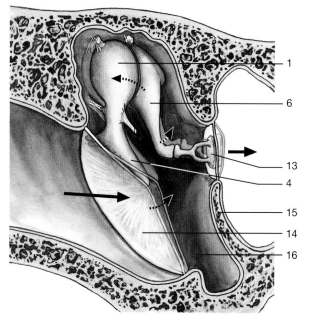

1
6
13
4
15
14
16

**Position and movements of the auditory ossicles.**

**Malleus**
1 Head
2 Neck
3 Lateral process
4 Handle

**Incus**
5 Articular facet for malleus
6 Long crus
7 Short crus
8 Body
9 Lenticular process

**Stapes**
10 Head
11 Neck
12 Anterior and posterior crura
13 Base

**Walls of tympanic cavity**
14 Tympanic membrane
15 Promontory
16 Hypotympanic recess
  of tympanic cavity

**Internal ear (labyrinth)**
17 Lateral semicircular duct
18 Anterior semicircular duct
19 Posterior semicircular duct
20 Common crus
21 Ampulla
22 Beginning of endolymphatic
  duct
23 Utricular prominence
24 Saccular prominence
25 Incus
26 Malleus
27 Stapes
28 Cochlea

**Tympanic cavity**
29 Epitympanic recess
30 Mastoid antrum
31 Chorda tympani
32 Tendon of stapedius muscle
33 Round window
  (fenestra cochleae)

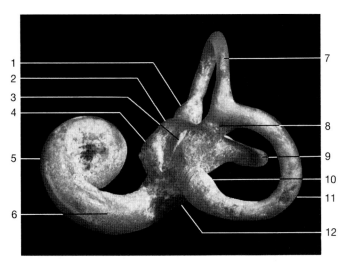

1  Ampulla
   (anterior semicircular canal)
2  Elliptical recess
3  Aqueduct of the vestibule
4  Spherical recess
5  Cochlea
6  Base of cochlea
7  Anterior semicircular canal
8  Crus commune or
   common limb
9  Lateral semicircular canal
10 Posterior bony ampulla
11 Posterior semicircular canal
   (posterior canal)
12 Fenestra cochleae
13 Bony ampulla
14 Fenestra vestibuli
15 Cupula of cochlea

16 External acoustic meatus
17 Mastoid air cells
18 Tympanic cavity and
   fenestra cochleae (probe)
19 External acoustic meatus
20 Facial canal
21 Base of cochlea and
   musculotubal canal
22 Malleus and incus
23 Stapes
24 Tympanic membrane
25 Tympanic cavity
26 Aqueduct of cochlea
27 Endolymphatic sac
28 Endolymphatic duct
29 Macula of utricle
30 Macula of saccule

**Cast of the right labyrinth** (postero-medial aspect).

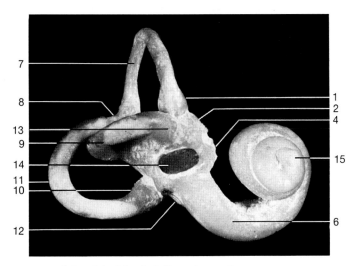

**Cast of the right labyrinth** (lateral aspect).

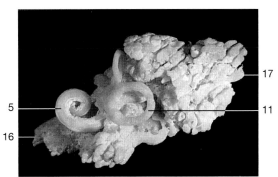

**Cast of the labyrinth and mastoid cells** (posterior aspect). Life size.

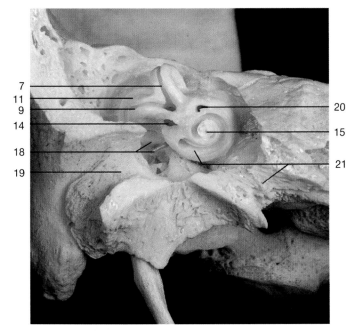

**Dissection of bony labyrinth in situ.** Semicircular canals and cochlear duct opened.

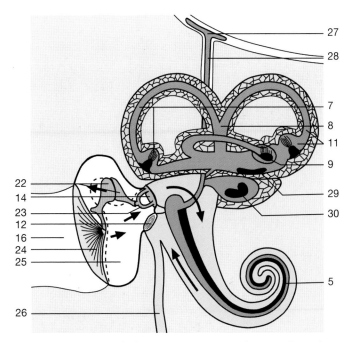

**Auditory and vestibular apparatus.** Arrows: direction of sound waves; blue = perilymphatic ducts.

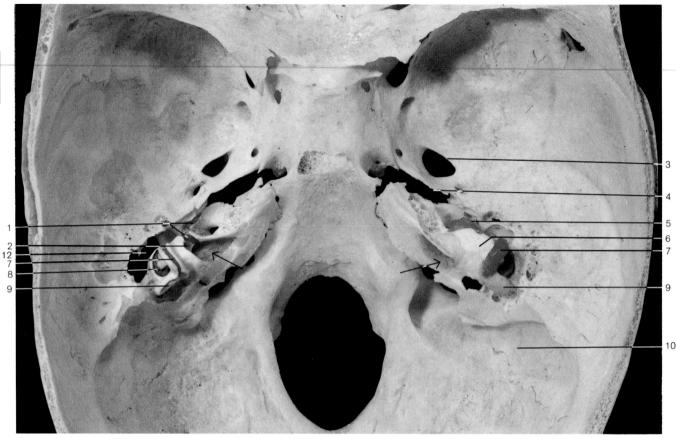

**Bony labyrinth, petrous part of the temporal bone** (from above). Left: semicircular canals opened; right: semicircular canals closed. Arrows: internal acoustic meatus.

| | | |
|---|---|---|
| 1 Facial canal and semicanal of auditory tube | 9 Posterior semicircular canal | 17 Fenestra vestibuli |
| 2 Superior vestibular area | 10 Groove for sigmoid sinus | 18 Promontory |
| 3 Foramen ovale | 11 Sigmoid sinus | 19 Zygomatic process |
| 4 Foramen lacerum | 12 Tympanic cavity | 20 Fenestra cochleae |
| 5 Cochlea | 13 Auditory tube | 21 Mastoid process |
| 6 Vestibule | 14 Mastoid air cells | |
| 7 Anterior semicircular canal | 15 Facial, vestibulocochlear, and intermediate nerves | |
| 8 Lateral semicircular canal | 16 Temporal fossa | |

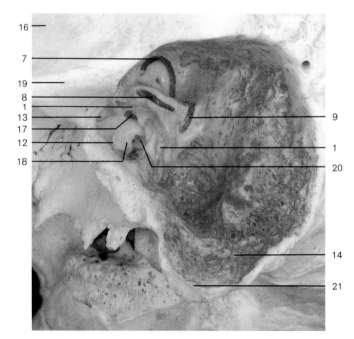

**Bony labyrinth** (left lateral aspect). Temporal and tympanic bone partly removed, semicircular canals opened.

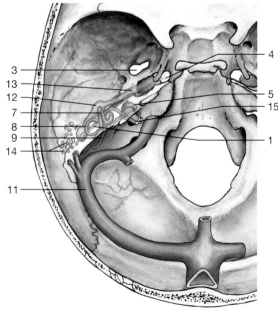

**Internal ear** (from above). Diagram showing the position of the membranous labyrinth and the tympanic cavity.

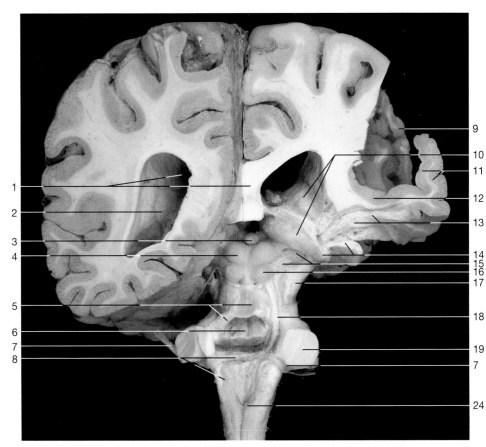

1   Left lateral ventricle
    and corpus callosum
2   Thalamus
3   Pineal gland (epiphysis)
4   Superior colliculus
5   Superior medullary velum and
    superior cerebellar peduncle
6   Rhomboid fossa
7   Vestibulocochlear nerve (n. VIII)
8   Dorsal acoustic striae and
    inferior cerebellar peduncle
9   Insular lobe
10  Caudate nucleus and thalamus
11  Temporal lobe (superior temporal
    gyrus) (area of acoustic centers)
12  Transverse temporal gyri of Heschl
    (area of primary acoustic centers)
13  Acoustic radiation
    of internal capsule
14  Lateral geniculate body and
    optic radiation (cut)
15  Medial geniculate body and
    brachium of inferior colliculus
16  Inferior colliculus
17  Cerebral peduncle
18  Lateral lemniscus
19  Middle cerebellar peduncle
20  Dorsal (posterior) cochlear
    nucleus
21  Ventral (anterior) cochlear
    nucleus
22  Inferior olive with olivo-
    cochlear tract of Rasmussen (red)
23  Ganglion spirale
24  Obex
25  Frontal lobe
26  Temporal lobe
27  Middle temporal gyrus
    (area of tertiary acoustic centers)
28  Trapezoid body

**Dissection of the brain stem showing the auditory pathway** (posterior aspect). Cerebellum and posterior part of the two hemispheres have been removed.

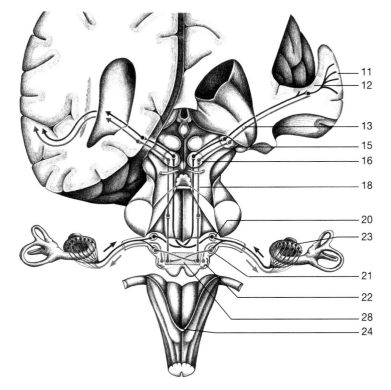

**Auditory pathway** (compare with the dissection above).
Red = descending (efferent) pathway (olivocochlear tract of Rasmussen); green and blue = ascending (afferent) pathways.

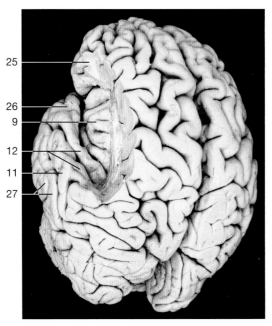

**Auditory areas in the left hemisphere** (supero-lateral aspect). Parts of the frontal and parietal lobes have been removed.

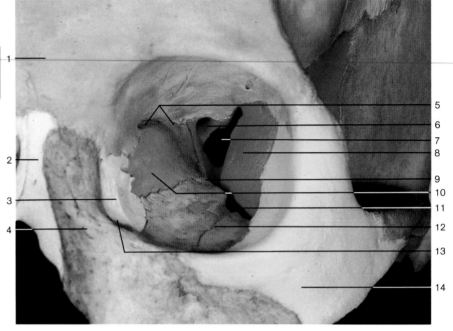

1  Frontal bone
2  Nasal bone
3  Lacrimal bone
4  Maxilla (frontal process)
5  Ethmoidal foramina
6  Lesser wing of sphenoid bone
   and optic canal
7  Superior orbital fissure
8  Greater wing of sphenoid bone
9  Orbital process of palatine bone
10  Orbital plate of ethmoid bone
11  Inferior orbital fissure
12  Infra-orbital sulcus
13  Nasolacrimal canal
14  Zygomatic bone
15  Levator palpebrae superioris muscle
16  Superior rectus muscle
17  Superior oblique muscle
18  Lateral rectus muscle
19  Medial rectus muscle
20  Inferior rectus muscle
21  Optic nerve (n. II)
22  Nasal septum
23  Middle nasal concha
24  Maxillary sinus
25  Inferior nasal concha
26  Sclera
27  Ophthalmic artery
28  Orbital fatty tissue
29  Tenon's space
30  Periorbita and maxilla
31  Frontal sinus
32  Superior conjunctival fornix
33  Cornea
34  Superior tarsal plate
35  Lens
36  Inferior tarsal plate
37  Inferior conjunctival fornix
38  Inferior oblique muscle

**Bones of the left orbit** (indicated by different colors).

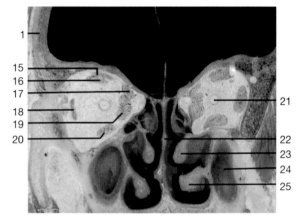

**Frontal section through the posterior part of the orbit.**

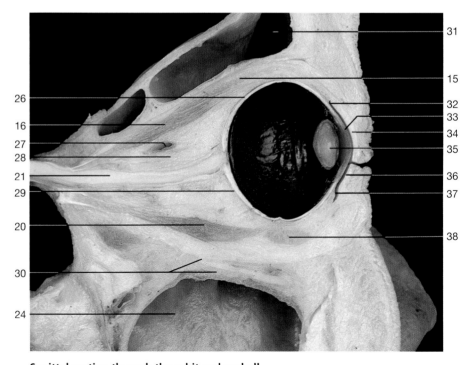

**Sagittal section through the orbit and eyeball.**

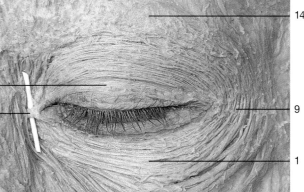

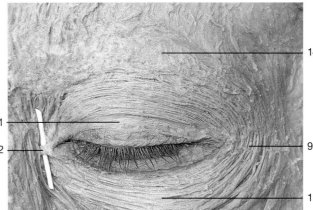

**Lids and lacrimal apparatus of the left eye** (anterior aspect). Parts of the eyelids have been removed to reveal the underlying eyeball. The maxillary sinus has been opened.

**Facial muscles of the left eye** (anterior aspect). The orbicularis oculi muscle and its connection to the superior labial muscles are shown. Note the medial palpebral ligament (probe).

| | |
|---|---|
| 1 Orbicularis oculi muscle | 10 Infra-orbital artery and nerve |
| 2 Superior lacrimal canaliculus | 11 Maxillary sinus |
| 3 Lacrimal sac | 12 Medial palpebral ligament |
| 4 Inferior lacrimal canaliculus | 13 Levator labii superioris muscle |
| 5 Nasolacrimal duct | 14 Frontal belly of occipitofrontalis muscle |
| 6 Inferior nasal concha | 15 Aponeurosis of levator palpebrae superioris muscle |
| 7 Upper eyelid | 16 Lacrimal gland |
| 8 Eyeball | 17 Palpebral portion of orbicularis oculi muscle |
| 9 Lateral palpebral ligament | 18 Infra-orbital foramen |

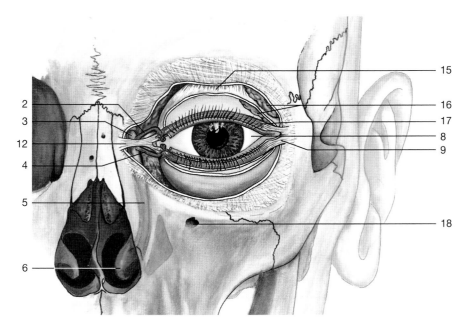

**Lacrimal apparatus of the left eye** (anterior aspect).
Red = Palpebral portion of the orbicularis oculi muscle.

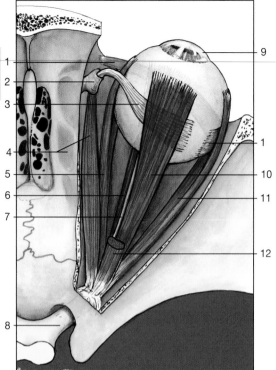

**Right orbit with eyeball and extra-ocular muscles** (from above). Levator palpebrae superioris muscle has been severed.

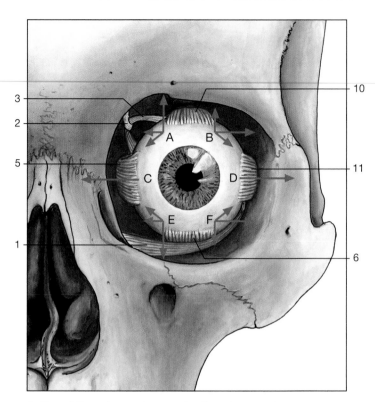

**Action of the extra-ocular muscles** (anterior aspect).

A = Superior rectus muscle
B = Inferior oblique muscle
C = Medial rectus muscle
D = Lateral rectus muscle
E = Inferior rectus muscle
F = Superior oblique muscle

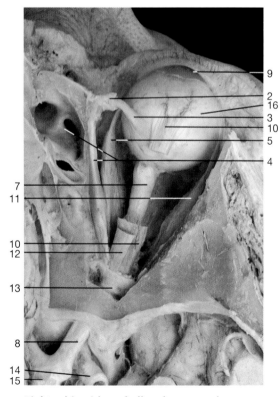

**Right orbit with eyeball and extra-ocular muscles** (from above). The roof of the orbit has been removed, the superior rectus muscle and the levator palpebrae superioris muscle have been severed.

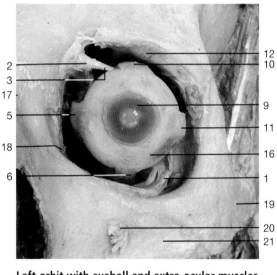

**Left orbit with eyeball and extra-ocular muscles** (anterior aspect). Lids, conjunctiva, and lacrimal apparatus have been removed.

1  Inferior oblique muscle
2  Trochlea
3  Tendon of superior oblique muscle
4  Superior oblique muscle and ethmoid air cells
5  Medial rectus muscle
6  Inferior rectus muscle
7  Optic nerve (extracranial part)
8  Optic nerve (intracranial part)
9  Cornea
10  Superior rectus muscle
11  Lateral rectus muscle
12  Levator palpebrae superioris muscle
13  Common annular tendon
14  Internal carotid artery
15  Optic chiasma
16  Sclera
17  Nasal bone
18  Nasolacrimal duct
19  Zygomatic bone
20  Infra-orbital nerves
21  Maxilla

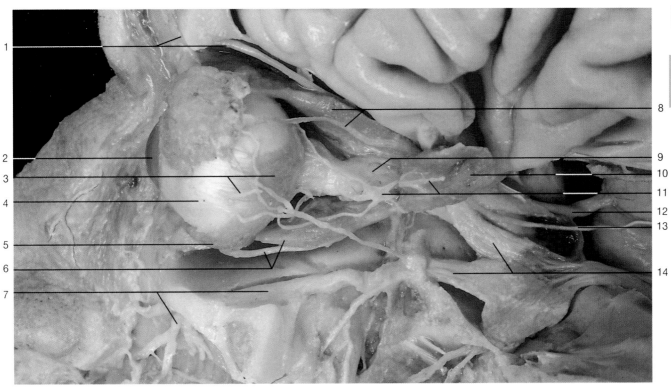

**Extra-ocular muscles and their nerves** (lateral aspect of the left eye). Lateral rectus muscle divided and reflected.

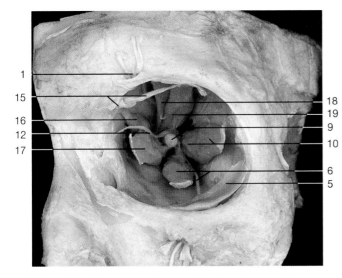

**Left orbit with extra-ocular muscles** (anterior aspect). Eyeball removed.

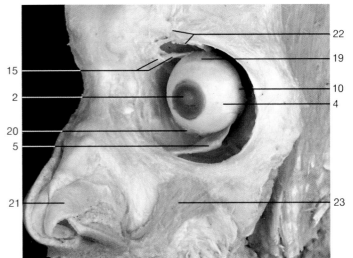

**Extra-ocular muscles** (antero-lateral aspect).

| | | | |
|---|---|---|---|
| 1 | Supra-orbital nerve | 12 | Oculomotor nerve (n. III) |
| 2 | Cornea | 13 | Trochlear nerve (n. IV) |
| 3 | Insertion of lateral rectus muscle | 14 | Ophthalmic nerve (n. V₁) and maxillary nerve (n. V₂) |
| 4 | Eyeball (sclera) | 15 | Trochlea and tendon of superior oblique muscle |
| 5 | Inferior oblique muscle | 16 | Superior oblique muscle |
| 6 | Inferior rectus muscle and inferior branch of oculomotor nerve | 17 | Medial rectus muscle |
| | | 18 | Levator palpebrae superioris muscle |
| 7 | Infra-orbital nerve | 19 | Superior rectus muscle |
| 8 | Superior rectus muscle and lacrimal nerve | 20 | Inferior rectus muscle |
| 9 | Optic nerve (n. II) | 21 | Greater alar cartilage |
| 10 | Lateral rectus muscle | 22 | Supra-orbital nerve and levator palpebrae superioris muscle |
| 11 | Ciliary ganglion and abducens nerve (n. VI) | 23 | Levator labii superioris muscle |

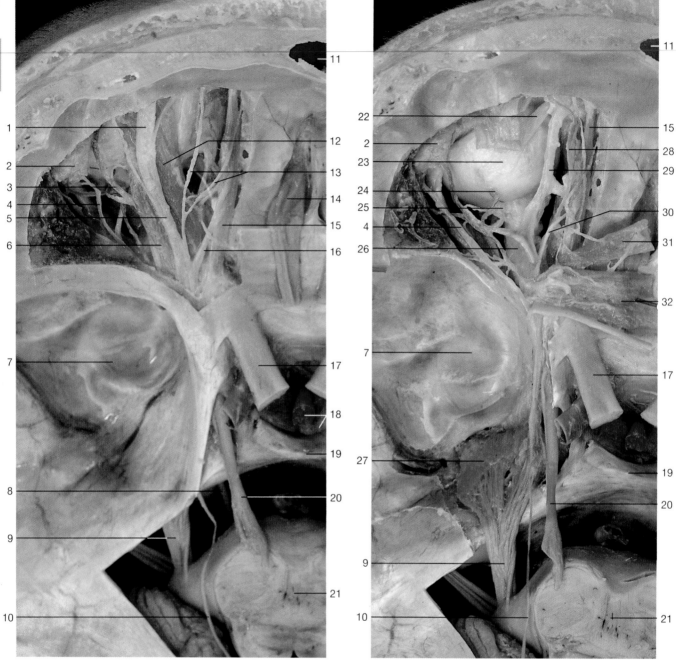

**Superficial layer of the left orbit** (superior aspect). The roof of the orbit and a portion of the left tentorium have been removed.

**Middle layer of the left orbit** (superior aspect). The roof of the orbit has been removed and the superior extra-ocular muscles have been divided and reflected.

| | | | |
|---|---|---|---|
| 1 | Lateral branch of frontal nerve | 10 | Trochlear nerve (intracranial part) |
| 2 | Lacrimal gland | 11 | Frontal sinus |
| 3 | Lacrimal vein | 12 | Levator palpebrae superioris muscle |
| 4 | Lacrimal nerve | 13 | Branches of supratrochlear nerve |
| 5 | Frontal nerve | 14 | Olfactory bulb |
| 6 | Superior rectus | 15 | Superior oblique muscle |
| 7 | Middle cranial fossa | 16 | Trochlear nerve (intra-orbital part) |
| 8 | Abducent nerve (n. VI) | 17 | Optic nerve (intracranial part) |
| 9 | Trigeminal nerve (n. V) | 18 | Pituitary gland and infundibulum |

| | |
|---|---|
| 19 | Dorsum sellae |
| 20 | Oculomotor nerve (n. III) |
| 21 | Midbrain |
| 22 | Tendon of superior oblique muscle |
| 23 | Eyeball |
| 24 | Vena vorticosa |
| 25 | Short ciliary nerves |
| 26 | Optic nerve (extracranial part) |
| 27 | Trigeminal ganglion |

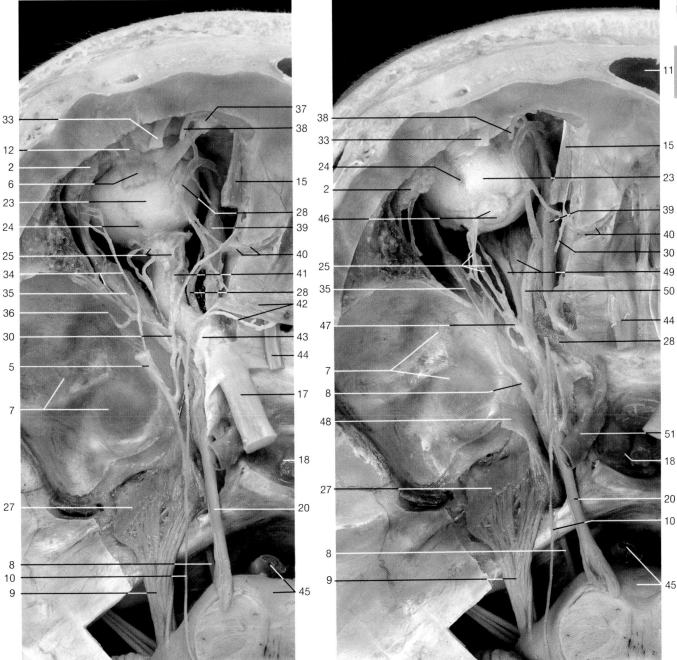

**Middle layer of the left orbit** (superior aspect). The roof of the orbit and the superior extra-ocular muscles have been removed.

**Deeper layer of the left orbit** (superior aspect). The optic nerve has now been removed.

| | |
|---|---|
| 28 | Ophthalmic artery |
| 29 | Superior ophthalmic vein |
| 30 | Nasociliary nerve |
| 31 | Levator palpebrae superioris muscle (reflected) |
| 32 | Superior rectus muscle (reflected) |
| 33 | Lateral branch of supra-orbital nerve |
| 34 | Lacrimal nerve and artery |
| 35 | Lateral rectus muscle |
| 36 | Meningolacrimal artery (anastomosing with middle meningeal artery) |
| 37 | Trochlea |
| 38 | Medial branch of supra-orbital nerve |
| 39 | Medial rectus muscle |
| 40 | Anterior ethmoidal artery and nerve |
| 41 | Long ciliary nerve |
| 42 | Superior oblique muscle and trochlear nerve |
| 43 | Common tendinous ring |
| 44 | Olfactory tract |
| 45 | Basilar artery and pons |
| 46 | Optic nerve (external sheath of optic nerve, divided) |
| 47 | Ciliary ganglion |
| 48 | Ophthalmic nerve (divided, reflected) |
| 49 | Inferior branch of oculomotor nerve and inferior rectus muscle |
| 50 | Superior branch of oculomotor nerve |
| 51 | Internal carotid artery |

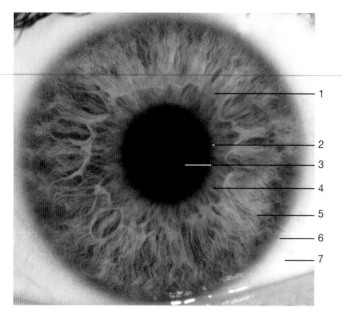

**Anterior segment of the human eye.** Note the colored iris and the location of the lens behind the iris.

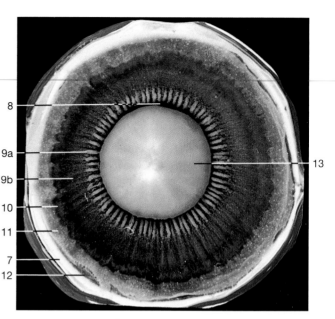

**Anterior segment of the eyeball** (posterior aspect). The opacity of the lens is an artifact.

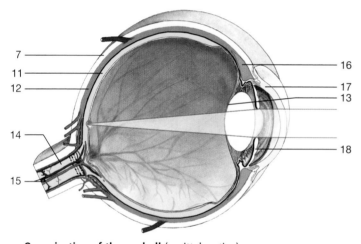

**Organization of the eyeball** (sagittal section).
Red lines = projection of the light on the fovea centralis.

1   Fold of iris
2   Pupillary margin of iris
3   Anterior surface of the lens
4   Inner border of iris
5   Outer border of iris
6   Corneal limbus
7   Sclera
8   Zonular fibers
9   Ciliary body
   a   Ciliary processes (pars plicata)
   b   Ciliary ring (pars plana)
10  Ora serrata
11  Retina
12  Choroid
13  Posterior surface of the lens
14  Optic nerve (n. II)
15  Central retinal artery and vein
16  Ciliary muscle
17  Cornea
18  Iris
19  Orbital bone
20  Superior rectus muscle
21  Vitreous body
22  Lens
23  Inferior rectus muscle
24  Maxillary sinus

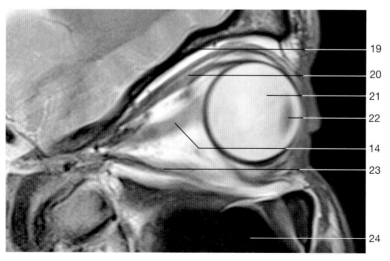

**Sagittal section through the orbit and eyeball** (MRI scan).
(Prof. Uder, Dept. of Radiology, Univ. Erlangen-Nuremberg, Germany.)

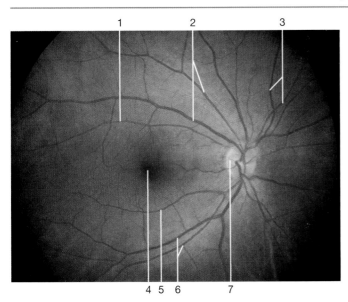

1  Superior macular artery
2  Superior temporal artery and vein of retina
3  Medial artery and vein of retina
4  Fovea centralis and macula lutea
5  Inferior macular artery
6  Inferior temporal artery and vein of retina
7  Optic disc
8  Superior temporal artery of retina
9  Superior nasal artery of retina
10  Inferior temporal artery of retina
11  Inferior nasal artery of retina
12  Posterior and anterior ethmoidal arteries
13  Long and short posterior ciliary arteries
14  Optic nerve (n. II) and ophthalmic artery
15  Central retinal artery
16  Retinal arteries
17  Supratrochlear artery
18  Supra-orbital artery
19  Anterior ciliary artery
20  Dorsal nasal artery
21  Iridial arteries
22  Lens

**Fundus of a normal right eye.** Notice, the arteries are smaller and lighter than the veins. (Courtesy of Prof. Okamura, Eye Dept., Univ. Kumamoto, Japan.)

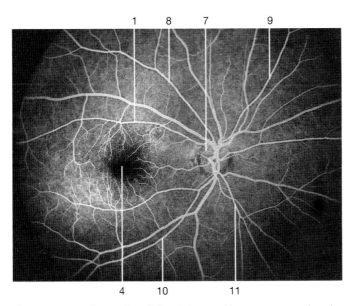

**Fluorescent angiography of the right eye** (the same eye as above). The retinal vessels are shown. (Courtesy of Prof. Okamura, Eye Dept., Univ. Kumamoto, Japan.)

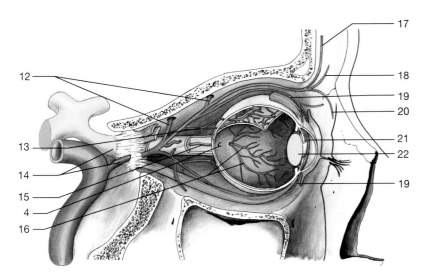

**Orbit with eyeball, optic nerve, and vessels of the eye.** The ophthalmic artery and its branches are shown.

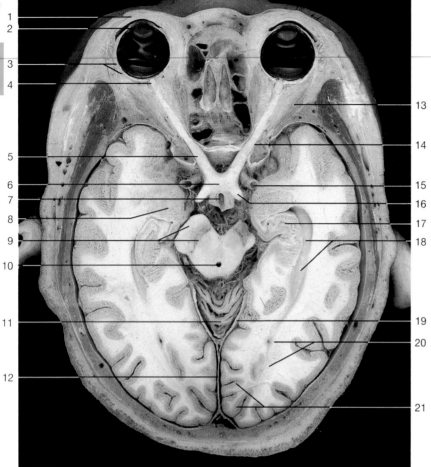

1  Upper lid
2  Cornea
3  Eyeball (sclera, retina)
4  Head of optic nerve
5  Optic nerve
6  Optic chiasma
7  Infundibular recess of hypothalamus
8  Amygdaloid body
9  Substantia nigra and crus cerebri
10  Cerebral aqueduct
11  Vermis of cerebellum
12  Falx cerebri
13  Lateral rectus muscle
14  Optic canal
15  Internal carotid artery
16  Optic tract
17  Hippocampus
18  Inferior horn of lateral ventricle
19  Cerebellar tentorium
20  Optic radiation of Gratiolet
21  Visual cortex
     (area calcarina, striate cortex)
22  Lens
23  Eyeball
24  Medial rectus muscle
25  Cerebral peduncle
26  Ethmoidal cells
27  Optic nerve (n. II) with dura sheath
28  Temporal muscle
29  Oculomotor nerve (n. III) and
     pituitary gland (hypophysis)

**Horizontal section through the head** at the level of optic chiasma and striate cortex (superior aspect). Note the relationship of hypothalamic infundibulum to optic chiasma.

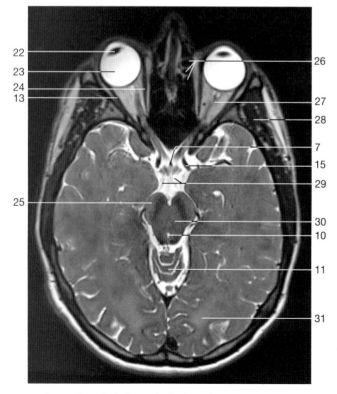

**Horizontal section through the head** at the level of sella turcica (MRI scan). (Prof. Uder, Dept. of Radiology, Univ. Erlangen-Nuremberg, Germany.)

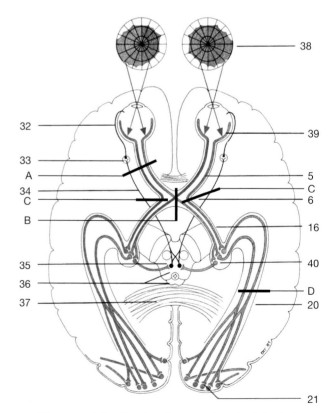

**Diagram of the visual pathway and path of the light reflex.**

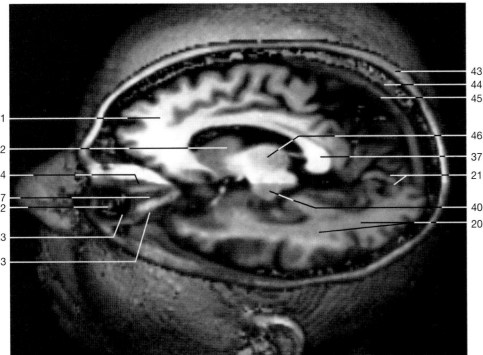

30 Midbrain
31 Occipital lobe
32 Long and short ciliary nerves
33 Ciliary ganglion
34 Oculomotor nerve (n. III)
   within the cavernous sinus
35 Accessory oculomotor nuclei
36 Colliculi of midbrain
37 Corpus callosum
38 Visual field
39 Retina
40 Lateral geniculate body
41 Frontal lobe
42 Caudate nucleus
43 Skin of scalp
44 Diploe of the skull
45 Dura mater
46 Thalamus
47 Anterior cerebral artery
48 Frontal sinus
49 Internal capsule
50 Lentiform nucleus (putamen)
51 Hippocampus
52 Temporal lobe
   of the left hemisphere

**3-D reconstruction of the human visual pathway** (MRI scan). (Prof. Huk, Univ. Erlangen-Nuremberg, Germany.)

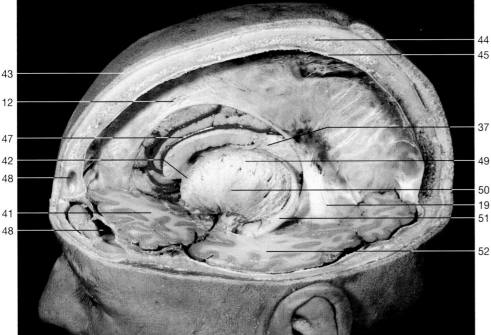

**Dissection of brain stem in situ.** Left hemisphere has been partly removed (compare with the MRI scan above).

In **binocular vision** the visual field (38) is projected upon portions of both retinae (blue and red in the drawing). In the chiasma the fibers from the two retinal portions are combined to form the left optic tract. The fibers of the two eyes remain separated from each other throughout the entire visual pathway up to their final termination in the visual cortex (21). **Injuries on the optic pathway** produce visual defects whose nature depends on the location of the injury. Destruction of one optic nerve (A) produces **blindness in the corresponding eye** with loss of pupillary light reflex. If **lesions of the chiasma** destroy the crossing fibers of the nasal portions of the retina (B), both temporal fields of vision are lost **(bitemporal hemianopsia)**. If both lateral angles of the chiasma are compressed (C), the nondecussating fibers from the temporal retinae are affected, resulting in loss of nasal visual fields **(binasal hemianopsia)**. Lesions posterior to the chiasma (D) (i.e., optic tract, lateral geniculate body, optic radiation, or visual cortex) result in a loss of the entire opposite field of vision **(homonymous hemianopsia)**.

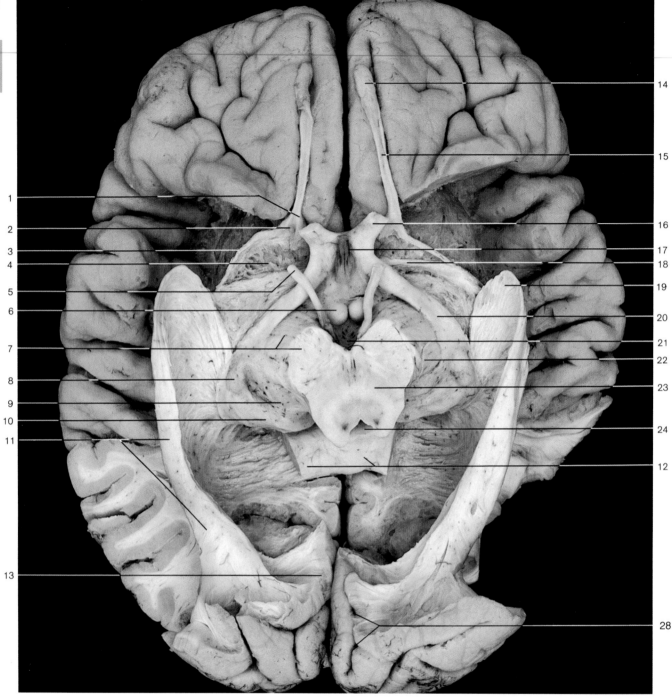

**Dissection of the visual pathway** (inferior aspect). The midbrain is divided. Frontal pole at the top.

1   Medial olfactory stria
2   Olfactory trigone
3   Lateral olfactory stria
4   Anterior perforated substance
5   Oculomotor nerve (n. III)
6   Mamillary body
7   Cerebral peduncle
8   Lateral geniculate body
9   Medial geniculate body
10  Pulvinar of thalamus
11  Optic radiation
12  Splenium of the corpus callosum
    (commissural fibers)
13  Cuneus
14  Olfactory bulb

15  Olfactory tract
16  Optic nerve (n. II)
17  Infundibulum
18  Anterior commissure
19  Genu of optic radiation
20  Optic tract
21  Interpeduncular fossa and
    posterior perforated substance
22  Trochlear nerve (n. IV)
23  Substantia nigra
24  Cerebral aqueduct
25  Visual cortex
26  Line of Gennari
27  Gyrus of striate cortex
28  Calcarine sulcus

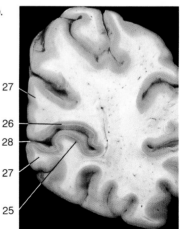

**Frontal section of the striate cortex** at the level of the striate area in the occipital lobe.

# 2.5 Nasal and Oral Cavities

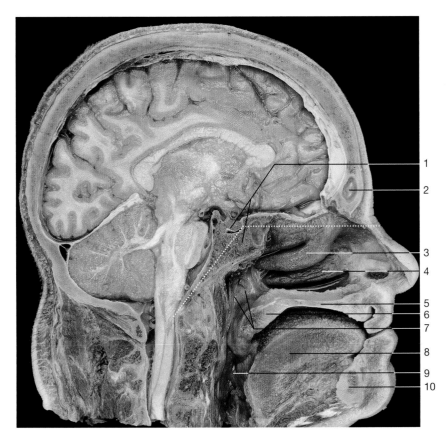

**Median sagittal section through the head.** The palate separates nasal and oral cavities. The base of the skull forms an angle of about 150° at the sella turcica (dotted line).

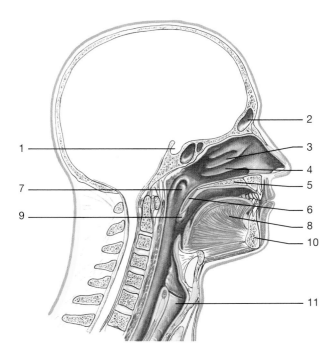

1 Hypophysis within hypophysial fossa
2 Frontal sinus
3 Middle nasal concha
4 Inferior nasal concha
5 Hard palate
6 Soft palate
7 Pharynx with auditory tube
8 Tongue
9 Pharynx with palatine tonsil
10 Mandible
11 Larynx

**Median sagittal section through the head.** The tongue has been disposed to show the connection of the oral cavity with the pharynx and the position of the palatine tonsil.

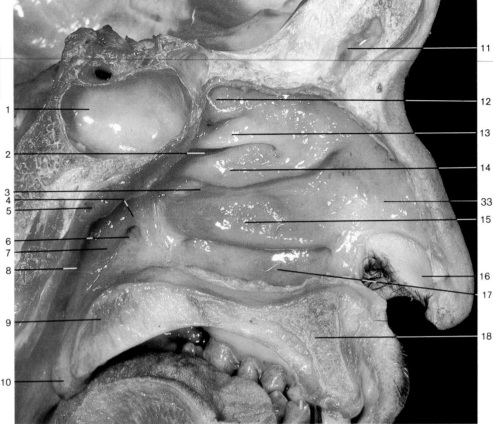

1  Sphenoidal sinus
2  Superior meatus
3  Middle meatus
4  Tubal elevation
5  Pharyngeal tonsil
6  Pharyngeal orifice
   of auditory tube
7  Salpingopharyngeal fold
8  Pharyngeal recess
9  Soft palate
10 Uvula
11 Frontal sinus
12 Spheno-ethmoidal recess
13 Superior nasal concha
14 Middle nasal concha
15 Inferior nasal concha
16 Vestibule
17 Inferior meatus
18 Hard palate
19 Grooves for the middle
   meningeal artery and
   parietal bone (yellow)
20 Maxillary hiatus
21 Perpendicular process
   of palatine bone
22 Openings of ethmoidal air cells
23 Nasofrontal duct
24 Medial pterygoid plate (red)
25 Horizontal plate
   of palatine process
26 Ethmoidal air cells
27 Maxillary sinus
28 Nasal septum
29 Pterygoid hamulus
30 Nasal bone (white)
31 Frontal process of maxilla
   (violet)
32 Palatine process of maxilla
   (violet)
33 Nasal atrium

**Lateral wall of the nasal cavity.** Septum removed.

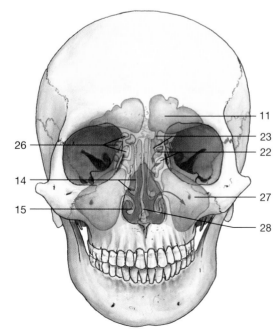

**Bones of the left nasal cavity** (medial aspect).

**Paranasal sinuses and their connections with the nasal cavity.** Openings indicated by arrows.

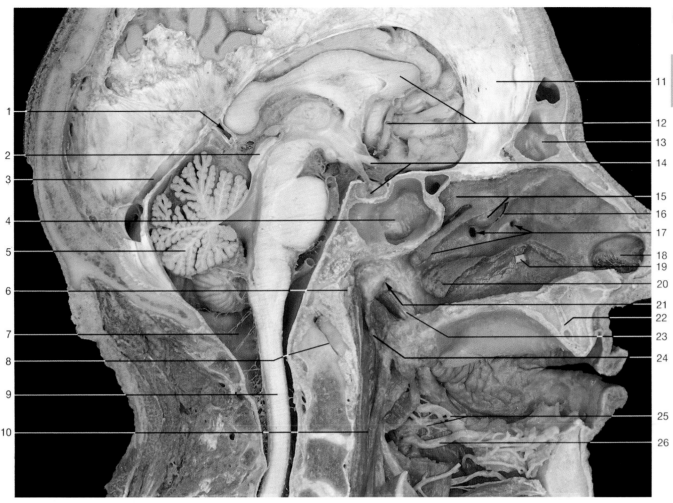

**Median section through the head with nasal and oral cavities.** The middle and inferior nasal conchae have been partly removed to show the openings of paranasal sinuses.

1 Great cerebral vein (Galen's vein)
2 Tectum of midbrain
3 Straight sinus
4 Sphenoidal sinus
5 Cerebellum
6 Pharyngeal tonsil
7 Cerebellomedullary cistern
8 Median atlanto-axial joint
9 Spinal cord
10 Oral part of pharynx
11 Falx cerebri
12 Corpus callosum and anterior cerebral artery
13 Frontal sinus
14 Optic chiasm and pituitary gland
15 Superior nasal concha and ethmoidal bulla
16 Semilunar hiatus
17 Accessory openings to maxillary sinus
   and cut edge of middle nasal concha
18 Vestibule
19 Opening of nasolacrimal duct
20 Inferior nasal concha (cut)
21 Opening of auditory tube
22 Incisive canal
23 Levator veli palatini muscle
24 Salpingopharyngeal fold
25 Lingual nerve and submandibular ganglion
26 Submandibular duct
27 Spheno-ethmoidal recess
28 Superior nasal meatus
29 Salpingopalatine fold
30 Nasofrontal duct
31 Nasolacrimal duct

**Lateral wall of the nasal cavity.** Openings indicated by arrows.

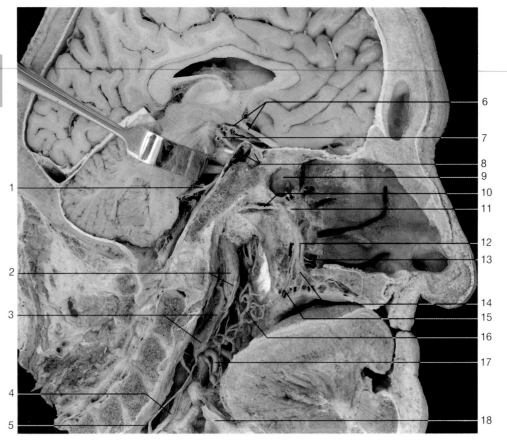

| | |
|---|---|
| 1 | Facial nerve |
| 2 | Internal carotid artery and internal carotid plexus |
| 3 | Superior cervical ganglion |
| 4 | Vagus nerve (n. X) |
| 5 | Sympathetic trunk |
| 6 | Optic nerve (n. II) and ophthalmic artery |
| 7 | Oculomotor nerve (n. III) |
| 8 | Internal carotid artery and cavernous sinus |
| 9 | Sphenoidal sinus |
| 10 | Nerve of the pterygoid canal |
| 11 | Pterygopalatine ganglion |
| 12 | Descending palatine artery |
| 13 | Lateral inferior posterior nasal branches and lateral posterior nasal and septal arteries |
| 14 | Greater palatine nerves and artery |
| 15 | Lesser palatine nerves and arteries |
| 16 | Branches of ascending pharyngeal artery |
| 17 | Lingual artery |
| 18 | Epiglottis |
| 19 | Anterior ethmoidal artery |
| 20 | Olfactory bulb |
| 21 | Olfactory tract |
| 22 | Nasopalatine nerve |
| 23 | Choanae |
| 24 | Frontal sinus |
| 25 | Crista galli |
| 26 | Anterior ethmoidal artery and nerve, and nasal branch of anterior ethmoidal artery |
| 27 | Nasal septum |
| 28 | Septal artery |
| 29 | Crest of nasal septum |
| 30 | Hard palate |
| 31 | Cerebellar tentorium |
| 32 | Trochlear nerve (n. IV) |
| 33 | Trigeminal nerve (n. V) with motor root |
| 34 | Internal carotid plexus |
| 35 | Lingual nerve with chorda tympani |
| 36 | Medial pterygoid muscle and medial pterygoid plate |
| 37 | Inferior alveolar nerve |
| 38 | Sympathetic trunk |
| 39 | Greater petrosal nerve |
| 40 | Palatine nerves |
| 41 | Tongue |
| 42 | Olfactory bulb |
| 43 | Ophthalmic nerve (n. $V_1$) |
| 44 | Trigeminal ganglion |

**Nerves of the lateral wall of nasal cavity** (sagittal section through the head). Mucous membranes partly removed, pterygoid canal opened.

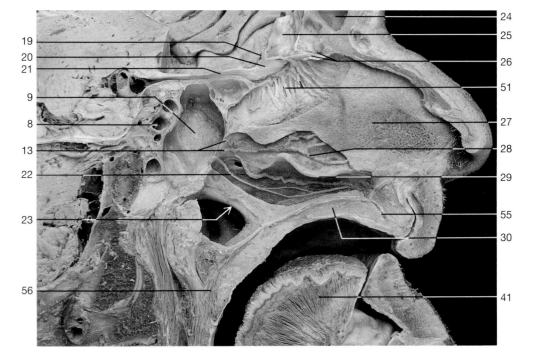

**Nasal septum.** Dissection of nerves and vessels.

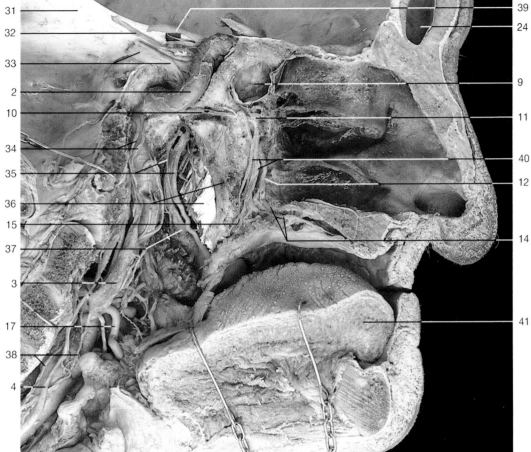
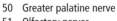

| 45 | Maxillary nerve (n. V$_2$) |
|---|---|
| 46 | Mandibular nerve (n. V$_3$) |
| 47 | Deep petrosal nerve |
| 48 | Medial pterygoid muscle |
| 49 | Tensor veli palatine muscle |
| 50 | Greater palatine nerve |
| 51 | Olfactory nerves |
| 52 | Internal and medial nasal branches of anterior ethmoidal nerve |
| 53 | Lateral superior posterior nasal branches |
| 54 | Lateral inferior posterior nasal branches |
| 55 | Incisive canal with nasopalatine nerve |
| 56 | Uvula |

**Nerves of the lateral wall of nasal cavity** (sagittal section through the head). Carotid canal opened, mucous membranes of pharynx and nasal cavity partly removed.

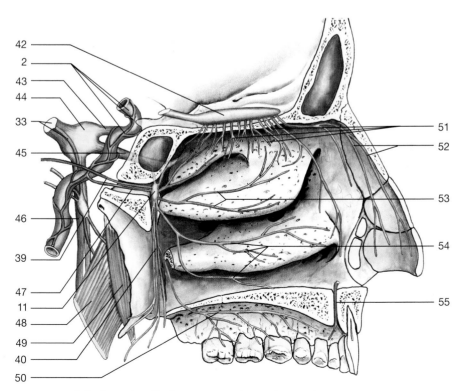

**Nerves of the lateral wall of nasal cavity** (sagittal section).

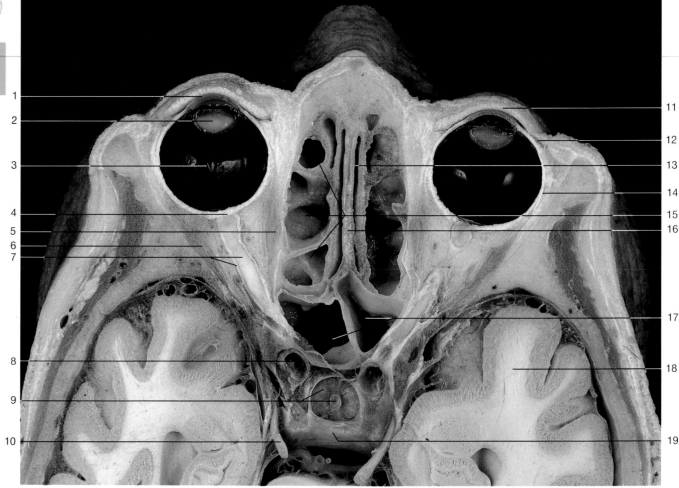

**Horizontal section through the nasal cavity, the orbits, and temporal lobes of the brain** at the level of pituitary gland.

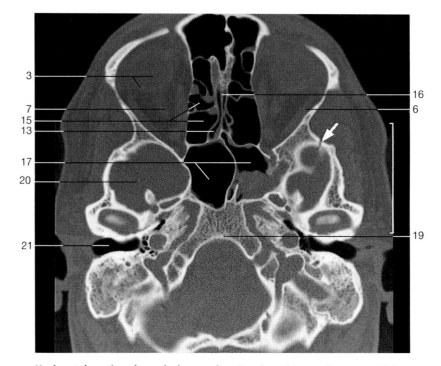

**Horizontal section through the nasal cavity, the orbits, and temporal lobes of the brain** (CT scan). Bar = 2 cm. Arrow: fracture.

1  Cornea
2  Lens
3  Vitreous body (eyeball)
4  Head of optic nerve
5  Medial rectus muscle
6  Lateral rectus muscle
7  Optic nerve with dural sheath
8  Internal carotid artery
9  Pituitary gland and infundibulum
10  Oculomotor nerve
11  Superior tarsal plate of eyelid
12  Fornix of conjunctiva
13  Nasal cavity
14  Sclera
15  Ethmoidal sinus
16  Nasal septum
17  Sphenoidal sinus
18  Temporal lobe
19  Clivus
20  Middle cranial fossa
21  External acoustic meatus
22  Superior sagittal sinus
23  Falx cerebri
24  Superior rectus and levator
    palpebrae superioris muscles
25  Eyeball and lacrimal gland
26  Inferior rectus and inferior oblique muscles
27  Zygomatic bone
28  Maxillary sinus
29  Inferior nasal concha
30  Hard palate

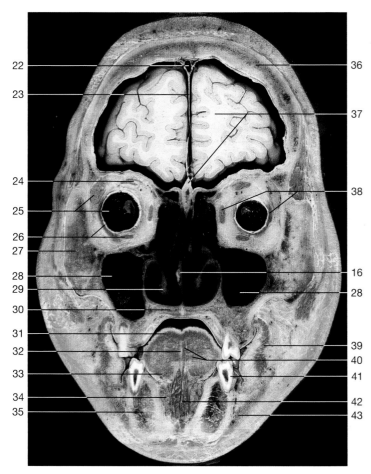

**Coronal section through the head** at the level of the second premolar of the mandible.

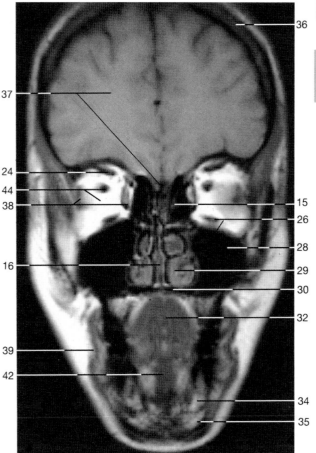

**Coronal section through the head** (MRI scan).
(Prof. Heuck, Munich, Germany.) Note the situation of the head cavities.

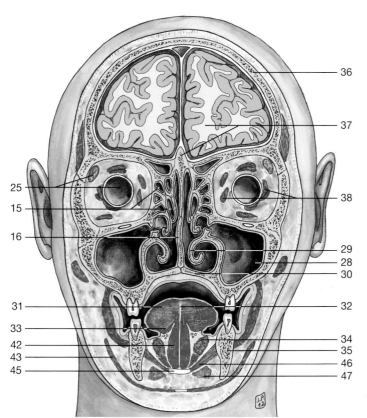

31    Superior longitudinal muscle of tongue
32    Lingual septum
33    Inferior longitudinal muscle of tongue
34    Sublingual gland
35    Mandible
36    Calvaria
37    Frontal lobe of brain and crista galli
38    Lateral and medial rectus muscles
39    Buccinator muscle
40    Vertical and transverse muscles of tongue
41    Second premolar of the mandible
42    Genioglossus muscle
43    Platysma muscle
44    Orbit and optic nerve (n. II)
45    Hyoid bone
46    Mylohyoid muscle
47    Submandibular gland

◁  **Coronal section through the head** at the level of the second premolar of the mandible.

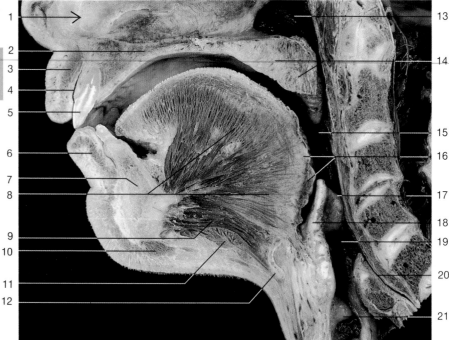

1   Nasal cavity
2   Hard palate
3   Upper lip and
    orbicularis oris muscle
4   Vestibule of oral cavity
5   First incisor
6   Lower lip and
    orbicularis oris muscle
7   Mandible
8   Genioglossus muscle
9   Geniohyoid muscle
10  Anterior belly of diagastric muscle
11  Mylohyoid muscle
12  Hyoid bone
13  Nasopharynx
14  Soft palate and uvula
15  Oropharynx
16  Root of tongue and lingual tonsil
17  Laryngopharynx
18  Epiglottis
19  Ary-epiglottic fold
20  Laryngopharynx
    continuous with esophagus
21  Larynx

**Median sagittal section through the oral cavity and pharynx.**

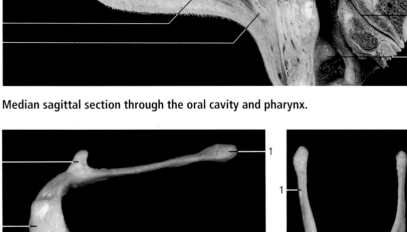

1   Greater cornu ⎤
2   Lesser cornu  ⎬ of hyoid bone
3   Body          ⎦

**Hyoid bone** (oblique-lateral aspect).          **Hyoid bone** (anterior aspect).

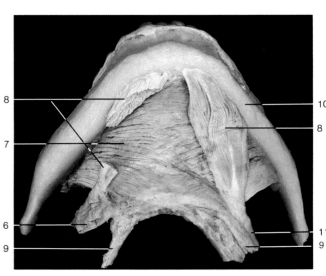

**Muscles of the floor of the oral cavity** (superior aspect).

1   Lesser cornu and body of hyoid bone
2   Hyoglossus muscle (divided)
3   Ramus of mandible and inferior alveolar nerve
4   Geniohyoid muscle
5   Genioglossus muscle (divided)
6   Stylohyoid muscle (divided)

**Muscles of the floor of the oral cavity** (inferior aspect). Cut on the base.

7   Mylohyoid muscle
8   Anterior belly of digastric muscle
9   Hyoid bone
10  Mandible
11  Intermediate tendon of digastric muscle

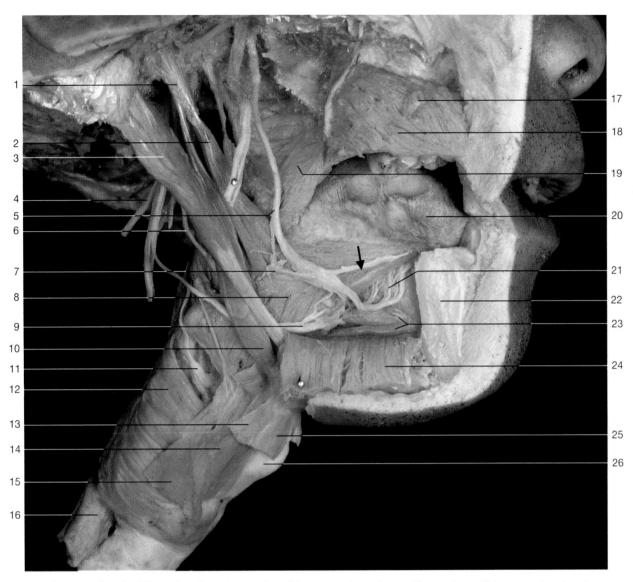

**Parapharyngeal and sublingual regions.** Innervation of the tongue. Lateral part of face and mandible removed, oral cavity opened. Arrow: submandibular duct.

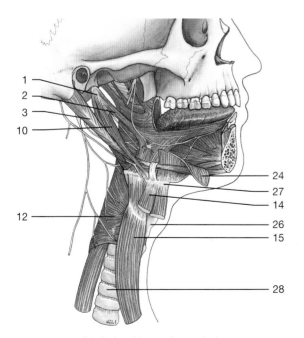

**Supra- and infrahyoid muscles and pharynx.**

| | | | |
|---|---|---|---|
| 1 | Styloid process | 14 | Thyrohyoid muscle |
| 2 | Styloglossus muscle | 15 | Sternothyroid muscle |
| 3 | Posterior belly of digastric muscle | 16 | Esophagus |
| 4 | Vagus nerve (n. X) | 17 | Parotid duct (divided) |
| 5 | Lingual nerve (n. V$_3$) | 18 | Buccinator muscle |
| 6 | Glossopharyngeal nerve (n. IX) | 19 | Superior constrictor muscle of pharynx |
| 7 | Submandibular ganglion | 20 | Tongue |
| 8 | Hyoglossus muscle | 21 | Terminal branches of lingual nerve |
| 9 | Hypoglossal nerve (n. XII) | 22 | Mandible (divided) |
| 10 | Stylohyoid muscle | 23 | Genioglossus and geniohyoid muscles |
| 11 | Internal branch of superior laryngeal nerve (branch of vagus nerve, not visible) | 24 | Mylohyoid muscle (divided and reflected) |
| 12 | Middle constrictor muscle of pharynx | 25 | Sternohyoid muscle (divided) |
| | | 26 | Thyroid cartilage |
| 13 | Omohyoid muscle (divided) | 27 | Hyoid bone |
| | | 28 | Trachea |

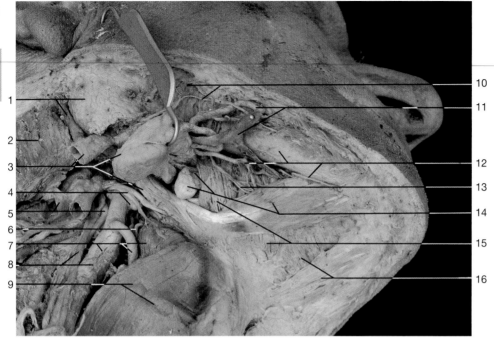

| | |
|---|---|
| 1 | Parotid gland and retromandibular vein |
| 2 | Sternocleidomastoid muscle |
| 3 | Retromandibular vein, submandibular gland, and stylohyoid muscle |
| 4 | Hypoglossal nerve and lingual artery |
| 5 | Vagus nerve and internal jugular vein |
| 6 | Superior laryngeal artery |
| 7 | External carotid artery, thyrohyoid muscle, and superior thyroid artery |
| 8 | Common carotid artery and superior root of ansa cervicalis |
| 9 | Omohyoid and sternohyoid muscles |
| 10 | Masseter muscle and marginal mandibular branch of facial nerve |
| 11 | Facial artery and vein |
| 12 | Mandible and submental artery and vein |
| 13 | Mylohyoid nerve |
| 14 | Submandibular duct, sublingual gland, and anterior belly of digastric muscle |
| 15 | Mylohyoid muscle |
| 16 | Mylohyoid muscle and anterior belly of left digastric muscle |
| 17 | Hyoglossus muscle and lingual artery |
| 18 | Lingual nerve |
| 19 | Hypoglossal nerve |
| 20 | Geniohyoid muscle |
| 21 | Anterior belly of right digastric muscle |
| 22 | Submandibular gland and duct |

**Submandibular triangle,** superficial dissection. Right side (inferior aspect). Submandibular gland has been reflected.

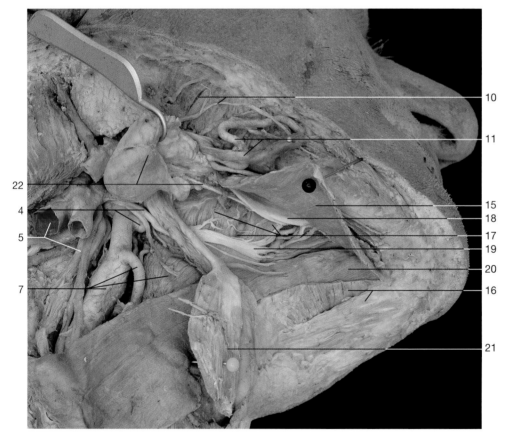

**Submandibular triangle,** deep dissection. Right side (inferior aspect). Mylohyoid muscle has been severed and reflected to display the lingual and hypoglossal nerves.

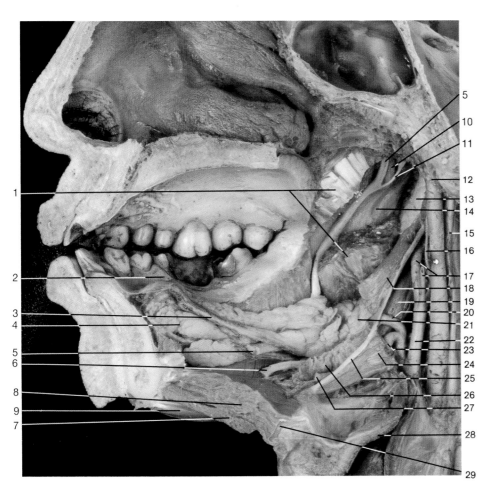

1. Medial pterygoid muscle
2. Sublingual papilla
3. Submandibular duct
4. Sublingual gland
5. Lingual nerve
6. Hypoglossal nerve
7. Mylohyoid muscle
8. Geniohyoid muscle
9. Anterior belly of digastric muscle
10. Inferior alveolar nerve
11. Chorda tympani
12. Internal carotid artery
13. Parotid gland
14. Sphenomandibular ligament
15. Vagus nerve
16. Glossopharyngeal nerve
17. Superficial temporal artery and ascending pharyngeal artery
18. Styloglossus muscle
19. Posterior belly of digastric muscle
20. Facial artery
21. Submandibular gland
22. External carotid artery
23. Lingual artery
24. Middle pharyngeal constrictor muscle
25. Stylohyoid ligament
26. Hyoglossus muscle
27. Deep lingual artery
28. Epiglottis
29. Hyoid bone
30. Buccinator muscle
31. Tongue
32. Mandible (divided)
33. Parotid duct
34. Masseter muscle
35. Right and left sublingual caruncle
36. Left sublingual caruncle

**Oral cavity** (internal aspect). Tongue and pharyngeal wall removed.

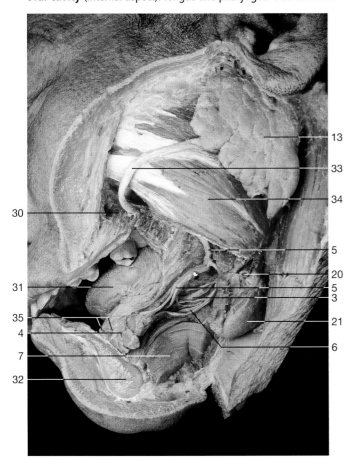

**Dissection of the major salivary glands** (infero-lateral aspect). Left mandible and buccinator muscle partly removed to view the oral cavity.

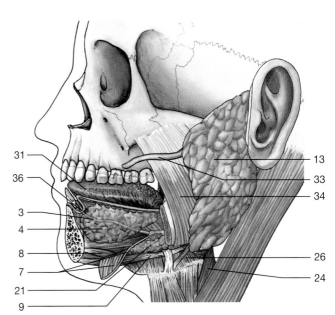

**Location of the major salivary glands** (lateral aspect) in relation to the oral cavity.

# 2.6 Neck and Organs of the Neck

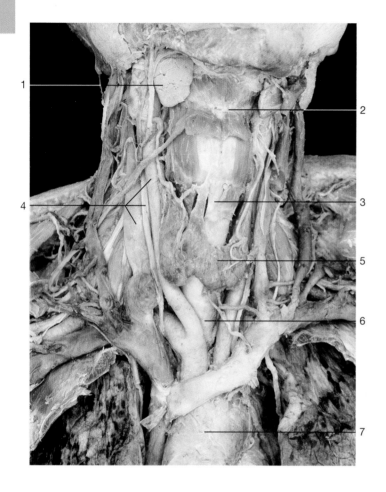

**Regional anatomy of the neck** (anterior aspect). The anteriorly located muscles and the thoracic wall have been removed.

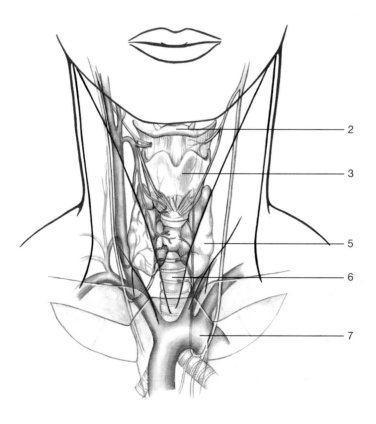

**Organs of the neck** (anterior aspect). The main arterial trunks are indicated in red.

1 Submandibular gland
2 Hyoid bone
3 Larynx (thyroid cartilage)
4 Nerves and vessels of the neck
  (carotid artery, internal jugular vein, and vagus nerve)
5 Thyroid gland
6 Trachea
7 Aortic arch

1   Nasal septum
2   Uvula
3   Genioglossus muscle
4   Mandible
5   Geniohyoid muscle
6   Mylohyoid muscle
7   Hyoid bone
8   Thyroid cartilage
9   Manubrium sterni
10  Sphenoidal sinus
11  Nasopharynx
12  Oropharynx
13  Epiglottis
14  Laryngopharynx
15  Arytenoid muscle
16  Vocal fold
17  Cricoid cartilage
18  Trachea
19  Left brachiocephalic vein
20  Thymus
21  Esophagus

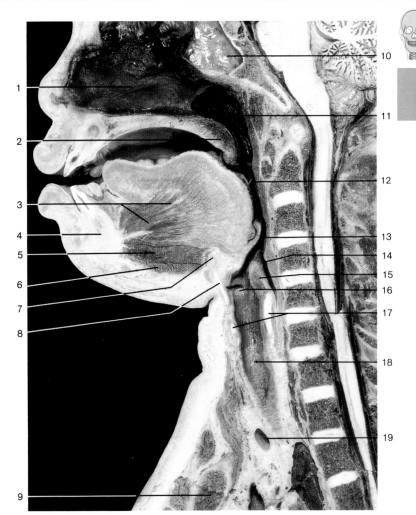

**Median section through adult head and neck.** Note the low position of the adult larynx when compared with that of the neonate (compare with the dissection below).

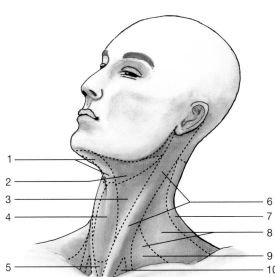

**Regions and triangles of the neck**
(oblique-lateral aspect).

1   Submental triangle ⎫
2   Submandibular triangle ⎬ Anterior cervical region
3   Carotid triangle ⎪
4   Muscular triangle ⎭
5   Jugular fossa
6   Sternocleidomastoid region
7   Posterior cervical region
8   Lateral cervical region
9   Greater supraclavicular fossa (supraclavicular triangle)
10  Lesser supraclavicular fossa

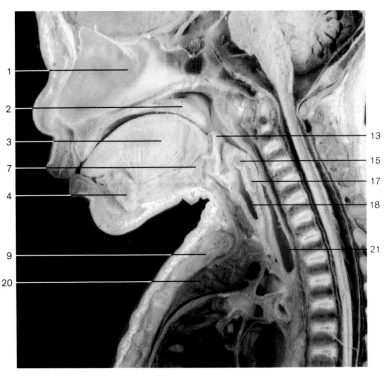

**Median section through neonate head and neck.** Note the high position of the larynx permitting the epiglottis to nearly reach the uvula (compare with the dissection above).

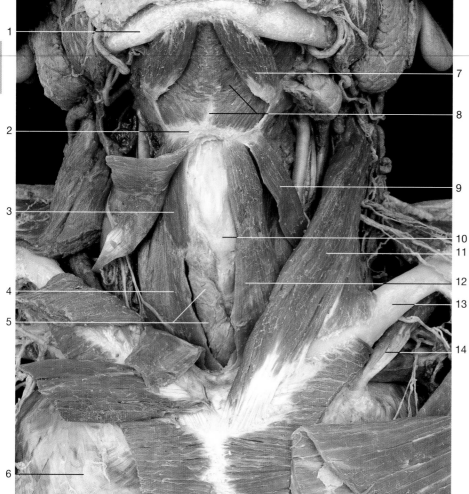

| | |
|---|---|
| 1 | Mandible |
| 2 | Hyoid bone |
| 3 | Thyrohyoid muscle |
| 4 | Sternothyroid muscle |
| 5 | Thyroid gland |
| 6 | Second rib |
| 7 | Anterior belly of digastric muscle |
| 8 | Mylohyoid muscle (and mylohyoid raphe) |
| 9 | Omohyoid muscle |
| 10 | Thyroid cartilage |
| 11 | Sternocleidomastoid muscle |
| 12 | Sternohyoid muscle |
| 13 | Clavicle |
| 14 | Subclavius muscle |
| 15 | Posterior belly of digastric muscle |
| 16 | Stylohyoid muscle |
| 17 | Scalene muscles |
| 18 | Trapezius muscle |
| 19 | First rib |
| 20 | Scapula |
| 21 | Trachea |
| 22 | Manubrium sterni |

**Muscles of the neck** (anterior aspect). Sternocleidomastoid and sternohyoid muscles on the right have been divided and reflected.

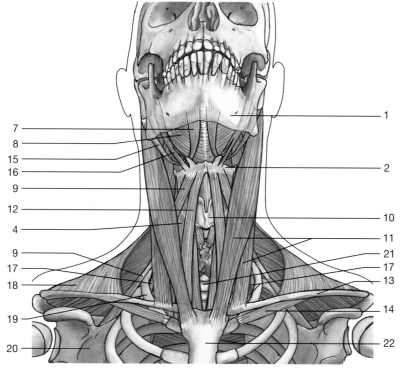

**Muscles of the neck** (anterior aspect).

The muscles of the neck are complex and highly sophisticated. There are two major groups of muscles to be distinguished according to their functional aspects. One group is constituted by muscles connecting head to the hyoid bone and the larynx. The second category of muscles links the head and the ribcage.

The sternocleidomastoid muscle represents the border between the anterior and posterior cervical triangle.

1   Sternohyoid and thyrohyoid
    muscles
2   Larynx
3   Cricoid cartilage
4   Internal jugular vein,
    common carotid artery, and
    vagus nerve
5   Esophagus
6   Body of cervical vertebra
7   Vertebral artery
8   Spinal cord
9   Posterior scalene muscle
10  Deep muscles of the neck
11  Trapezius muscle
12  Omohyoid muscle
13  Thyroid gland
14  Sternocleidomastoid muscle
15  Sympathetic trunk
16  Longus colli muscle
17  Anterior scalene muscle
18  Longissimus capitis muscle
19  Middle scalene muscle
20  Ventral and dorsal root
    of cervical spinal nerve
21  Trachea
22  Vertebral artery and vein,
    and foramen transversarium
23  Cervical spinal nerve
24  Superior facet of articular process
25  Spinous process
26  Sternohyoid and sternothyroid
    muscles

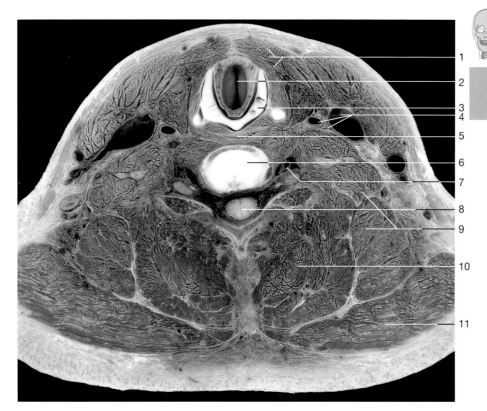

**Axial section through the neck** at the level of the intervertebral disc between the fifth and sixth cervical vertebrae (inferior aspect).

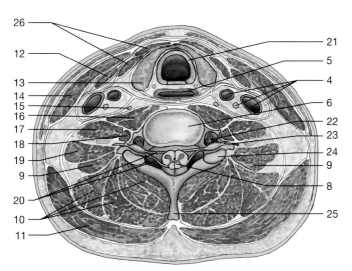

**Organization of the neck** (axial section at the level of the thyroid gland).

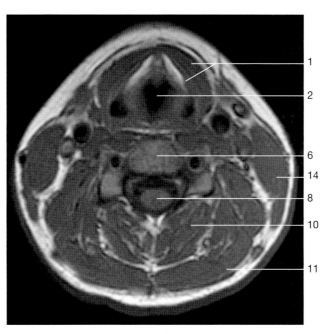

**Axial section through the neck** at the level of the fourth cervical vertebra (MRI scan). (From Heuck et al., MRT-Atlas, 2009.)

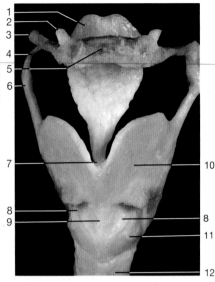

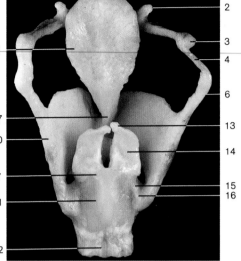

1 Epiglottis
2 Lesser cornu of hyoid bone
3 Greater cornu of hyoid bone
4 Lateral thyrohyoid ligament
5 Body of hyoid bone
6 Superior cornu
   of thyroid cartilage
7 Thyro-epiglottic ligament
8 Conus elasticus
9 Cricothyroid ligament
10 Thyroid cartilage
11 Cricoid cartilage
12 Trachea
13 Corniculate cartilage
14 Arytenoid cartilage
15 Posterior crico-arytenoid
    ligament
16 Cricothyroid joint
17 Crico-arytenoid joint

**Cartilages of the larynx and the hyoid bone** (anterior aspect).

**Cartilages of the larynx and the hyoid bone** (posterior aspect).

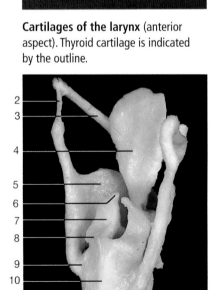

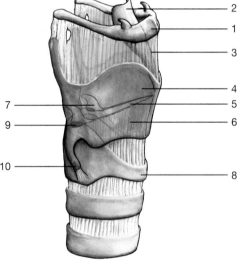

1 Hyoid bone
2 Epiglottis
3 Thyrohyoid membrane
4 Thyroid cartilage
5 Vocal ligament
6 Conus elasticus
7 Arytenoid cartilage
8 Cricoid cartilage
9 Crico-arytenoid joint
10 Cricothyroid joint
11 Tracheal cartilages
12 Corniculate cartilage
13 Muscular process
   of arytenoid cartilage
14 Vocal process
   of arytenoid cartilage
15 Lamina of cricoid cartilage
16 Arch of cricoid cartilage

**Cartilages of the larynx** (anterior aspect). Thyroid cartilage is indicated by the outline.

**Cartilages and ligaments of the larynx** (lateral aspect).

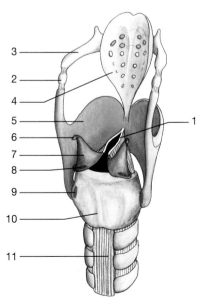

1 Vocal ligament
2 Lateral thyrohyoid ligament
3 Greater cornu of hyoid bone
4 Epiglottis
5 Thyroid cartilage
6 Corniculate cartilage
7 Arytenoid cartilage
8 Crico-arytenoid joint
9 Cricothyroid joint
10 Cricoid cartilage
11 Trachea

**Cartilages of the larynx** (oblique-posterior aspect).

**Cartilages of the larynx** (oblique-posterior aspect).

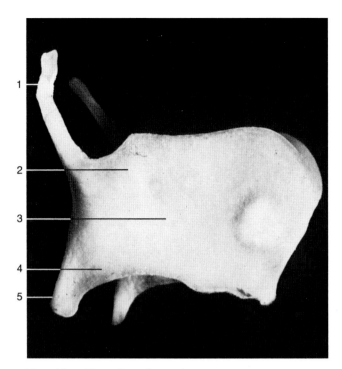

**Thyroid cartilage** (lateral aspect).

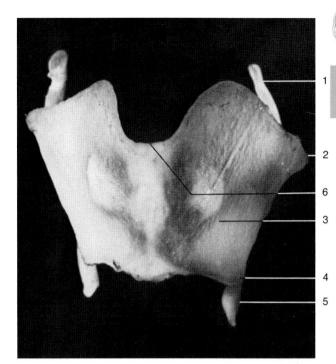

**Thyroid cartilage** (anterior aspect).

| | | | |
|---|---|---|---|
| 1 | Superior cornu | 4 | Inferior thyroid tubercle |
| 2 | Superior thyroid tubercle | 5 | Inferior cornu |
| 3 | Lamina of thyroid cartilage | 6 | Superior thyroid notch |

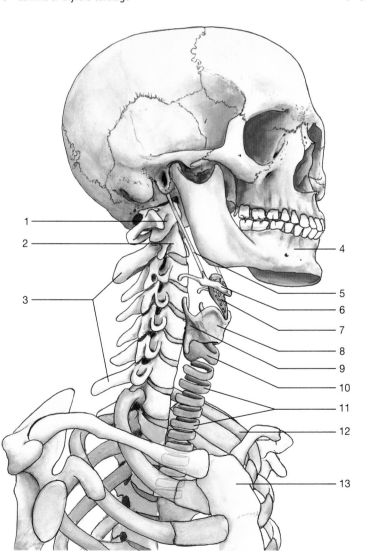

1  Atlas
2  Axis
3  Cervical vertebrae II–VII
4  Mandible
5  Stylohyoid ligament
6  Hyoid bone
7  Epiglottis
8  Thyroid cartilage
9  Arytenoid cartilage
10 Cricoid cartilage
11 Tracheal cartilages
12 First rib
13 Manubrium of sternum

**Position of the larynx and hyoid bone** in the neck (oblique-lateral aspect).

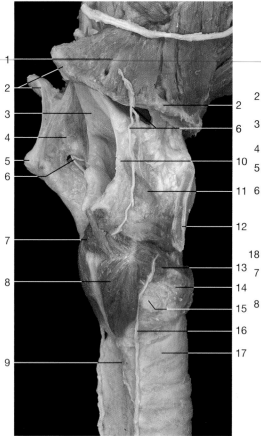

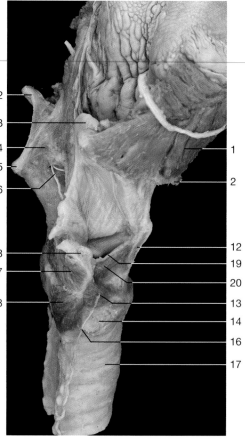

1   Hyoglossus muscle
2   Hyoid bone
3   Epiglottis
4   Thyrohyoid membrane
5   Superior cornu
    of thyroid cartilage
6   Superior laryngeal nerve
7   Transverse arytenoid
    muscle
8   Posterior crico-arytenoid
    muscle
9   Transverse muscle
    of trachea
10  Ary-epiglottic fold
11  Thyro-epiglottic muscle
12  Thyroid cartilage
13  Lateral crico-arytenoid
    muscle
14  Cricoid cartilage
15  Articular facet
    for thyroid cartilage
16  Inferior laryngeal nerve
    (branch of recurrent nerve)
17  Trachea
18  Arytenoid cartilage
19  Vocal ligament
20  Vocalis muscle (part of
    thyro-arytenoid muscle)
21  Thyrohyoideus muscle
22  Cricothyroideus muscle
23  Root of tongue
24  Cuneiform tubercle
25  Corniculate tubercle
26  Ary-epiglottic muscle

**Laryngeal muscles** (lateral aspect).
Thyroid cartilage and thyro-arytenoid muscle
have been partly removed.

**Laryngeal muscles** (lateral aspect).
Half of the thyroid cartilage has been removed.
Dissection of the vocal ligament.

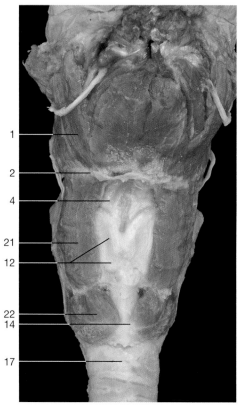

**Laryngeal muscles and larynx**
(anterior aspect).

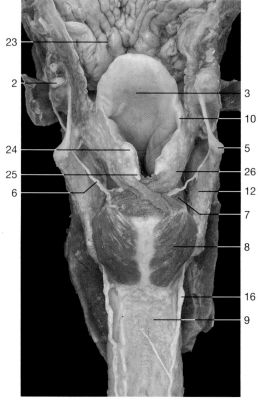

**Laryngeal muscles and larynx**
(posterior aspect).

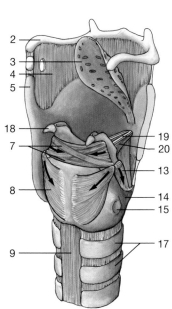

**Action of internal muscles
of the larynx.**

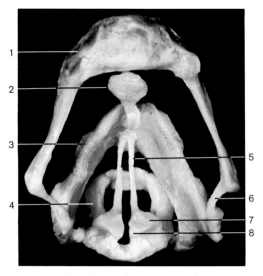

**Laryngeal cartilages** (superior aspect).

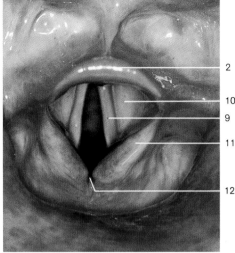

**Glottis in vivo** (superior aspect).

1 Hyoid bone
2 Epiglottis
3 Thyroid cartilage
4 Cricoid cartilage
5 Vocal ligament
6 Thyrohyoid ligament
7 Arytenoid cartilage
8 Corniculate cartilage
9 Vocal fold
10 Vestibular fold
11 Ary-epiglottic fold
12 Interarytenoid notch
13 Mandible
14 Anterior belly
    of digastric muscle
15 Mylohyoid muscle
16 Pyramidal lobe
    of thyroid gland
17 Sternohyoid and
    sternothyroid muscles
18 Common carotid artery
19 Internal jugular vein
20 Rima glottidis
21 Sternocleidomastoid
    muscle
22 Transverse arytenoid
    muscle
23 Pharynx and inferior
    constrictor muscle
24 Ventricle of larynx
25 Vocalis muscle
26 Trachea
27 Superior cornu
    of thyroid cartilage
28 Root of tongue
    (lingual tonsil)
29 Piriform recess
30 Vocalis muscle
31 Lateral crico-arytenoid
    muscle
32 Thyroid gland

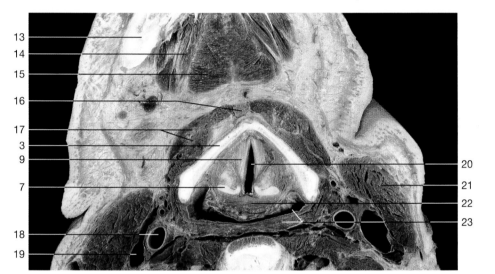

**Horizontal section through the larynx** at the level of the vocal folds (superior aspect).

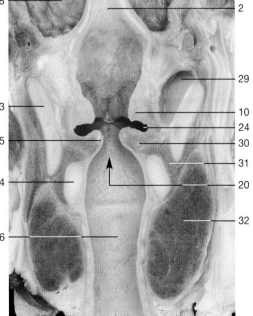

**Sagittal section through larynx and trachea.**

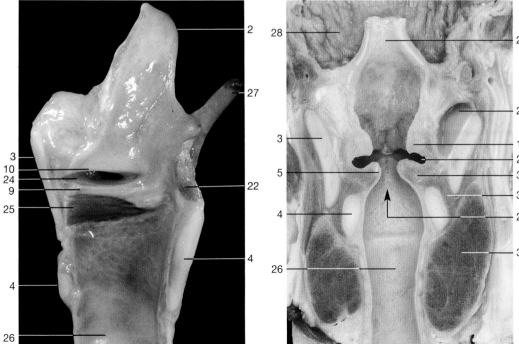

**Coronal section through larynx and trachea.**

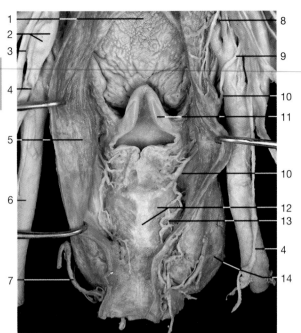

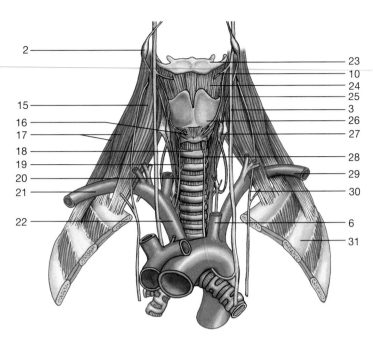

**Innervation of the larynx** (posterior aspect).
Dissection of superior and inferior laryngeal nerves.
Pharynx has been opened.

**Innervation of the larynx** (anterior aspect).

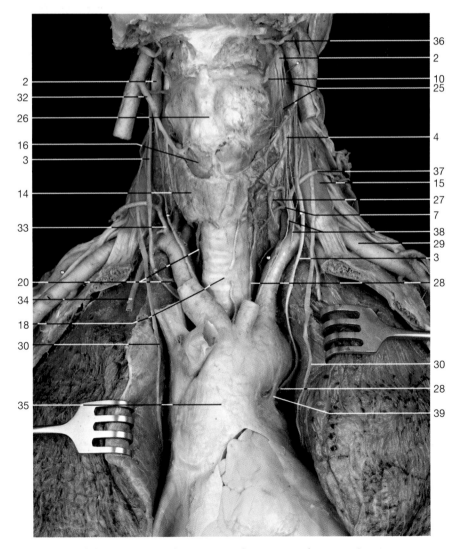

**Larynx and thoracic organs** (anterior aspect). Dissection of vagus and recurrent laryngeal nerves.

1   Tongue
2   Superior cervical ganglion
3   Vagus nerve (n. X)
4   Sympathetic trunk
5   Inferior constrictor muscle of pharynx
6   Left common carotid artery
7   Inferior thyroid artery
8   Glossopharyngeal nerve (n. IX)
9   Superior laryngeal nerve
10  Internal branch of superior laryngeal nerve
11  Epiglottis
12  Posterior crico-arytenoid muscle and
    cricoid cartilage
13  Recurrent laryngeal nerve
14  Thyroid gland
15  Anterior scalene muscle
16  Cricothyroid muscle
17  Middle and posterior scalene muscles
18  Trachea
19  Longus capitis muscle
20  Right recurrent laryngeal nerve
21  Right subclavian artery
22  Brachiocephalic trunk
23  Hyoid bone
24  Thyrohyoid membrane
25  External branch of superior laryngeal nerve
26  Thyroid cartilage
27  Middle cervical ganglion
28  Left recurrent laryngeal nerve
29  Left subclavian artery
30  Phrenic nerve
31  Second rib
32  Superior thyroid artery
33  Thyrocervical trunk
34  Internal thoracic artery
35  Aortic arch
36  Hypoglossal nerve (n. XII)
37  Transverse cervical artery
38  Inferior cervical cardiac nerves
    (branches of sympathetic trunk)
39  Ligamentum arteriosum

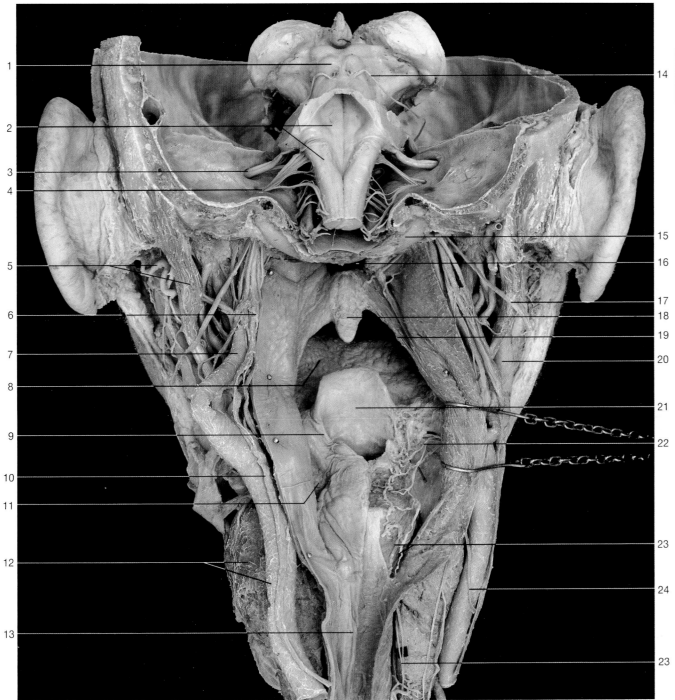

**Larynx and oral cavity** (posterior aspect). Mucous membrane on the right half of pharynx has been removed.

| | | |
|---|---|---|
| 1 Midbrain (inferior colliculus) | 9 Ary-epiglottic fold | 18 Uvula and soft palate |
| 2 Rhomboid fossa and medulla oblongata | 10 Vagus nerve | 19 Palatopharyngeus muscle |
| 3 Vestibulocochlear and facial nerve | 11 Piriform recess | 20 External carotid artery |
| 4 Glossopharyngeal, vagus, and accessory nerves | 12 Thyroid gland and common carotid artery | 21 Epiglottis |
| 5 Occipital artery and posterior belly of digastric muscle | 13 Esophagus | 22 Internal branch of superior laryngeal nerve |
| 6 Superior cervical ganglion | 14 Trochlear nerve | 23 Inferior laryngeal nerve |
| 7 Internal carotid artery | 15 Occipital condyle | 24 Ansa cervicalis |
| 8 Oral cavity (tongue) | 16 Nasal cavity (choana) | |
| | 17 Accessory nerve | |

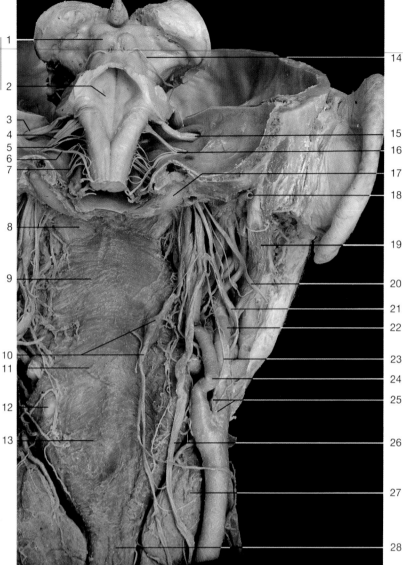

1  Inferior colliculus of midbrain
2  Facial colliculus in floor of rhomboid fossa
3  Vestibulocochlear and facial nerves
4  Glossopharyngeal nerve
5  Vagus nerve
6  Accessory nerve
7  Hypoglossal nerve
8  Pharyngobasilar fascia
9  Superior constrictor muscle of pharynx
10 Sympathetic trunk and superior cervical ganglion (medially displaced)
11 Middle constrictor muscle of pharynx
12 Greater cornu of hyoid bone
13 Inferior constrictor muscle of pharynx
14 Trochlear nerve
15 Internal acoustic meatus with facial and vestibulocochlear nerves
16 Jugular foramen with glossopharyngeal, vagus, and assessory nerves
17 Occipital condyle
18 Occipital artery
19 Posterior belly of digastric muscle
20 Accessory nerve (extracranial part)
21 Hypoglossal nerve (extracranial part)
22 External carotid artery
23 Carotid sinus nerve
24 Internal carotid artery
25 Carotid sinus and carotid body
26 Vagus nerve
27 Thyroid gland
28 Esophagus
29 Choanae
30 Medial pterygoid plate
31 Foramen lacerum
32 Pharyngeal tubercle
33 Hard palate
34 Greater and lesser palatine foramen
35 Pterygoid hamulus
36 Lateral pterygoid plate
37 Foramen ovale
38 Mandibular fossa
39 Carotid canal
40 Styloid process and stylomastoid foramen
41 Jugular foramen

**Pharynx and parapharyngeal nerves in connection with the brain stem** (posterior aspect).

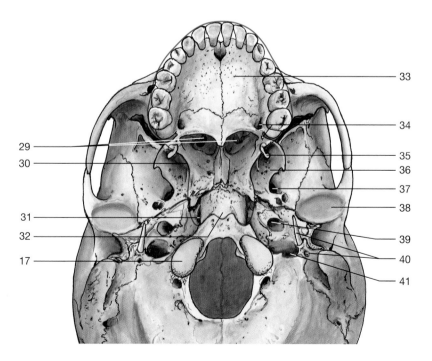

**Base of the skull** (inferior aspect).
Red line = outline of superior constrictor muscle in continuation with buccinator and orbicularis oris muscles.

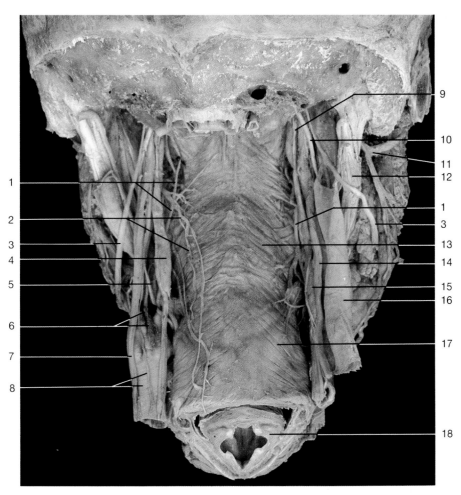

| | |
|---|---|
| 1 | Ascending pharyngeal artery |
| 2 | Pharyngeal plexus |
| 3 | Accessory nerve |
| 4 | Superior cervical ganglion of sympathetic trunk |
| 5 | Superior laryngeal nerve |
| 6 | Carotid body and carotid sinus nerve |
| 7 | Left vagus nerve |
| 8 | Common carotid artery and cardiac branch of vagus nerve |
| 9 | Glossopharyngeal nerve |
| 10 | Hypoglossal nerve |
| 11 | Facial nerve |
| 12 | Posterior belly of digastric muscle |
| 13 | Middle constrictor muscle of pharynx |
| 14 | Right vagus nerve |
| 15 | Sympathetic trunk |
| 16 | Internal jugular vein |
| 17 | Inferior constrictor muscle of pharynx |
| 18 | Larynx |
| 19 | Buccinator muscle |
| 20 | Soft palate and palatine glands |
| 21 | Palatine tonsil |
| 22 | Uvula of palate |
| 23 | Pharynx (oral part) |
| 24 | Parotid gland |
| 25 | Longus capitis muscle |
| 26 | Median atlanto-axial joint and anterior arch of atlas |
| 27 | Dens of axis |
| 28 | Spinal cord |
| 29 | Dura mater |
| 30 | Incisive papilla |
| 31 | Oral vestibule |
| 32 | Masseter muscle |
| 33 | Mandible |
| 34 | Mandibular canal with vessels and nerve |
| 35 | Medial pterygoid muscle |
| 36 | External carotid artery |
| 37 | Internal carotid artery |
| 38 | Atlas |
| 39 | Vertebral artery |
| 40 | Splenius capitis muscle |
| 41 | Semispinalis capitis muscle |

**Pharynx with parapharyngeal nerves and vessels** (posterior aspect).

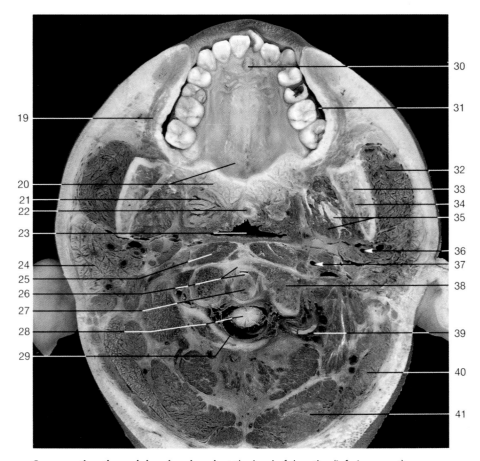

**Cross section through head and neck** at the level of the atlas (inferior aspect).

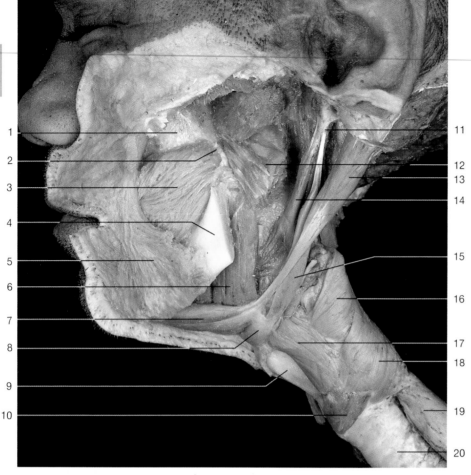

| | |
|---|---|
| 1 | Maxilla |
| 2 | Pterygomandibular raphe |
| 3 | Buccinator muscle |
| 4 | Mandible (divided) |
| 5 | Depressor anguli oris muscle |
| 6 | Mylohyoid muscle |
| 7 | Anterior belly of digastric muscle |
| 8 | Hyoid bone |
| 9 | Thyroid cartilage |
| 10 | Cricothyroid muscle |
| 11 | Styloid process |
| 12 | Medial pterygoid muscle (divided) |
| 13 | Posterior belly of digastric muscle |
| 14 | Styloglossus muscle |
| 15 | Stylohyoid muscle |
| 16 | Thyropharyngeal part of inferior constrictor muscle of pharynx |
| 17 | Thyrohyoid muscle |
| 18 | Cricopharyngeal part of inferior constrictor muscle of pharynx |
| 19 | Esophagus |
| 20 | Trachea |
| 21 | First molar of maxilla |
| 22 | Tongue |
| 23 | Inferior longitudinal muscle of tongue |
| 24 | Genioglossus muscle |
| 25 | Superior constrictor muscle of pharynx |
| 26 | Hypoglossal nerve |
| 27 | Hyoglossus muscle |
| 28 | Superior laryngeal nerve and superior laryngeal artery |

**Dissection of pharynx, supra-, and infrahyoid muscles** (lateral aspect). Mandible partly removed.

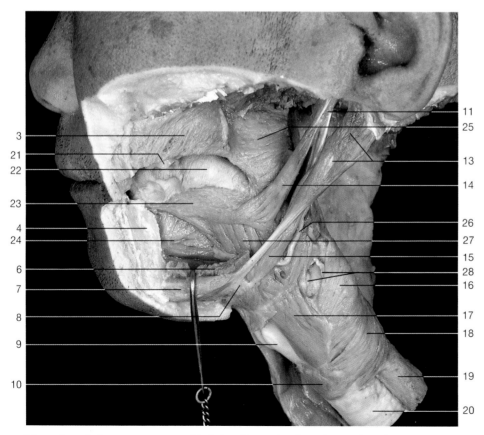

**Dissection of pharynx, supra-, and infrahyoid muscles** (lateral aspect). Oral cavity opened.

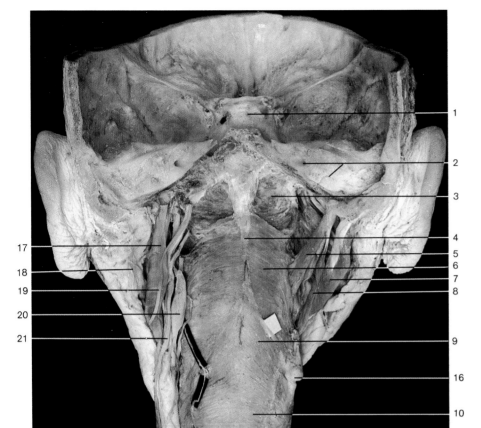

1 Sella turcica
2 Internal acoustic meatus and petrous part of temporal bone
3 Pharyngobasilar fascia
4 Fibrous raphe of pharynx
5 Stylopharyngeal muscle
6 Superior constrictor muscle of pharynx
7 Posterior belly of digastric muscle
8 Stylohyoid muscle
9 Middle constrictor muscle of pharynx
10 Inferior constrictor muscle of pharynx
11 Muscle-free area (Killian's triangle)
12 Esophagus
13 Trachea
14 Thyroid and parathyroid glands
15 Medial pterygoid muscle
16 Greater horn of hyoid bone
17 Internal jugular vein
18 Parotid gland
19 Accessory nerve
20 Superior cervical ganglion of sympathetic trunk
21 Vagus nerve
22 Laimer's triangle (area prone to developing diverticula)
23 Orbicularis oculi muscle
24 Nasalis muscle
25 Levator labii superioris and levator labii alaeque nasi muscles
26 Levator anguli oris muscle
27 Orbicularis oris muscle
28 Buccinator muscle
29 Depressor labii inferioris muscle
30 Hyoglossus muscle
31 Thyrohyoid muscle
32 Thyroid cartilage
33 Cricothyroid muscle
34 Pterygomandibular raphe
35 Tensor veli palatini muscle
36 Levator veli palatini muscle
37 Depressor anguli oris muscle
38 Mentalis muscle
39 Styloglossus muscle

**Muscles of the pharynx** (posterior aspect).

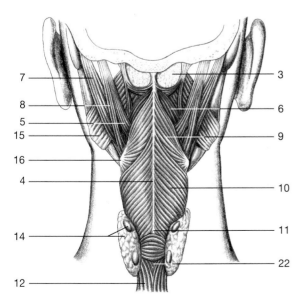

**Muscles of the pharynx** (posterior aspect).

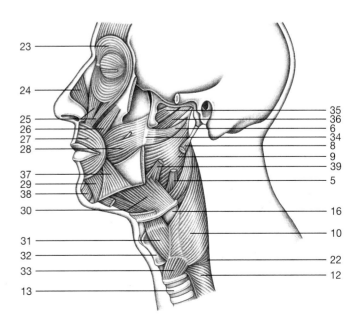

**Muscles of the pharynx** (lateral aspect).

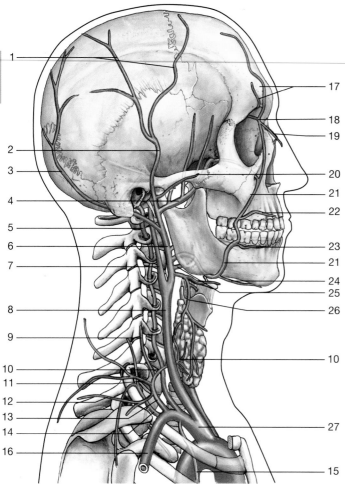

1 Frontal and parietal branches
  of superficial temporal artery
2 Superficial temporal artery
3 Occipital artery
4 Maxillary artery
5 Vertebral artery
6 External carotid artery
7 Internal carotid artery
8 Common carotid artery (divided)
9 Ascending cervical artery
10 Inferior thyroid artery
11 Transverse cervical artery with two branches
   (superficial cervical artery and
   descending scapular artery)
12 Suprascapular artery
13 Thyrocervical trunk
14 Costocervical trunk with two branches
   (deep cervical artery and supreme intercostal artery)
15 Internal thoracic artery
16 Axillary artery
17 Supra-orbital and supratrochlear arteries
18 Angular artery
19 Dorsal nasal artery
20 Transverse facial artery
21 Facial artery
22 Superior labial artery
23 Inferior labial artery
24 Submental artery
25 Lingual artery
26 Superior thyroid artery
27 Brachiocephalic trunk

**Arteries of head and neck** (lateral aspect). Diagram of the main
branches of external carotid and subclavian arteries.

▷ **To page 171:**

1 Galea aponeurotica
2 Frontal branch ⎤ of superficial
3 Parietal branch ⎦ temporal artery
4 Superior auricular muscle
5 Superficial temporal artery and vein
6 Middle temporal artery
7 Auriculotemporal nerve
8 Branches of facial nerve
9 Facial nerve
10 External carotid artery
   within the retromandibular fossa
11 Posterior belly of digastric muscle
12 Sternocleidomastoid artery
13 Sympathetic trunk and superior cervical ganglion
14 Sternocleidomastoid muscle (divided and reflected)
15 Clavicle (divided)
16 Transverse cervical artery
17 Ascending cervical artery and phrenic nerve
18 Anterior scalene muscle
19 Suprascapular artery

20 Dorsal scapular artery
21 Brachial plexus and axillary artery
22 Thoraco-acromial artery
23 Lateral thoracic artery
24 Median nerve (displaced) and
   pectoralis minor muscle (reflected)
25 Frontal belly of occipitofrontalis muscle
26 Orbital part of orbicularis oculi muscle
27 Angular artery and vein
28 Facial artery
29 Superior labial artery
30 Zygomaticus major muscle
31 Inferior labial artery
32 Parotid duct
33 Buccal fat pad
34 Maxillary artery
35 Masseter muscle
36 Facial artery and mandible
37 Submental artery
38 Anterior belly of digastric muscle

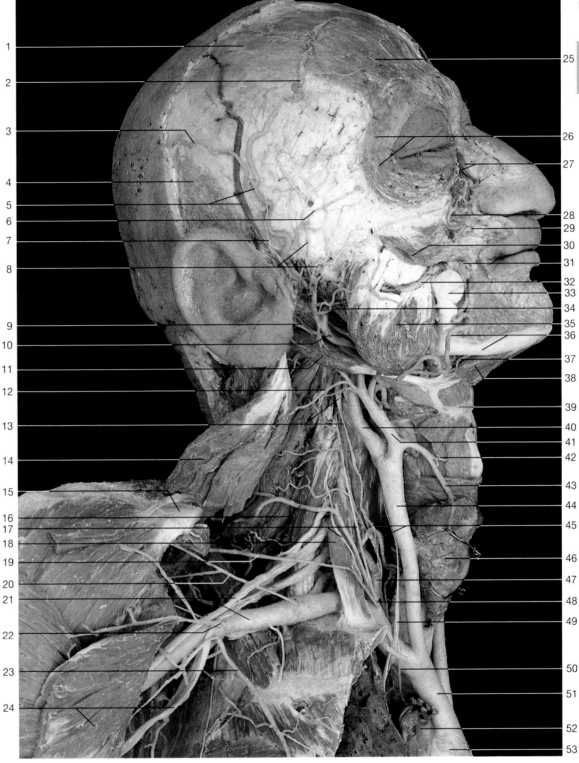

**Main branches of head and neck arteries** (lateral aspect). Anterior thoracic wall and clavicle partly removed; pectoralis muscles have been reflected to display the subclavian and axillary arteries.

39 Hyoid bone
40 Internal carotid artery
41 External carotid artery
42 Superior laryngeal artery
43 Superior thyroid artery
44 Common carotid artery
45 Thyroid ansa of sympathetic trunk and inferior thyroid artery

46 Thyroid gland (right lobe)
47 Vertebral artery
48 Thyrocervical trunk
49 Vagus nerve
50 Ansa subclavia of sympathetic trunk
51 Brachiocephalic trunk
52 Superior vena cava (divided)
53 Aortic arch

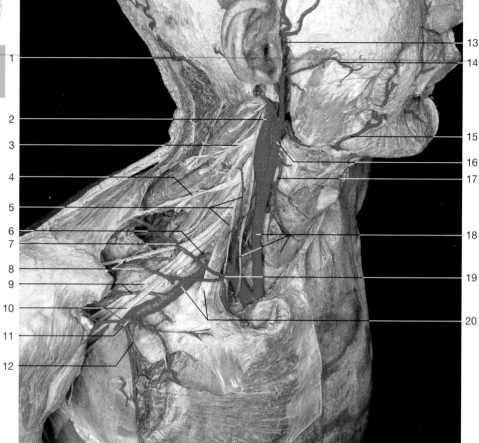

1   Occipital branch of occipital artery
2   Internal carotid artery
3   Cervical plexus
4   Supraclavicular nerve
5   Phrenic nerve and
     ascending cervical artery
     on anterior scalene muscle
6   Transverse cervical artery
7   Superficial cervical artery
8   Suprascapular artery and nerve
9   Brachial plexus and
     transverse cervical artery
10  Lateral cord of brachial plexus
11  Thoraco-acromial artery
12  Lateral thoracic artery
13  Superficial temporal artery
14  Transverse facial artery
15  Facial artery
16  External carotid artery
17  Superior thyroid artery
18  Common carotid artery,
     vagus nerve, and thyroid gland
19  Thyrocervical trunk
20  Subclavian artery and
     anterior scalene muscle
21  Occipital vein
22  Superficial temporal vein
23  Sternocleidomastoid muscle
24  Trapezius muscle
25  Internal jugular vein
26  External jugular vein
27  Subclavian vein
28  Cephalic vein
29  Axillary vein and artery
30  Supra-orbital veins
31  Angular vein
32  Superior labial vein
33  Inferior labial vein
34  Facial vein
35  Submental vein
36  Superior thyroid vein
37  Anterior jugular vein
38  Thoracic duct
39  Inferior thyroid vein
40  Superior vena cava
41  Parotid gland and facial nerve
42  Great auricular nerve
43  External jugular vein
44  Brachial plexus
45  Cephalic vein
     within the deltopectoral triangle
46  Right brachiocephalic vein
47  Superior vena cava
48  Right lung (reflected)
49  Superficial temporal artery and vein
50  Facial artery and vein
51  Cervical branch of facial nerve and
     submandibular gland
52  Internal jugular vein,
     common carotid artery, and
     omohyoid muscle
53  Anterior jugular vein and
     thyroid gland
54  Jugular venous arch
55  Left brachiocephalic vein
56  Pericardium of heart
     (location of right atrium)

**Arteries of head and neck** (antero-lateral aspect). Clavicle, sternocleidomastoid muscle, and veins have been partly removed. Arteries have been colored red.

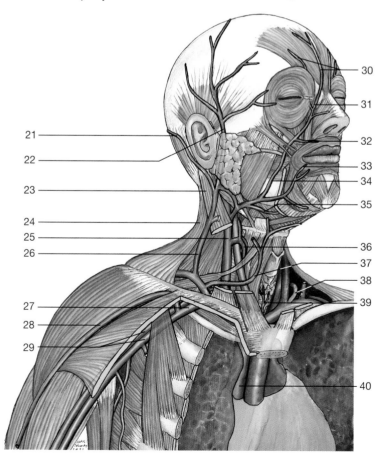

**Veins of head, neck, and shoulder** (anterior aspect). Sternocleidomastoid muscle and anterior thoracic wall partly removed. Note the venous connection with the superior vena cava.

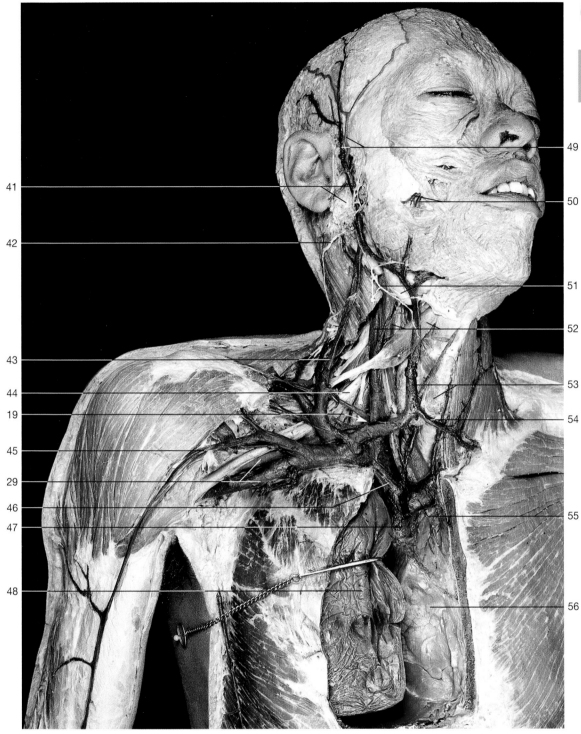

**Veins of head, neck, and shoulder** (anterior aspect). Part of the thoracic wall, clavicle, and sternocleidomastoid muscle have been removed. Veins have been colored blue; arteries have been colored red.

The **internal jugular vein** is the continuation of the sigmoid sinus, which drains most of the venous blood from the brain together with the external cerebrospinal fluid. By joining the subclavian vein, it forms the right brachiocephalic vein, which continues on the right side directly into the superior vena cava. The common way to introduce the lead from a pacemaker device into the heart is by way of the cephalic vein. On the left side, the thoracic duct joins the internal jugular vein at the point where the subclavian vein and the internal jugular vein form the left brachiocephalic vein. Note that the subclavian vein lies in front of the anterior scalene muscle, whereas the subclavian artery and the brachial plexus lie posterior to that muscle. The **cephalic vein** joins the axillary vein by passing into the deltopectoral triangle. **The subclavian vein** is strongly fixed to the first rib, so it can be punctured with a needle at that point (underneath the sternal end of the clavicle) to introduce a catheter (subclavian line).

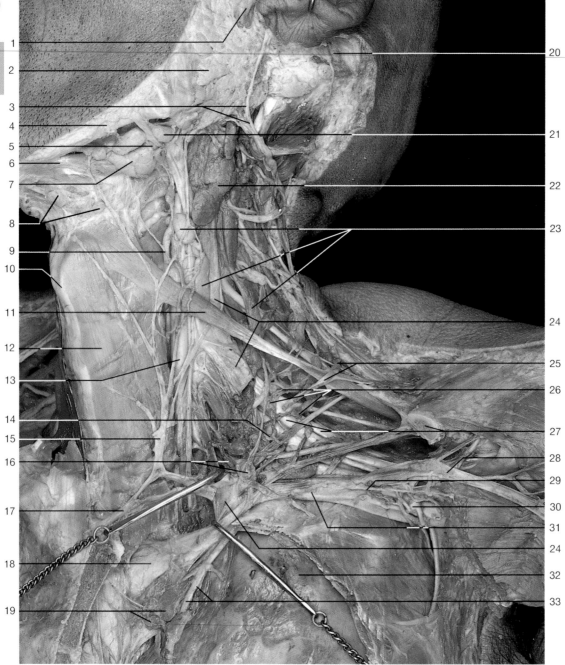

**Lymph nodes and lymph vessels of the neck,** left side (oblique-lateral aspect). The sternocleidomastoid muscle and the left half of the thoracic wall have been removed. Lower part of the internal jugular vein has been cut and laterally displaced to show the thoracic duct.

| | | |
|---|---|---|
| 1 Superficial parotid lymph node | 13 Common carotid artery | 24 Internal jugular vein |
| 2 Parotid gland | 14 Supraclavicular lymph nodes | 25 External jugular vein |
| 3 Great auricular nerve | 15 Anterior jugular vein | 26 Jugulo-omohyoid lymph nodes |
| 4 Mandible | 16 Thoracic duct and internal jugular vein | 27 Brachial plexus |
| 5 Facial vein | 17 Jugular venous arch | 28 Cephalic vein |
| 6 Anterior belly of digastric muscle | 18 Left brachiocephalic vein | 29 Subclavian trunk |
| 7 Submandibular gland | 19 Superior mediastinal lymph nodes | 30 Infraclavicular lymph nodes |
| 8 Submental lymph nodes | 20 Retro-auricular lymph nodes | 31 Subclavian vein |
| 9 Superior thyroid artery | 21 Submandibular nodes | 32 Lung |
| 10 Thyroid cartilage | 22 Superficial cervical lymph nodes | 33 Internal thoracic artery and vein |
| 11 Omohyoid muscle | 23 Jugulodigastric lymph nodes and jugular trunk | |
| 12 Sternohyoid muscle | | |

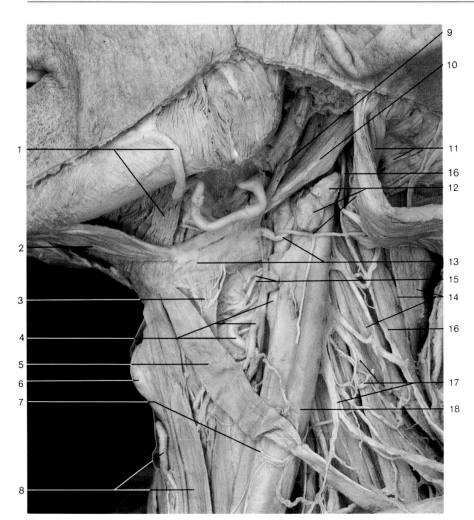

**Carotid triangle**, left side (lateral aspect). Sternocleidomastoid muscle reflected.

1  Mylohyoid muscle and facial artery
2  Anterior belly of digastric muscle
3  Thyrohyoid muscle
4  External carotid artery,
   superior thyroid artery, and vein
5  Omohyoid muscle
6  Thyroid cartilage
7  Ansa cervicalis
8  Sternohyoid muscle and
   superior thyroid artery
9  Stylohyoid muscle
10 Posterior belly of digastric muscle
11 Sternocleidomastoid muscle (reflected)
12 Superior cervical lymph nodes and
   sternocleidomastoid artery
13 Hyoid bone and hypoglossal nerve (n. XII)
14 Splenius capitis and
   levator scapulae muscles
15 Superior laryngeal artery and
   internal branch of
   superior laryngeal nerve
16 Accessory nerve
17 Cervical plexus
18 Internal jugular vein
19 Facial vein
20 Submandibular lymph nodes
21 Submental lymph nodes
22 Thoracic duct
23 Retro-auricular lymph nodes
24 Occipital lymph nodes
25 Parotid lymph nodes
26 Jugulodigastric lymph node
27 Deep cervical lymph nodes
28 External jugular vein
29 Jugulo-omohyoid lymph node
30 Jugular trunk
31 Subclavian trunk
32 Infraclavicular lymph nodes

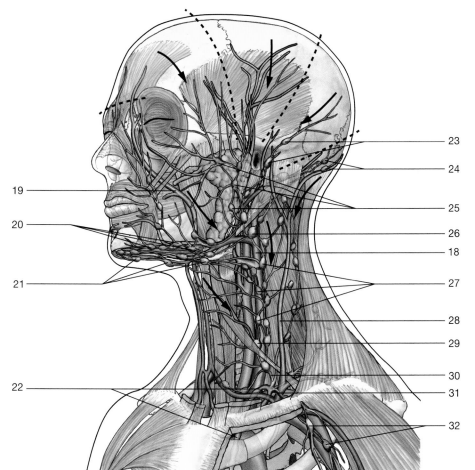

**Lymph nodes and veins of head and neck** (oblique-lateral aspect). Dotted lines = border between irrigation areas; arrows: direction of lymph flow.

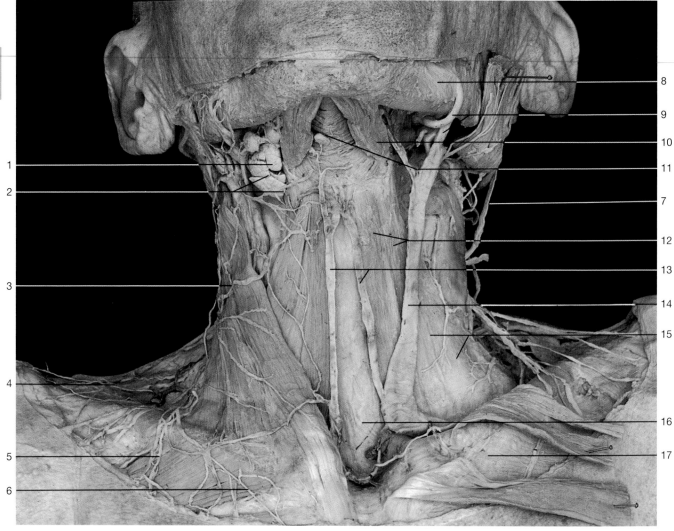

**Anterior region of the neck** (superficial layer). The superficial fascia has been removed.

1  Submandibular gland
2  Cervical branch of facial nerve
3  Transverse cervical nerve ⎫
4  Lateral supraclavicular nerves ⎪ Cutaneous
5  Middle supraclavicular nerves ⎬ branches of
6  Medial supraclavicular nerves ⎪ cervical plexus
7  Great auricular nerve ⎭

8  Mandible
9  Facial artery and vein
10 Anterior belly of digastric muscle
11 Mylohyoid muscle
12 Infrahyoid muscles
   (sternohyoid, sternothyroid, and
   omohyoid muscles)

13 Anterior jugular veins
14 External jugular vein
15 Pretracheal lamina of cervical fascia
16 Thyroid gland
17 Clavicle
18 Superficial lamina of cervical fascia
19 Carotid sheath with common carotid artery,
   internal jugular vein, and vagus nerve
20 Carotid sheath
21 Cervical part of sympathetic trunk
22 Prevertebral lamina of cervical fascia
23 Platysma muscle
24 Sternocleidomastoid muscle
25 Vertebral artery and vein
26 Scalene muscles
27 Trapezius muscle

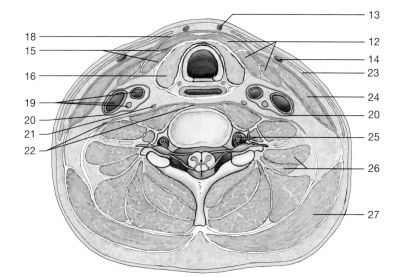

◁ **Cross section through the neck** at the level of the
thyroid gland. Notice the position of the three
laminae of cervical fascia (blue colored).

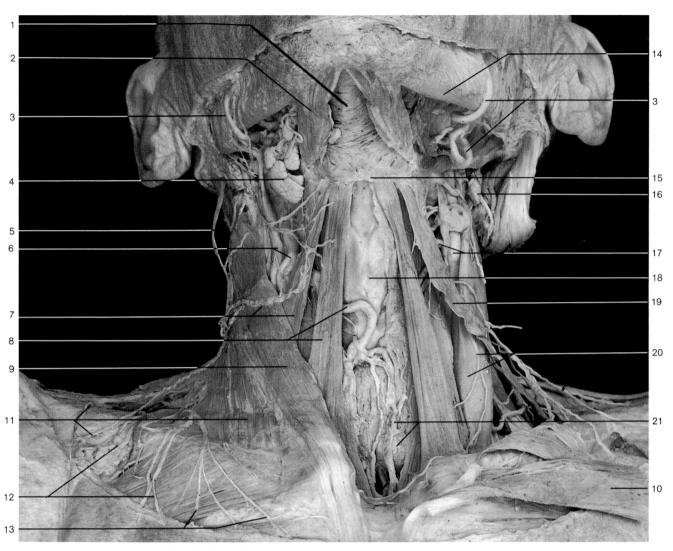

**Anterior region of the neck** with anterior triangle (right side: superficial layer, left side: deeper layer). The pretracheal lamina of cervical fascia and left sternocleidomastoid muscle have been removed.

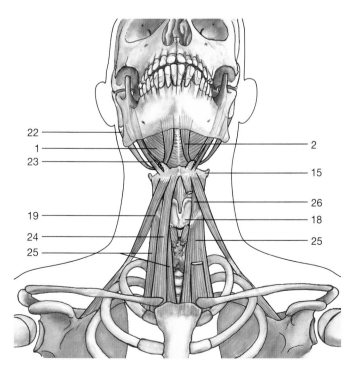

**Supra- and infrahyoid muscles** (anterior aspect).

1  Mylohyoid muscle
2  Anterior belly of digastric muscle
3  Facial artery
4  Submandibular gland
5  Great auricular nerve
6  Internal jugular vein and common carotid artery
7  Transverse cervical nerve and omohyoid muscle
8  Sternohyoid muscle and superior thyroid artery
9  Sternocleidomastoid muscle (sternal head)
10 Left sternocleidomastoid muscle (reflected)
11 Sternocleidomastoid muscle (clavicular head)
   and lateral supraclavicular nerves
12 Middle supraclavicular nerves
13 Medial supraclavicular nerves
14 Mandible
15 Hyoid bone
16 Superficial cervical lymph nodes
17 Left superior thyroid artery and
   external carotid artery
18 Thyroid cartilage
19 Superior belly of omohyoid muscle
20 Internal jugular vein and branches of ansa cervicalis
21 Thyroid gland and unpaired inferior thyroid vein
22 Posterior belly of digastric muscle
23 Stylohyoid muscle
24 Sternohyoid muscle
25 Sternothyroid muscle
26 Thyrohyoid muscle

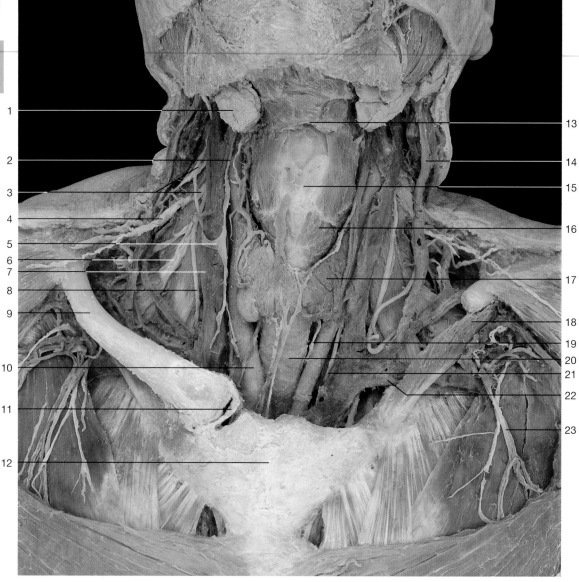

**Anterior region of the neck** (deep layer). Sternocleidomastoid muscles and left clavicle have been removed. Thyroid gland in relation to trachea, larynx, and vessels of the neck is shown.

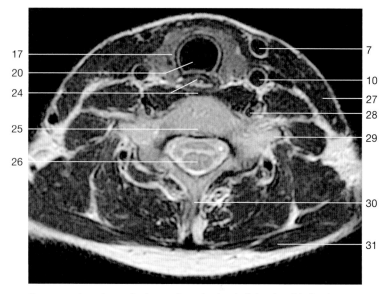

**Cross section through the neck** at the level of the thyroid gland (MRI scan). (Courtesy of Prof. Heuck, Munich, Germany.)

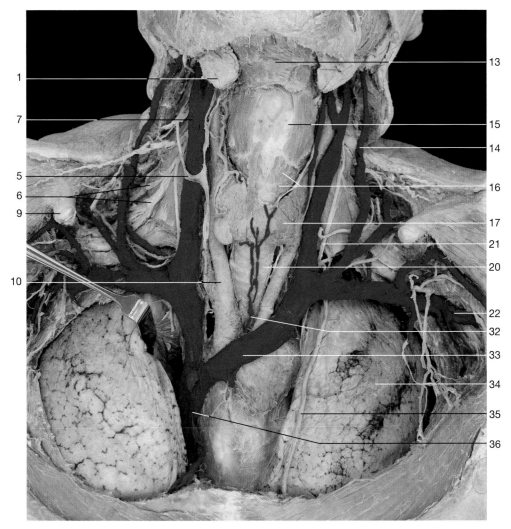

1. Submandibular gland
2. Cervical branch of facial nerve (n. VII)
3. Cervical plexus
4. Middle supraclavicular nerves
5. Ansa cervicalis
6. Brachial plexus
7. Internal jugular vein
8. Phrenic nerve
9. Clavicle
10. Common carotid artery
11. Sternoclavicular joint with articular disc
12. Manubrium of sternum
13. Hyoid bone
14. External jugular vein
15. Thyroid cartilage
16. Cricothyroid muscle
17. Thyroid gland
18. Subclavius muscle
19. Recurrent laryngeal nerve
20. Trachea
21. Vagus nerve (n. X)
22. Subclavian vein
23. Middle pectoral nerve
24. Esophagus
25. Body of cervical vertebra
26. Spinal cord
27. Sternocleidomastoid muscle
28. Vertebral artery
29. Transverse process of cervical vertebra
30. Spinous process of cervical vertebra
31. Trapezius muscle
32. Inferior thyroid vein
33. Left brachiocephalic vein
34. Superior lobe of left lung
35. Internal thoracic artery
36. Superior vena cava
37. Superior thyroid artery
38. Inferior thyroid artery
39. Thyrocervical trunk
40. Subclavian artery
41. Aortic arch

**Anterior region of the neck** and thoracic cavity (deeper layer). Both clavicles, sternum, and ribs have been removed. Main veins have been colored blue.

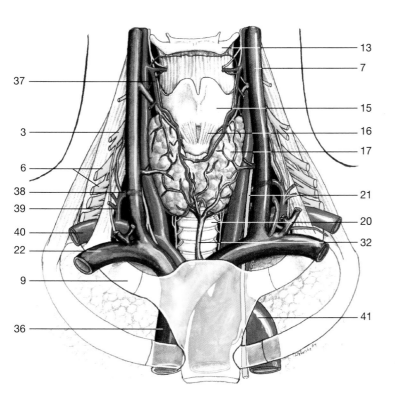

**Anterior region of the neck.** Regional anatomy of the thyroid gland with related blood vessels.

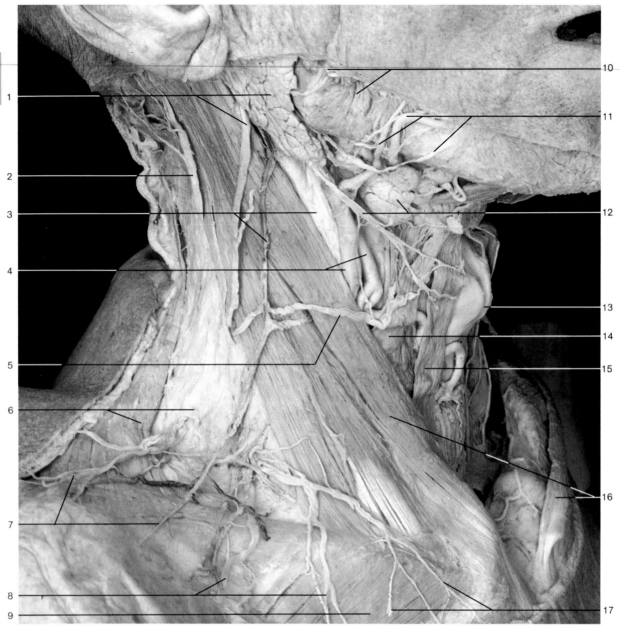

**Lateral region of the neck** with posterior and carotid triangles (superficial layer).

1  Parotid gland and great auricular nerve
2  Lesser occipital nerve
3  Internal and external jugular veins
4  Retromandibular vein and external carotid artery
5  Transverse cervical nerve with communicating branch to cervical branch of facial nerve
6  Trapezius muscle and superficial lamina of cervical fascia
7  Lateral supraclavicular nerves
8  Middle supraclavicular nerves
9  Pectoralis major muscle

10  Buccal branch of facial nerve and masseter muscle
11  Facial artery and vein and mandibular branch of facial nerve
12  Cervical branch of facial nerve and submandibular gland (only in the dissection)
13  Thyroid cartilage
14  Omohyoid muscle
15  Sternohyoid muscle
16  Sternocleidomastoid muscle
17  Medial supraclavicular nerves
18  Mandibular branch of facial nerve

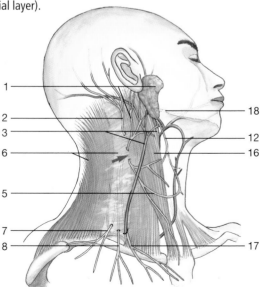

**Cutaneous branches of cervical plexus** (lateral region). Erb's point is indicated by an arrowhead.

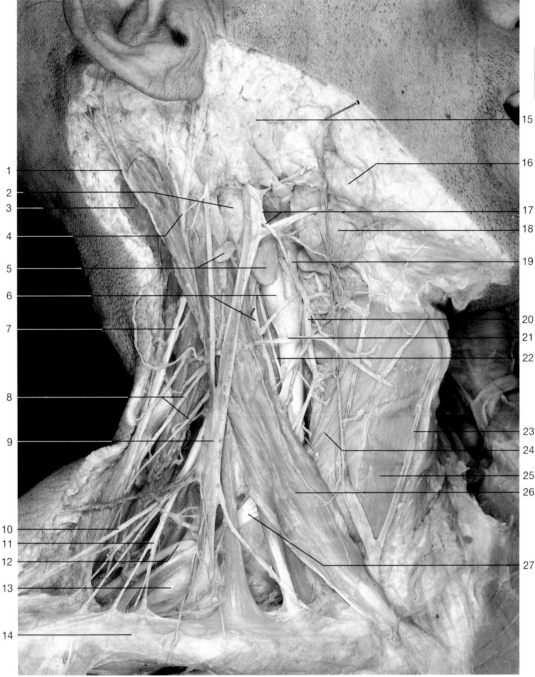

**Lateral region of the neck** with posterior and carotid triangles (superficial layer). The superficial lamina of cervical fascia has been removed to display the cutaneous branches of the cervical plexus and subcutaneous veins.

| | | | |
|---|---|---|---|
| 1 | Lesser occipital nerve | 15 | Parotid gland |
| 2 | Internal jugular vein | 16 | Mandible |
| 3 | Splenius capitis muscle | 17 | Cervical branch of facial nerve |
| 4 | Great auricular nerve | 18 | Submandibular gland |
| 5 | Submandibular nodes | 19 | External carotid artery |
| 6 | Internal carotid artery and vagus nerve | 20 | Superior thyroid artery |
| 7 | Accessory nerve | 21 | Transverse cervical nerve |
| 8 | Muscular branches of cervical plexus | 22 | Superior root of ansa cervicalis |
| 9 | External jugular vein | 23 | Anterior jugular vein |
| 10 | Posterior supraclavicular nerves | 24 | Omohyoid muscle |
| 11 | Middle supraclavicular nerves | 25 | Sternohyoid muscle |
| 12 | Suprascapular artery | 26 | Sternocleidomastoid muscle |
| 13 | Pretracheal lamina of fascia of neck | 27 | Intermediate tendon of omohyoid muscle |
| 14 | Clavicle | | |

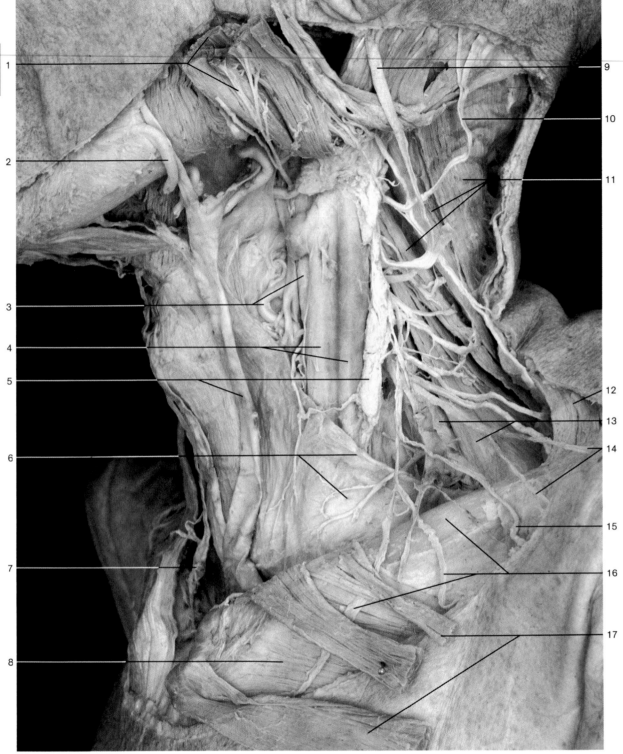

**Lateral region of the neck** (deep layer). Sternocleidomastoid muscle has been cut and reflected to display the pretracheal lamina of the cervical fascia.

1   Sternocleidomastoid muscle (reflected) and
    branch of accessory nerve
2   Facial artery
3   External carotid artery and superior thyroid artery
4   Internal jugular vein
5   Deep cervical lymph nodes and external jugular vein
6   Omohyoid muscle and pretracheal lamina of cervical fascia
7   Anterior jugular vein
8   Pectoralis major muscle

9   Great auricular nerve
10  Lesser occipital nerve
11  Splenius capitis and levator scapulae muscles
12  Trapezius muscle
13  Middle scalene muscle and brachial plexus
14  Posterior supraclavicular nerves
15  Middle supraclavicular nerve
16  Clavicle and anterior supraclavicular nerves
17  Sternocleidomastoid muscle (reflected)

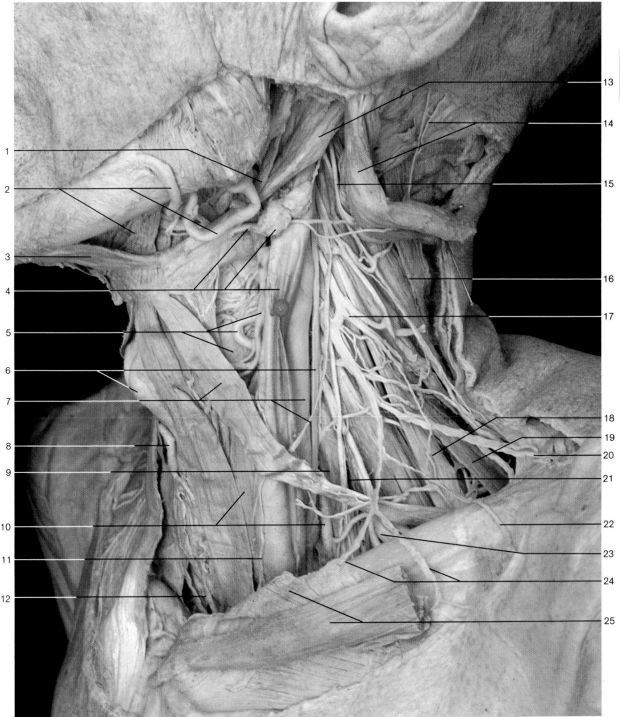

**Lateral region of the neck** (deep layer). The internal jugular vein has been reflected to expose the carotid artery and vagus nerve.

1 Stylohyoid muscle
2 Facial artery and mylohyoid muscle
3 Anterior belly of digastric muscle
4 Internal jugular vein, hypoglossal nerve, and superficial cervical lymph nodes
5 Superior thyroid artery and vein and inferior pharyngeal constrictor muscle
6 Thyroid cartilage and vagus nerve
7 Ansa cervicalis, omohyoid muscle, and common carotid artery
8 Right superior thyroid artery
9 Anterior scalene muscle
10 Sternothyroid muscle and inferior thyroid artery
11 Muscular branches of ansa cervicalis to the infrahyoid muscles
12 Inferior thyroid vein

13 Posterior belly of digastric muscle
14 Sternocleidomastoid muscle and lesser occipital nerve
15 Accessory nerve
16 Splenius capitis muscle
17 Cervical plexus
18 Posterior scalene muscle
19 Levator scapulae muscle
20 Posterior supraclavicular nerves
21 Phrenic nerve
22 Middle supraclavicular nerve
23 Brachial plexus
24 Anterior supraclavicular nerves
25 Sternocleidomastoid muscle

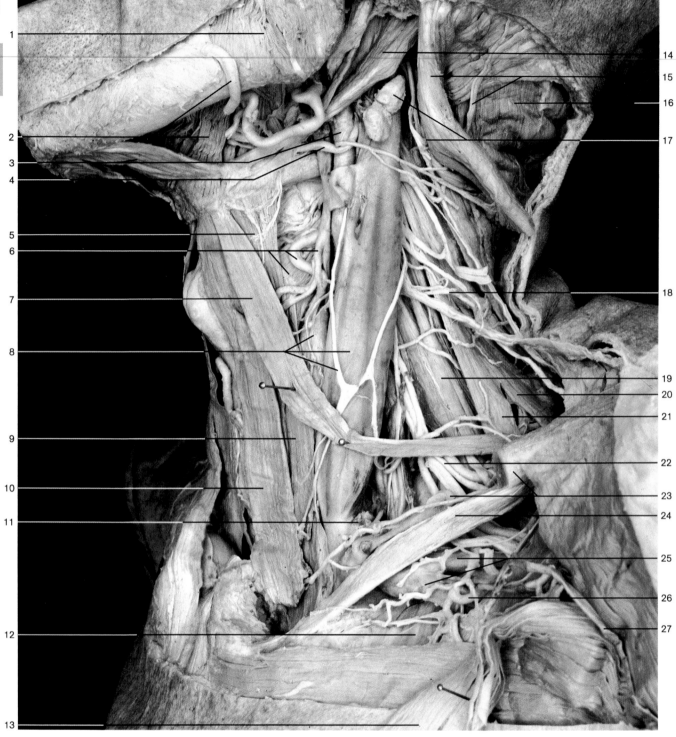

**Lateral region of the neck** with ansa cervicalis (deeper layer). The cervical fascia and the clavicle are partly removed. Ansa cervicalis and infrahyoid muscles are displayed.

1  Masseter muscle
2  Mylohyoid muscle and facial artery
3  External carotid artery and anterior belly of digastric muscle
4  Hypoglossal nerve
5  Thyrohyoid muscle
6  Superior thyroid artery and vein and inferior pharyngeal constrictor muscle
7  Superior belly of omohyoid muscle
8  Ansa cervicalis, thyroid gland, and internal jugular vein
9  Sternothyroid muscle
10  Sternohyoid muscle
11  Thoracic duct
12  Pectoralis minor muscle
13  Pectoralis major muscle
14  Posterior belly of digastric muscle
15  Sternocleidomastoid muscle and lesser occipital nerve
16  Splenius capitis muscle
17  Superficial cervical lymph nodes and accessory nerve
18  Cervical plexus
19  Middle scalene muscle
20  Levator scapulae muscle
21  Posterior scalene muscle
22  Brachial plexus
23  Transverse cervical artery and clavicle
24  Subclavius muscle
25  Subclavian artery and vein
26  Thoraco-acromial artery
27  Cephalic vein

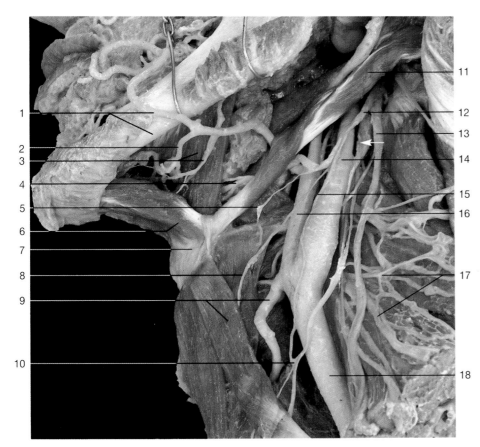

1  Facial artery and mandible
2  Submental artery
3  Mylohyoid muscle and nerve
4  Hypoglossal nerve
   (lingual branches)
5  Thyrohyoid branch
   of hypoglossal nerve (n. XII)
6  Anterior belly of digastric muscle
7  Hyoid bone
8  Omohyoid branch
   of hypoglossal nerve (n. XII)
9  Omohyoid muscle and
   superior thyroid artery
10 Ansa cervicalis
11 Posterior belly of digastric muscle
12 Hypoglossal nerve (n. XII)
13 Vagus nerve (n. X)
14 Internal carotid artery
15 Superior root of ansa cervicalis
16 External carotid artery
17 Cervical plexus
18 Common carotid artery
19 Facial artery and vein
20 Omohyoid muscle
21 Internal jugular vein
22 Sternohyoid and sternothyroid
   muscles
23 Clavicle
24 Superficial temporal artery and vein
25 Occipital artery
26 Spinal nerves ($C_3$ and $C_4$)
27 Spinal processes
   of cervical vertebrae ($C_4$ and $C_5$)
28 Scapula

**Lateral region of the neck and submandibular region** with hypoglossal nerve (n. XII).
Mandible slightly elevated. Arrow: superior cervical ganglion.

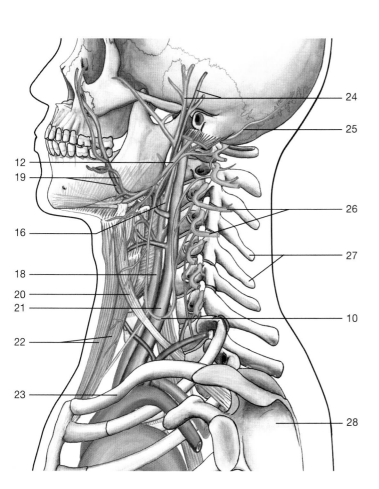

**Nerves and vessels of the neck** (lateral aspect).
The ansa cervicalis with its connection to the spinal nerves
is depicted.

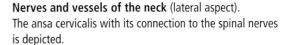

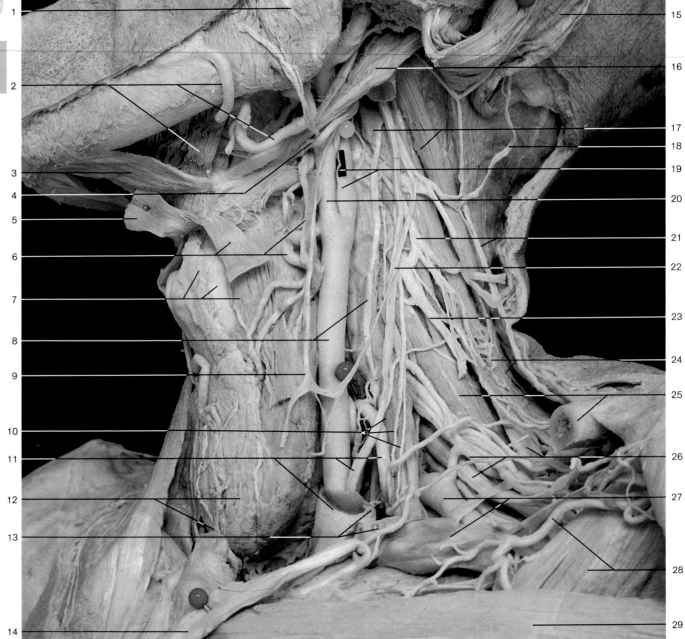

**Lateral region of the neck** (deeper layer). Clavicle partly removed to show the slit between the scalene muscles. Internal jugular vein removed.

1   Masseter muscle
2   Mylohyoid muscle and facial artery
3   Anterior belly of digastric muscle
4   Hypoglossal nerve
5   Sternohyoid muscle
6   Omohyoid muscle, superior thyroid artery and vein
7   Sternothyroid muscle, thyroid cartilage, and pyramidal lobe of thyroid gland
8   Common carotid artery and sympathetic trunk
9   Ansa cervicalis
10  Phrenic nerve, ascending cervical artery, and anterior scalene muscle

11  Inferior thyroid artery, vagus nerve, and internal jugular vein (cut)
12  Thyroid gland and unpaired inferior thyroid venous plexus
13  Thoracic duct and left subclavian trunk
14  Subclavius muscle (reflected)
15  Sternocleidomastoid muscle (reflected)
16  Posterior belly of digastric muscle
17  Superior cervical ganglion and splenius muscle
18  Lesser occipital nerve
19  Internal carotid artery and branch of the glossopharyngeal nerve to the carotid body
20  External carotid artery

21  Cervical plexus and accessory nerve
22  Inferior root of ansa cervicalis
23  Supraclavicular nerve
24  Levator scapulae muscle
25  Middle scalene muscle and clavicle
26  Transverse cervical artery, brachial plexus, and posterior scalene muscle
27  Subclavian artery and vein
28  Thoraco-acromial artery and pectoralis minor muscle
29  Pectoralis major muscle

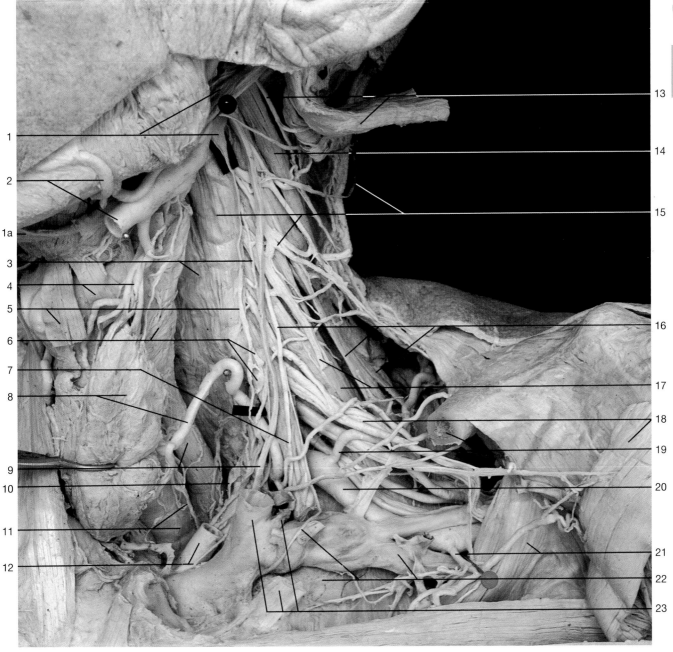

**Lateral region of the neck** (deepest layer). Thyroid gland reflected to expose the esophagus and the recurrent laryngeal nerve.

1 Superior cervical ganglion of sympathetic trunk and posterior belly of digastric muscle
1a Anterior belly of digastric muscle
2 Facial artery and common carotid artery (reflected anteriorly)
3 Ascending cervical artery and longus colli muscle
4 Omohyoid muscle and superior thyroid artery
5 Sympathetic trunk and sternohyoid muscle
6 Middle cervical ganglion and inferior pharyngeal constrictor muscle
7 Anterior scalene muscle and phrenic nerve
8 Thyroid gland and inferior thyroid artery
9 Vagus nerve and esophagus
10 Stellate ganglion
11 Recurrent laryngeal nerve and trachea

12 Common carotid artery and cervical cardiac branch of vagus nerve
13 Sternocleidomastoid muscle and accessory nerve
14 Splenius capitis muscle
15 Lesser occipital nerve, longus capitis muscle, and cervical plexus
16 Phrenic nerve, posterior scalene muscle, and levator scapulae muscle
17 Supraclavicular nerves and middle scalene muscle
18 Brachial plexus and pectoralis major muscle (clavicular head)
19 Transverse cervical artery and clavicle
20 Subclavian artery
21 Thoraco-acromial artery and pectoralis minor muscle
22 First rib, accessory phrenic nerve, and subclavian vein
23 Internal jugular vein, thoracic duct, and subclavius muscle

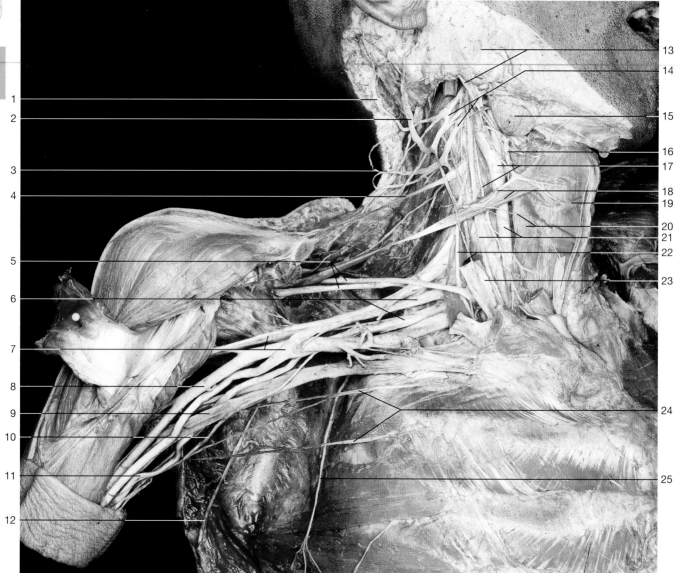

**Lateral region of the neck and shoulder** (deepest layer). Cervical and brachial plexuses and their relation to the blood vessels are shown. Note the location and content of scalene triangle. Sternocleidomastoid muscle and clavicle have been removed; the internal jugular vein was divided to display the roots of cervical and brachial plexuses.

1  Lesser occipital nerve
2  Great auricular nerve
3  Cutaneous branches of cervical plexus
4  Supraclavicular nerve
5  Suprascapular nerve and artery
6  Brachial plexus
7  Median nerve (with two roots) and musculocutaneous nerve
8  Axillary artery
9  Axillary vein
10  Medial brachial cutaneous nerve
11  Ulnar nerve
12  Thoracodorsal nerve
13  Parotid gland and facial nerve (cervical branch)
14  Cervical plexus

15  Submandibular gland
16  Superior thyroid artery
17  Common carotid artery dividing in internal and external carotid artery and superior root of ansa cervicalis
18  Omohyoid muscle and cervical branch of facial nerve joining the transverse cervical nerve ($C_2$, $C_3$)
19  Sternohyoid muscle
20  Transverse cervical nerve and sternothyroid muscle
21  Common carotid artery and vagus nerve
22  Phrenic nerve and anterior scalene muscle
23  Internal jugular vein
24  Intercostobrachial nerves
25  Long thoracic nerve

# 3 Trunk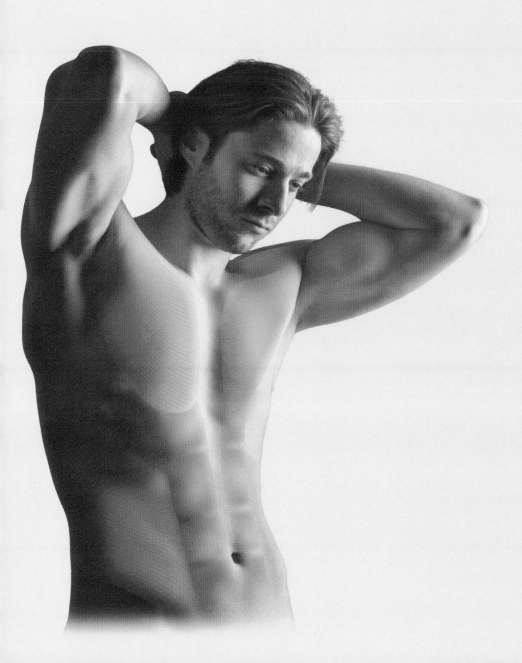

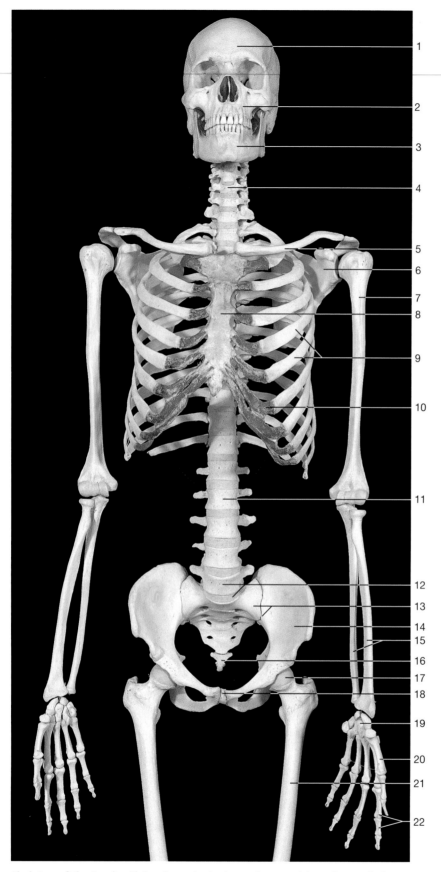

1   Frontal bone
2   Maxilla
3   Mandible
4   Cervical vertebrae
5   Clavicle
6   Scapula
7   Humerus
8   Sternum
9   Ribs
10  Costal cartilage
11  Lumbar vertebrae
12  Lumbar vertebra (L$_5$) and promontory
13  Sacrum
14  Hip bone
15  Radius and ulna
16  Coccyx
17  Head of femur
18  Pubic symphysis
19  Carpal bones
20  Metacarpal bones
21  Femur
22  Phalanges

**Skeleton of the trunk** with head, vertebral column, thorax, pelvis, and upper limb (anterior aspect).

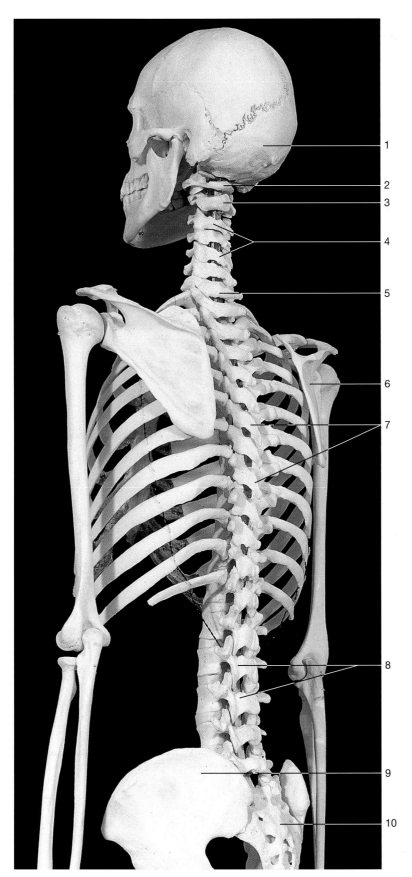

1 Occipital bone
2 Atlas
3 Axis
4 Cervical vertebrae
5 Vertebra prominens (C₇)
6 Scapula
7 Thoracic vertebrae
8 Lumbar vertebrae
9 Hip bone
10 Sacrum

**Skeleton of the trunk** with head, vertebral column, thorax, pelvis, and shoulder girdle (oblique-posterior aspect).

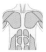

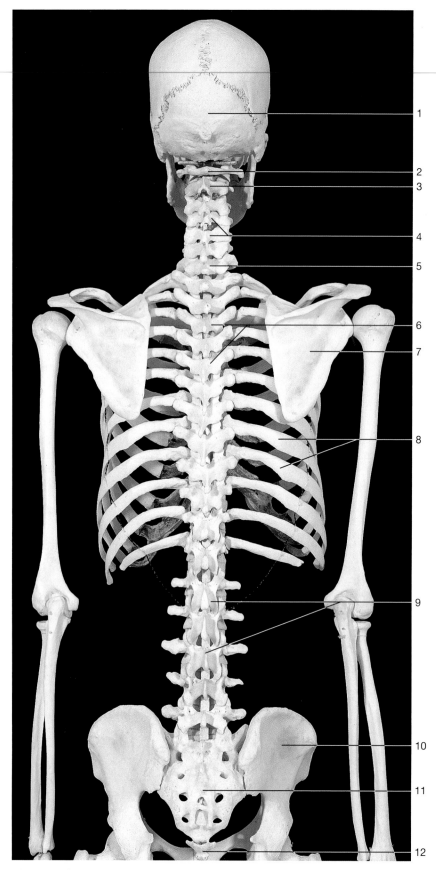

1   Occipital bone
2   Atlas
3   Axis
4   Cervical vertebrae
5   Vertebra prominens (C₇)
6   Thoracic vertebrae
7   Scapula
8   Ribs
9   Lumbar vertebrae
10  Hip bone
11  Sacrum
12  Coccyx

**Skeleton of the trunk** with head, vertebral column, thorax, pelvis, and shoulder girdle (posterior aspect).

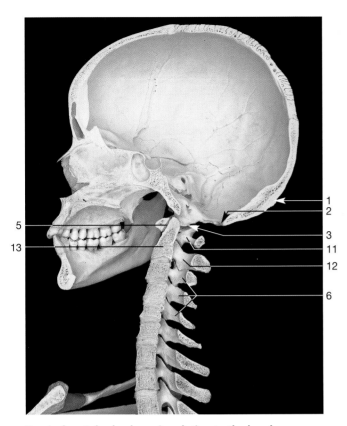

**Cervical vertebral column in relation to the head** (midsagittal section, medial aspect).

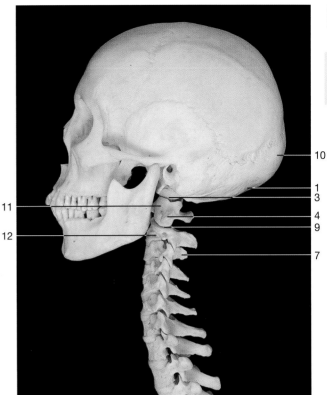

**Atlas and axis in relation to the head** (lateral aspect).

1   External occipital protuberance
2   Foramen magnum
3   Atlanto-occipital joint
4   Transverse process of atlas
5   Median atlanto-axial joint
6   Vertebral canal
7   Spinous process of third cervical vertebra
8   Occipital condyle

9    Lateral atlanto-axial joint
10   Occipital bone
11   Atlas
12   Axis
13   Dens of axis
14   Hypoglossal canal
15   Spinous process of axis

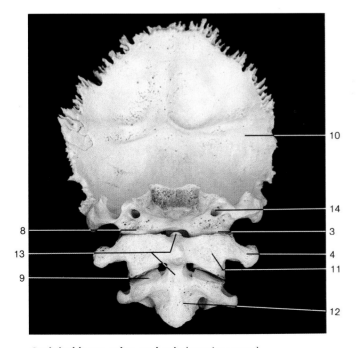

**Occipital bone, atlas, and axis** (anterior aspect).

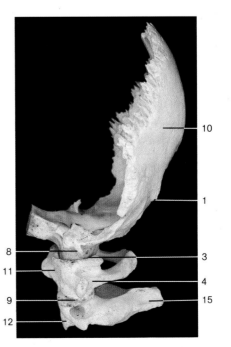

**Occipital bone, atlas, and axis** (left lateral aspect).

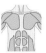

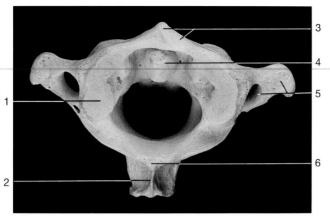

**Atlas and axis** (from above).

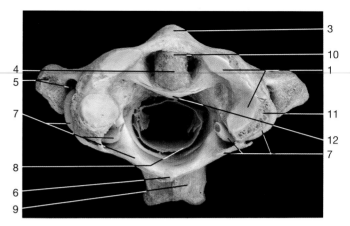

**Median atlanto-axial joint and transverse ligament of atlas** (from above). Dens of axis partly severed.

| | |
|---|---|
| 1 Superior articular facet of atlas | 13 Superior articular facet of axis |
| 2 Spinous process | 14 Inferior articular process |
| 3 Anterior arch of atlas with anterior tubercle | 15 Body of axis |
| 4 Dens of axis | 16 Pedicle and lamina of axis |
| 5 Transverse foramen and process | 17 Superior longitudinal band of cruciform ligament |
| 6 Posterior tubercle of atlas | 18 Alar ligaments |
| 7 Posterior arch of atlas and vertebral artery | 19 Transverse ligament of atlas |
| 8 Dura mater | 20 Inferior longitudinal band of cruciform ligament |
| 9 Spinous process of axis | 21 Occipital bone |
| 10 Median atlanto-axial joint (anterior part) | 22 Atlanto-occipital joint |
| 11 Articular capsule of atlanto-occipital joint | 23 Lateral atlanto-axial joint |
| 12 Transverse ligament of atlas | 24 Third cervical vertebra (C₃) |

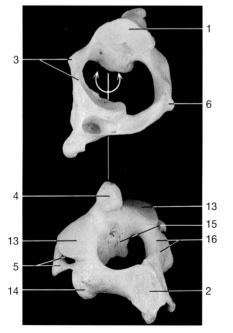

**Atlas and axis** (left oblique postero-lateral aspect, demonstrating the articulation of the dens of axis with the atlas [arrows]).

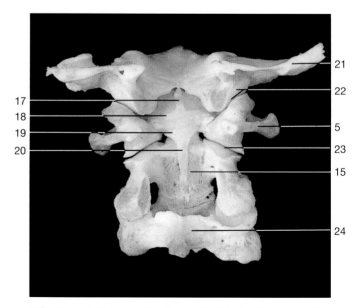

**Atlanto-occipital and atlanto-axial joints** (posterior aspect). Posterior part of occipital bone, posterior arch of atlas, and axis have been removed to show the cruciform ligament.

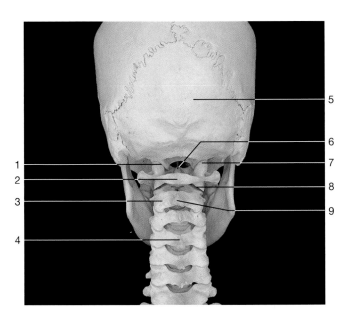

1  Superior articular facet
2  Posterior tubercle of atlas
3  Pedicle and lamina of axis
4  Spinous process of cervical vertebra
5  Occipital bone
6  Dens of axis
7  Atlanto-occipital joint
8  Lateral atlanto-axial joint
9  Spinous process of axis
10  External occipital protuberance
11  Foramen magnum
12  Transverse process of atlas
13  Posterior longitudinal ligament
14  Occipital condyle
15  Tectorial membrane
16  Dorsum sellae
17  Clivus
18  Axis
19  Sella turcica
20  Superior orbital fissure
21  Internal acoustic meatus
22  Jugular foramen
23  Hypoglossal canal
24  Superior longitudinal band of cruciform ligament
25  Alar ligaments
26  Transverse ligament of atlas

**Cervical vertebral column and skull** (posterior aspect). Note the location of the atlanto-occipital and atlanto-axial joints.

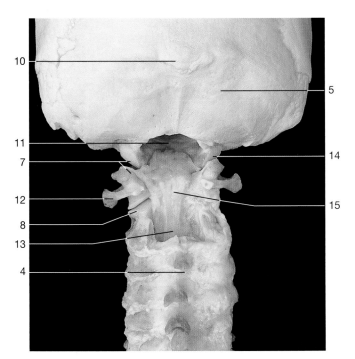

**Cervical vertebral column and skull with ligaments** (posterior aspect). Posterior arches of atlas and axis have been removed to show the tectorial membrane.

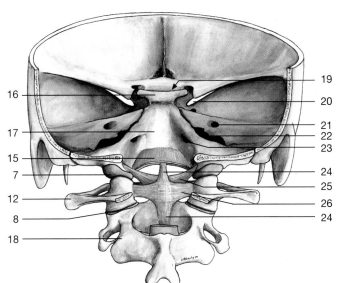

**Atlanto-occipital and atlanto-axial joints with ligaments** (posterior aspect). Posterior part of occipital bone and posterior arch of atlas have been removed to show the cruciform ligament.

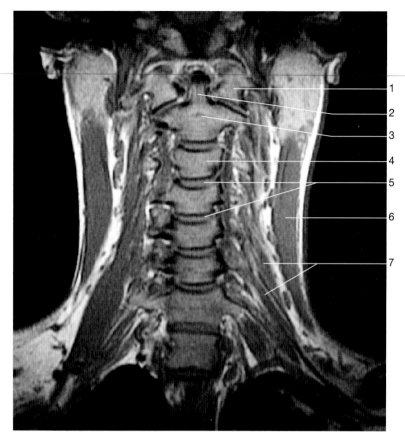

1   Atlas
2   Dens of axis
3   Axis
4   Body of cervical vertebra (C₃)
5   Intervertebral discs
6   Sternocleidomastoid muscle
7   Scalene muscles

**Coronal section through the cervical vertebral column** at the level of the vertical bodies (MRI scan). (Courtesy of Prof. Heuck, Munich, Germany.)

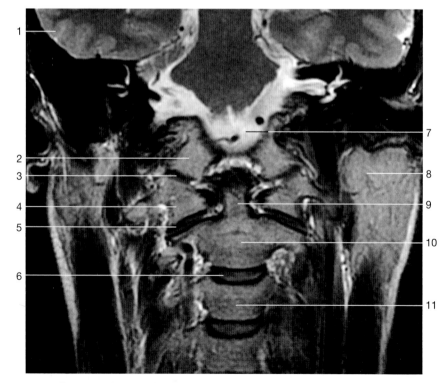

1   Cerebellum
2   Occipital condyle
3   Atlanto-occipital joint
4   Atlas
5   Lateral atlanto-axial joint
6   Intervertebral disc
7   Cistern of pons
8   Head of mandible
9   Dens of axis
10  Axis
11  Body of cervical vertebra (C₃)

**Coronal section through the cervical vertebral column** at the level of the dens of axis (MRI scan). (Courtesy of Prof. Heuck, Munich, Germany.)

1  Pons
2  Base of skull (clivus)
3  Medulla oblongata
4  Atlas (anterior arch)
5  Dens of axis
6  Intervertebral disc
7  Body of cervical vertebra (C₄)
8  Site of larynx
9  Trachea
10  Cerebellum
11  Cerebellomedullary cistern
12  Spinal cord
13  Trapezius muscle
14  Muscles of the neck
15  Spinous process of cervical vertebra (C₇)
16  Internal jugular vein
17  Common carotid artery
18  Vagus nerve (n. X)
19  Larynx
20  Body of cervical vertebra
21  Vertebral artery
22  Spinal nerve with spinal ganglion
23  Transverse process of cervical vertebra
24  Spinous process of cervical vertebra

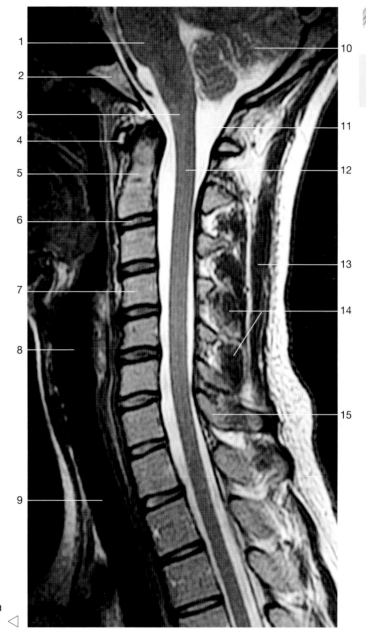

**Midsagittal section through the cervical vertebral column**
showing the spinal cord in connection with the medulla oblongata
(MRI scan). (Courtesy of Prof. Heuck, Munich, Germany.) ◁

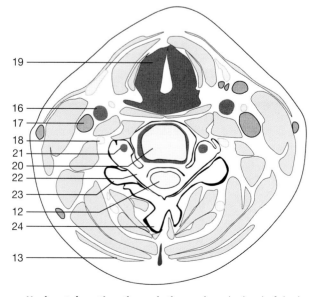

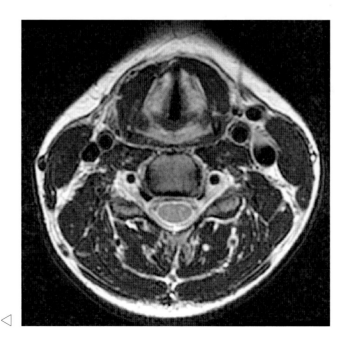

**Horizontal section through the neck** at the level of the larynx
(MRI scan). (Courtesy of Prof. Heuck, Munich, Germany.)
Compare with the schematic drawing. ◁

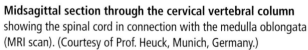

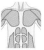

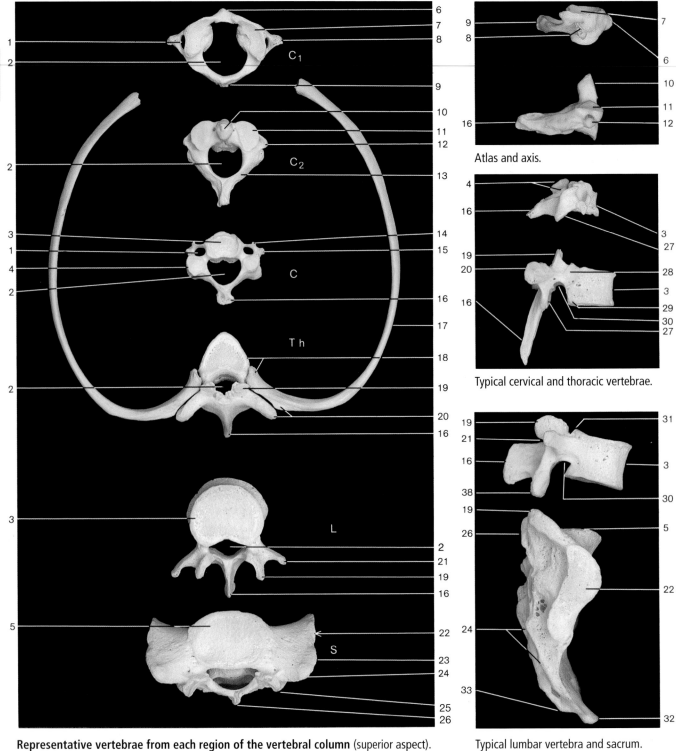

Atlas and axis.

Typical cervical and thoracic vertebrae.

**Representative vertebrae from each region of the vertebral column** (superior aspect). From top to bottom: atlas (C₁), axis (C₂), cervical vertebra (C), thoracic vertebra (Th), lumbar vertebra (L), and sacrum (S).

Typical lumbar vertebra and sacrum.

△

**Representative vertebrae from each region of the vertebral column** (lateral aspect, ventral surface on the right).

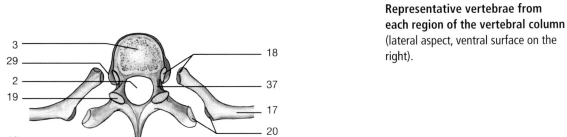

**General organization of ribs and vertebrae.**

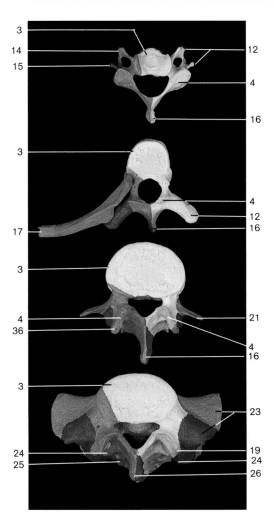

**General characteristics of the vertebrae.**
Typical cervical, thoracic, and lumbar vertebrae and sacrum.

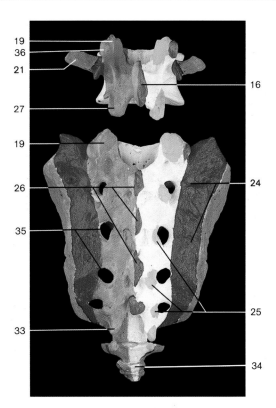

**General characteristics of lumbar vertebrae and sacrum** (posterior aspect).

| | | |
|---|---|---|
| Green | = | Ribs or homologous processes |
| Red | = | Muscular processes (transverse and spinous processes) |
| Orange | = | Laminae and articular processes |
| Yellow and blue | = | Articular facets |

| | |
|---|---|
| 1 | Foramen transversarium |
| 2 | Vertebral foramen |
| 3 | Body of vertebra |
| 4 | Superior articular facet |
| 5 | Base of sacrum |
| 6 | Anterior tubercle of atlas |
| 7 | Superior articular facet of atlas |
| 8 | Transverse process |
| 9 | Posterior tubercle of atlas |
| 10 | Dens of axis |
| 11 | Superior articular surface |
| 12 | Transverse process |
| 13 | Arch of vertebra |
| 14 | Anterior tubercle of transverse process |
| 15 | Posterior tubercle of transverse process |
| 16 | Spinous process |
| 17 | Shaft of rib |
| 18 | Body of vertebra and head of rib articulating with each other (costovertebral joint) |
| 19 | Superior articular process |
| 20 | Transverse process and tubercle of rib articulating with each other (costotransverse joint) |
| 21 | Costal process |
| 22 | Auricular surface |
| 23 | Lateral part of sacrum |
| 24 | Lateral sacral crest |
| 25 | Intermediate sacral crest |
| 26 | Median sacral crest |
| 27 | Inferior articular facet |
| 28 | Superior demifacet for head of rib |
| 29 | Inferior demifacet for head of rib |
| 30 | Inferior vertebral notch |
| 31 | Superior vertebral notch |
| 32 | Apex of the sacrum |
| 33 | Sacral cornu |
| 34 | Coccyx |
| 35 | Dorsal sacral foramina |
| 36 | Mamillary process |
| 37 | Pedicle |
| 38 | Inferior articular process |

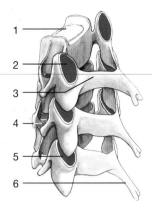

**Cervical vertebrae** (lateral aspect, blue = articular facets).

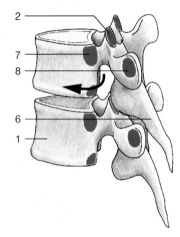

**Thoracic vertebrae** (lateral aspect, blue = articular facets).

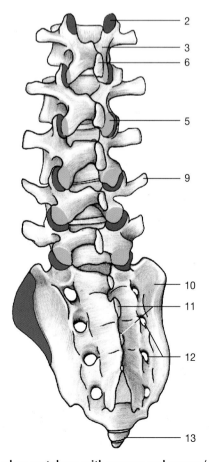

**Lumbar vertebrae with sacrum and coccyx** (posterior aspect, blue = articular facets).

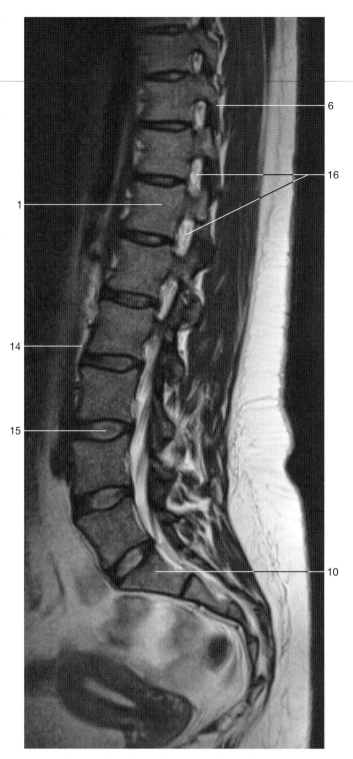

**Paramedian section through the vertebral column** with pelvic cavity (MRI scan). (Prof. Uder, Dept. of Radiology, Univ. Erlangen-Nuremberg, Germany.)

| | |
|---|---|
| 1   Body of vertebra | 8   Transverse process |
| 2   Superior articular facet |     with articular facet |
| 3   Vertebral arch |     of costotransverse joint |
| 4   Transverse process of vertebra | 9   Costal process of lumbar vertebra |
| 5   Zygapophysial joint | 10  Sacrum |
| 6   Spinous process | 11  Median sacral crest |
| 7   Superior articular facet | 12  Dorsal sacral foramina |
|     of articulation with head of ribs | 13  Coccyx |
| | 14  Anterior longitudinal ligament |
| | 15  Intervertebral disc |
| | 16  Vertebral canal |

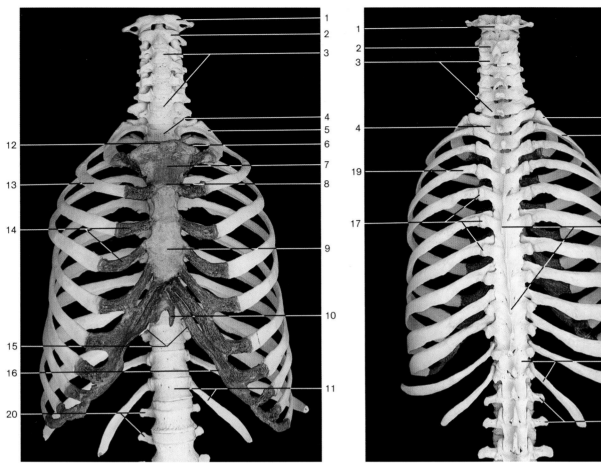

**Skeleton of the thorax** (anterior aspect).

**Skeleton of the thorax** (posterior aspect).

1 Atlas
2 Axis
3 Cervical vertebrae
4 First thoracic vertebra
5 First rib
6 Facet for clavicle and clavicular notch
7 Manubrium sterni
8 Sternal angle
9 Body of sternum
10 Xiphoid process
11 Twelfth thoracic vertebra and rib
12 Jugular notch
13 Second rib
14 Costal cartilages
15 Infrasternal angle
16 Costal arch
17 Costotransverse joints between the transverse processes of thoracic vertebrae and the tubercles of the ribs
18 Spinous processes
19 Costal angle
20 Costal processes of lumbar vertebrae

**Disarticulated skeleton of the thorax.** The twelve ribs (I–XII) are arranged in a craniocaudal direction.

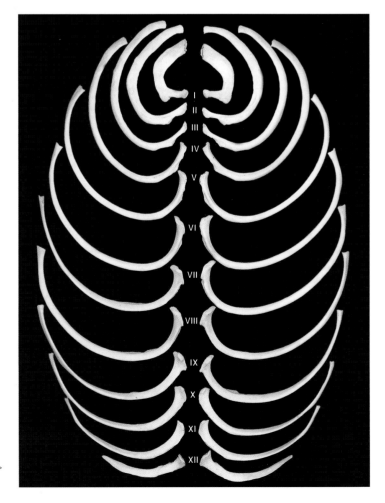

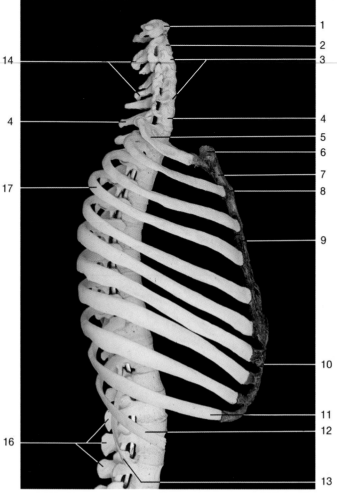

**Skeleton of the thorax** (right lateral aspect).

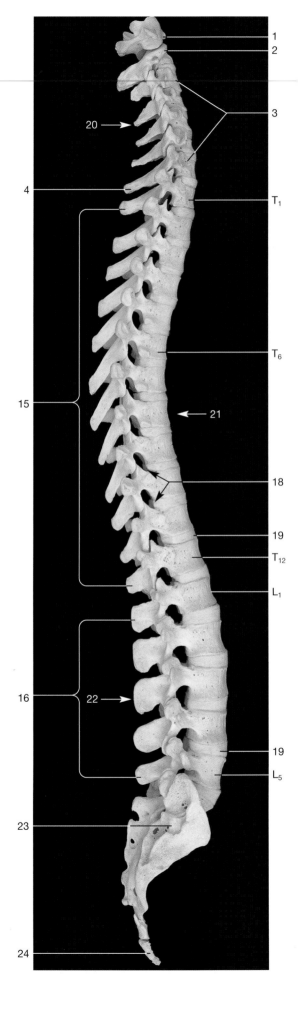

1  Atlas
2  Axis
3  Cervical vertebrae
4  Vertebra prominens (C₇)
5  First rib
6  Facet for clavicle
7  Manubrium sterni
8  Sternal angle
9  Body of sternum
10 Costal arch
11 Tenth rib
12 Eleventh rib
13 Twelfth rib
14 Spinous processes of cervical vertebrae
15 Spinous processes of thoracic vertebrae
16 Spinous processes of lumbar vertebrae
17 Costal angle
18 Intervertebral foramina
19 Intervertebral discs
20 Cervical curvature
21 Thoracic curvature
22 Lumbar curvature
23 Sacrum
24 Coccyx

**Vertebral column**
(right lateral aspect).

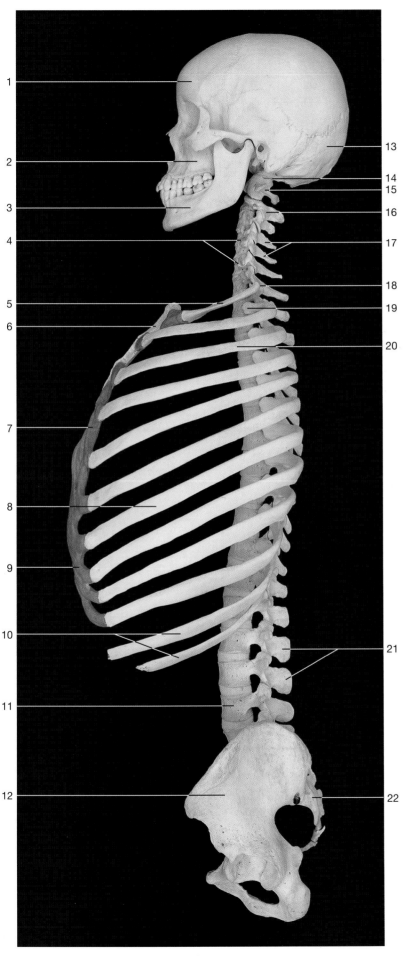

1  Frontal bone
2  Maxilla
3  Mandible
4  Bodies of cervical vertebrae
5  First rib
6  Manubrium of sternum
7  Sternum (corpus sterni)
8  Seventh rib (last of the true ribs)
9  Costal arch
10  Floating ribs (costae fluctuantes)
11  Body of fourth lumbar vertebra
12  Pelvis
13  Occipital bone
14  Atlanto-occipital joint
15  Atlas
16  Axis
17  Spinous processes of cervical vertebrae (C$_4$, C$_5$)
18  Costotransverse joint of first rib
19  Head of second rib
20  Third rib
21  Spinous processes of lumbar vertebrae (L$_2$, L$_3$)
22  Sacrum

**Vertebral column and thorax** in connection with head and pelvis (lateral aspect).

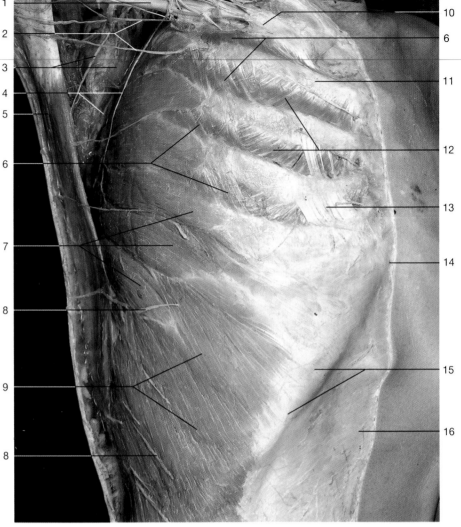

1   Axillary vein
2   Intercostobrachial nerves
3   Subscapularis muscle and
    thoracodorsal nerve
4   Long thoracic nerve,
    lateral thoracic artery and vein
5   Latissimus dorsi muscle
6   External intercostal muscles
7   Serratus anterior muscle
8   Lateral cutaneous branches
    of intercostal nerves
9   External abdominal oblique muscle
10  Clavicle (divided)
11  Second rib
    (costochondral junction)
12  Internal intercostal muscles
13  External intercostal membrane
14  Position of xiphoid process
15  Costal arch or margin
16  Anterior layer of rectus sheath

**Muscles of the thorax,** superficial layer (lateral aspect). Upper limb elevated.
Pectoralis major and minor muscles have been removed.

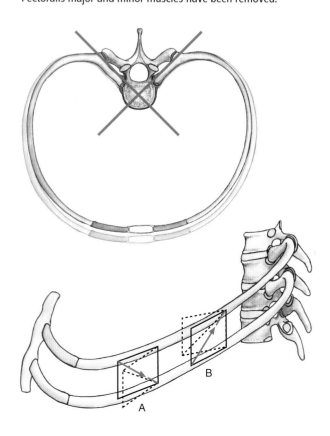

**Effect of intercostal muscles on the costovertebral and
costotransverse joints.** Axes of movement indicated by red lines;
direction of movements indicated by red arrows.
A = Action of internal intercostal muscles (expiration);
B = Action of external intercostal muscles (inspiration).

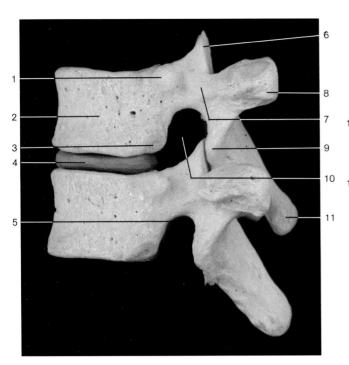

**Two thoracic vertebrae** (left lateral aspect).

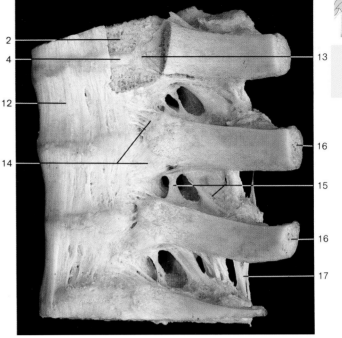

**Ligaments of thoracic vertebrae and costovertebral joints** (left antero-lateral aspect).

| | | | |
|---|---|---|---|
| 1 | Superior demifacet for head of rib | 9 | Inferior articular process |
| 2 | Body of vertebra | 10 | Intervertebral foramen |
| 3 | Inferior demifacet for head of rib | 11 | Spinous process |
| 4 | Intervertebral disc | 12 | Anterior longitudinal ligament |
| 5 | Inferior vertebral notch | 13 | Intra-articular ligament |
| 6 | Superior articular facet and superior articular process | 14 | Radiate ligament |
| 7 | Pedicle | 15 | Superior costotransverse ligament |
| 8 | Transverse process and facet for tubercle of rib | 16 | Body of rib |

| | | | |
|---|---|---|---|
| 17 | Intertransverse ligament | 23 | Vertebral canal |
| 18 | Articulation of head of rib with two vertebrae | 24 | Inferior facet of articulation with head of rib |
| 19 | Angle of costotransverse joint (articular facet) | 25 | Head of rib |
| 20 | Costotransverse joint | 26 | Superior articular process |
| 21 | Tubercle of rib | 27 | Facets of articulation with costotransverse joint |
| 22 | Costal angle of rib | | |

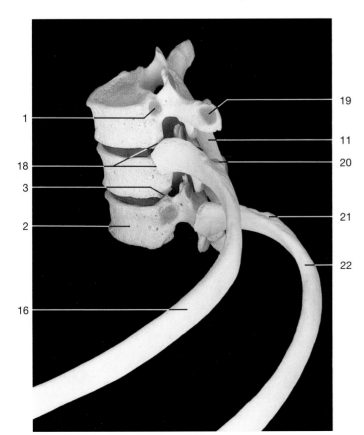

**Costovertebral joints** (lateral aspect).

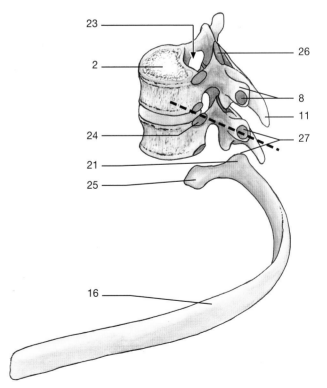

**Costovertebral joints** (lateral aspect). Two thoracic vertebrae with an articulating rib (separated). Axis of movement indicated by dashed line. Blue = articular facets.

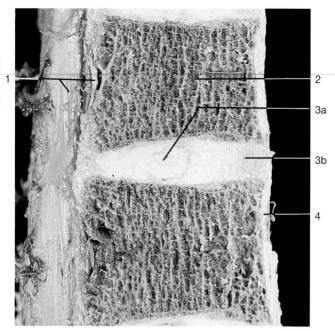

**Median sagittal section through the bodies of lumbar vertebrae,** showing the intervertebral discs, each of which consists of an outer laminated portion and an inner core.

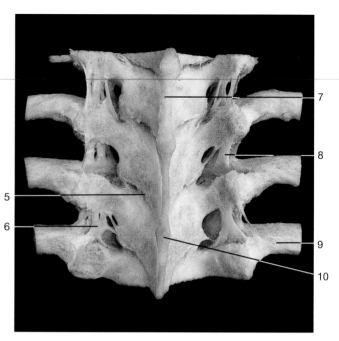

**Ligaments of the thoracic vertebrae** (posterior aspect).

1  Posterior longitudinal ligament and spinal dura mater
2  Body of vertebra
3  Intervertebral disc
   a  Inner core (nucleus pulposus)
   b  Outer portion (anulus fibrosus)
4  Anterior longitudinal ligament
5  Ligamentum flavum
6  Intertransverse ligament
7  Supraspinous ligament

8  Superior costotransverse ligament
9  Rib
10  Spinous process
11  Costal process of lumbar vertebra
12  Sacrum
13  Intervertebral foramen
14  Interspinous ligament
15  Transverse process of thoracic vertebra

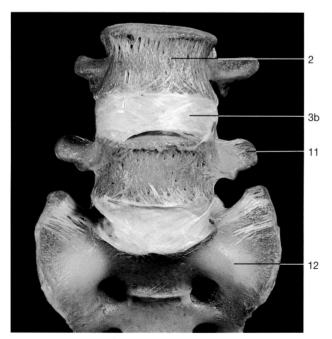

**Two caudal lumbar vertebrae and sacrum with their intervertebral discs** (anterior aspect). Anterior longitudinal ligament removed.

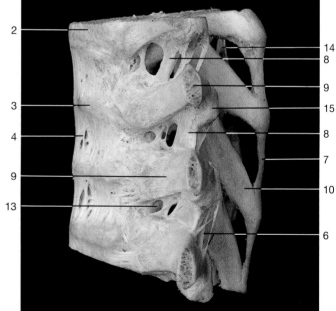

**Ligaments of the thoracic vertebrae** (left lateral aspect).

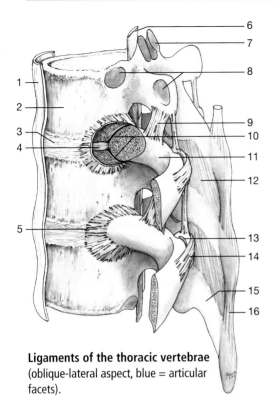

**Ligaments of the thoracic vertebrae**
(oblique-lateral aspect, blue = articular facets).

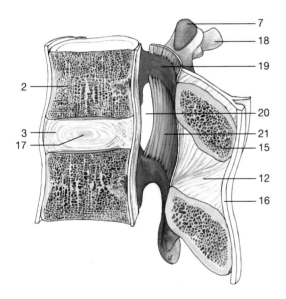

**Ligaments of the lumbar vertebrae**
(median sagittal section, blue = articular facets).

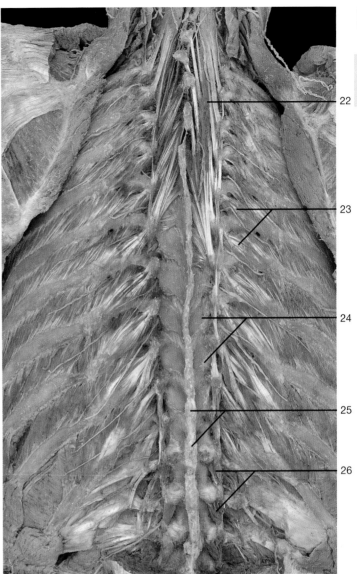

**Vertebral column and ribs** (posterior aspect). Muscles of the back has been widely removed to display the ligaments.

| | | | |
|---|---|---|---|
| 1 | Anterior longitudinal ligament | 10 | Joint of head of rib |
| 2 | Body of vertebra | 11 | Rib |
| 3 | Intervertebral disc | 12 | Interspinal ligament |
| 4 | Intra-articular ligament | 13 | Costotransverse joint |
| 5 | Radiate ligament | 14 | Lateral costotransverse ligament |
| 6 | Posterior longitudinal ligament | 15 | Spinous process |
| 7 | Superior articular facet | 16 | Supraspinal ligament |
| 8 | Articular facets of joint of head of rib and costotransverse joint | 17 | Nucleus pulposus |
| | | 18 | Costal process |
| 9 | Superior costotransverse ligament | 19 | Vertebral arch |

| | |
|---|---|
| 20 | Intervertebral foramen |
| 21 | Intertransverse ligament |
| 22 | Semispinalis cervicis muscle |
| 23 | Levatores costarum muscles |
| 24 | Bodies of lumbar vertebrae |
| 25 | Spinous processes of lumbar vertebrae and supraspinal ligaments |
| 26 | Intertransversarii muscles |

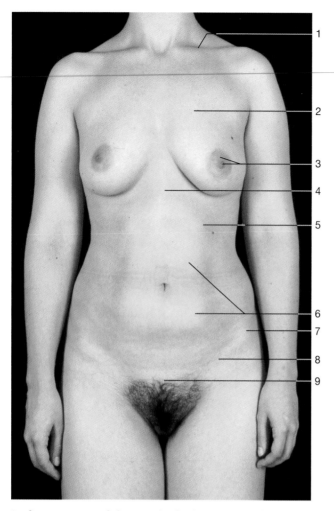

| | |
|---|---|
| 1 | Clavicle |
| 2 | Pectoralis major muscle |
| 3 | Areola and nipple |
| 4 | Infrasternal angle |
| 5 | Costal arch |
| 6 | Rectus abdominis muscle |
| 7 | Anterior superior iliac spine |
| 8 | Inguinal ligament |
| 9 | Mons pubis |
| 10 | External abdominal oblique muscle |
| 11 | Spermatic cord |
| 12 | Deltoid muscle |
| 13 | External intercostal muscle |
| 14 | Internal abdominal oblique muscle |
| 15 | Transverse abdominal muscle |
| 16 | Rectus sheath |
| 17 | Pectoralis minor muscle |
| 18 | Anterior serratus muscle |
| 19 | Linea alba |

**Surface anatomy of the anterior body wall in the female.**
Note the differences of hairiness between the regions.

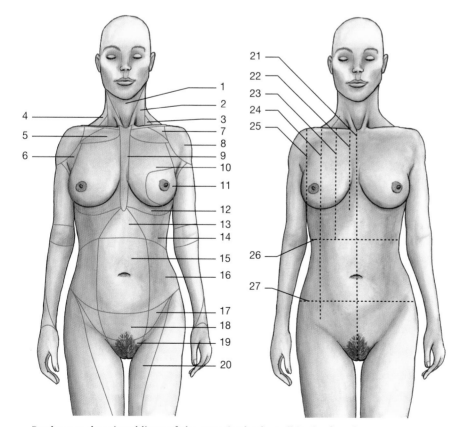

| | |
|---|---|
| 1 | Anterior cervical region |
| 2 | Sternocleidomastoid region |
| 3 | Omoclavicular triangle |
| 4 | Lateral cervical region |
| 5 | Infraclavicular fossa |
| 6 | Axillary region |
| 7 | Clavipectoral triangle |
| 8 | Deltoid region |
| 9 | Presternal region |
| 10 | Inframammary region |
| 11 | Mammary region |
| 12 | Pectoral region |
| 13 | Epigastric region |
| 14 | Hypochondriac region |
| 15 | Umbilical region |
| 16 | Lateral abdominal region |
| 17 | Inguinal region |
| 18 | Pubic region |
| 19 | Urogenital region |
| 20 | Femoral triangle |
| 21 | Anterior median line |
| 22 | Sternal line |
| 23 | Parasternal line |
| 24 | Mammillary line (medioclavicular line) |
| 25 | Axillary line |
| 26 | Horizontal plane at the level of the inferior thoracic aperture |
| 27 | Horizontal plane at the level of the anterior superior iliac spine |

**Regions and regional lines of the anterior body wall in the female.**

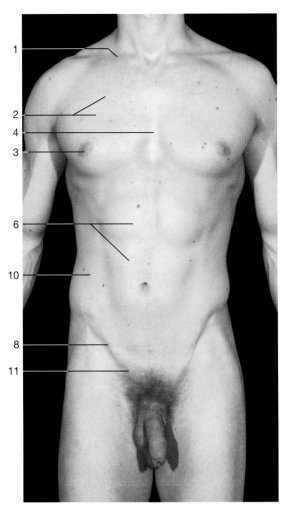

**Surface anatomy of the anterior body wall in the male.** Localization and structure of the muscles can be identified.

**Muscles of the anterior body wall.**

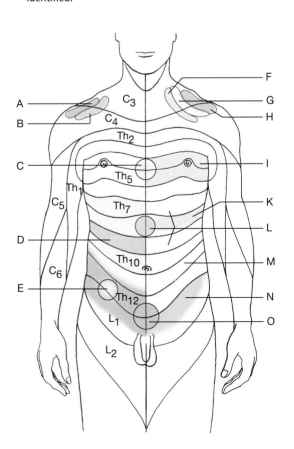

◁ **Segments of the anterior body wall.**
Head's zones are indicated.

**Head's zones**

A = Duodenum
B = Gallbladder, liver ($C_3$–$C_4$)
C = Esophagus ($Th_4$, $Th_5$)
D = Liver, gallbladder ($Th_6$–$Th_{11}$)
E = Colon, vermiform appendix ($Th_{11}$–$T_{12}$, $L_1$)
F = Heart
G = Pancreas
H = Stomach ($C_3$, $C_4$)
I = Heart ($Th_3$, $Th_4$)
K = Pancreas ($Th_8$)
L = Stomach ($Th_6$–$Th_9$)
M = Small intestine ($Th_{10}$–$L_1$)
N = Kidney, ureter, testis ($Th_{10}$–$L_1$)
O = Urinary bladder ($Th_{11}$–$L_1$)

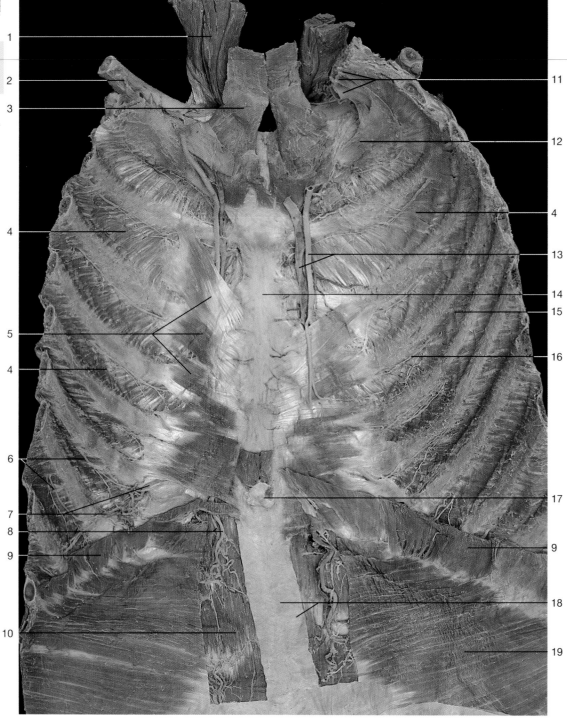

**Anterior thoracic wall** (posterior aspect). Diaphragm partly removed, posterior layer of rectus sheath fenestrated on both sides.

1 Sternocleidomastoid muscle (divided)
2 Clavicle
3 Sternothyroid muscle
4 Internal intercostal muscle
5 Transversus thoracis muscle
6 Intercostal arteries and nerves
7 Musculophrenic artery
8 Superior epigastric artery and vein
9 Diaphragm (divided)
10 Rectus abdominis muscle

11 Subclavian artery and brachial plexus
12 First rib
13 Internal thoracic artery and vein
14 Sternum
15 Innermost intercostal muscle
16 Intercostal artery and vein
17 Xiphoid process
18 Linea alba and
    posterior layer of rectus sheath
19 Transverse abdominal muscle

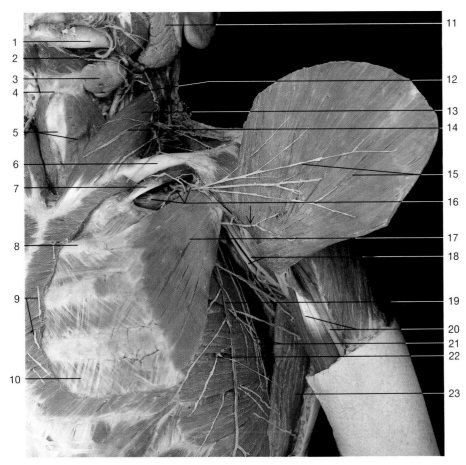

1 Mandible
2 Facial artery
3 Submandibular gland
4 Hyoid bone
5 Thyroid cartilage and sternohyoid muscle
6 Clavicle
7 Subclavius muscle
8 Second rib
9 Anterior cutaneous branches of intercostal nerves
10 External intercostal membrane
11 Parotid gland
12 External carotid artery
13 Sternocleidomastoid muscle and cutaneous branches of cervical plexus
14 Supraclavicular nerves
15 Pectoralis major muscle and lateral pectoral nerves
16 Thoraco-acromial artery and subclavian vein
17 Pectoralis minor muscle
18 Median and ulnar nerve
19 Thoraco-epigastric vein
20 Cephalic vein and long head of biceps brachii muscle
21 Lateral thoracic artery and long thoracic nerve
22 Lateral cutaneous branches of intercostal nerve
23 Latissimus dorsi muscle
24 Median nerve
25 Axillary artery
26 Intercostobrachial nerves
27 Thoracodorsal nerve
28 Long thoracic nerve
29 Latissimus dorsi muscle
30 Serratus anterior muscle
31 Thoraco-acromial artery
32 Clavicle
33 External intercostal muscle
34 Third rib
35 Internal intercostal muscle
36 Anterior intercostal artery and vein, and intercostal nerve
37 Costal arch or margin

**Thoracic wall** (anterior aspect). Left pectoralis major muscle has been divided and reflected. Note the connection of the cephalic vein with the subclavian vein.
Arrow: medial pectoral nerve.

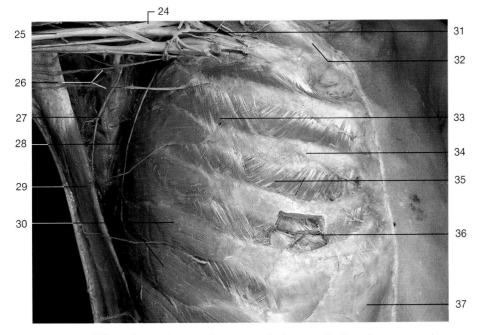

**Thoracic wall** (lateral aspect). Pectoralis major and minor muscles have been removed. A section of the fourth rib has been cut and removed to display the intercostal vessels and nerve.

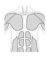

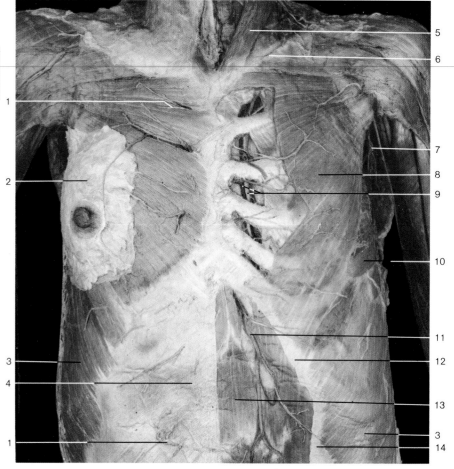

1   Anterior perforating branches
    of intercostal nerve
2   Mammary gland
3   External abdominal oblique muscle
4   Rectus sheath (anterior layer)
5   Sternocleidomastoid muscle
6   Clavicle
7   Lateral thoracic artery and vein
8   Pectoralis major muscle
9   Internal thoracic artery and vein
10  Serratus anterior muscle
11  Superior epigastric artery and vein
12  Costal margin
13  Rectus abdominis muscle
14  Cut edge of the anterior layer
    of the rectus sheath
15  Subclavian artery
16  Highest intercostal artery
17  Internal thoracic artery
18  Musculophrenic artery
19  Superficial epigastric artery
20  Deep circumflex iliac artery
21  Superior epigastric artery
22  Inferior epigastric artery
23  Superficial circumflex iliac artery

**Thoracic and abdominal walls** (anterior aspect). Dissection of the internal thoracic artery and vein. Left pectoralis major muscle partly removed. Anterior lamina of the rectus sheath on the left side has been removed.

**Main arteries of thoracic and abdominal walls** (anterior aspect).

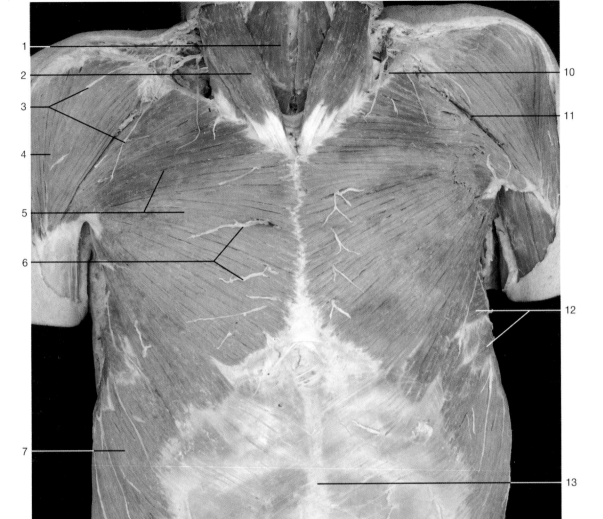

**Thoracic and abdominal walls with superficial muscles** (anterior aspect). The fascia of pectoralis major muscle and the abdominal wall have been removed; the anterior layer of the sheath of the rectus abdominis muscle is displayed.

1 Sternohyoid muscle
2 Sternocleidomastoid muscle
3 Supraclavicular nerves (branches of cervical plexus)
4 Deltoid muscle
5 Pectoralis major muscle
6 Anterior cutaneous branches of intercostal nerves
7 External abdominal oblique muscle
8 Lateral cutaneous branches of intercostal nerves

9 Umbilicus and umbilical ring
10 Clavicle
11 Cephalic vein
12 Serratus anterior muscle
13 Linea alba
14 Sheath of rectus abdominis muscle (anterior layer)
15 Inguinal ligament

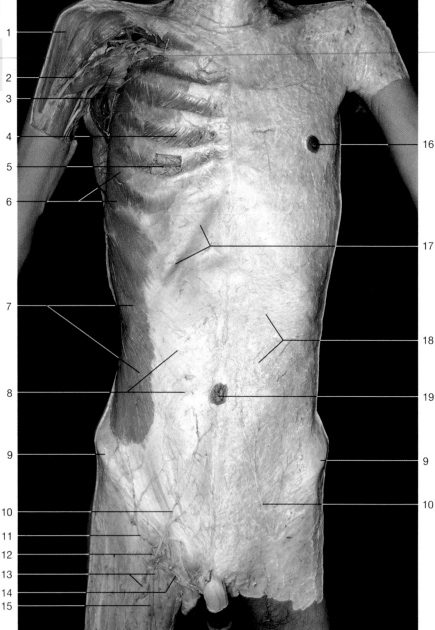

1 Deltoid muscle
2 Cephalic vein
3 Pectoralis major muscle (divided)
4 Internal intercostal muscle
5 Intercostal artery and vein (intercostal space, fenestrated)
6 Serratus anterior muscle
7 External abdominal oblique muscle
8 Anterior layer of rectus sheath
9 Iliac crest
10 Superficial epigastric vein
11 Superficial circumflex iliac vein
12 Saphenous opening
13 Superficial inguinal lymph nodes
14 Superficial external pudendal veins
15 Great saphenous vein
16 Nipple
17 Costal margin
18 Subcutaneous fatty tissue
19 Umbilicus
20 Anterior layer of rectus sheath
21 Rectus abdominis muscle
22 Posterior layer of rectus sheath
23 Internal abdominal oblique muscle
24 External abdominal oblique muscle (cut)
25 Transverse abdominal muscle
26 Transversalis fascia and peritoneum
27 Psoas major muscle
28 Body of lumbar vertebra ($L_4$)
29 Quadratus lumborum muscle
30 Medial tract of erector spinae muscle
31 Lateral tract of erector spinae muscle (longissimus and iliocostalis muscles)
32 Small intestine
33 Left ureter
34 Abdominal aorta
35 Inferior vena cava
36 Descending colon
37 Spinous process

**Thoracic and abdominal walls** (anterior aspect). Right pectoralis major and minor muscles are divided. Muscles of thoracic and abdominal walls on the right side are displayed.

**Horizontal section through the trunk** at the level of the umbilicus, superior to arcuate line (inferior aspect).

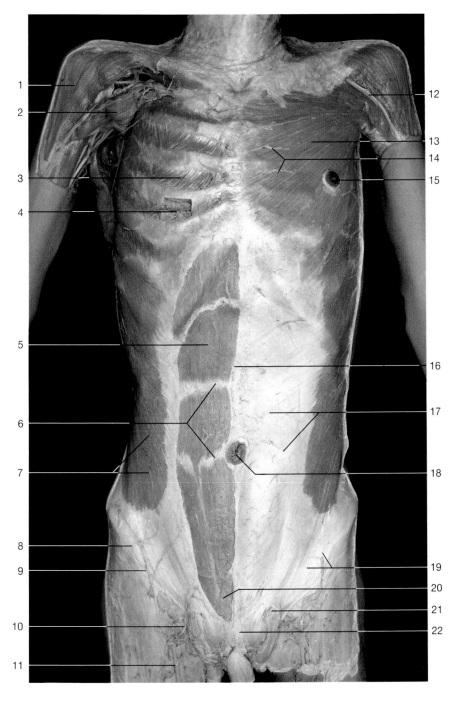

1  Deltoid muscle
2  Pectoralis major muscle (divided)
3  Internal intercostal muscle
4  Intercostal artery and vein
5  Rectus abdominis muscle
6  Tendinous intersections
7  External abdominal oblique muscle
8  Anterior superior iliac spine
9  Superficial circumflex iliac vein
10  Superficial epigastric vein
11  Great saphenous vein
12  Cephalic vein
13  Pectoralis major muscle
14  Anterior cutaneous branches
   of intercostal nerves
15  Nipple
16  Linea alba
17  Anterior layer of rectus sheath
18  Umbilicus
19  Inguinal ligament
20  Pyramidal muscle
21  Superficial inguinal ring and
   spermatic cord
22  Fundiform ligament of penis
23  Common iliac arteries
24  Small intestine
25  Inferior vena cava
26  Body of lumbar vertebra (L$_4$)
27  Psoas major muscle
28  Spinous process
29  Internal abdominal oblique muscle
30  Transverse abdominal muscle
31  Descending colon
32  Ilium
33  Multifidus muscle
34  Longissimus and iliocostalis muscles

**Thoracic and abdominal walls** (anterior aspect). Right pectoralis major and minor muscles and anterior layer of rectus sheath have been removed on the right side.

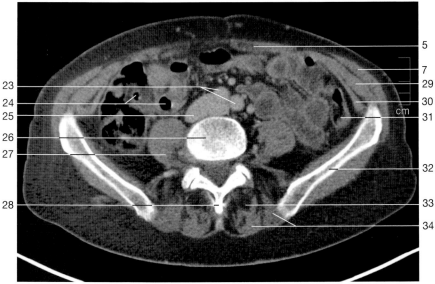

**Horizontal section through the trunk** at the level of fourth lumbar vertebra (inferior aspect, CT scan).

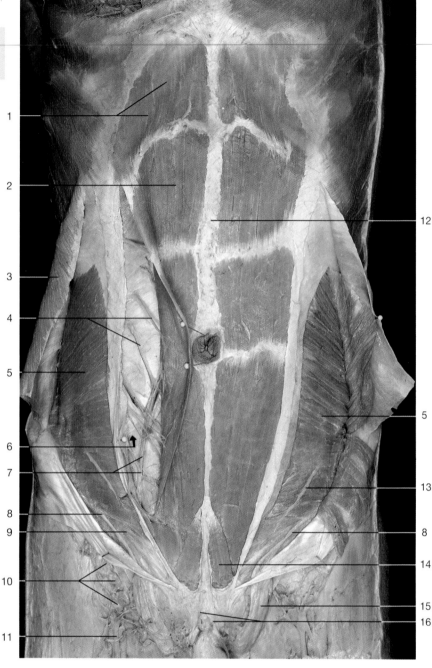

1　Costal margin
2　Rectus abdominis muscle
3　External abdominal oblique muscle (reflected)
4　Thoraco-abdominal (intercostal) nerves with accompanying vessels
5　Internal abdominal oblique muscle
6　Arcuate line (arrow)
7　Inferior epigastric artery and vein
8　Ilio-inguinal nerve
9　Position of deep inguinal ring
10　Superficial inguinal lymph nodes
11　Great saphenous vein
12　Linea alba
13　Iliohypogastric nerve
14　Pyramidal muscle
15　Spermatic cord
16　Fundiform ligament of penis

**Thoracic and abdominal walls** (anterior aspect). External abdominal oblique muscle has been divided and reflected on both sides. The right rectus muscle has been reflected medially to display the posterior layer of rectus sheath. Arrow: location of arcuate line.

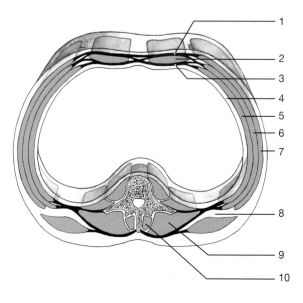

1　Anterior layer of rectus sheath
2　Rectus abdominis muscle
3　Posterior layer of rectus sheath
4　Transversalis fascia
5　Transverse abdominal muscle
6　Internal abdominal oblique muscle
7　External abdominal oblique muscle
8　Thoracolumbar fascia with superficial and deep layer
9　Lateral column of erector spinae muscle
10　Medial column of erector spinae muscle

**Horizontal section through the trunk,** superior to arcuate line (inferior aspect).

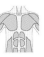

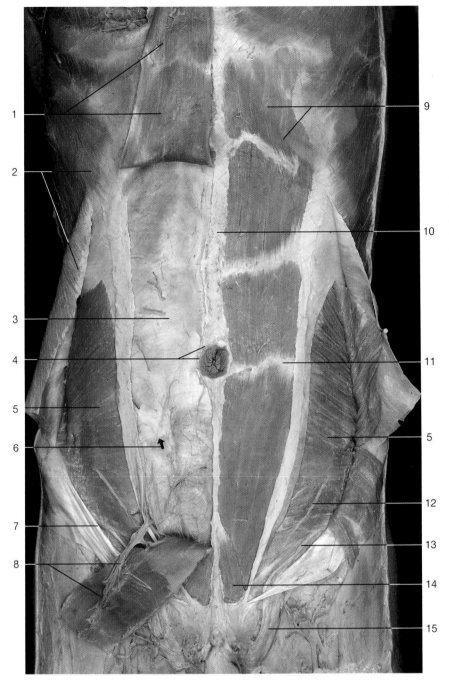

1   Rectus abdominis muscle (reflected)
2   External abdominal oblique muscle (divided)
3   Posterior layer of rectus sheath
4   Umbilical ring
5   Internal abdominal oblique muscle
6   Arcuate line (arrow)
7   Inguinal ligament
8   Inferior epigastric artery and vein and rectus abdominis muscle (divided and reflected)
9   Costal margin
10  Linea alba
11  Tendinous intersection
12  Iliohypogastric nerve
13  Ilio-inguinal nerve
14  Pyramidal muscle
15  Spermatic cord

**Thoracic and abdominal walls** (anterior aspect). External abdominal oblique muscle has been divided and reflected on both sides. The right rectus muscle has been cut and reflected to display the posterior layer of rectus sheath. Arrow: location of arcuate line.

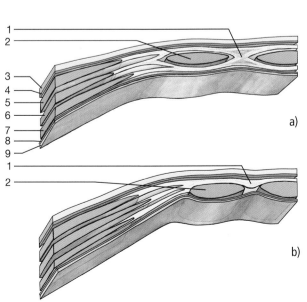

1   Linea alba
2   Rectus abdominis muscle
3   Epidermis
4   Fascia of external abdominal oblique muscle (green)
5   External abdominal oblique muscle
6   Internal abdominal oblique muscle
7   Transverse abdominal muscle
8   Transversalis fascia (green)
9   Peritoneum

**Transverse sections through the abdominal wall**
a) superior and
b) inferior
to arcuate line.

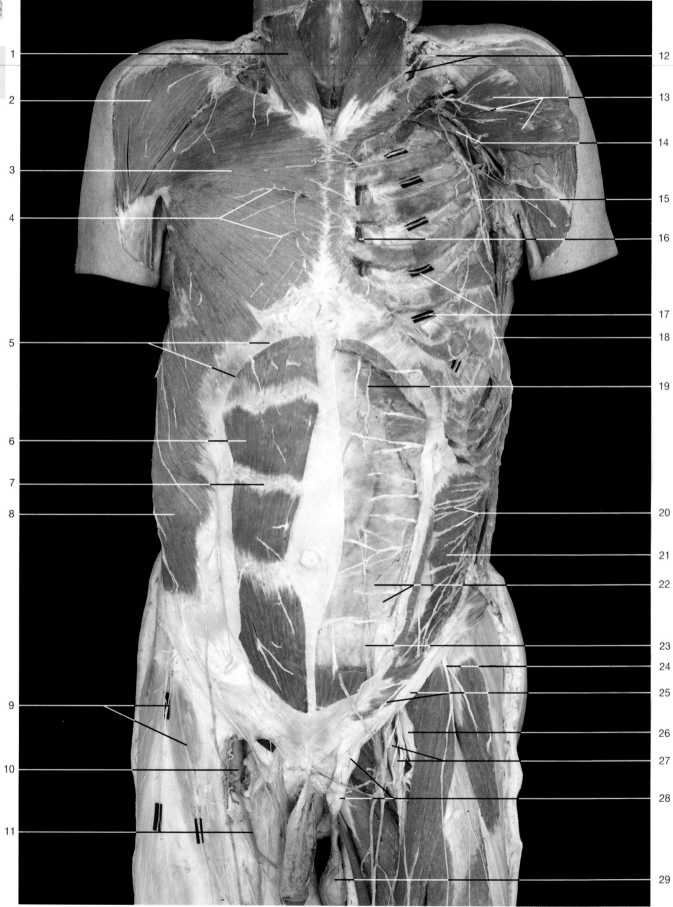

**Thoracic and abdominal walls with vessels and nerves** (anterior aspect). Right side: superficial layers; left side: deeper layers. Pectoralis major and minor muscles and the external and internal intercostal muscles on the left side have been removed to display the intercostal nerves. The anterior layer of rectus sheath, the left rectus abdominis muscle, and the external and internal abdominal oblique muscles have been removed to show the thoraco-abdominal nerves within the abdominal wall.

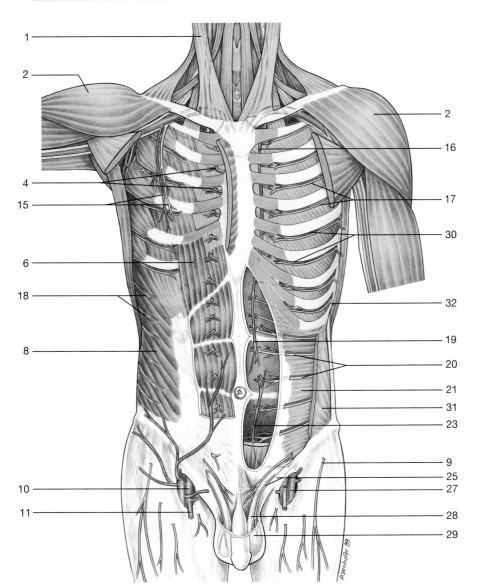

1  Sternocleidomastoid muscle
2  Deltoid muscle
3  Pectoralis major muscle
4  Anterior cutaneous branches
   of intercostal nerves
5  Cut edge of anterior layer
   of rectus sheath
6  Rectus abdominis muscle
7  Tendinous intersection
8  External abdominal oblique muscle
9  Lateral femoral cutaneous nerve
10 Femoral vein
11 Great saphenous vein
12 Medial supraclavicular nerves
13 Pectoralis minor muscle (reflected)
   and medial pectoral nerves
14 Axillary vein
15 Long thoracic nerve and
   lateral thoracic artery
16 Internal thoracic artery
17 Intercostal nerves
18 Lateral cutaneous branches
   of intercostal nerves
19 Superior epigastric artery
20 Thoraco-abdominal (intercostal) nerves
21 Transverse abdominal muscle
22 Posterior layer of rectus sheath
23 Inferior epigastric artery
24 Lateral femoral cutaneous nerve
25 Inguinal ligament and ilio-inguinal nerve
26 Femoral nerve
27 Femoral artery
28 Spermatic cord
29 Testis
30 Posterior intercostal arteries
31 Internal abdominal oblique muscle
32 Lateral cutaneous branch
   of intercostal nerve
33 Dorsal branch of spinal nerve
34 Latissimus dorsi muscle
35 Deep muscles of the back
   (medial and lateral tract)
36 Anterior layer of rectus sheath
37 Posterior layer of rectus sheath
38 Thoracolumbar fascia
39 Spinal cord
40 Aorta
41 Ventral root ⎫ of spinal
42 Dorsal root ⎭ nerve

**Thoracic and abdominal walls with vessels and nerves** (anterior aspect). Right side: superficial layers; left side: deeper layers. Note the segmental organization of the blood vessels and nerves.

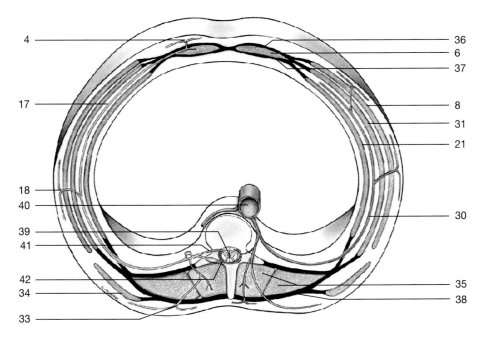

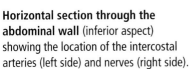

**Horizontal section through the abdominal wall** (inferior aspect) showing the location of the intercostal arteries (left side) and nerves (right side).

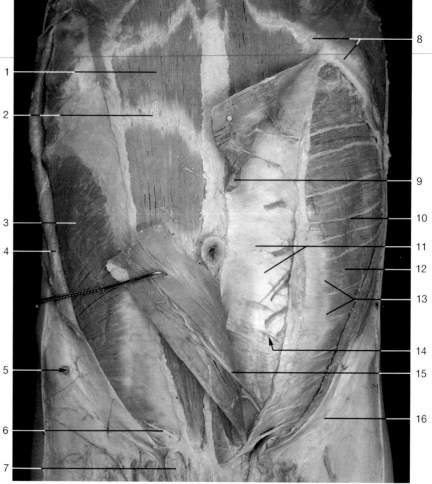

1   Rectus abdominis muscle
2   Tendinous intersection
3   Internal abdominal oblique muscle
4   External abdominal oblique muscle
    (reflected)
5   Anterior superior iliac spine
6   Ilio-inguinal nerve
7   Spermatic cord
8   Costal margin
9   Superior epigastric artery
10  Thoraco-abdominal (intercostal) nerves
11  Posterior layer of rectus sheath
12  Transverse abdominal muscle
13  Semilunar line
14  Arcuate line
15  Inferior epigastric artery
16  Inguinal ligament

**Abdominal wall with vessels and nerves** (anterior aspect). The left rectus abdominis muscle has been divided and reflected to display the inferior epigastric vessels. The left internal abdominal oblique muscle has been removed to show the thoraco-abdominal nerves.

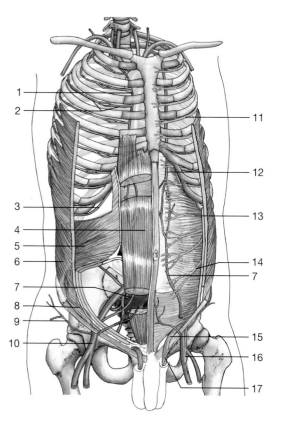

1   Internal thoracic artery
2   Intercostal artery
3   Musculophrenic artery
4   Rectus abdominis muscle
5   Internal abdominal oblique muscle
6   External abdominal oblique muscle
7   Inferior epigastric artery
8   Deep circumflex iliac artery
9   Superficial circumflex iliac artery
10  Femoral artery
11  Intercostal nerve
12  Superior epigastric artery
13  Intercostal nerve
14  Iliohypogastric nerve ($L_1$)
15  Spermatic cord
16  Femoral branch of genitofemoral nerve
17  Genital branch of genitofemoral nerve

**Thoracic and abdominal walls with arteries and nerves** (anterior aspect).

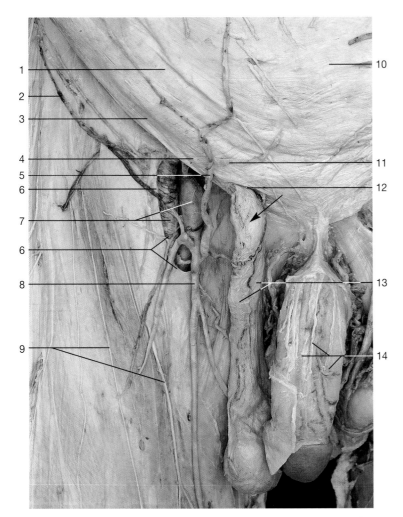

1 Aponeurosis of external abdominal oblique muscle
2 Superficial circumflex iliac vein
3 Inguinal ligament
4 Lateral crus of inguinal ring
5 Superficial epigastric vein
6 Saphenous opening
7 Femoral artery and vein
8 Great saphenous vein
9 Anterior cutaneous branches of femoral nerve
10 Anterior layer of rectus sheath
11 Intercrural fibers
12 Superficial inguinal ring
13 Spermatic cord and genital branch
   of genitofemoral nerve
14 Penis with dorsal nerves and
   deep dorsal vein of penis
15 Aponeurosis of external abdominal oblique muscle
   (divided and reflected)
16 Internal abdominal oblique muscle
17 Ilio-inguinal nerve
18 Anterior cutaneous branches
   of iliohypogastric nerve
19 Superficial external pudendal veins

**Inguinal canal in the male,** right side (superficial layer, anterior aspect). There is a small inguinal hernia (arrow).

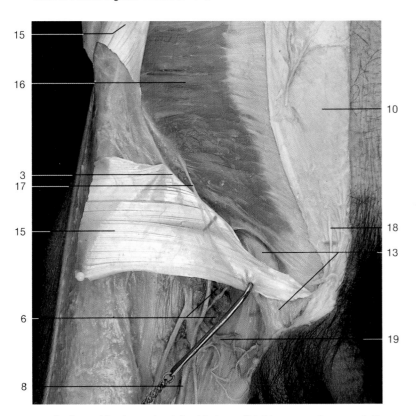

**Inguinal canal in the male,** right side (superficial layer, anterior aspect). The external abdominal oblique muscle has been divided to display the inguinal canal.

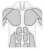

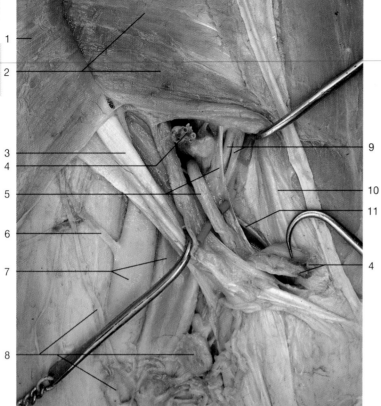

1   Internal abdominal oblique muscle (reflected)
2   Transverse abdominal muscle
3   Inguinal ligament
4   Spermatic cord
    with the exception of the ductus deferens
    (divided and reflected)
5   Ductus deferens and interfoveolar ligament
6   Superficial circumflex iliac artery
7   Femoral artery and vein
8   Superficial inguinal lymph nodes and
    inguinal lymph vessel
9   Inferior epigastric artery and vein
10  Falx inguinalis or conjoint tendon (cut)
11  Pubic branch of inferior epigastric artery
12  Iliacus muscle
13  Ureter
14  Ductus deferens (in situ)
15  Femoral nerve
16  Spermatic cord with ductus deferens and
    external spermatic fascia
17  Cremaster muscle
18  Internal spermatic fascia
19  Tunica vaginalis testis
20  Testis and epididymis
21  Rectum
22  Anterior layer of rectus sheath
23  Intercrural fibrae
24  Urinary bladder
25  Superficial inguinal ring
26  Saphenous opening with great saphenous vein
27  Deep dorsal vein of penis
28  Penis
29  Glans of penis
30  Rectus abdominis muscle
31  Deep inguinal ring
32  Pampiniform venous plexus and testicular artery
33  Fascia lata and sartorius muscle
34  Anterior superior iliac spine
35  Inferior epigastric artery
36  Lateral femoral cutaneous nerve
37  Ilioinguinal nerve
38  Suspensory ligament of penis
39  Sartorius muscle
40  External abdominal oblique muscle
41  Dartos fascia and scrotal skin
42  Ductus deferens
43  Vaginal process
44  Peritoneum

**Inguinal canal in the male,** right side (deep layer, anterior aspect).
Spermatic cord with exception of ductus deferens (probe) has been divided
and reflected.

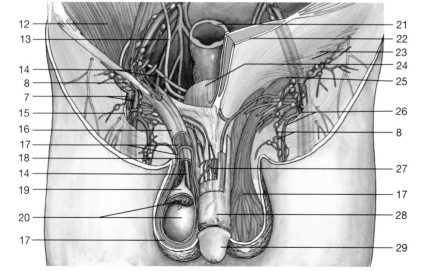

**General characteristics of lower part of anterior abdominal wall and
inguinal canal.**

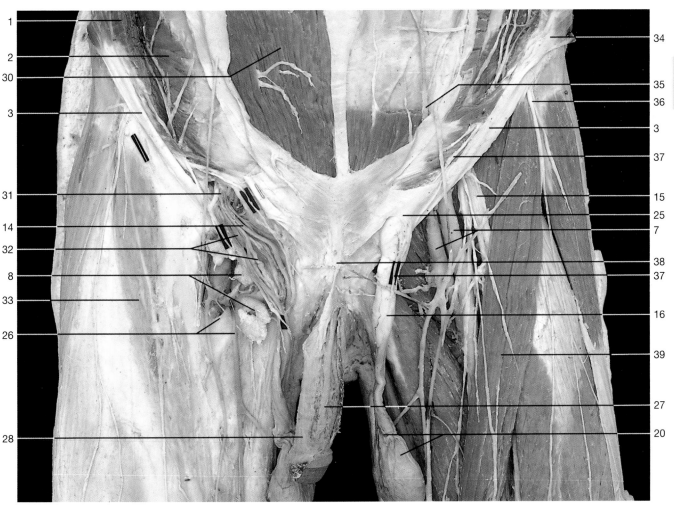

**Inguinal and femoral regions in the male** (anterior aspect). On the right, the spermatic cord was dissected to display the ductus deferens and the accompanying vessels and nerves. The fascia lata on the left side has been removed.

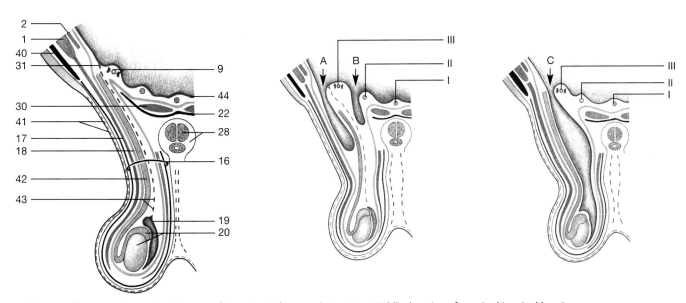

**Layers of spermatic cord and types of hernias.** Left: normal situation. Middle: location of acquired inguinal hernias:
A = indirect inguinal hernia; B = direct inguinal hernia. Right: congenital indirect inguinal hernia (C); the vaginal process remained open.
I   = Median umbilical fold containing urachus chord.
II  = Medial umbilical fold with remnants of umbilical artery.
III = Lateral umbilical fold with inferior epigastric artery and vein.

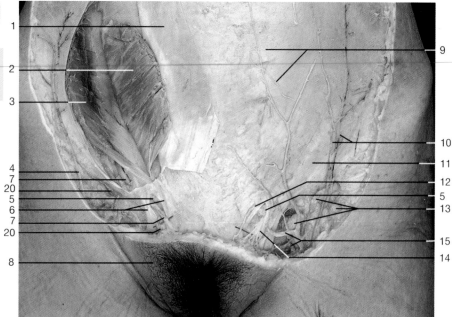

1 Aponeurosis of external abdominal oblique muscle
2 Internal abdominal oblique muscle (divided and reflected)
3 Transverse abdominal muscle
4 Superficial circumflex iliac artery and vein
5 Superficial inguinal ring with fat pad
6 Medial and lateral crural fibers
7 Round ligament (ligamentum teres uteri)
8 Labium majus pudendi
9 Anterior layer of rectus sheath
10 Superficial epigastric artery and vein
11 Inguinal ligament
12 Cutaneous branch of ilio-inguinal nerve
13 Superficial inguinal lymph nodes
14 Entrance of round ligament into the labium majus
15 External pudendal artery and vein
16 Position of deep inguinal ring
17 Ilio-inguinal nerve
18 Internal abdominal oblique muscle
19 Pubic branch of inferior epigastric artery
20 Genital branch of genitofemoral nerve
21 Fat pad of inguinal canal
22 Ilio-inguinal nerve
23 Sheath of round ligament (inguinal canal)
24 Transversalis fascia

**Inguinal region in the female** (anterior aspect). Left side: superficial layer; right side: external and internal abdominal oblique muscles divided and reflected.

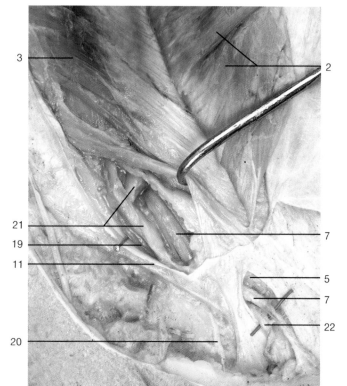

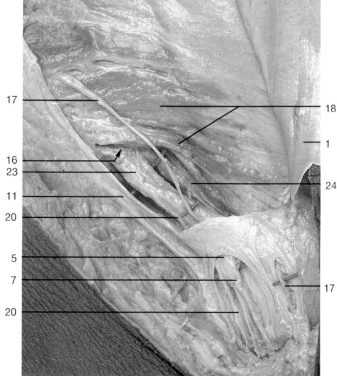

**Inguinal canal in the female,** right side (anterior aspect). The external abdominal oblique muscle has been divided and reflected to display the ilio-inguinal nerve and the round ligament.

**Inguinal canal in the female,** right side (anterior aspect). The external and internal abdominal oblique muscles have been divided and reflected to show the content of the inguinal canal.

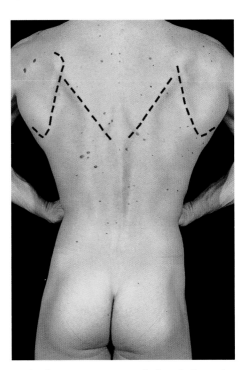

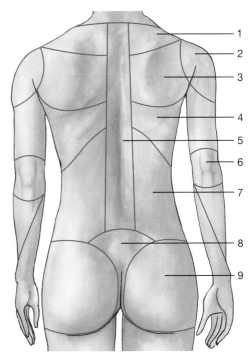

**Back of a strong man.** Borderlines indicate the scapula and the trapezius muscle.

**Regions of the back in the female.**

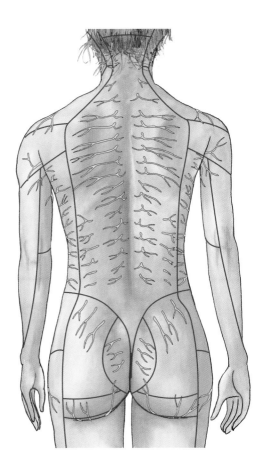

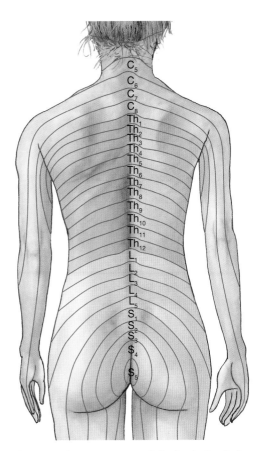

**Innervation of the back.** The dorsal branches of the spinal nerves display a segmental arrangement. The segmental innervation regions of the back are indicated.

**Segmental arrangement of the back.** Cervical (C$_1$–C$_8$; only shown are C$_5$–C$_8$), thoracal (Th$_1$–Th$_{12}$), lumbar (L$_1$–L$_5$), and sacral (S$_1$–S$_5$) segments are colored different.

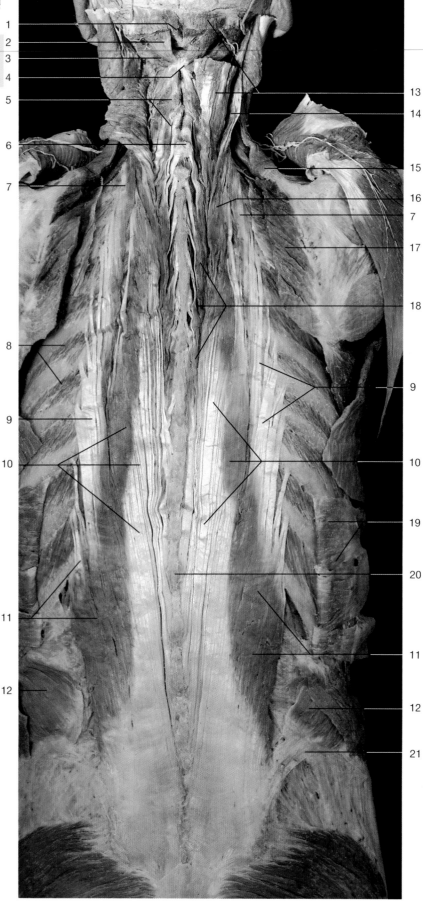

**Muscles of the back.** Dissection of the erector spinae muscle (lateral column of the intrinsic back muscles).

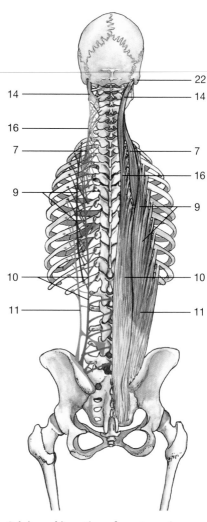

**Origin and insertion of erector spinae muscle** (sacrospinal system).

1   Rectus capitis posterior minor muscle
2   Rectus capitis posterior major muscle
3   Obliquus capitis inferior muscle
4   Spinous process of axis
5   Semispinalis cervicis muscle
6   Spinous process
    of seventh cervical vertebra
7   Iliocostalis cervicis muscle
8   External intercostal muscles
9   Iliocostalis thoracis muscle
10   Longissimus thoracis muscle
11   Iliocostalis lumborum muscle
12   Internal abdominal oblique muscle
13   Semispinalis capitis muscle (divided)
14   Longissimus capitis muscle
15   Levator scapulae muscle
16   Longissimus cervicis muscle
17   Rhomboid major muscle
18   Spinalis thoracis muscle
19   Serratus posterior inferior muscle
    (reflected)
20   Spinous process
    of second lumbar vertebra
21   Iliac crest
22   Mastoid process

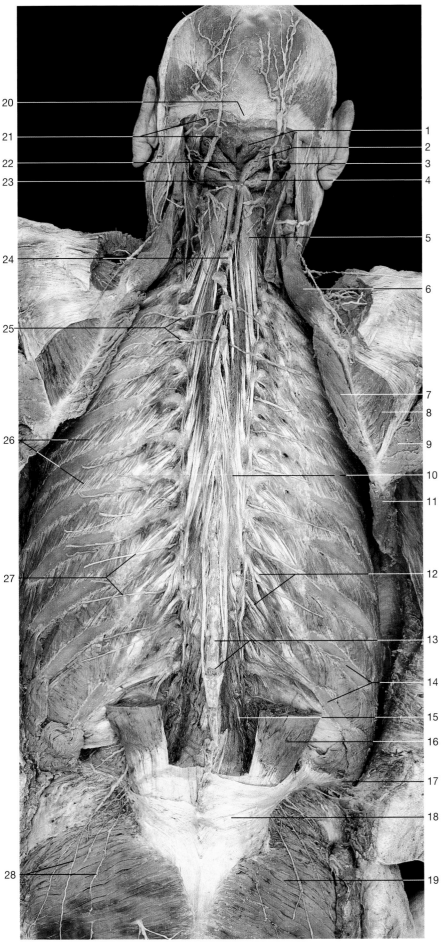

1  Rectus capitis posterior minor muscle
2  Rectus capitis posterior major muscle
3  Obliquus capitis superior muscle
4  Obliquus capitis inferior muscle
5  Semispinalis cervicis muscle
6  Levator scapulae muscle
7  Rhomboideus major muscle
8  Scapula with infraspinatus muscle
9  Teres major muscle
10  Spinalis muscle
11  Latissimus dorsi muscle
12  Levatores costarum muscles
13  Spinous processes of lumbar vertebrae
14  Ribs ($Th_{11}$, $Th_{12}$)
15  Multifidus muscle
16  Longissimus and iliocostalis muscles (cut)
17  Iliac crest (lumbar triangle)
18  Thoracolumbar fascia
19  Gluteus maximus muscle
20  External occipital protuberance
21  Occipital artery and
    greater occipital nerve ($C_2$)
22  Posterior tubercle of atlas
23  Spinous process of axis
24  Spinous process
    of seventh cervical vertebra
    (vertebra prominens)
25  Medial branches of dorsal branches
    of spinal nerves
26  External intercostal muscles
27  Lateral branches of dorsal branches
    of spinal nerves
28  Superior cluneal nerves

**Muscles of the back.** Dissection of the deeper layer of the intrinsic back muscles.
Longissimus and iliocostalis muscles are cut.

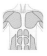

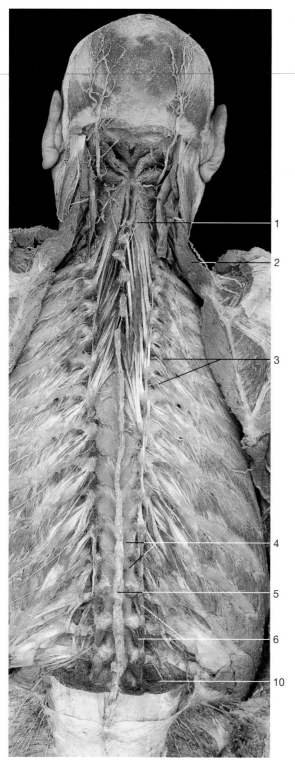

**Muscles of the back** (deepest layer).

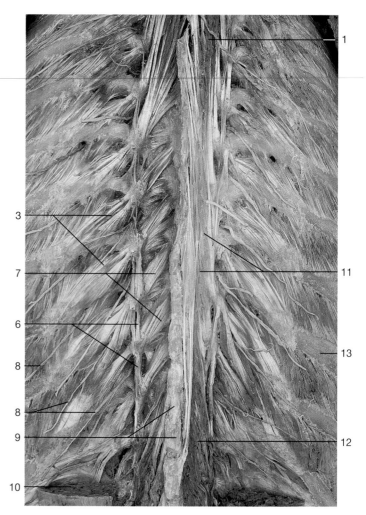

**Muscles of the back** (deepest layer). Lumbar region (higher magnification).

1    Semispinalis cervicis muscle
2    Levator scapulae muscle
3    Levatores costarum muscles
4    Vertebral arches of lumbar vertebrae
5    Supraspinal ligaments
6    Intertransverse lumbar muscles
7    Lumbar rotator muscles
8    Cutaneous branches of spinal nerves
9    Lumbar interspinal muscles
10   Longissimus and iliocostalis muscles (cut)
11   Spinal muscle of the back
12   Multifidus muscle
13   Tenth rib ($T_{10}$)

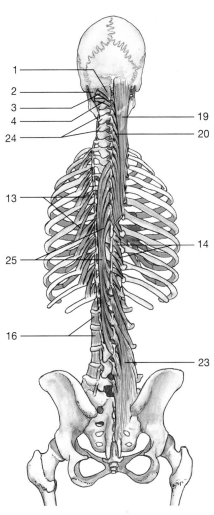

**Origin and insertion of erector spinae muscle, medial column** (transversospinal and intertransversal system).

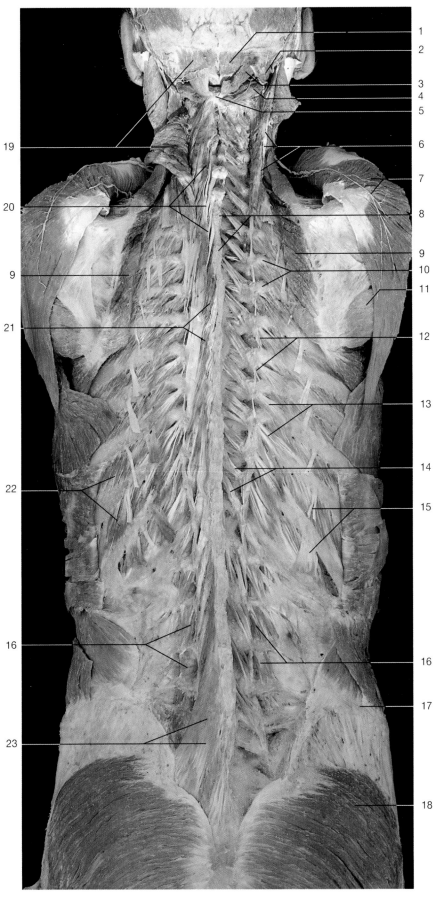

**Muscles of the back.** Transversospinal muscles, deepest layer on the right, where all parts of semispinalis and multifidus muscles have been removed.

1 Rectus capitis posterior minor muscle
2 Obliquus capitis superior muscle
3 Rectus capitis posterior major muscle
4 Obliquus capitis inferior muscle
5 Spinous process of axis
6 Longissimus capitis muscle
7 Trapezius muscle (reflected) and accessory nerve (n. XI)
8 Spinous processes
9 Rhomboid major muscle
10 Transverse processes of thoracic vertebrae
11 Teres major muscle
12 Intertransverse ligaments
13 Levatores costarum muscles
14 Rotatores muscles
15 Tendons of iliocostalis muscle
16 Intertransversarii laterales lumborum muscles
17 Iliac crest
18 Gluteus maximus muscle
19 Semispinalis capitis muscle
20 Semispinalis cervicis muscle
21 Semispinalis thoracis muscle
22 External intercostal muscles
23 Multifidus muscle
24 Posterior cervical intertransversarii muscles
25 Spinalis thoracis muscle

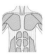

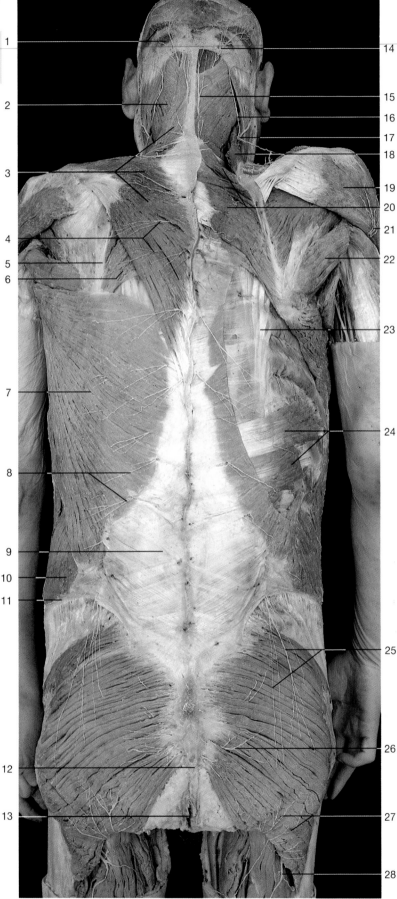

1   Occipital belly of occipitofrontalis muscle
2   Splenius capitis muscle
3   Trapezius muscle
4   Medial cutaneous branches of dorsal rami
    of spinal nerves
5   Medial margin of scapula
6   Rhomboid major muscle
7   Latissimus dorsi muscle
8   Lateral cutaneous branches of dorsal rami
    of spinal nerves
9   Thoracolumbar fascia
10  External abdominal oblique muscle
11  Iliac crest
12  Last coccygeal vertebra
13  Anus
14  Greater occipital nerve
15  Third occipital nerve
16  Lesser occipital nerve
17  Cutaneous branches of cervical plexus
18  Levator scapulae muscle
19  Deltoid muscle
20  Rhomboid major and minor muscles
21  Upper lateral cutaneous nerve of arm
    (branch of axillary nerve)
22  Teres major muscle
23  Iliocostalis thoracis muscle
24  Serratus posterior inferior muscle
25  Superior cluneal nerves
26  Middle cluneal nerves
27  Inferior cluneal nerves
28  Posterior femoral cutaneous nerve

**Innervation of the back** (superficial [left] and deeper [right] layers).
Right trapezius and latissimus dorsi muscles have been removed.

▷   **To page 231:**

1   Trapezius muscle
2   Infraspinatus muscle
3   Left latissimus dorsi muscle
4   Thoracolumbar fascia
5   Splenius cervicis muscle
6   Serratus posterior superior muscle
7   Medial branches of dorsal rami
    of thoracic spinal nerves
8   Lateral branches of dorsal rami
    of thoracic spinal nerves
9   Iliocostalis muscle
10  Serratus posterior inferior muscle
11  Latissimus dorsi muscle (reflected)

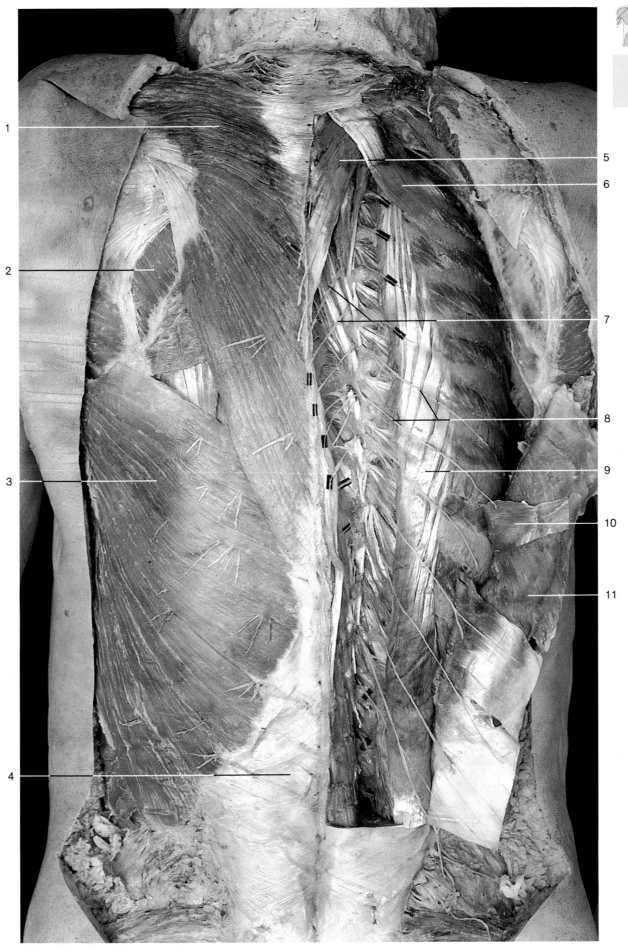

**Innervation of the back.** Dissection of the dorsal branches of the spinal nerves. On the right, longissimus thoracis muscle has been removed and iliocostalis muscle laterally reflected.

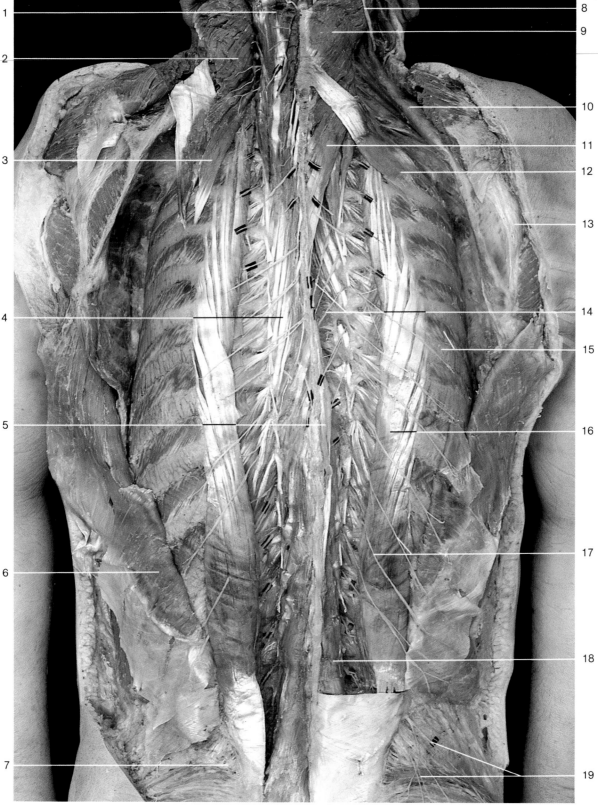

**Innervation of the back** (deeper layer).

1 Semispinalis capitis muscle
2 Left splenius capitis muscle
(cut and reflected)
3 Left splenius cervicis muscle
(cut and reflected)
4 Semispinalis thoracis muscle
5 Spinalis thoracis muscle
6 Latissimus dorsi muscle (reflected)

7 Iliac crest
8 Lesser occipital nerve
9 Splenius capitis muscle
10 Levator scapulae muscle
11 Splenius cervicis muscle
12 Serratus posterior superior muscle
13 Scapula

14 Medial branches of dorsal rami
of spinal nerves
15 Rib and external intercostal muscle
16 Iliocostalis thoracis muscle
17 Lateral branches of dorsal rami
of spinal nerves
18 Multifidus muscle
19 Superior cluneal nerves

1 Greater occipital nerve ($C_2$)
2 Suboccipital nerve ($C_1$)
3 Medial branches of dorsal rami of spinal nerves
4 Lateral branches of dorsal rami of spinal nerves
5 Superior cluneal nerves ($L_1$–$L_3$)
6 Middle cluneal nerves ($S_1$–$S_3$)
7 Inferior cluneal nerves
   (derived from branches of the sacral plexus, ventral rami)
8 Lesser occipital nerve
9 Great auricular nerve
10 Trapezius muscle
11 Deltoid muscle
12 Latissimus dorsi muscle
13 Gluteus maximus muscle
14 External intercostal muscle
15 Internal intercostal muscle
16 Innermost intercostal muscle
17 Dorsal ramus of spinal nerve
18 Spinal nerve and spinal ganglion
19 Sympathetic trunk with ganglion
20 Intercostal nerve
21 Lateral cutaneous branch ⎫ of intercostal nerve
22 Anterior cutaneous branch ⎭
23 Longissimus thoracis muscle
24 Spinal cord
25 Aorta
26 Esophagus
27 Body of rib
28 Thoracic rib
29 Thoracic duct
30 Azygos vein

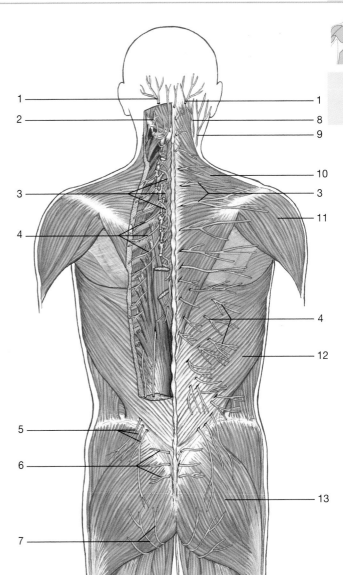

**General characteristics of the innervation of the back.**
Distribution of dorsal branches of spinal nerves. Note the segmental arrangement of the innervation of the dorsal part of the trunk.

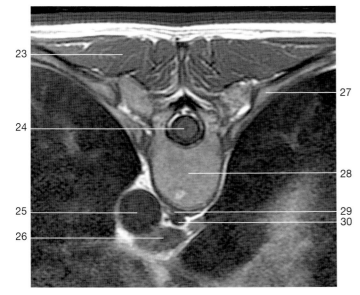

**Horizontal section through the posterior part of the thoracic wall** (MRI scan). (From Heuck et al., MRT-Atlas, 2009.)

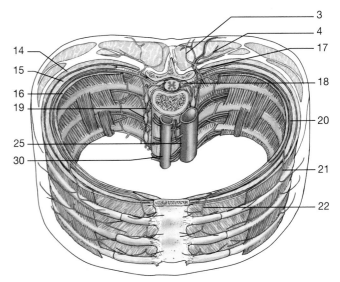

**Horizontal section through the anterior and posterior parts of the thoracic wall.** Position and branches of spinal nerves and vessels in one thoracic segment are shown.

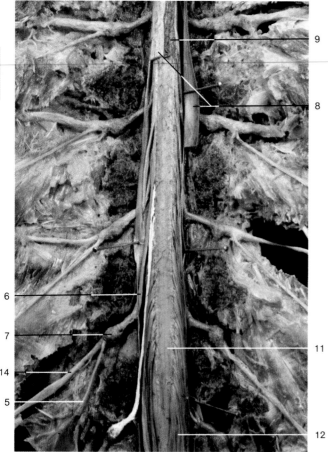

**Lumbar part of spinal cord** (posterior aspect). Note the relation between the nervous and muscular segments.

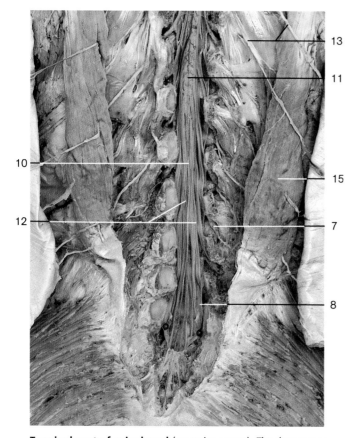

**Terminal part of spinal cord** (posterior aspect). The dura mater has been removed.

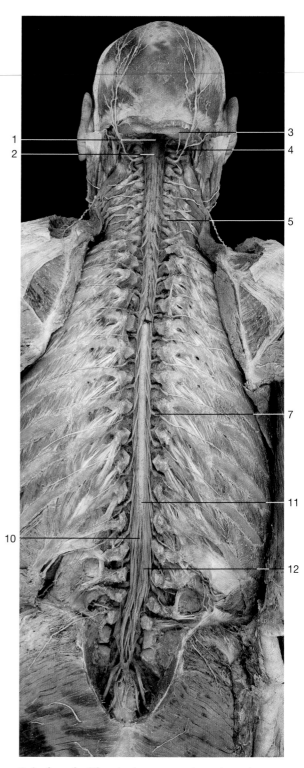

**Spinal cord with spinal nerves and meningeal coverings.** The vertebral canal has been opened. Longissimus dorsi and iliocostal muscles have been removed.

| | |
|---|---|
| 1 Cerebellomedullary cistern | 9 Spinal arachnoid mater |
| 2 Medulla oblongata | 10 Filum terminale |
| 3 Third cervical nerve (C$_3$) | 11 Conus medullaris |
| 4 Greater occipital nerve (C$_2$) | 12 Cauda equina |
| 5 Dorsal primary ramus | 13 Lateral branch of dorsal ramus of spinal nerve |
| 6 Dorsal roots | |
| 7 Spinal ganglion | 14 Ventral ramus of spinal nerve (intercostal nerve) |
| 8 Spinal dura mater | 15 Iliocostalis muscle |

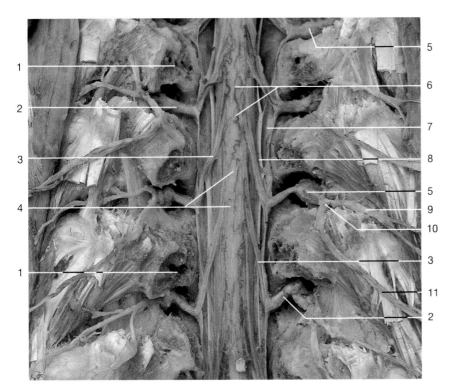

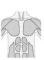

1 Arch of vertebra (divided)
2 Spinal nerve with meningeal coverings
3 Dorsal roots of thoracic spinal nerves
4 Spinal cord (thoracic portion)
5 Spinal ganglia with meningeal coverings
6 Pia mater with blood vessels
7 Dura mater (opened)
8 Denticulate ligament
9 Lateral branch of dorsal ramus of spinal nerve
10 Dorsal ramus of spinal nerve
   (dividing into a medial and lateral branch)
11 Medial branch of dorsal ramus of spinal nerve
12 Spinal dura mater
13 Spinal nerves of sacral segments
14 Filum terminale

**Thoracic part of spinal cord** (posterior aspect). Vertebral canal and dura mater have been opened.

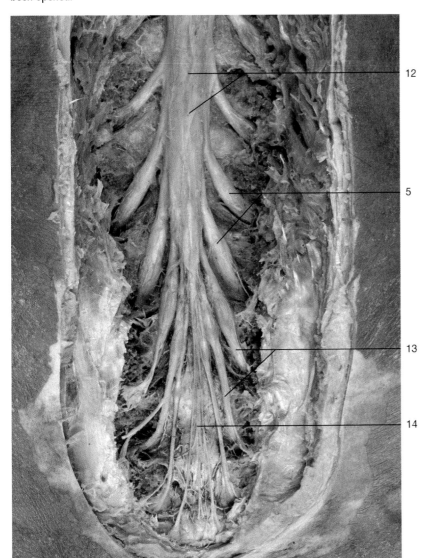

**Terminal part of spinal cord with dura mater** (posterior aspect). Dorsal part of sacrum has been removed.

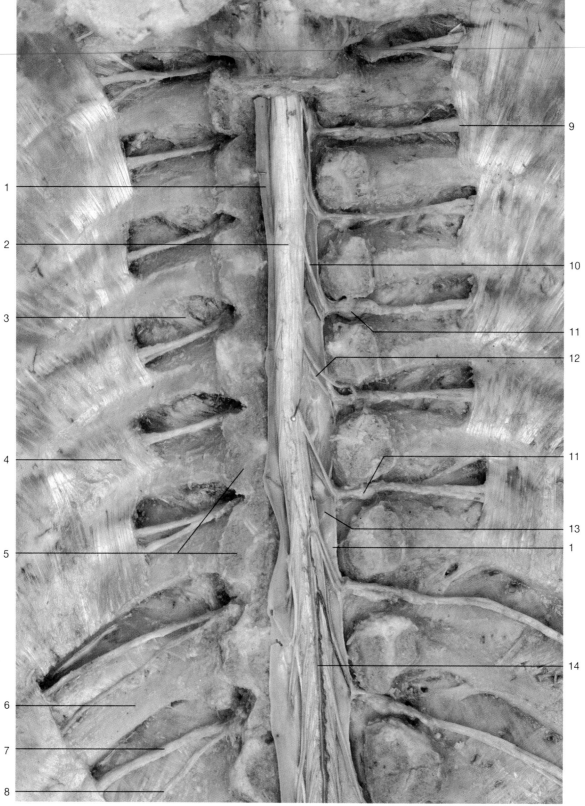

**Spinal cord with intercostal nerves.** Inferior thoracic region (anterior aspect). Anterior portion of thoracic vertebrae removed, dural sheath opened, and spinal cord slightly reflected to the right to display the dorsal and ventral roots.

1  Dura mater
2  Spinal cord
3  Costotransverse ligament
4  Innermost intercostal muscle
5  Vertebral arches (cut surfaces)

6  Eleventh rib
7  Intercostal nerve
8  Collateral branch of intercostal nerve
9  Intercostal nerve
   (entering the intermuscular interval)

10  Anterior root filaments
11  Spinal (dorsal root) ganglion
12  Posterior root filaments
13  Arachnoid mater and denticulate ligament
14  Anterior spinal artery

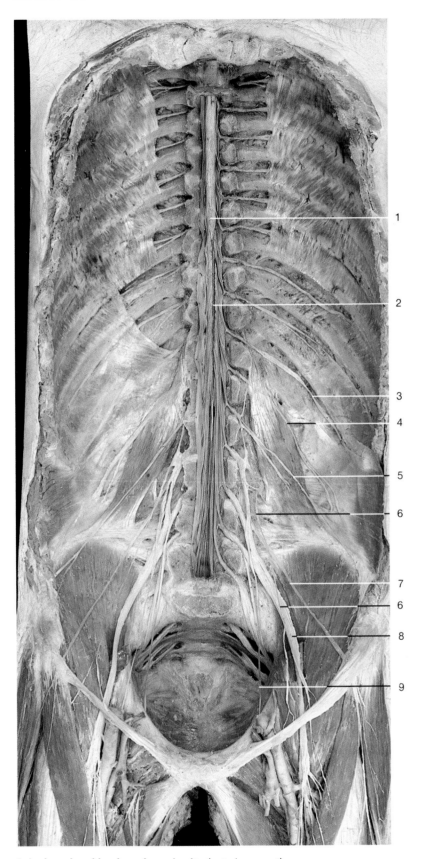

**Spinal cord and lumbar plexus in situ** (anterior aspect).

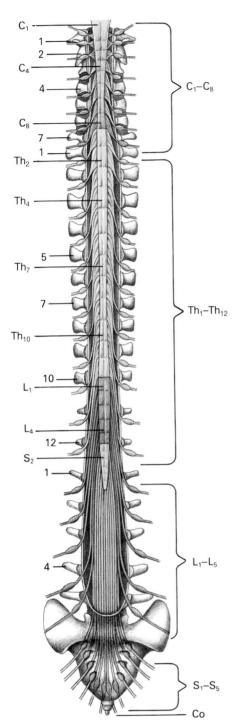

**Organization of spinal cord segments in relation to the vertebral column** (anterior aspect).
C = cervical; Th = thoracic; L = lumbar; S = sacral segments; Co = coccygeal bone. Numbers indicate the related vertebrae.

| | |
|---|---|
| 1 Conus medullaris | 6 Genitofemoral nerve |
| 2 Filum terminale | 7 Lateral femoral cutaneous nerve |
| 3 Subcostal nerve | 8 Femoral nerve |
| 4 Iliohypogastric nerve | 9 Obturator nerve |
| 5 Ilio-inguinal nerve | |

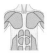

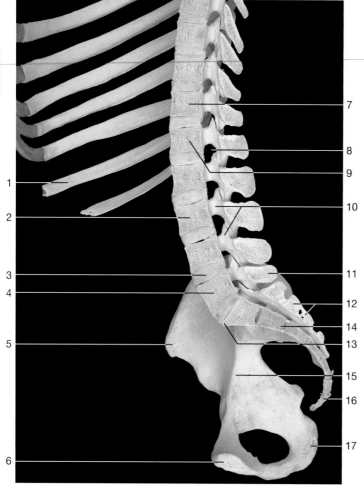

**Lumbar part of vertebral column with pelvis and lower thoracic part** (sagittal section, medial aspect).

1 Eleventh rib
2 Body of third lumbar vertebra
3 Intervertebral disc
4 Body of fifth lumbar vertebra
5 Anterior superior iliac spine
6 Symphysial surface
7 Body of twelfth thoracic vertebra
8 Intervertebral foramen
9 Body of first lumbar vertebra
10 Vertebral canal
11 Spinous process of fifth lumbar vertebra
12 Sacrum (median sacral crest)
13 Promontory (promontorium)
14 Sacrum
15 Arcuate line
16 Coccyx
17 Ischial tuberosity
18 Sympathetic trunk with ganglia
19 Ureter
20 Iliohypogastric nerve ($Th_{12}$, $L_1$)
21 Ilio-inguinal nerve ($L_1$)
22 Femoral nerve ($L_1$–$L_4$)
23 Genitofemoral nerve ($L_1$, $L_2$)
24 Inferior hypogastric plexus
25 Ductus deferens
26 Urinary bladder
27 Medullary cone of spinal cord
28 Root filaments of spinal nerves
29 Subarachnoid space
   (filled with cerebrospinal fluid) (blue)
30 Terminal filament of spinal cord
31 Sacral plexus
32 Pelvic splanchnic nerves (nervi erigentes)
33 Rectum

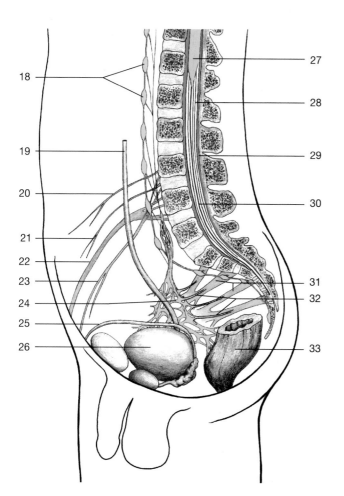

**Lumbar part of vertebral column with spinal cord and root filaments** (sagittal section). Note the high location of the medullary cone. Sacral plexus and inferior hypogastric plexus are schematically shown.

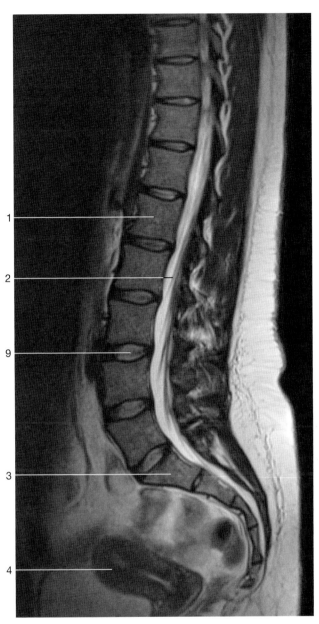

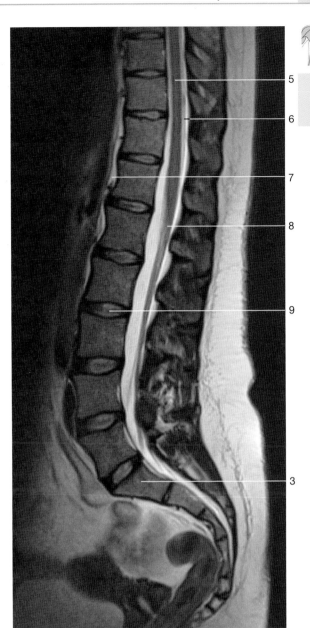

**Paramedian section through the lumbar part of vertebral column with vertebral canal and spinal cord**
(dashed line in the schematic drawing; MRI scan).
(Prof. Uder, Dept. of Radiology, Univ. Erlangen-Nuremberg, Germany.)

**Median section through the lumbar part of vertebral column with vertebral canal and spinal cord**
(continuous line in the schematic drawing; MRI scan).
(Prof. Uder, Dept. of Radiology, Univ. Erlangen-Nuremberg, Germany.)

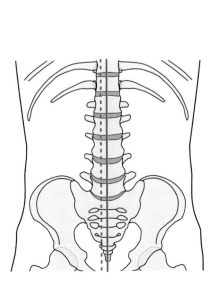

1  First lumbar vertebra (L₁)
2  Root filaments of spinal nerves
3  Sacrum
4  Uterus
5  Spinal cord
6  Dura mater of spinal cord
7  Anterior longitudinal ligament
8  Medullary cone of spinal cord
9  Intervertebral disc of lumbar vertebra

**Localization of the sections** (red lines).

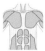

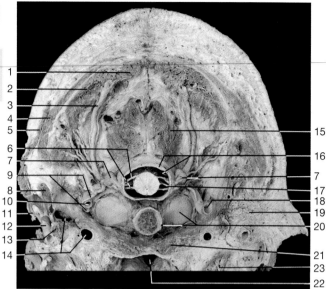

**Horizontal section through the neck.** Dissection of the second cervical spinal nerve. Posterior surface at top of figure.

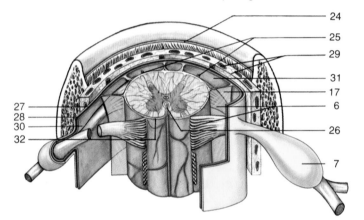

**Spinal cord with meningeal coverings** (anterior aspect).

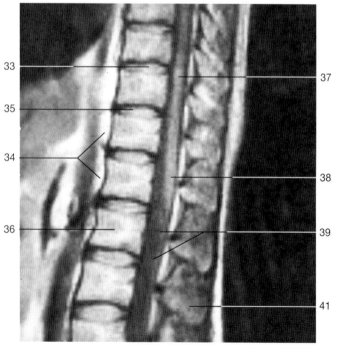

**Sagittal section through the vertebral canal** (Th₉–L₂). (MRI scan).

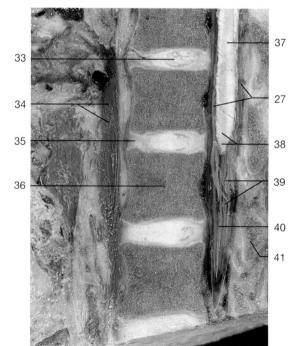

**Sagittal section through the vertebral canal** (Th₁₂–L₂). Note the red bone marrow (unfixed).

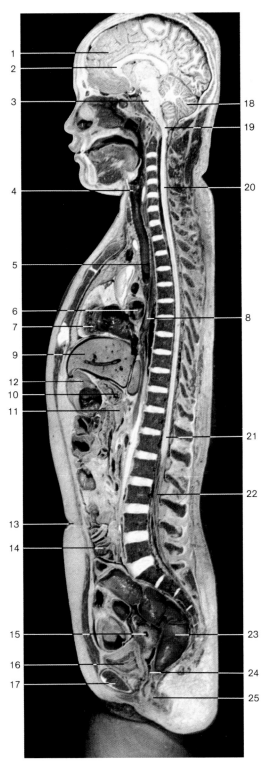

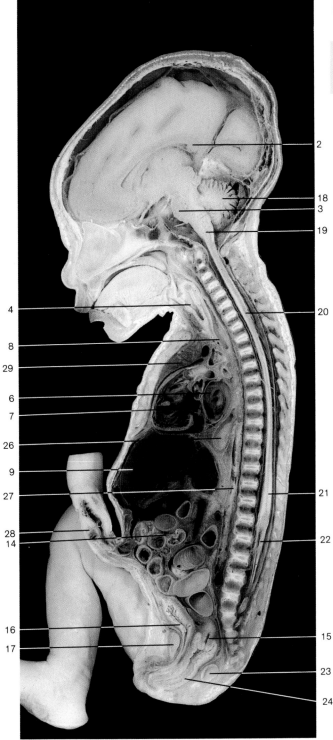

**Median section through the head and trunk in the adult** (female). The conus medullaris of the spinal cord is located at the level of L₁.

**Median section through the head and trunk in the neonate.**
Note that in the neonate the conus medullaris of the spinal cord extends far more caudally than in the adult.

| | | | | | |
|---|---|---|---|---|---|
| 1 | Cerebrum | 11 | Pancreas | 21 | Conus medullaris |
| 2 | Corpus callosum | 12 | Transverse colon | 22 | Cauda equina |
| 3 | Pons | 13 | Umbilicus | 23 | Rectum |
| 4 | Larynx | 14 | Small intestine | 24 | Vagina |
| 5 | Trachea | 15 | Uterus | 25 | Anus |
| 6 | Left atrium | 16 | Urinary bladder | 26 | Inferior vena cava |
| 7 | Right ventricle | 17 | Pubic symphysis | 27 | Aorta |
| 8 | Esophagus | 18 | Cerebellum | 28 | Umbilical cord |
| 9 | Liver | 19 | Medulla oblongata | 29 | Thymus |
| 10 | Stomach | 20 | Spinal cord | | |

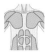

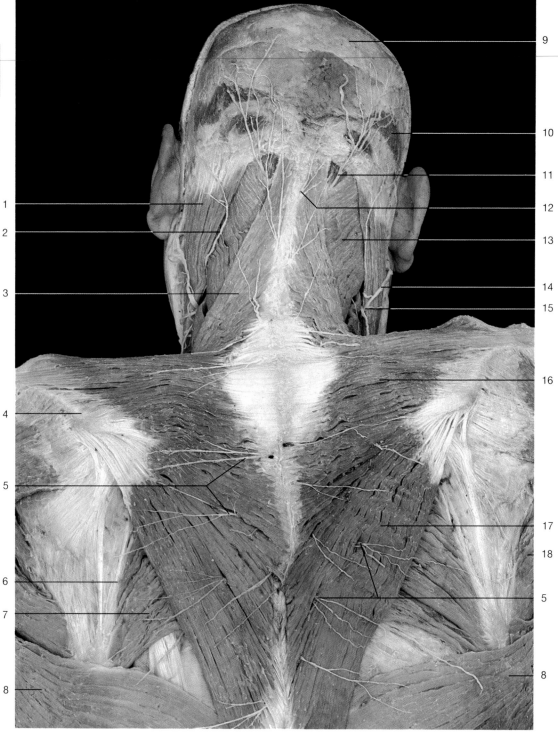

**Posterior aspect of the neck** (superficial layer). Dissection of the trapezius muscle and the cutaneous branches of the dorsal branches of spinal nerves.

| | |
|---|---|
| 1 Sternocleidomastoid muscle | 10 Occipital belly of occipitofrontalis muscle |
| 2 Lesser occipital nerve | 11 Greater occipital nerve |
| 3 Descending fibers of trapezius muscle | 12 Third occipital nerve |
| 4 Spine of scapula | 13 Splenius capitis muscle |
| 5 Medial cutaneous branches of dorsal rami of spinal nerves | 14 Great auricular nerve |
| 6 Medial margin of scapula | 15 Cutaneous nerves of cervical plexus |
| 7 Rhomboid major muscle | 16 Transverse fibers of trapezius muscle |
| 8 Latissimus dorsi muscle | 17 Ascending fibers of trapezius muscle |
| 9 Galea aponeurotica | 18 Teres major muscle |

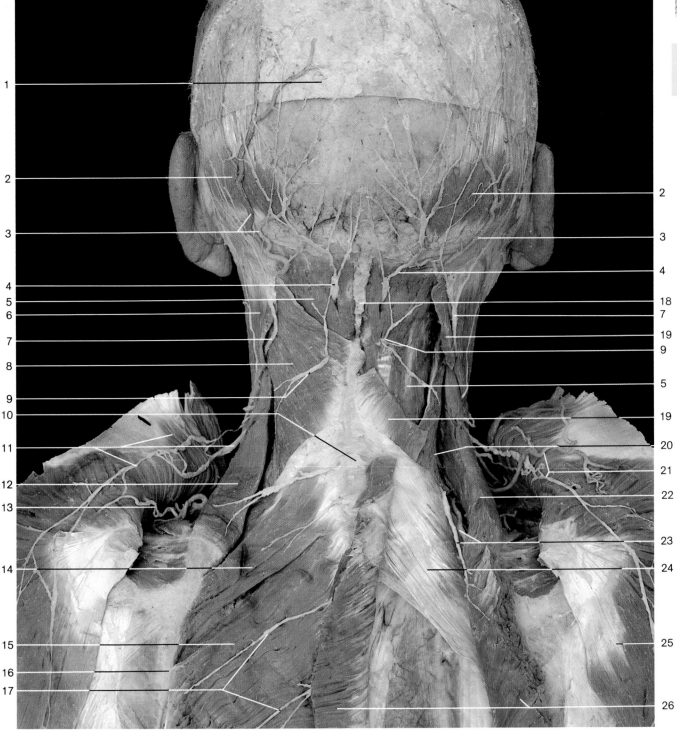

**Posterior aspect of the neck** (deeper layer). The left trapezius muscle has been divided and reflected. On the right, trapezius, rhomboid, and splenius muscles have been divided. The right levator scapulae muscle has been slightly reflected.

1   Galea aponeurotica
2   Occipital belly of occipitofrontalis muscle
3   Occipital artery
4   Greater occipital nerve (C₂)
5   Semispinalis capitis muscle
6   Sternocleidomastoid muscle
7   Lesser occipital nerve
8   Left splenius capitis muscle
9   Third occipital nerve (C₃)
10  Spinous process
      of vertebra prominens (C₇)

11  Left trapezius muscle and accessory nerve
12  Levator scapulae muscle
13  Superficial branch
      of transverse cervical artery
14  Rhomboid minor muscle
15  Rhomboid major muscle
16  Medial margin of scapula
17  Medial branches of dorsal rami
      of spinal nerves
18  Ligamentum nuchae
19  Splenius capitis muscle (divided)

20  Splenius cervicis muscle
21  Right accessory nerve and superficial
      branch of transverse cervical artery
22  Right levator scapulae muscle
23  Dorsal scapular nerve and
      deep branch of transverse cervical artery
24  Serratus posterior superior muscle
25  Right trapezius muscle
      (divided and reflected)
26  Right rhomboid major muscle
      (divided and reflected)

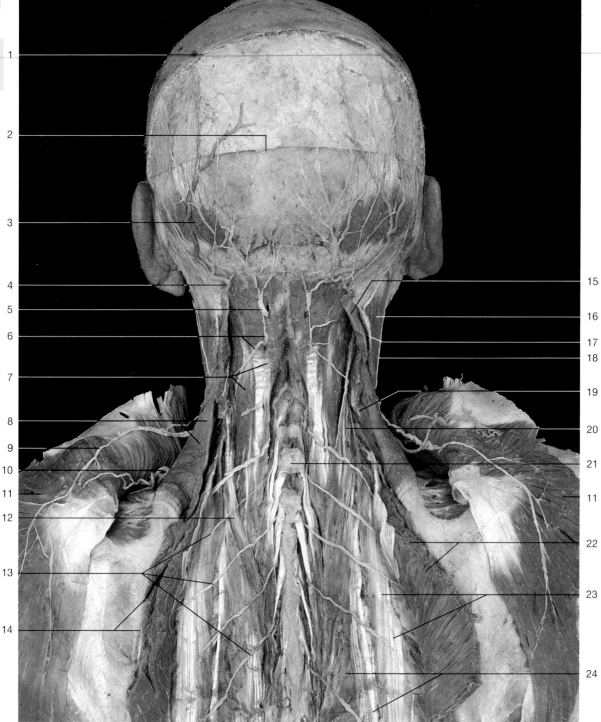

**Posterior aspect of the neck** (deepest layer). Trapezius, splenius capitis, and cervicis muscles have been divided and partly removed or reflected.

| | | | |
|---|---|---|---|
| 1 | Skin of scalp | 9 | Accessory nerve (n. XI) |
| 2 | Galea aponeurotica | 10 | Superficial cervical artery |
| 3 | Occipital belly | 11 | Trapezius muscle (reflected) |
| | of occipitofrontalis muscle | 12 | Longissimus cervicis muscle |
| 4 | Occipital artery | 13 | Medial cutaneous branches |
| 5 | Greater occipital nerve | | of dorsal rami of spinal nerves |
| 6 | Third occipital nerve | 14 | Medial margin of scapula |
| 7 | Semispinalis capitis muscle | 15 | Splenius capitis muscle (divided) |
| 8 | Levator scapulae muscle | 16 | Sternocleidomastoid muscle |

| | |
|---|---|
| 17 | Lesser occipital nerve |
| 18 | Great auricular nerve |
| 19 | Splenius cervicis muscle |
| 20 | Longissimus cervicis muscle |
| 21 | Spinous process |
| | of vertebra prominens (C$_7$) |
| 22 | Rhomboid muscles (divided) |
| 23 | Iliocostalis thoracis muscle |
| 24 | Longissimus thoracis muscle |

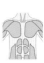

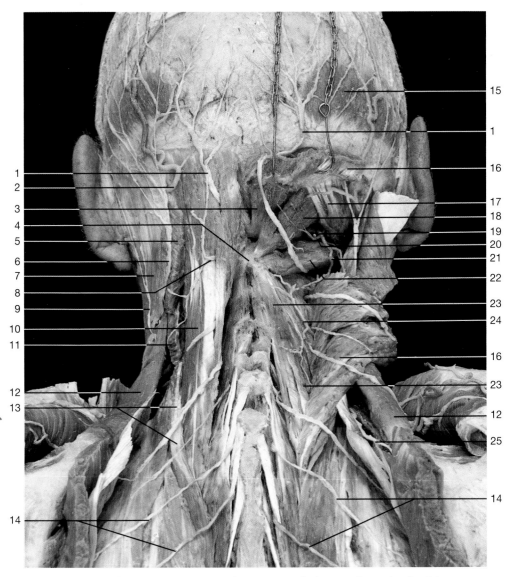

1   Greater occipital nerve
2   Occipital artery
3   Rectus capitis posterior
    minor muscle
4   Spinous process of axis
5   Left splenius capitis muscle
    (cut)
6   Lesser occipital nerve
7   Left sternocleidomastoid
    muscle
8   Third occipital nerve (C₃)
9   Great auricular nerve
10  Left semispinalis capitis
    muscle
11  Left semispinalis cervicis
    muscle (cut)
12  Levator scapulae muscle
13  Left longissimus cervicis
    muscle
14  Medial branches
    of dorsal rami
    of spinal nerves
15  Occipital belly
    of occipitofrontalis muscle
16  Semispinalis capitis muscle
    (cut)
17  Obliquus capitis superior
    muscle
18  Rectus capitis posterior major
    muscle
19  Vertebral artery
20  Suboccipital nerve (C₁)
21  Muscular branch
    of vertebral artery
22  Obliquus capitis inferior
    muscle
23  Right semispinalis cervicis
    muscle
24  Deep cervical artery
25  Dorsal scapular nerve
26  External occipital
    protuberance
27  Trapezius muscle (cut)
28  Cervical vertebra (C₃)
29  Mastoid process and
    splenius capitis muscle
30  Atlas
31  Axis
32  Spinous process
    of third cervical vertebra

**Posterior aspect of the neck** (deepest layer). Dissection of suboccipital triangle. The right semispinalis capitis muscle has been divided and reflected.

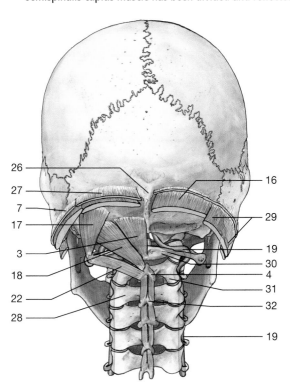

**Suboccipital triangle and position of the vertebral artery.**

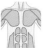

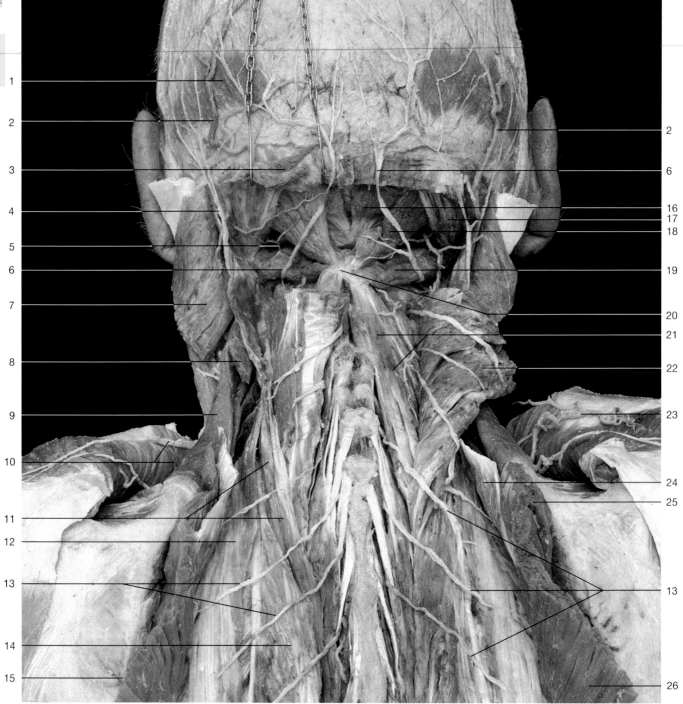

**Posterior aspect of the neck** (deepest layer). Dissection of suboccipital triangle on both sides.

1   Occipital belly of occipitofrontalis muscle
2   Occipital artery
3   Insertion of semispinalis capitis muscle (divided)
4   Lesser occipital nerve
     (from cervical plexus)
5   Suboccipital nerve (C$_1$)
6   Greater occipital nerve (C$_2$)
7   Splenius capitis muscle (reflected)
8   Splenius cervicis muscle
9   Levator scapulae muscle
10  Accessory nerve (n. XI) and trapezius muscle

11  Longissimus cervicis muscle
12  Iliocostalis cervicis muscle
13  Medial cutaneus branches of dorsal rami
     of spinal nerves (C$_7$, C$_8$)
14  Longissimus thoracis muscle
15  Medial margin of scapula
16  Rectus capitis posterior minor muscle
17  Obliquus capitis superior muscle
18  Rectus capitis posterior major muscle
19  Obliquus capitis inferior muscle
20  Spinous process of axis

21  Semispinalis cervicis muscle
22  Semispinalis capitis muscle
     (divided and reflected)
23  Transverse cervical artery
     (superficial branch)
24  Serratus posterior superior muscle
     (divided and reflected)
25  Rhomboid minor muscle
     (divided and reflected)
26  Rhomboid major muscle
     (divided and reflected)

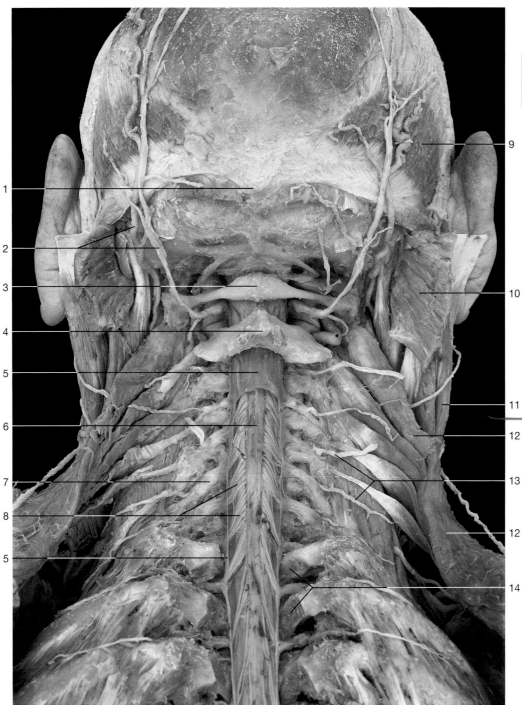

**Posterior aspect of the neck** (deepest layer). The vertebral canal caudally of the atlas and axis has been opened to show the spinal cord. The dura mater has been partly removed.

| | | | |
|---|---|---|---|
| 1 | External occipital protuberance | 8 | Posterior root filaments (fila radicularia posterior) |
| 2 | Greater occipital nerve (C$_2$) and occipital artery | 9 | Occipital belly of occipitofrontalis muscle |
| 3 | Atlas (posterior arch) | 10 | Splenius capitis muscle (cut and reflected) |
| 4 | Axis (posterior arch) | 11 | Sternocleidomastoid muscle |
| 5 | Spinal dura mater | 12 | Levator scapulae muscle |
| 6 | Spinal cord | 13 | Posterior branches of spinal nerves |
| 7 | Spinal ganglion | 14 | Arches of cervical vertebrae (cut) |

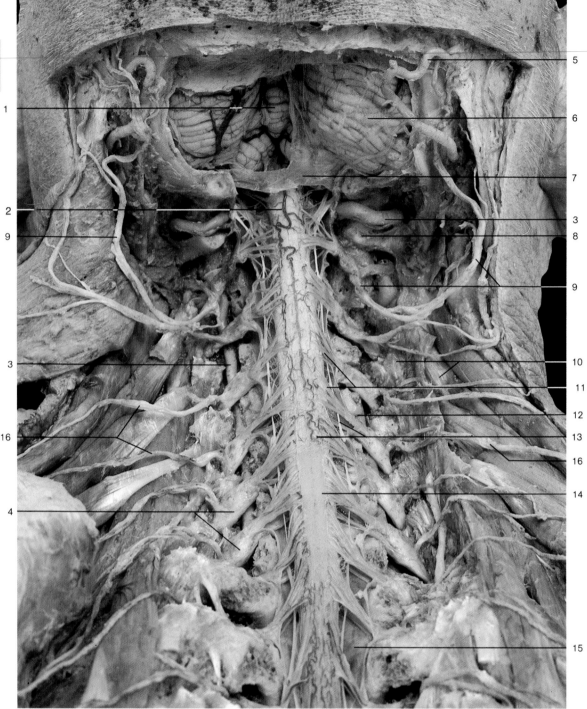

**Posterior aspect of the neck** (deepest layer). Dissection of medulla oblongata and spinal cord. The cranial cavity has been opened.

| | | | |
|---|---|---|---|
| 1 | Vermis of the cerebellum | 9 | Greater occipital nerve (C₂) |
| 2 | Medulla oblongata and posterior spinal artery | 10 | Levator scapulae muscle and intertransverse ligament |
| 3 | Vertebral artery | 11 | Dorsal roots of spinal nerves |
| 4 | Spinal ganglion | 12 | Vertebral arch |
| 5 | Occipital artery | 13 | Denticulate ligament and arachnoid mater |
| 6 | Cerebellum | 14 | Area where pia mater has been removed |
| 7 | Cerebellomedullary cistern | 15 | Spinal dura mater |
| 8 | Posterior arch of atlas | 16 | Dorsal rami of spinal nerves |

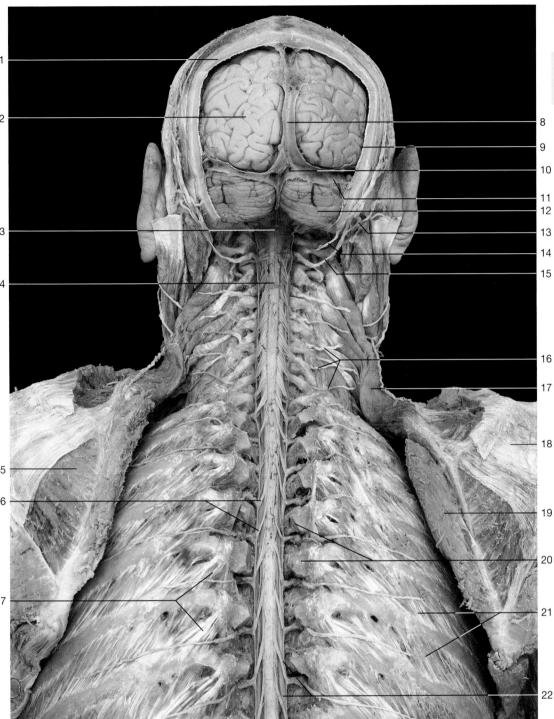

**Posterior aspect of the neck** (deepest layer). Dissection of medulla oblongata and spinal cord in relation to the brain.

| | | | |
|---|---|---|---|
| 1 | Calvaria | 12 | Cerebellum |
| 2 | Left hemisphere of the brain | 13 | Occipital artery |
| 3 | Cerebellomedullary cistern | 14 | Suboccipital nerve (C$_1$) |
| 4 | Spinal cord | 15 | Greater occipital nerve (C$_2$) |
| 5 | Scapula with infraspinous muscle | 16 | Posterior branches of spinal nerves |
| 6 | Posterior root filaments (fila radicularia posterior) | 17 | Levator scapulae muscle |
| 7 | Levatores costarum muscles | 18 | Deltoid muscle |
| 8 | Falx cerebri with sinus sagittalis superior | 19 | Rhomboid muscles |
| 9 | Subarachnoidal space | 20 | Vertebral arches (cut) |
| 10 | Confluens sinuum | 21 | External intercostal muscles |
| 11 | Transverse sinus | 22 | Spinal dura mater |

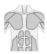

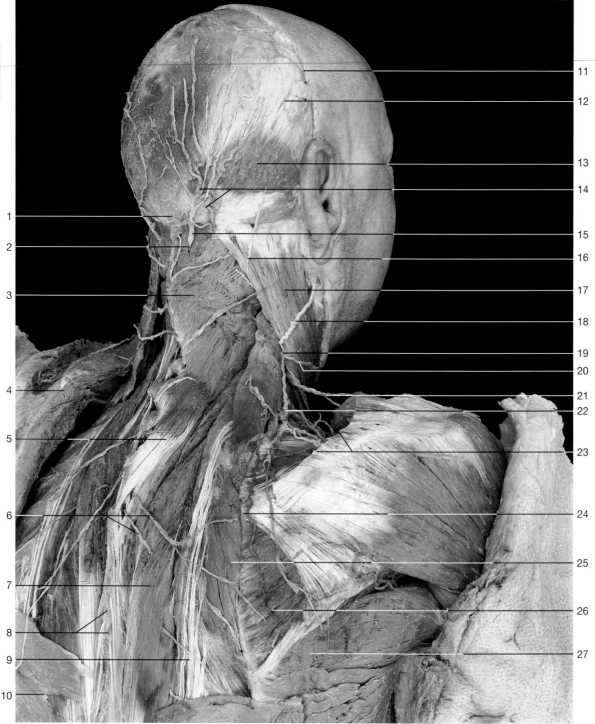

**Oblique-lateral aspect of the neck** (deeper layer). The trapezius muscle has been removed.

1 External occipital protuberance
2 Semispinalis capitis muscle
3 Splenius capitis muscle
4 Scapula
5 Splenius cervicis muscle
6 Posterior branches of spinal nerves
7 Longissimus muscle
8 Spinous processes of thoracic vertebrae
9 Iliocostalis muscle
10 Latissimus dorsi muscle
11 Epidermis of the head (scalp)
12 Galea aponeurotica
13 Occipital belly of occipitofrontalis muscle
14 Occipital artery

15 Greater occipital nerve (C$_2$)
16 Lesser occipital nerve
17 Sternocleidomastoid muscle
18 Great auricular nerve
19 Punctum nervosum
20 Transverse cervical nerve
21 Supraclavicular nerves
22 Accessory nerve (n. XI)
23 Trapezius muscle (cut edge)
24 Medial margin of scapula
25 Rhomboid major muscle
26 Infraspinous muscle
27 Teres major muscle

# 4 Thoracic Organs

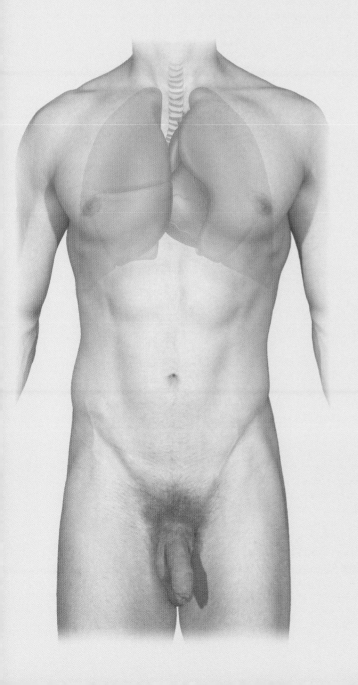

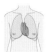

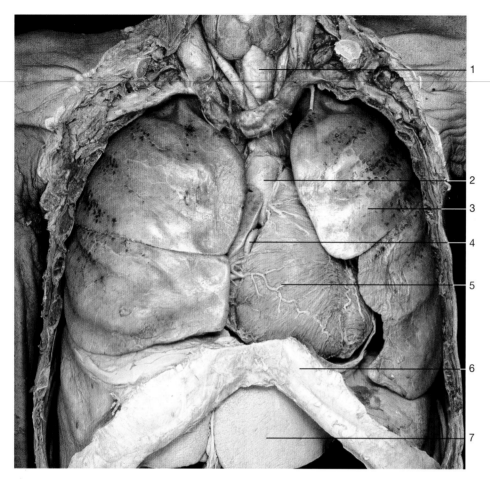

1 Trachea
2 Ascending aorta
3 Upper lobe of left lung
4 Right coronary artery
5 Right ventricle of the heart
6 Costal margin
7 Liver
8 Sternum
9 Right auricle of the heart
10 Middle lobe of right lung
11 Right atrium of the heart
12 Main bronchus
13 Azygos vein
14 Left ventricle of the heart and bulb of aorta
15 Esophagus
16 Descending aorta
17 Spinal cord

**Thoracic organs in situ** (anterior aspect). The anterior thoracic wall has been removed.

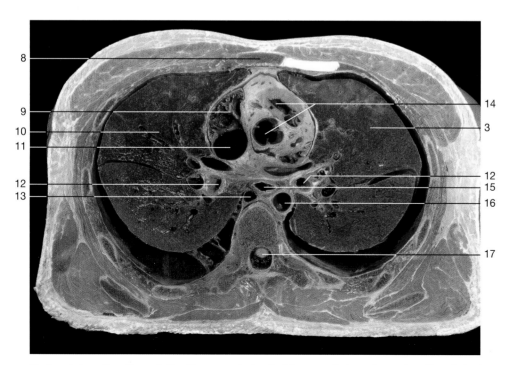

**Horizontal section through the thorax** at the level of the seventh thoracic vertebra (from below).

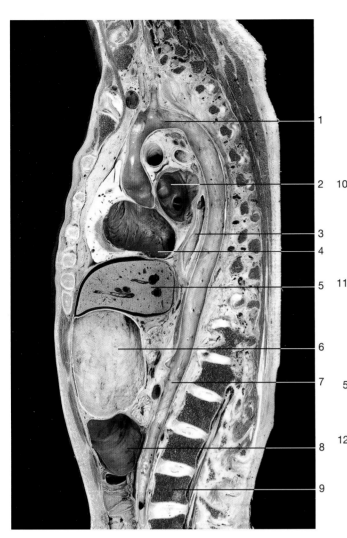

**Sagittal section through the thoracic and abdominal cavities.**

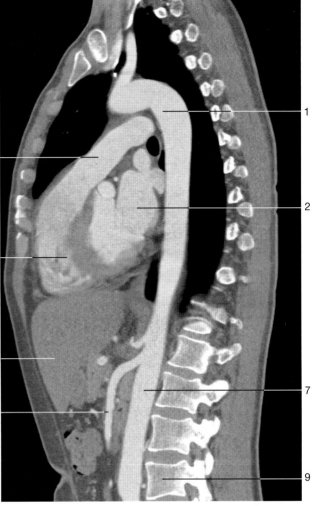

**Sagittal section through the thoracic and abdominal cavities** (MRI scan). (Prof. Uder, Dept. of Radiology, Univ. Erlangen-Nuremberg.)

| | | |
|---|---|---|
| 1 | Aortic arch | 4 | Right atrium |
| 2 | Left atrium | | of the heart |
| | of the heart | 5 | Liver |
| 3 | Esophagus | 6 | Stomach |

| | |
|---|---|
| 7 | Abdominal aorta |
| 8 | Transverse colon (dilated) |
| 9 | Body of lumbar vertebra |

| | |
|---|---|
| 10 | Pulmonary trunk |
| 11 | Right ventricle of the heart |
| 12 | Superior mesenteric artery |
| 13 | Trachea |

| | |
|---|---|
| 14 | Remaining parts of thymus gland |
| 15 | Ascending aorta |
| 16 | Pericardium |

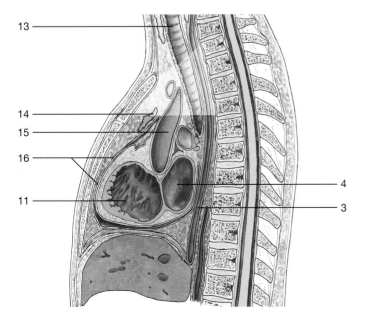

**Sagittal section through the thoracic cavity.** The parts of the mediastinum are indicated by colors (compare with the table).

| Parts of mediastinum | Content |
|---|---|
| Superior mediastinum (yellow) | Trachea, brachiocephalic veins, thymus, aortic arch, esophagus, thoracic duct |
| Middle mediastinum (blue) | Heart, ascending aorta, pulmonary trunk, pulmonary veins, phrenic nerves |
| Posterior mediastinum (orange) | Esophagus with vagus nerves, descending aorta, thoracic duct, sympathetic trunks |
| Anterior mediastinum (pink) | Smaller vessels and nerves, fat and connective tissue, thymus (only in the child) |

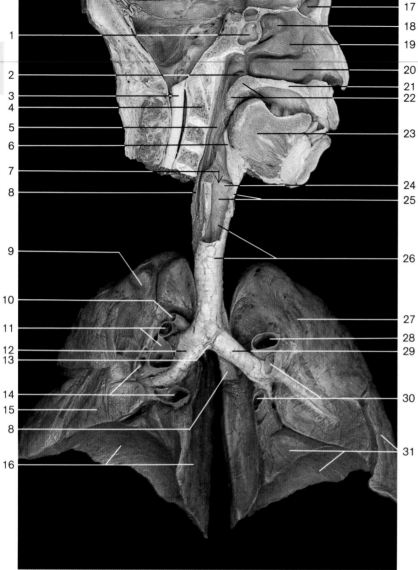

1   Sphenoid sinus
2   Pharyngeal opening of auditory tube
3   Spinal cord
4   Dens of axis
5   Oropharynx (oropharyngeal isthmus)
6   Epiglottis
7   Entrance of larynx
8   Esophagus
9   Upper lobe of right lung
10  Azygos vein
11  Branches of pulmonary artery
12  Right main bronchus
13  Bifurcation of trachea
14  Tributaries of right pulmonary veins
15  Middle lobe of right lung
16  Lower lobe of right lung
17  Frontal sinus
18  Superior nasal concha
19  Middle nasal concha
20  Inferior nasal concha
21  Hard palate
22  Soft palate with uvula
23  Tongue
24  Vocal fold
25  Larynx
26  Trachea
27  Upper lobe of left lung
28  Left pulmonary artery
29  Left main bronchus
30  Left pulmonary veins
31  Lower lobe of left lung

**Respiratory system.** The lungs have been fixed in expiration and turned laterally. Head bisected and turned laterally.

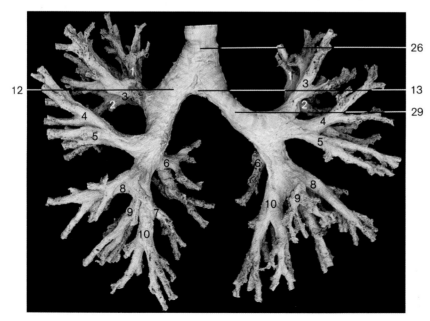

**Bronchial tree** (anterior aspect). The lung tissue has been removed. The bronchopulmonary segments are numbered 1–10.

▷  **To page 255:**

1   Nasal cavity
2   Pharynx
3   Larynx (thyroid cartilage)
4   Trachea
5   Upper lobe of right lung
6   Bifurcation of trachea
7   Right main bronchus
8   Horizontal fissure of right lung
9   Middle lobe of right lung
10  Oblique fissures of lungs
11  Lower lobe of right lung
12  Clavicle
13  Upper lobe of left lung
14  Left main bronchus
15  Bronchi supplying bronchopulmonary segments
16  Lower lobe of left lung
17  Costal margin
18  Hyoid bone
19  Right superior lobe bronchus
20  Right middle lobe bronchus
21  Right inferior lobe bronchus
22  Left superior lobe bronchus
23  Left inferior lobe bronchus
24  Segmental bronchi
25  Branches of pulmonary arteries
26  Branches of pulmonary veins

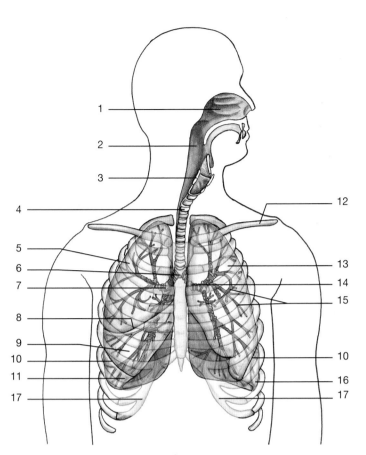

**Organization and positions of the respiratory organs** (anterior aspect).

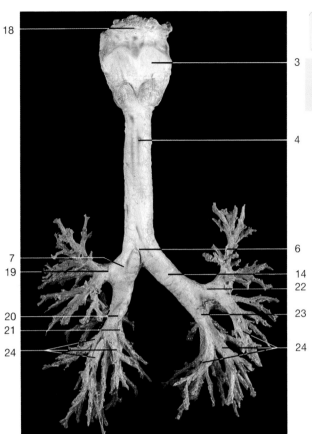

**Larynx, trachea, and bronchial tree** (anterior aspect).

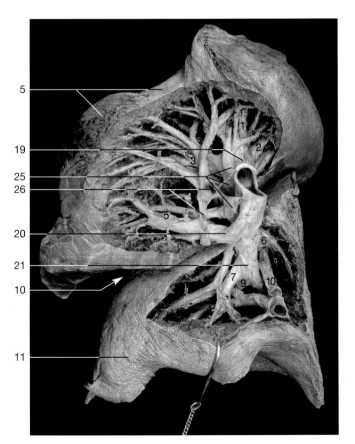

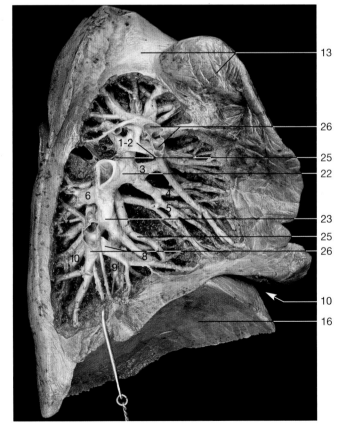

**Mediastinal dissection of the bronchial tree, pulmonary veins, and pulmonary arteries** of right lung (left) and left lung (right) (medial aspect). The bronchopulmonary segments are numbered 1–10.

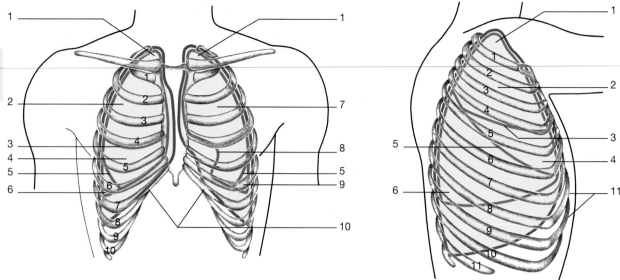

**Surface projections of lungs and pleura on the thoracic wall.** Left: anterior aspect; right: right-lateral aspect. Red = margins of the lung; blue = margins of pleura. The numbers indicate the ribs.

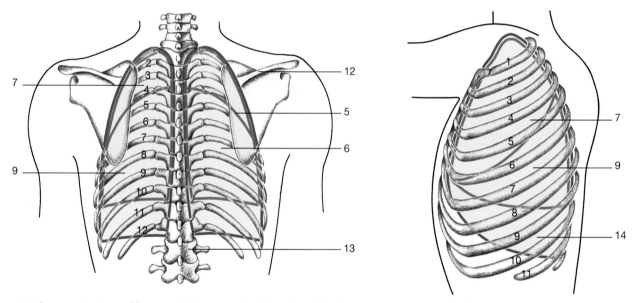

**Surface projections of lungs and pleura on the thoracic wall.** Left: posterior aspect; right: left-lateral aspect. Red = margins of lung; blue = margins of pleura. The numbers indicate the ribs.

| | | |
|---|---|---|
| 1  Apex of lung | 6  Lower lobe of right lung | 11  Costal margin |
| 2  Upper lobe of right lung | 7  Upper lobe of left lung | 12  Spine of scapula |
| 3  Horizontal fissure of right lung | 8  Cardiac notch of left lung | 13  First lumbar vertebra |
| 4  Middle lobe of right lung | 9  Lower lobe of left lung | 14  Space between border of lung and pleura |
| 5  Oblique fissures of lungs | 10  Infrasternal angle |      (costodiaphragmatic recess) |

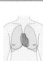

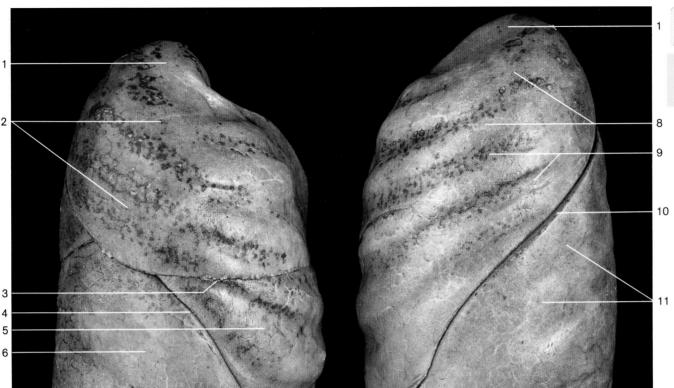

**Right lung** (lateral aspect).

**Left lung** (lateral aspect).

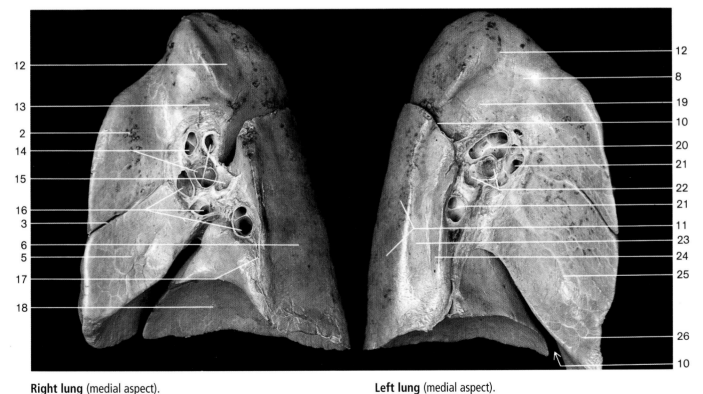

**Right lung** (medial aspect).

**Left lung** (medial aspect).

| | | | |
|---|---|---|---|
| 1 | Apex of lung | 8 | Upper lobe of left lung |
| 2 | Upper lobe of right lung | 9 | Impressions of ribs |
| 3 | Horizontal fissure of right lung | 10 | Oblique fissure of left lung |
| 4 | Oblique fissure of right lung | 11 | Lower lobe of left lung |
| 5 | Middle lobe of right lung | 12 | Groove of subclavian artery |
| 6 | Lower lobe of right lung | 13 | Groove of azygos arch |
| 7 | Inferior border | 14 | Branches of right pulmonary artery |

| | | | |
|---|---|---|---|
| 15 | Bronchi | 22 | Left secondary bronchi |
| 16 | Right pulmonary veins | 23 | Groove of thoracic aorta |
| 17 | Pulmonary ligament | 24 | Groove of esophagus |
| 18 | Diaphragmatic surface | 25 | Cardiac impression |
| 19 | Groove of aortic arch | 26 | Lingula |
| 20 | Left pulmonary artery | | |
| 21 | Branches of left pulmonary veins | | |

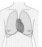

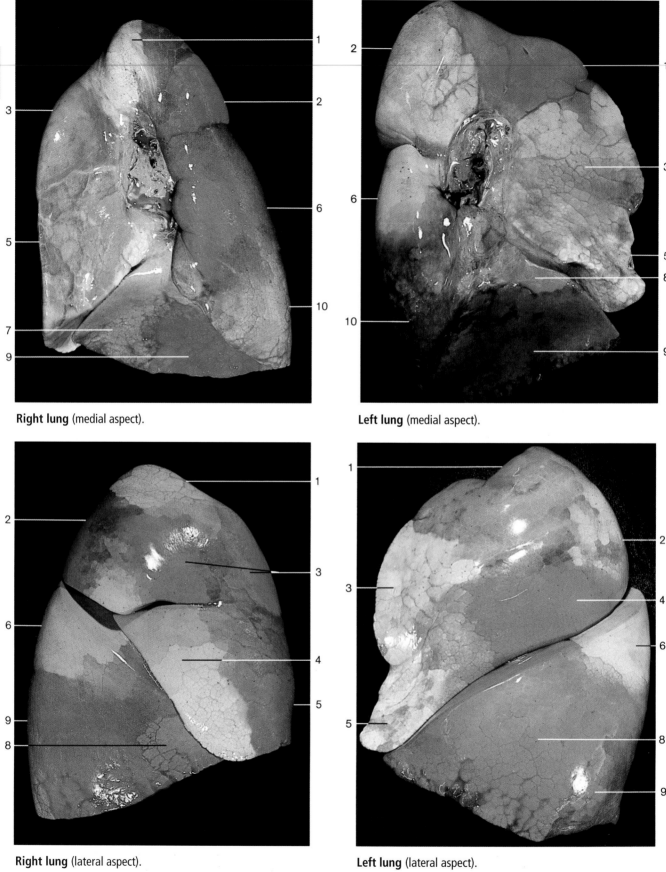

**Right lung** (medial aspect).

**Left lung** (medial aspect).

**Right lung** (lateral aspect).

**Left lung** (lateral aspect).

The bronchopulmonary segments of the lungs are differentiated by the various colors. Notice that there is no segment in the left lung that corresponds to the seventh segment of the right lung. Compare with the schematic drawing on the facing page.

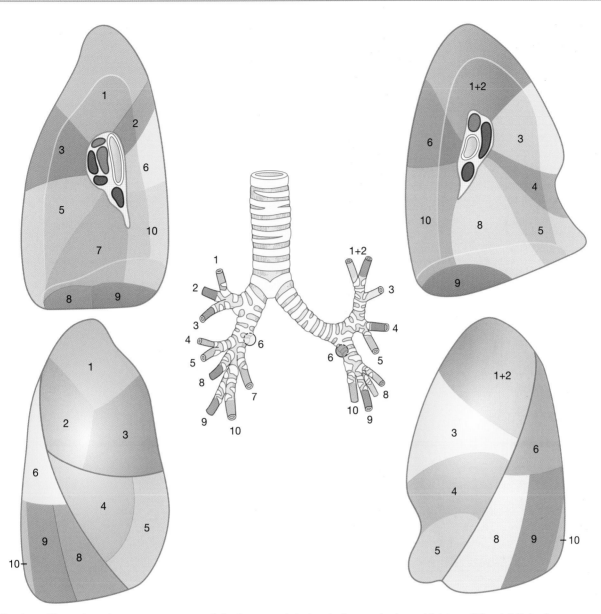

**Distribution of bronchopulmonary segments of the lungs and their relation to the bronchial tree.** (After J. F. Huber.)

The bronchopulmonary segments are morphologically and functionally separate, independent respiratory units of the lung tissue. Each segment is surrounded by connective tissue that is continuous with the visceral pleura. The segmental bronchi are centrally located in each segment and are closely accompanied by branches of the pulmonary arteries, whereas the tributaries of the pulmonary veins run **between** the segments. Thus, the veins serve two adjacent segments that drain for the most part into more than one vein. A bronchopulmonary segment is therefore not a complete vascular unit, but segmentation is the result of a specific architecture of the lung vasculature.

| Right lung | | | Left lung | | | |
|---|---|---|---|---|---|---|
| 1 Apical segment | Upper lobe bronchus | | 1+2 Apicoposterior segment | Superior division | Upper lobe bronchus | |
| 2 Posterior segment | | | | | | |
| 3 Anterior segment | | | 3 Anterior segment | | | |
| | | | 4 Superior lingular segment | Inferior division | | |
| 4 Lateral segment | Middle lobe bronchus | | 5 Inferior lingular segment | | | |
| 5 Medial segment | | | | | | |
| 6 Superior (apical) segment | Lower lobe bronchus | | 6 Superior (apical) segment | Lower lobe bronchus | | |
| 7 Medial basal segment | | | 7 Absent | | | |
| 8 Anterior basal segment | | | 8 Anteromedial basal segment | | | |
| 9 Lateral basal segment | | | 9 Lateral basal segment | | | |
| 10 Posterior basal segment | | | 10 Posterior basal segment | | | |

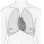

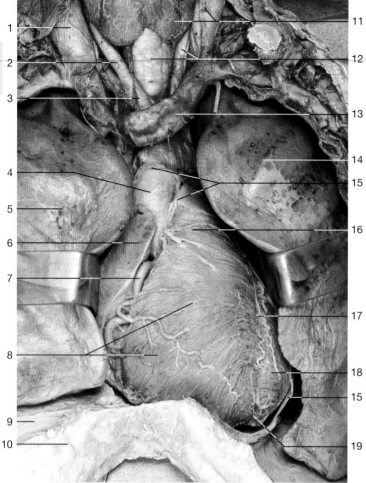

1  Internal jugular vein
2  Common carotid artery
3  Brachiocephalic trunk
4  Ascending aorta
5  Right lung
6  Right auricle
7  Right coronary artery
8  Myocardium of right ventricle
9  Diaphragm
10 Costal margin
11 Thyroid gland and internal jugular vein
12 Trachea and left common carotid artery
13 Left brachiocephalic vein
14 Left lung
15 Pericardium (cut edge)
16 Pulmonary trunk
17 Anterior interventricular artery
18 Myocardium of left ventricle
19 Apex of the heart

**Heart and related vessels in situ** (anterior aspect). Myocardium and coronary arteries have been displayed.

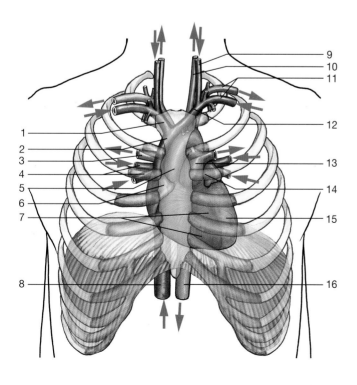

1  Right brachiocephalic vein
2  Superior vena cava
3  Right pulmonary artery
4  Right pulmonary veins
5  Ascending aorta
6  Right atrium
7  Right ventricle
8  Inferior vena cava
9  Left internal jugular vein
10 Left common carotid artery
11 Left axillary artery and vein
12 Left brachiocephalic vein
13 Pulmonary trunk
14 Left atrium
15 Left ventricle
16 Descending aorta

**Position of heart and related vessels in the thoracic cavity** (anterior aspect). Blue = regions of heart and vessels with venous blood flow; red = regions of heart and vessels with arterial blood flow; blue arrows: veins; red arrows: arteries.

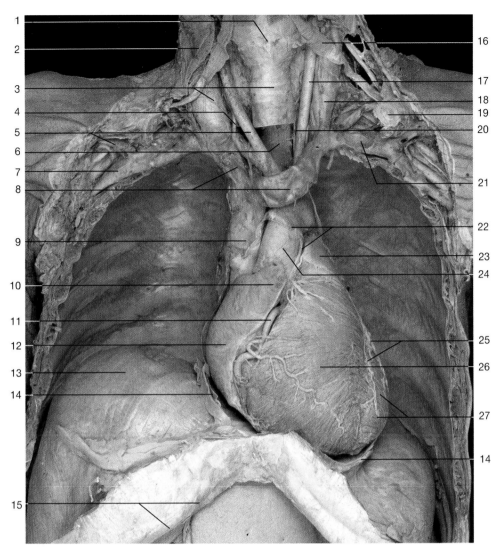

1  Larynx (thyroid cartilage)
2  Sternocleidomastoid muscle
   (divided)
3  Trachea (divided) and
   right internal jugular vein
4  Vagus nerve
5  Right common carotid artery
   and cephalic vein
6  Esophagus
7  Right axillary vein
8  Right and left
   brachiocephalic veins
9  Superior vena cava
10 Right auricle
11 Right coronary artery
12 Right atrium
13 Diaphragm
14 Pericardium (cut edges)
15 Costal margin
16 Omohyoid muscle
17 Left common carotid artery
18 Left internal jugular vein
19 Clavicle (divided)
20 Left recurrent laryngeal nerve
21 Subclavian vein
22 Pericardial reflection
23 Pulmonary trunk
24 Ascending aorta
25 Anterior interventricular sulcus and
   anterior interventricular branch
   of left coronary artery
26 Right ventricle
27 Left ventricle
28 Aortic valve
29 Tricuspid or right
   atrioventricular valve
30 Inferior vena cava
31 Pulmonary veins
32 Pulmonary valve
33 Left atrioventricular
   (bicuspid or mitral) valve

**Heart and related vessels in situ** (anterior aspect). Anterior thoracic wall, pericardium, and epicardium have been removed, the trachea has been divided.

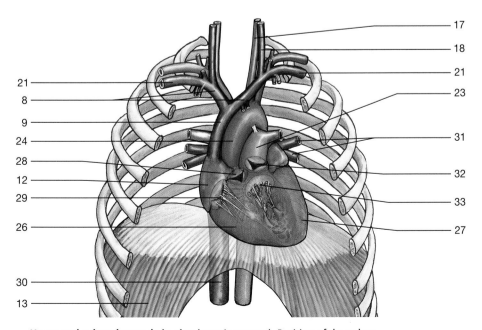

**Heart and related vessels in situ** (anterior aspect). Position of the valves.

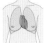

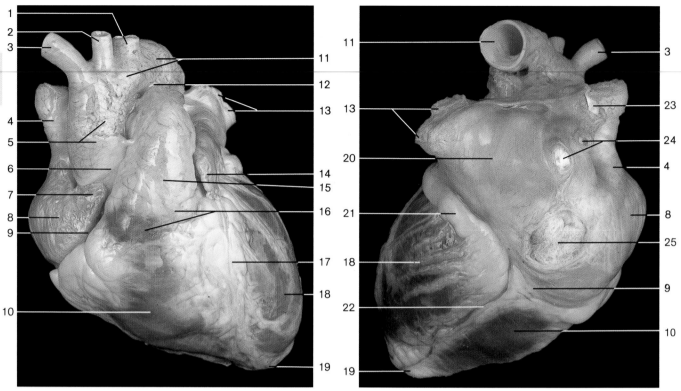

**Heart** of 30-year-old woman (anterior aspect).

**Heart** of 30-year-old woman (oblique-posterior aspect).

| | | | |
|---|---|---|---|
| 1 | Left subclavian artery | 10 | Right ventricle |
| 2 | Left common carotid artery | 11 | Aortic arch |
| 3 | Brachiocephalic trunk | 12 | Ligamentum arteriosum |
| 4 | Superior vena cava | 13 | Left pulmonary veins |
| 5 | Ascending aorta | 14 | Left auricle |
| 6 | Bulb of the aorta | 15 | Pulmonary trunk |
| 7 | Right auricle | 16 | Sinus of pulmonary trunk |
| 8 | Right atrium | 17 | Anterior interventricular sulcus |
| 9 | Coronary sulcus | 18 | Left ventricle |

| | |
|---|---|
| 19 | Apex of the heart |
| 20 | Left atrium |
| 21 | Epicardial fat overlying coronary sinus |
| 22 | Posterior interventricular sulcus |
| 23 | Pulmonary artery |
| 24 | Right pulmonary veins |
| 25 | Inferior vena cava |
| 26 | Pulmonary veins |

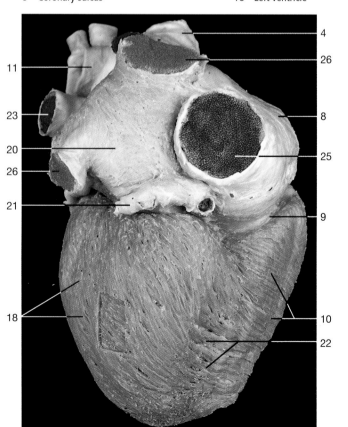

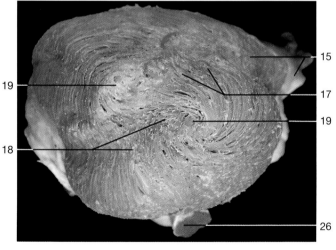

**Vortex of cardiac muscle fibers** (inferior aspect).

**Heart** (posterior aspect). The myocardium of the left ventricle has been fenestrated to show the muscle fiber bundles of the deeper layer with their more circular course.

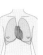

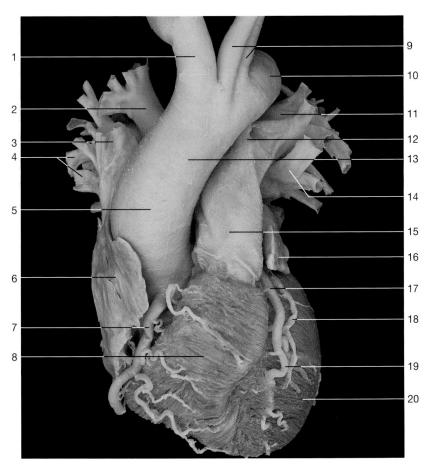

1   Brachiocephalic trunk
2   Right pulmonary artery
3   Superior vena cava
4   Right pulmonary veins
5   Ascending aorta
6   Right atrium
7   Right coronary artery
8   Right ventricle
9   Left common carotid artery and
    left subclavian artery
10  Descending aorta (thoracic part)
11  Ligamentum arteriosum
    (remnant of ductus arteriosus Botalli)
12  Left pulmonary artery
13  Aortic arch
14  Left pulmonary veins
15  Pulmonary trunk
16  Left atrium
17  Left coronary artery
18  Diagonal branch
    of anterior interventricular vein
19  Interventricular branch
    of left coronary artery
20  Left ventricle
21  Left brachiocephalic vein
22  Thoracic wall
23  Liver
24  Aortic valve
25  Chordae tendineae
26  Papillary muscles
27  Stomach

**Heart with coronary arteries** (anterior aspect, systolic phase of heart action).

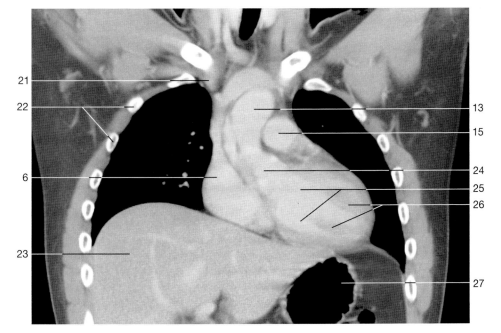

**Coronal section through the thorax** at the level of the ascending aorta (MRI scan).
(Prof. Uder, Dept. of Radiology, Univ. Erlangen-Nuremberg, Germany.)

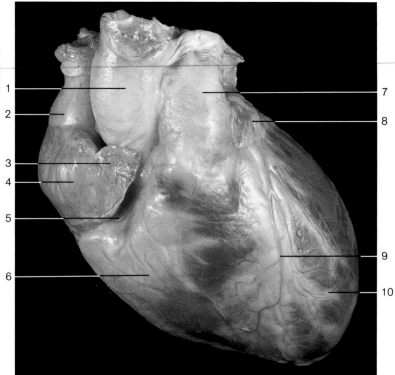

1  Ascending aorta
2  Superior vena cava
3  Right auricle
4  Right atrium
5  Coronary sulcus
6  Right ventricle
7  Pulmonary trunk
8  Left auricle
9  Anterior interventricular sulcus
10  Left ventricle
11  Right pulmonary artery
12  Sulcus terminalis with sinu-atrial node
13  Line indicating plane of position of valves
14  Myocardium of right atrium
15  Inferior vena cava
16  Valve of pulmonary trunk
17  Right tricuspid valve
18  Myocardium of right ventricle

**Heart, fixed in diastole** (anterior aspect). The ventricles are relaxed, atria contracted.

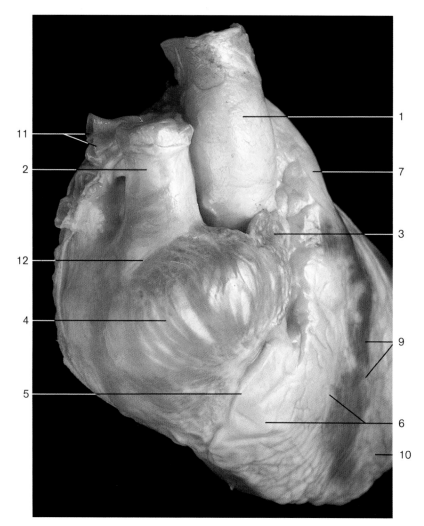

**Heart, fixed in systole** (antero-lateral aspect). The ventricles are contracted, atria dilated.

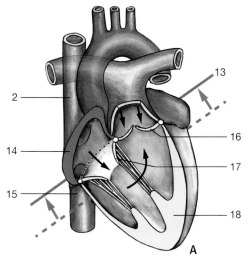

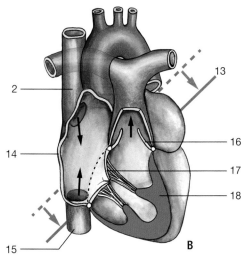

**Morphological changes during heart movements.**
Note the changes in position of the valves (red arrows).
Contracted portions of heart are indicated in dark gray.
A = **Diastole:** muscles of the ventricles relaxed,
atrioventricular valves open, semilunar valves closed.
B = **Systole:** muscles of ventricles contracted,
atrioventricular valves closed, semilunar valves open.

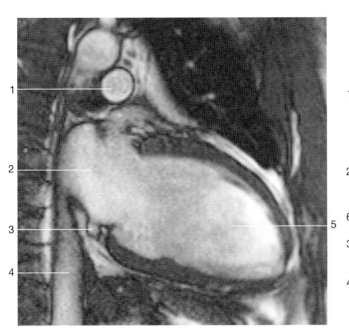

**Coronal section through the thorax at the level of the left ventricle in dilation** (MRI scan). (Prof. Uder, Dept. of Radiology, Univ. Erlangen-Nuremberg, Germany.)

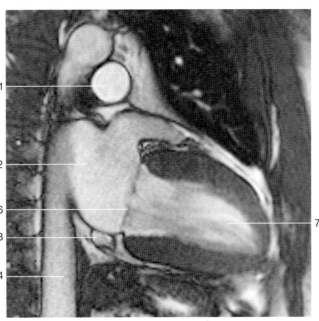

**Coronal section through the thorax at the level of the left ventricle in contraction** (MRI scan). (Prof. Uder, Dept. of Radiology, Univ. Erlangen-Nuremberg, Germany.)

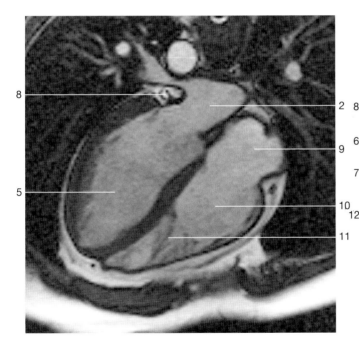

**Coronal section through the human heart in the process of dilation** (MRI scan). (Prof. Uder, Dept. of Radiology, Univ. Erlangen-Nuremberg, Germany.)

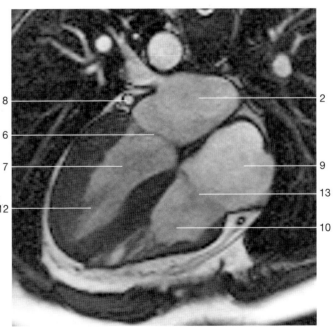

**Coronal section through the human heart in the process of contraction** (MRI scan). (Prof. Uder, Dept. of Radiology, Univ. Erlangen-Nuremberg, Germany.)

1  Pulmonary artery
2  Left atrium
3  Coronary sinus
4  Inferior vena cava
5  Left ventricle (dilated)
6  Left atrioventricular (mitral) valve
7  Left ventricle (contracted)

8  Great cardiac vein (left coronary vein)
9  Right atrium
10  Right ventricle
11  Septomarginal trabecula
12  Papillary muscle
13  Right atrioventricular (tricuspid) valve

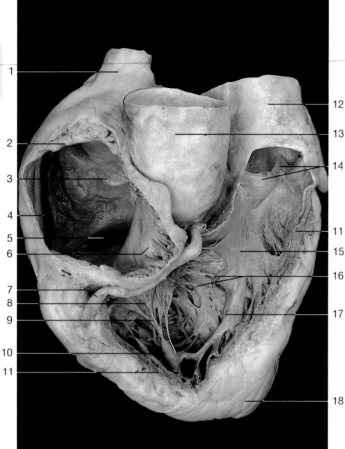

1   Superior vena cava
2   Crista terminalis
3   Fossa ovalis
4   Opening of inferior vena cava
5   Opening of coronary sinus
6   Right auricle
7   Right coronary artery and coronary sulcus
8   Anterior cusp of tricuspid valve
9   Chordae tendineae
10  Anterior papillary muscle
11  Myocardium
12  Pulmonary trunk
13  Ascending aorta
14  Pulmonic valve
15  Conus arteriosus (interventricular septum)
16  Septal papillary muscles
17  Septomarginal trabecula or moderator band
18  Apex of heart
19  Left auricle
20  Aortic valve
21  Left ventricle
22  Pulmonary veins
23  Position of fossa ovalis
24  Left atrium
25  Left atrioventricular (bicuspid or mitral) valve
26  Right atrium
27  Pericardium
28  Posterior papillary muscle
29  Right ventricle
30  Interventricular septum

**Right heart** (anterior aspect). Anterior wall of right atrium and ventricle removed.

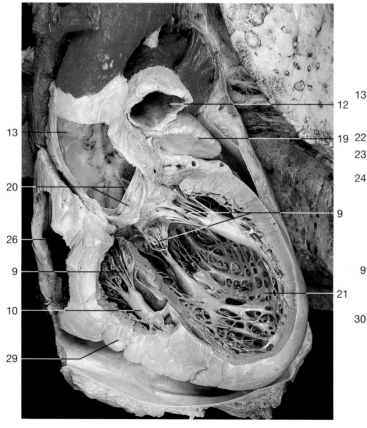

**Heart, left ventricle with mitral valve, papillary muscles, and aortic valve.** Anterior portion of the heart removed.

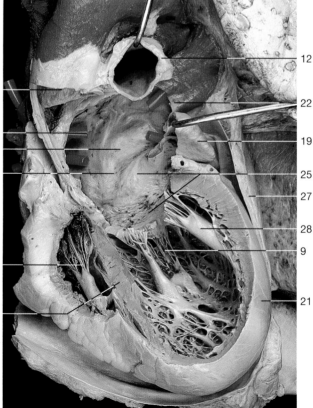

**Heart, left ventricle with posterior part of mitral valve and papillary muscles.** Atrium opened.

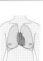

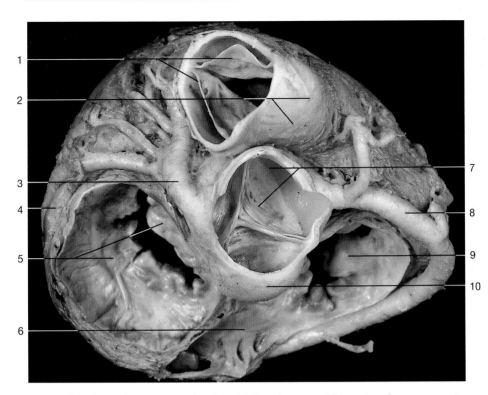

| | |
|---|---|
| 1 | Pulmonic valve |
| 2 | Sinus of pulmonary trunk |
| 3 | Left coronary artery |
| 4 | Great cardiac vein |
| 5 | Left atrioventricular (mitral) valve |
| 6 | Coronary sinus |
| 7 | Aortic valve |
| 8 | Right coronary artery |
| 9 | Right atrioventricular (tricuspid) valve |
| 10 | Bulb of aorta |
| 11 | Anterior semilunar cusp of pulmonic valve |
| 12 | Left semilunar cusp of pulmonic valve |
| 13 | Right semilunar cusp of pulmonic valve |
| 14 | Left semilunar cusp of aortic valve |
| 15 | Right semilunar cusp of aortic valve |
| 16 | Posterior semilunar cusp of aortic valve |
| 17 | Pulmonary artery |
| 18 | Right atrium |
| 19 | Left atrium with pulmonary veins |
| 20 | Ascending aorta with aortic valve |

**Valves of the heart** (superior aspect). Left and right atria removed. Dissection of coronary arteries. Anterior wall of the heart at the top.

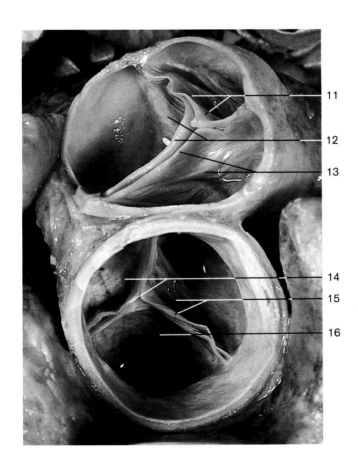

**Pulmonic and aortic valves** (superior aspect). Both valves are closed. Anterior wall of the heart at the top.

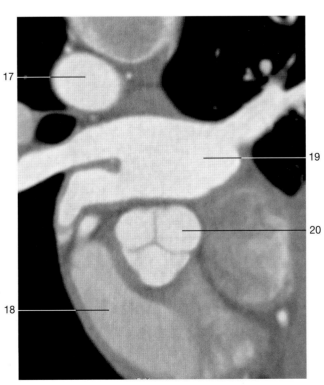

**Horizontal section through the heart** at the level of the aortic valve (MRI scan). (Prof. Uder, Dept. of Radiology, Univ. Erlangen-Nuremberg, Germany.)

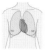

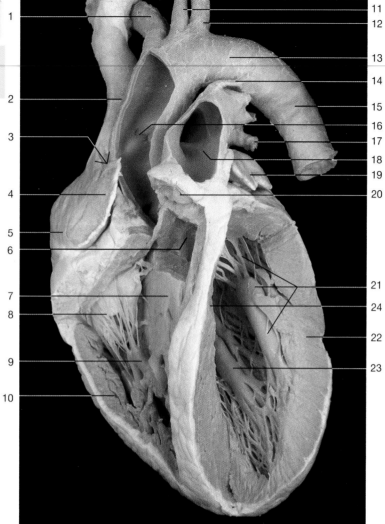

1 Brachiocephalic trunk
2 Superior vena cava
3 Sulcus terminalis
4 Right auricle
5 Right atrium
6 Aortic valve
7 Conus arteriosus (interventricular septum)
8 Right atrioventricular (tricuspid) valve
9 Anterior papillary muscle
10 Myocardium of right ventricle
11 Left common carotid artery
12 Left subclavian artery
13 Aortic arch
14 Ligamentum arteriosum
   (remnant of ductus arteriosus)
15 Thoracic aorta (descending aorta)
16 Ascending aorta
17 Left pulmonary vein
18 Pulmonary trunk
19 Left auricle
20 Pulmonic valve
21 Anterior papillary muscle
   with chordae tendineae
22 Myocardium of left ventricle
23 Posterior papillary muscle
24 Interventricular septum
25 Brachiocephalic veins
26 Chordae tendineae
27 Papillary muscles of right ventricle
28 Left atrium
29 Left atrioventricular (bicuspid or mitral) valve and
   chordae tendineae
30 Apex of the heart
31 Left coronary artery
32 Left ventricle

**Heart** (anterior aspect). Dissection of the four valves.

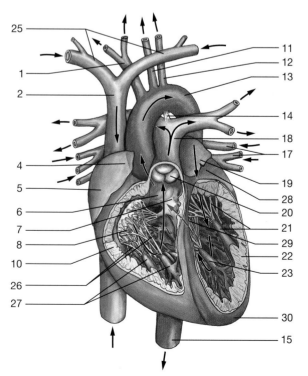

**Circulation within the heart** (anterior aspect).
Arrows: direction of blood flow.

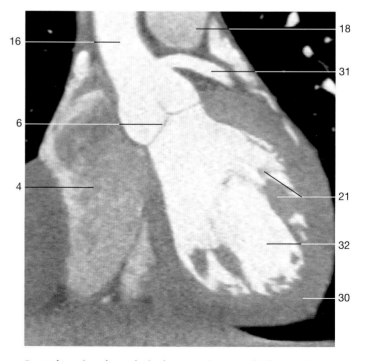

**Frontal section through the heart** at the level of left ventricle
and ascending aorta (MRI scan). (Prof. Uder, Dept. of Radiology,
Univ. Erlangen-Nuremberg, Germany.) Note the aortic valve.

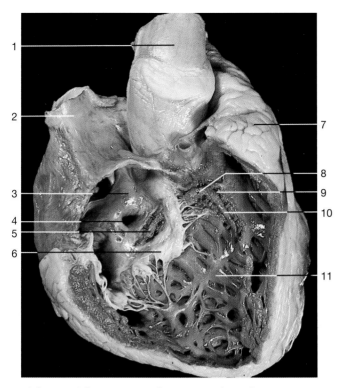

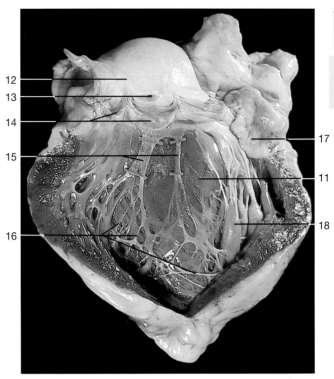

**Right ventricle.** Dissection of atrioventricular node, atrioventricular bundle (bundle of His), and right limb or bundle branch of conducting system (probes).

| | | | |
|---|---|---|---|
| 1 | Ascending aorta | 6 | Right atrioventricular valve |
| 2 | Superior vena cava | 7 | Pulmonary trunk |
| 3 | Right atrium | 8 | Atrioventricular bundle (bundle of His) |
| 4 | Opening of coronary sinus | 9 | Bifurcation of atrioventricular bundle |
| 5 | Atrioventricular node | 10 | Right bundle branch |

**Left ventricle.** Dissection of left limb or bundle branch of conducting system (probes).

11 Interventricular septum
12 Aortic sinus
13 Entrance of left coronary artery
14 Aortic valve
15 Branches of left bundle branch
16 Purkinje fibers
17 Left auricle
18 Anterior papillary muscles
19 Sulcus terminalis
20 Bulb of aorta
21 Sinu-atrial node (arrows)
22 Muscle fiber bundles of right atrium
23 Coronary sulcus (with right coronary artery)
24 Bundles of conducting system
25 Inferior vena cava
26 Papillary muscles with Purkinje fibers
27 Left atrium
28 Left bundle branch

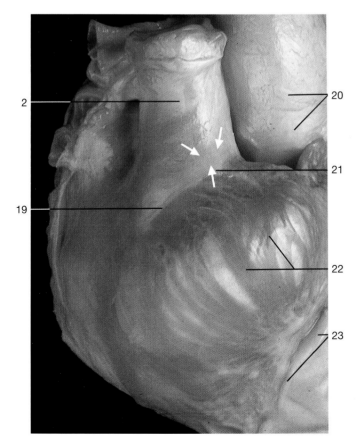

**Right atrium.** Anterior wall, showing the location of the sinu-atrial node (arrows).

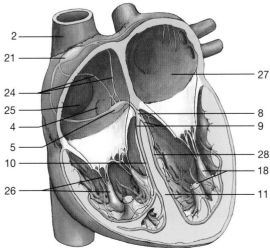

**Conducting system** (yellow) **of the heart.**

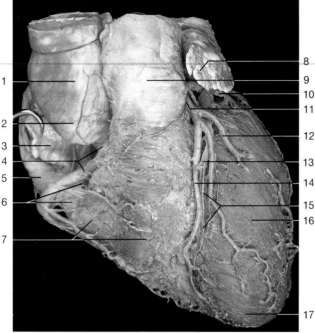

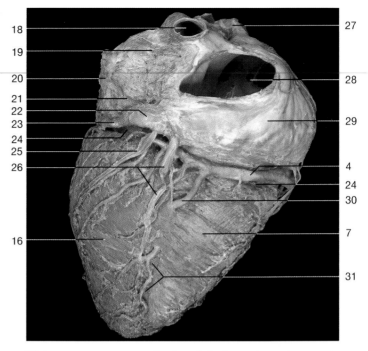

**Coronary arteries** (anterior aspect). The epicardium and subepicardial fatty tissue have been removed. The arteries have been injected with red resin from the aorta.

**Right coronary artery and veins of the heart** (posterior aspect). The epicardium and subepicardial fatty tissue have been removed. The arteries have been injected with red resin.

| | | | |
|---|---|---|---|
| 1 | Ascending aorta | 13 | Anterior interventricular vein |
| 2 | Aortic bulb and sinu-atrial branch of right coronary artery (in the dissection above) | 14 | Anterior interventricular artery |
| | | 15 | Anterior interventricular sulcus |
| | | 16 | Left ventricle |
| 3 | Right auricle | 17 | Apex of the heart |
| 4 | Right coronary artery | 18 | Right pulmonary vein |
| 5 | Right atrium | 19 | Left atrium |
| 6 | Coronary sulcus | 20 | Left pulmonary veins |
| 7 | Right ventricle | 21 | Oblique vein of left atrium (Marshall's vein) |
| 8 | Left auricle | 22 | Coronary sinus |
| 9 | Pulmonary trunk | 23 | Great cardiac vein |
| 10 | Circumflex branch of left coronary artery | 24 | Coronary sulcus (posterior part) |
| 11 | Left coronary artery | | |
| 12 | Diagonal branch of left coronary artery | | |

| | | | |
|---|---|---|---|
| 25 | Posterior vein of left ventricle | 33 | Right marginal branch of right coronary artery |
| 26 | Middle cardiac vein | 34 | Branch of sinu-atrial node |
| 27 | Left pulmonary artery | 35 | Minimal cardiac veins |
| 28 | Inferior vena cava | 36 | Small cardiac veins |
| 29 | Right atrium | 37 | Sternum |
| 30 | Posterior interventricular branch of right coronary artery | 38 | Left atrium with pulmonary veins |
| 31 | Posterior interventricular sulcus | 39 | Right marginal vein |
| 32 | Superior vena cava | | |

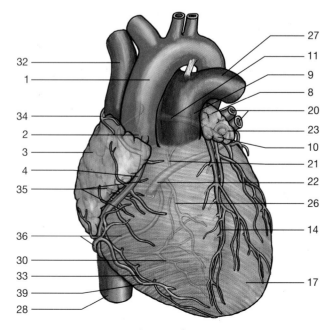

**Coronary arteries and veins of the heart** (anterior aspect).

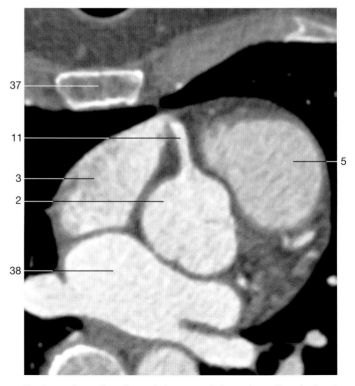

**Horizontal section through heart and thoracic wall** at the level of the aortic bulb (MRI scan). (Prof. Uder, Dept. of Radiology, Univ. Erlangen-Nuremberg, Germany.)

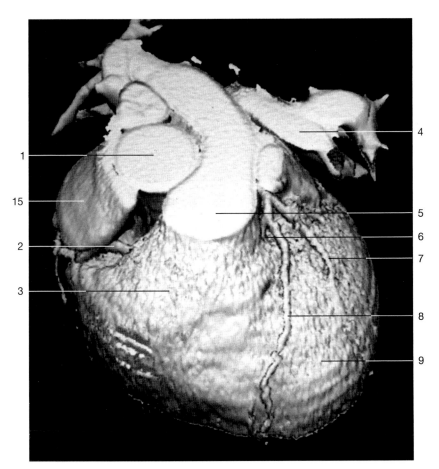

1 Ascending aorta
2 Right coronary artery
3 Right ventricle
4 Left atrium
5 Pulmonary trunk
6 Septal branch of left coronary artery
7 Diagonal branch of left coronary artery
8 Anterior interventricular branch
   of left coronary artery
9 Left ventricle
10 Aortic root
11 Right marginal branch of right coronary artery
12 Circumflex branch of left coronary artery
13 Apex of the heart
14 Superior vena cava
15 Right atrium

**Human heart** (3-D reconstruction of electron beam CT scans as "Shaded Surface Display").

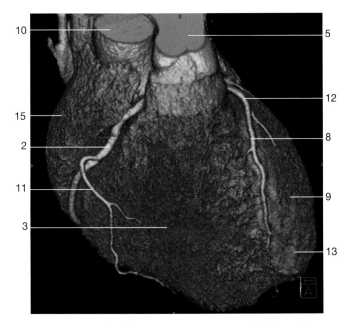

**Coronary arteries** (anterior aspect; stereoscopic MRI scan).
(Prof. Uder, Dept. of Radiology, Univ. Erlangen-Nuremberg, Germany.)

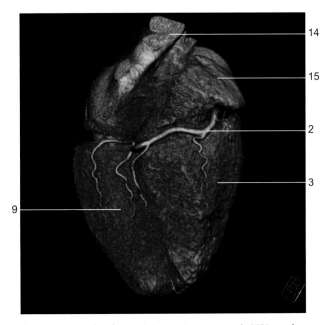

**Coronary arteries** (posterior aspect; stereoscopic MRI scan).
(Prof. Uder, Dept. of Radiology, Univ. Erlangen-Nuremberg, Germany.)

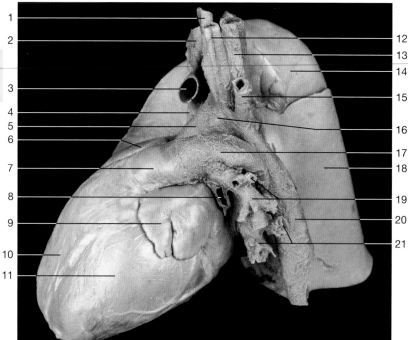

**Heart and right lung of the fetus** (viewed from left side). The left lung has been removed. Note the ductus arteriosus (Botalli).

**Heart of the fetus** (anterior aspect).
Right atrium and ventricle have been opened.

### Shunts in the fetal circulation system

| | | |
|---|---|---|
| 1. Ductus venosus (of Arantius) | between umbilical vein and inferior vena cava | bypass of liver circulation |
| 2. Foramen ovale | between right and left atrium | bypass of pulmonary circulation |
| 3. Ductus arteriosus (Botalli) | between pulmonary trunk and aorta | |

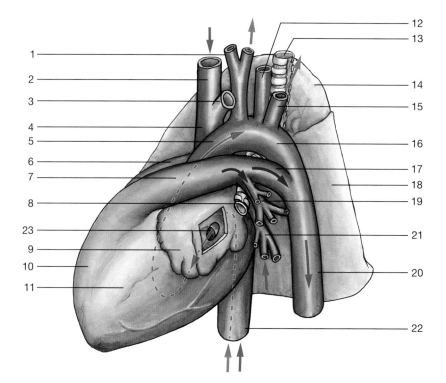

1   Right common carotid artery
2   Right brachiocephalic vein
3   Left brachiocephalic vein
4   Superior vena cava
5   Ascending aorta
6   Right auricle
7   Pulmonary trunk
8   Left primary bronchus
9   Left auricle
10  Right ventricle
11  Left ventricle
12  Left common carotid artery
13  Trachea
14  Superior lobe of right lung
15  Left subclavian artery
16  Aortic arch
17  Ductus arteriosus (Botalli)
18  Inferior lobe of right lung
19  Left pulmonary artery
    with branches to the left lung
20  Descending aorta
21  Left pulmonary veins
22  Inferior vena cava
23  Foramen ovale
24  Right atrium
25  Opening of inferior vena cava
26  Valve of inferior vena cava
    (Eustachian valve)
27  Opening of coronary sinus
28  Anterior papillary muscle of right ventricle

◁ **Heart and right lung of the fetus**
(compare with the dissection above).
Direction of blood flow indicated by arrows.
Note the change in oxygenation of blood
after ductus arteriosus entry into the aorta.

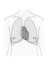

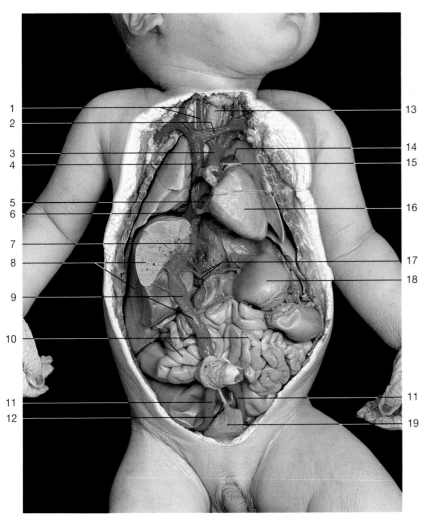

1   Internal jugular vein and
    right common carotid artery
2   Right and left brachiocephalic vein
3   Aortic arch
4   Superior vena cava
5   Foramen ovale
6   Inferior vena cava
7   Ductus venosus
8   Liver
9   Umbilical vein
10  Small intestine
11  Umbilical artery
12  Urachus
13  Trachea and left internal jugular vein
14  Left pulmonary artery
15  Ductus arteriosus (Botalli)
16  Right ventricle
17  Hepatic arteries (red) and
    portal vein (blue)
18  Stomach
19  Urinary bladder
20  Portal vein
21  Pulmonary veins
22  Descending aorta
23  Placenta

**Thoracic and abdominal organs in the newborn** (anterior aspect). The right atrium has been opened to show the foramen ovale. The left lobe of the liver has been removed.

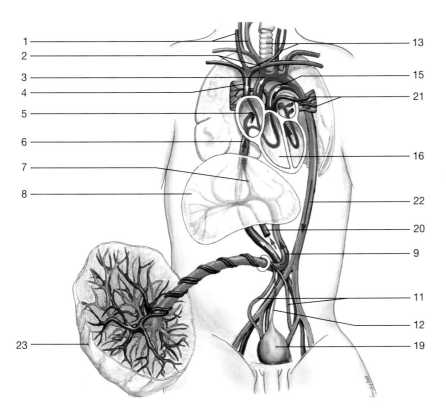

◁ **Fetal circulatory system.**
The oxygen gradient is indicated by color.

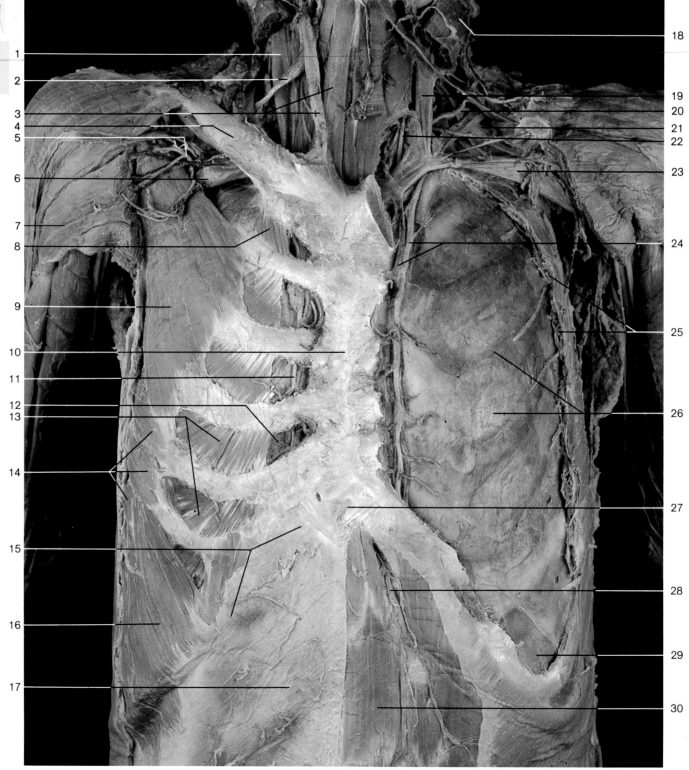

**Thoracic organs** (anterior aspect). The left clavicle and ribs have been partially removed, and the right intercostal spaces have been opened to show the internal thoracic vein and artery.

| | | | | | |
|---|---|---|---|---|---|
| 1 | Right internal jugular vein | 11 | Right internal thoracic artery and vein | 21 | Brachial plexus |
| 2 | Omohyoid muscle | 12 | Fascicles of transversus thoracis muscle | 22 | Vagus nerve |
| 3 | Sternohyoid muscle and external jugular vein | 13 | Internal intercostal muscles | 23 | Left axillary vein |
| 4 | Clavicle | 14 | Serratus anterior muscle | 24 | Left internal thoracic artery and vein |
| 5 | Thoraco-acromial artery | 15 | Costal margin | 25 | Ribs and thoracic wall (cut) |
| 6 | Right subclavian vein | 16 | External abdominal oblique muscle | 26 | Costal pleura |
| 7 | Pectoralis major muscle | 17 | Anterior sheath of rectus abdominis muscle | 27 | Xiphoid process |
| 8 | External intercostal muscle | 18 | Sternocleidomastoid muscle | 28 | Superior epigastric artery |
| 9 | Pectoralis minor muscle | 19 | Left internal jugular vein | 29 | Diaphragm |
| 10 | Body of sternum | 20 | Transverse cervical artery | 30 | Rectus abdominis muscle |

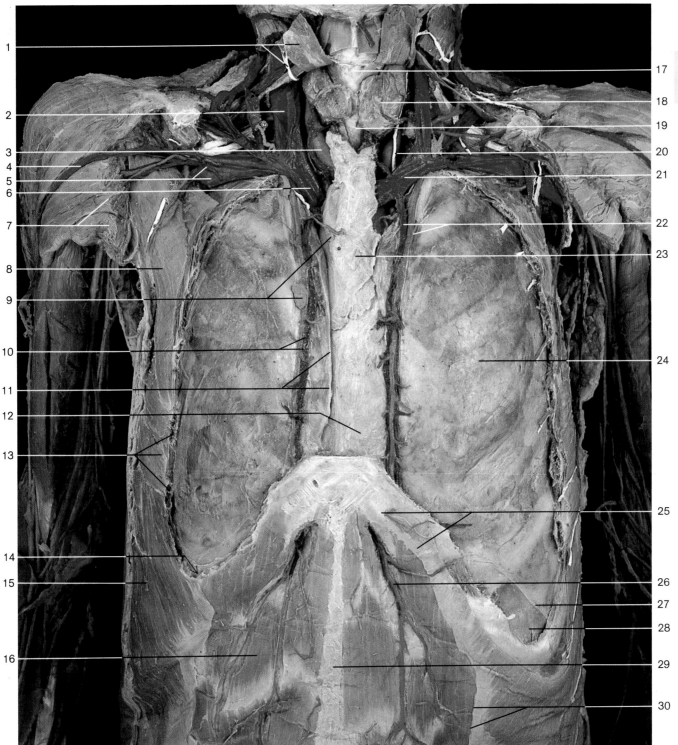

**Thoracic organs** (anterior aspect). Ribs, clavicle, and sternum have been partly removed to show anterior mediastinum and pleura. Red = arteries; blue = veins; green = lymph vessels and nodes.

| | | |
|---|---|---|
| 1 Sternothyroid muscle and its nerve (a branch of the ansa cervicalis) | 11 Anterior margin of costal pleura | 21 Left brachiocephalic vein |
| 2 Right internal jugular vein | 12 Pericardium | 22 Left internal thoracic artery and vein |
| 3 Right common carotid artery | 13 Fifth and sixth ribs (divided) and serratus anterior muscle | 23 Thymus |
| 4 Cephalic vein | 14 Costodiaphragmatic recess | 24 Costal pleura |
| 5 Right subclavian vein | 15 External abdominal oblique muscle | 25 Costal margin |
| 6 Right brachiocephalic vein | 16 Rectus abdominis muscle | 26 Superior epigastric artery |
| 7 Pectoralis major muscle (divided) | 17 Larynx (thyroid cartilage) | 27 Margin of costal pleura |
| 8 Pectoralis minor muscle (divided) | 18 Thyroid gland | 28 Diaphragm |
| 9 Parasternal lymph nodes | 19 Trachea | 29 Linea alba |
| 10 Internal thoracic artery and vein | 20 Left vagus nerve | 30 Cut edge of anterior sheath of rectus abdominis muscle |

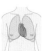

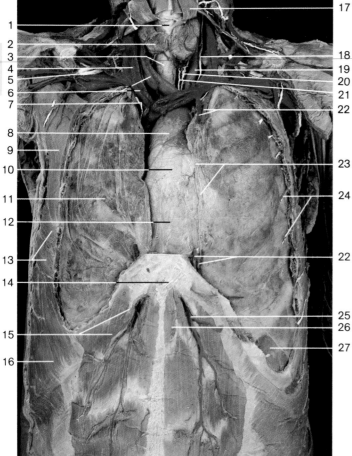

| | |
|---|---|
| 1 | Larynx (thyroid cartilage) |
| 2 | Thyroid gland |
| 3 | Trachea |
| 4 | Internal jugular vein |
| 5 | Brachial plexus |
| 6 | Right brachiocephalic vein and common carotid artery |
| 7 | Right phrenic nerve |
| 8 | Ascending aorta |
| 9 | Pectoralis minor muscle (divided) |
| 10 | Pulmonary trunk (covered by pericardium) |
| 11 | Costal pleura |
| 12 | Pericardium and heart |
| 13 | Serratus anterior muscle |
| 14 | Xiphoid process |
| 15 | Costal margin |
| 16 | External abdominal oblique muscle |
| 17 | Sternothyroid muscle (divided and reflected) |
| 18 | Vagus nerve |
| 19 | Left common carotid artery |
| 20 | Left sympathetic trunk |
| 21 | Left recurrent laryngeal nerve |
| 22 | Left internal thoracic artery and vein (divided) |
| 23 | Margin of costal pleura |
| 24 | Intercostal nerves and vessels |
| 25 | Superior epigastric artery |
| 26 | Rectus abdominis muscle |
| 27 | Diaphragm |
| 28 | Ansa cervicalis |
| 29 | Phrenic nerve and anterior scalene muscle |
| 30 | External jugular vein (divided) |
| 31 | Right subclavian vein |
| 32 | Right brachiocephalic vein |
| 33 | Internal thoracic artery (divided) |
| 34 | Internal thoracic vein (divided) |
| 35 | Right lung |
| 36 | Cricothyroid muscle |
| 37 | Omohyoid muscle |
| 38 | Thymus |
| 39 | Left lung |

**Thoracic organs** (anterior aspect). The internal thoracic vessels have been removed, and the anterior margins of the pleura and lungs have been slightly reflected to display the anterior and middle mediastinum, including the heart and great vessels. Red = arteries; blue = veins; green = lymph vessels and nodes.

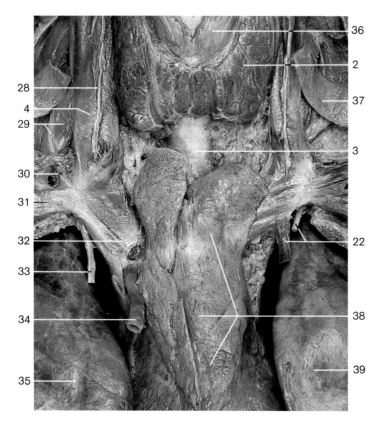

**Thoracic organs** (anterior aspect, enlarged details). The position (above the heart) and size of the thymus are shown.

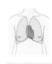

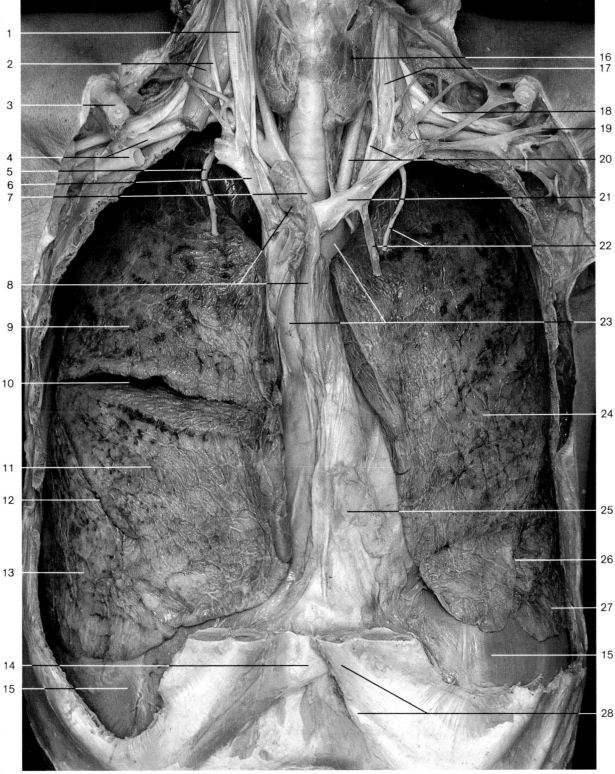

**Thoracic organs** (anterior aspect). The pleura has been opened and the lungs exposed. Remnants of the thymus and pericardium are seen.

| | | |
|---|---|---|
| 1 Right internal jugular vein | 11 Middle lobe of right lung | 20 Left common carotid artery and |
| 2 Phrenic nerve and anterior scalene muscle | 12 Oblique fissure of right lung | vagus nerve |
| 3 Clavicle (divided) | 13 Lower lobe of right lung | 21 Left brachiocephalic vein |
| 4 Right subclavian artery and vein | 14 Xiphoid process | 22 Internal thoracic artery and vein (divided) |
| 5 Internal thoracic artery | 15 Diaphragm | 23 Ascending aorta and aortic arch |
| 6 Right brachiocephalic vein | 16 Thyroid gland | 24 Upper lobe of left lung |
| 7 Brachiocephalic trunk | 17 Left internal jugular vein | 25 Pericardium |
| 8 Thymus (atrophic) | 18 Brachial plexus | 26 Oblique fissure of left lung |
| 9 Upper lobe of right lung | 19 Left cephalic vein | 27 Lower lobe of left lung |
| 10 Horizontal fissure of right lung (incomplete) | | 28 Costal margin |

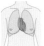

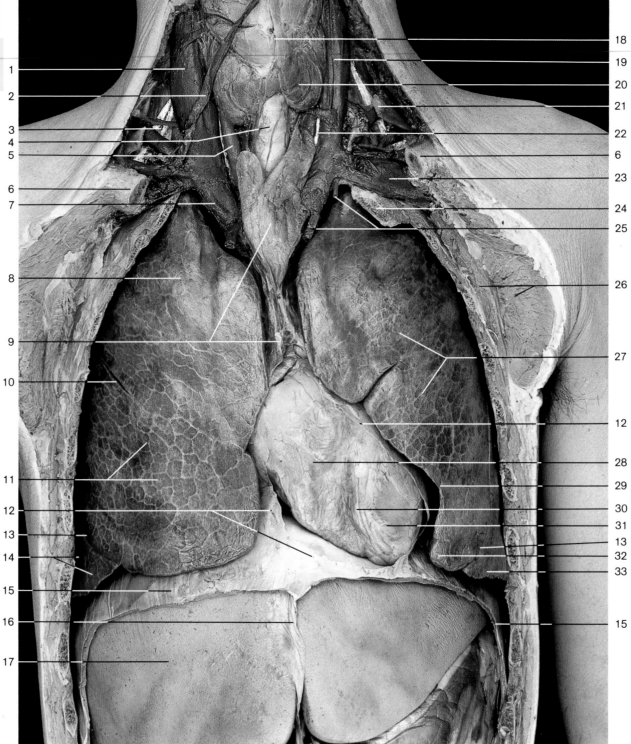

**Thoracic organs** (anterior aspect). The thoracic wall, costal pleura, pericardium, and diaphragm have been partly removed.
Red = arteries; blue = veins.

| | | | |
|---|---|---|---|
| 1 | Internal jugular vein | 13 | Oblique fissure of lung |
| 2 | External jugular vein (displaced medially) | 14 | Lower lobe of right lung |
| 3 | Brachial plexus | 15 | Diaphragm |
| 4 | Trachea | 16 | Falciform ligament |
| 5 | Right common carotid artery | 17 | Liver |
| 6 | Clavicle (divided) | 18 | Location of larynx |
| 7 | Right brachiocephalic vein | 19 | Left internal jugular vein |
| 8 | Upper lobe of right lung | 20 | Thyroid gland |
| 9 | Thymus (atrophic) | 21 | Omohyoid muscle (divided) |
| 10 | Horizontal fissure of right lung | 22 | Vagus nerve |
| 11 | Middle lobe of right lung | 23 | Left subclavian vein |
| 12 | Pericardium (cut edges) | 24 | First rib (divided) |

| | |
|---|---|
| 25 | Internal thoracic artery and vein |
| 26 | Pectoralis major and pectoralis minor muscles (cut edges) |
| 27 | Upper lobe of left lung |
| 28 | Right ventricle |
| 29 | Cardiac notch of left lung |
| 30 | Interventricular sulcus of heart |
| 31 | Left ventricle |
| 32 | Lingula |
| 33 | Lower lobe of left lung |

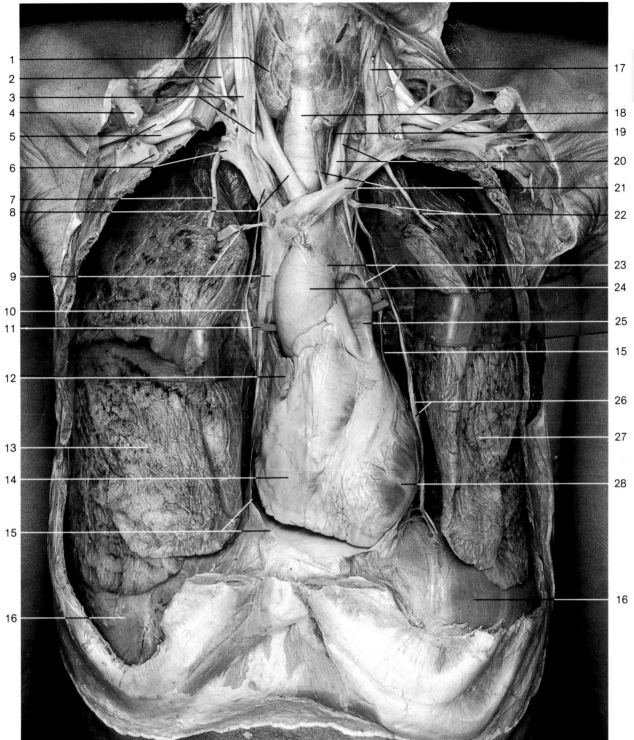
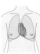

**Thoracic organs** (anterior aspect). Position of the heart and middle mediastinum. The anterior wall of the thorax, the costal pleura, and the pericardium have been removed and the lungs slightly reflected.

1  Thyroid gland
2  Phrenic nerve and anterior scalene muscle
3  Vagus nerve and internal jugular vein
4  Clavicle (divided)
5  Brachial plexus and subclavian artery
6  Subclavian vein
7  Internal thoracic artery
8  Brachiocephalic trunk and right brachiocephalic vein
9  Superior vena cava and thymic vein
10  Right phrenic nerve

11  Transverse pericardial sinus (probe)
12  Right auricle
13  Middle lobe of right lung
14  Right ventricle
15  Cut edge of pericardium
16  Diaphragm
17  Internal jugular vein
18  Trachea
19  Left recurrent laryngeal nerve
20  Left common carotid artery and vagus nerve

21  Left brachiocephalic vein and inferior thyroid vein
22  Left internal thoracic artery and vein (divided)
23  Upper margin of pericardial sac
24  Ascending aorta
25  Pulmonary trunk
26  Left phrenic nerve and left pericardiacophrenic artery and vein
27  Upper lobe of left lung
28  Left ventricle

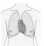

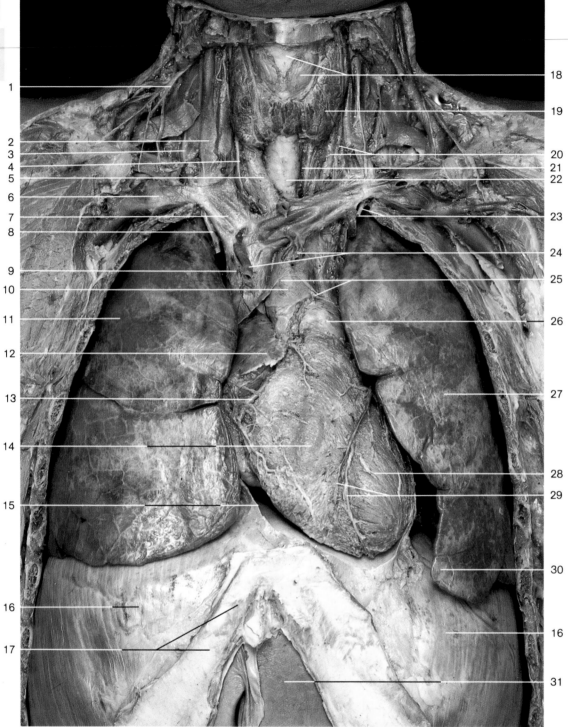

**Thoracic organs** (anterior aspect). Position of heart, dissection of coronary vessels in situ. The anterior wall of thorax, costal pleura, and pericardium have been removed.

| | |
|---|---|
| 1 | Intermediate supraclavicular nerve |
| 2 | Internal jugular vein |
| 3 | Right phrenic nerve |
| 4 | Right vagus nerve |
| 5 | Right common carotid artery |
| 6 | Right subclavian vein |
| 7 | Right brachiocephalic vein |
| 8 | Right internal thoracic artery |
| 9 | Superior vena cava |
| 10 | Ascending aorta |
| 11 | Right lung |
| 12 | Right atrium |
| 13 | Right coronary artery and small cardiac vein |
| 14 | Right ventricle |
| 15 | Cut edge of pericardium |
| 16 | Diaphragm |
| 17 | Costal margin |
| 18 | Larynx (cricothyroid muscle and thyroid cartilage) |
| 19 | Thyroid gland |
| 20 | Left common carotid artery and left vagus nerve |
| 21 | Left recurrent laryngeal nerve |
| 22 | Trachea |
| 23 | Left internal thoracic artery and vein (divided) |
| 24 | Thymic veins |
| 25 | Margin of pericardial sac |
| 26 | Pulmonary trunk |
| 27 | Left lung |
| 28 | Left ventricle |
| 29 | Anterior interventricular artery and vein |
| 30 | Lingula |
| 31 | Liver |

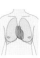

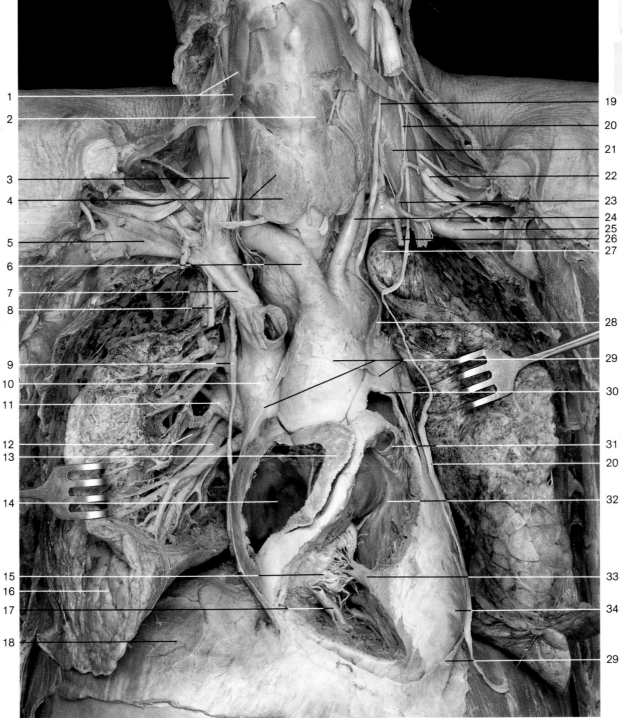

**Thoracic organs** (anterior aspect). Heart with valves in situ. Anterior wall of thorax, pleura, and anterior portion of pericardium have been removed. The right atrium and ventricle have been opened to show the right atrioventricular and pulmonary valves.

| | |
|---|---|
| 1 Omohyoid muscle | |
| 2 Pyramidal lobe of thyroid gland | |
| 3 Internal jugular vein | |
| 4 Thyroid gland | |
| 5 Right subclavian vein | |
| 6 Brachiocephalic trunk | |
| 7 Right brachiocephalic vein | |
| 8 Right internal thoracic artery | |
| 9 Right phrenic nerve | |
| 10 Superior vena cava | |
| 11 Pulmonary vein | |
| 12 Branches of pulmonary artery | |

| | |
|---|---|
| 13 Right auricle | |
| 14 Right atrium | |
| 15 Right atrioventricular (tricuspid) valve | |
| 16 Right lung | |
| 17 Posterior papillary muscle | |
| 18 Diaphragm | |
| 19 Left vagus nerve | |
| 20 Left phrenic nerve | |
| 21 Anterior scalene muscle | |
| 22 Brachial plexus | |
| 23 Thyrocervical trunk | |

| | |
|---|---|
| 24 Left common carotid artery | |
| 25 Left subclavian artery | |
| 26 Left internal thoracic artery | |
| 27 Apex of left lung | |
| 28 Left recurrent laryngeal nerve | |
| 29 Cut edge of pericardium | |
| 30 Pulmonary trunk (fenestrated) | |
| 31 Pulmonic valve | |
| 32 Supraventricular crest | |
| 33 Anterior papillary muscle | |
| 34 Left ventricle | |

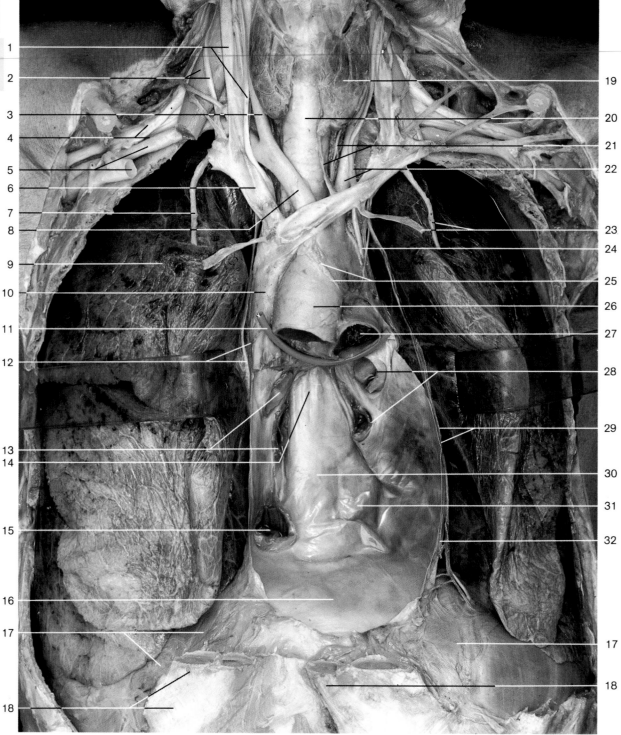

**Thoracic organs** (anterior aspect). Pericardium and mediastinum. Anterior wall of thorax and heart have been removed and the lungs slightly reflected. Note the probe within transverse pericardial sinus.

1  Right internal jugular vein and
   right vagus nerve
2  Right phrenic nerve and anterior scalene muscle
3  Right common carotid artery
4  Brachial plexus
5  Right subclavian artery and vein
6  Right brachiocephalic vein
7  Right internal thoracic artery (divided)
8  Brachiocephalic trunk
9  Upper lobe of right lung
10 Superior vena cava
11 Transverse pericardial sinus (probe)

12 Right phrenic nerve and right
   pericardiacophrenic artery and vein
13 Right pulmonary veins
14 Oblique sinus of pericardium
15 Inferior vena cava
16 Diaphragmatic part of pericardium
17 Diaphragm
18 Costal margin
19 Thyroid gland
20 Trachea
21 Left recurrent laryngeal nerve and
   inferior thyroid vein

22 Left common carotid artery and left vagus nerve
23 Left internal thoracic artery and vein (divided)
24 Vagus nerve at aortic arch
25 Cut edge of pericardium
26 Ascending aorta
27 Pulmonary trunk (divided)
28 Left pulmonary veins
29 Left phrenic nerve and
   left pericardiacophrenic artery and vein
30 Contour of esophagus beneath pericardium
31 Contour of aorta beneath pericardium
32 Pericardium (cut edge)

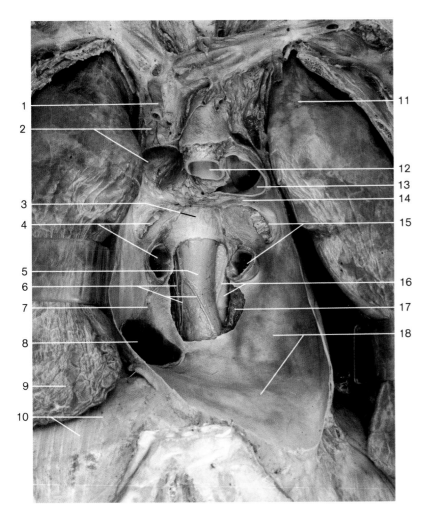

1   Internal thoracic vein
2   Superior vena cava
3   Oblique sinus of pericardium
4   Right pulmonary veins
5   Esophagus
6   Branches of right vagus nerve
7   Mesocardium
8   Inferior vena cava
9   Middle lobe of right lung
10  Diaphragm
11  Upper lobe of left lung
12  Ascending aorta
13  Pulmonary trunk
14  Transverse pericardial sinus
15  Left pulmonary veins
16  Descending aorta and left vagus nerve
17  Left lung (adjacent to pericardium)
18  Pericardium
19  Left subclavian artery
20  Vagus nerve
21  Left recurrent laryngeal nerve
22  Descending aorta
23  Pulmonary artery
24  Left atrium
25  Left ventricle
26  Coronary sinus
27  Left common carotid artery
28  Brachiocephalic trunk
29  Azygos arch
30  Right atrium
31  Right ventricle
32  Aortic arch

**Pericardial sac** (anterior aspect). The heart has been removed, and the posterior wall of the pericardium has been opened to show the adjacent esophagus and aorta.

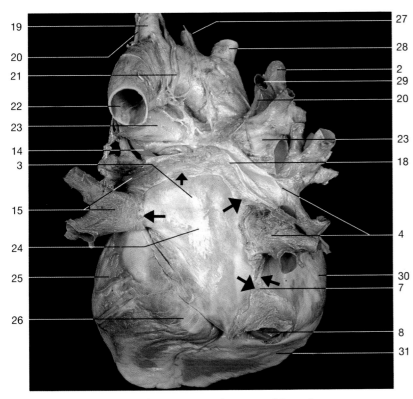

**Heart with epicardium** (posterior aspect). Arrows: oblique sinus.

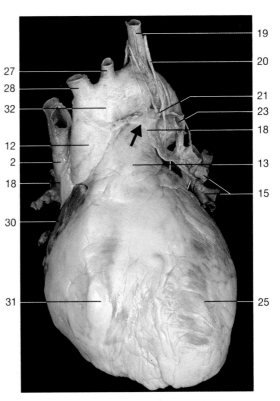

**Heart with epicardium** (anterior aspect). Arrow: pericardial reflection.

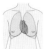

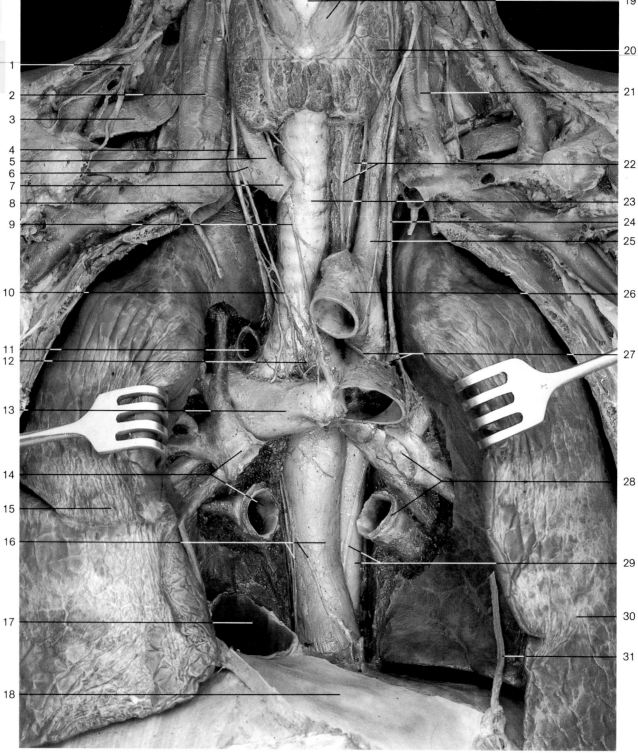

**Mediastinal organs** (anterior aspect). Heart and pericardium have been removed. Both lungs have been slightly reflected.

1 Supraclavicular nerves
2 Internal jugular vein
3 Omohyoid muscle
4 Right vagus nerve
5 Right common carotid artery
6 Right subclavian artery
7 Brachiocephalic trunk
8 Right brachiocephalic vein
9 Superior cervical cardiac branch of vagus nerve
10 Inferior cervical cardiac branches of vagus nerve

11 Azygos arch (divided)
12 Bifurcation of trachea
13 Right pulmonary artery
14 Right pulmonary veins
15 Right lung
16 Esophagus and branches of right vagus nerve
17 Inferior vena cava
18 Pericardium
19 Larynx (thyroid cartilage, cricothyroid muscle)
20 Thyroid gland
21 Internal jugular vein

22 Esophagus and left recurrent laryngeal nerve
23 Trachea
24 Left vagus nerve
25 Left common carotid artery
26 Aortic arch
27 Left recurrent laryngeal nerve branching off from vagus nerve
28 Left pulmonary veins
29 Thoracic aorta and left vagus nerve
30 Left lung
31 Left phrenic nerve (divided)

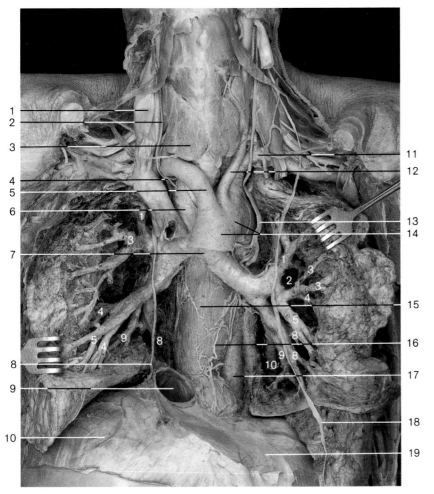

1   Internal jugular vein
2   Right vagus nerve
3   Thyroid gland
4   Right recurrent laryngeal nerve
5   Brachiocephalic trunk
6   Trachea
7   Bifurcation of trachea
8   Right phrenic nerve
9   Inferior vena cava
10  Diaphragm
11  Left subclavian artery
12  Left common carotid artery
13  Left vagus nerve
14  Aortic arch
15  Esophagus
16  Esophageal plexus
17  Thoracic aorta
18  Left phrenic nerve
19  Pericardium
    at the central tendon of diaphragm
20  Superior vena cava
21  Pulmonary veins and left atrium

**Bronchial tree in situ** (anterior aspect). Heart and pericardium have been removed. The bronchi of the bronchopulmonary segments are dissected.
1–10 = numbers of segments (compare with pages 254, 255, and 259).

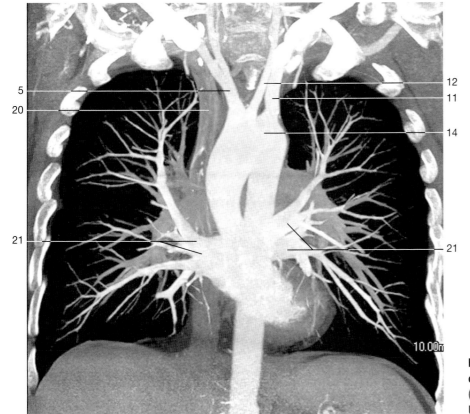

**Frontal section through the thoracic cavity** showing the mediastinal vessels (MRI scan). (Prof. Uder, Dept. of Radiology, Univ. Erlangen-Nuremberg, Germany.)

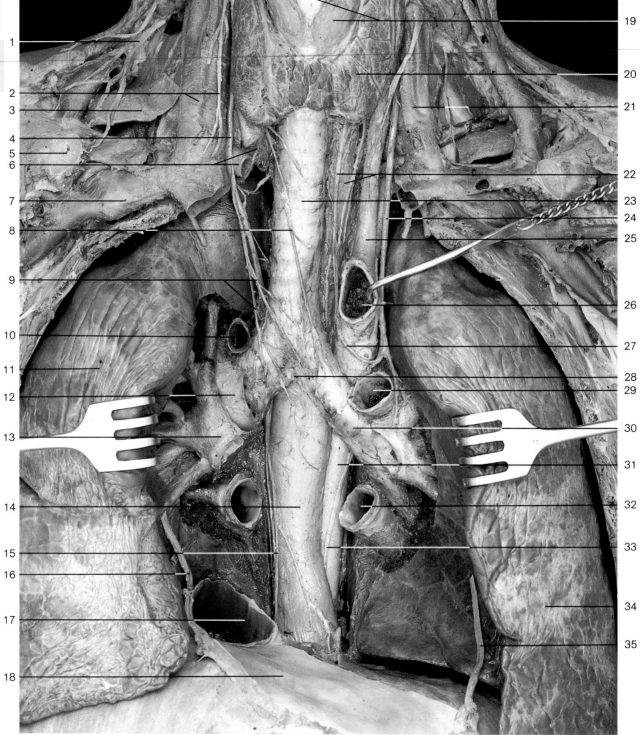

**Mediastinal organs** (anterior aspect). The heart with the pericardium has been removed, and the lungs and aortic arch have been slightly reflected to show the vagus nerves and their branches.

1   Supraclavicular nerves
2   Right internal jugular vein with ansa cervicalis
3   Omohyoid muscle
4   Right vagus nerve
5   Clavicle
6   Right subclavian artery and recurrent laryngeal nerve
7   Right subclavian vein
8   Superior cervical cardiac branch of vagus nerve
9   Inferior cervical cardiac branch of vagus nerve
10  Azygos arch (divided)
11  Right lung

12  Right pulmonary artery
13  Right pulmonary veins
14  Esophagus
15  Esophageal plexus
16  Right phrenic nerve (divided)
17  Inferior vena cava
18  Pericardium covering the diaphragm
19  Larynx (thyroid cartilage and cricothyroid muscle)
20  Thyroid gland
21  Left internal jugular vein
22  Esophagus and left recurrent laryngeal nerve
23  Trachea

24  Left vagus nerve
25  Left common carotid artery
26  Aortic arch
27  Left recurrent laryngeal nerve
28  Bifurcation of trachea
29  Left pulmonary artery
30  Left primary bronchus
31  Descending aorta
32  Left pulmonary veins
33  Branch of left vagus nerve
34  Left lung
35  Left phrenic nerve (divided)

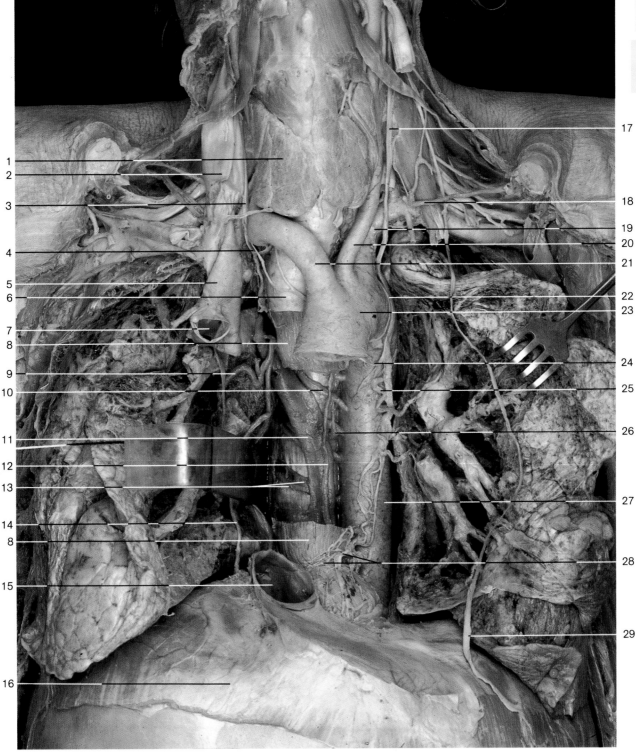

**Mediastinal organs** (anterior aspect). Heart and distal part of esophagus have been removed to display the vessels and nerves of the posterior mediastinum.

| | | |
|---|---|---|
| 1 Thyroid gland | 11 Azygos vein | 21 Brachiocephalic trunk |
| 2 Right internal jugular vein | 12 Thoracic duct | 22 Left vagus nerve |
| 3 Right vagus nerve | 13 Posterior intercostal artery and vein | 23 Aortic arch |
| 4 Point where right recurrent laryngeal nerve | (in front of the vertebral column) | 24 Left recurrent laryngeal nerve |
|   is branching off the vagus nerve | 14 Right phrenic nerve | 25 Left bronchial artery |
| 5 Right brachiocephalic vein | 15 Inferior vena cava | 26 Lymph node |
| 6 Trachea | 16 Diaphragm | 27 Thoracic aorta |
| 7 Left brachiocephalic vein (reflected) | 17 Left vagus nerve | 28 Esophageal plexus |
| 8 Esophagus | 18 Thyrocervical trunk | 29 Left phrenic nerve |
| 9 Right bronchial artery | 19 Left subclavian artery | |
| 10 Posterior intercostal artery | 20 Left common carotid artery | |

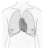

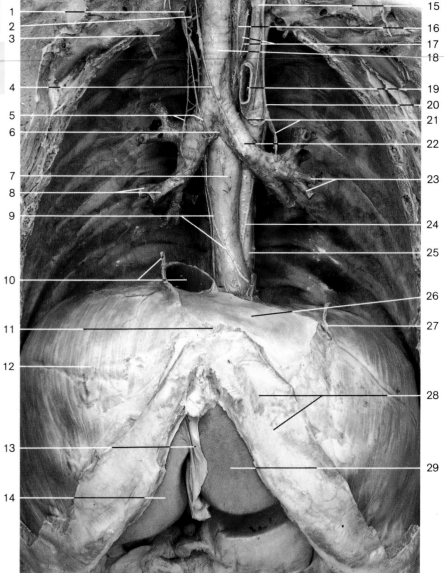

**Posterior mediastinal organs with diaphragm** (anterior aspect). Heart and lungs have been removed, the costal margin remains in place. Note the different courses of left and right vagus.

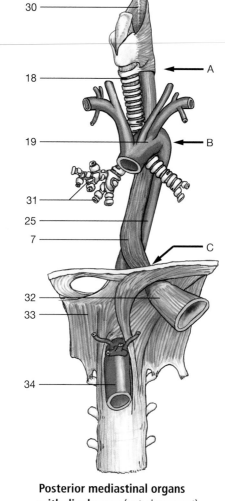

**Posterior mediastinal organs with diaphragm** (anterior aspect). Three regions in which the esophagus is narrowed are shown:

A = termed upper sphincter (at the level of the cricoid cartilage);
B = termed middle sphincter (at the level of the aortic arch);
C = termed lower sphincter (at the level of the diaphragm).

| | |
|---|---|
| 1 Right subclavian artery | 11 Sternal part of diaphragm |
| 2 Right recurrent laryngeal nerve | 12 Costal part of diaphragm |
| 3 Right brachiocephalic vein | 13 Falciform ligament of liver |
| 4 Superior cervical cardiac nerve | 14 Liver (quadrate lobe) |
| 5 Inferior cervical cardiac nerves and pulmonary branches | 15 Left common carotid artery |
| 6 Bifurcation of trachea | 16 Left recurrent laryngeal nerve |
| 7 Esophagus (thoracic part) | 17 Esophageal branches of left vagus nerve and esophagus |
| 8 Bronchi of lateral and medial segments of middle lobe | 18 Trachea |
| 9 Esophageal plexus and branches of right vagus nerve | 19 Aortic arch |
| 10 Inferior vena cava and right phrenic nerve (cut) | 20 Left vagus nerve |
| | 21 Left recurrent laryngeal nerve with inferior cardiac nerve |
| | 22 Left primary bronchus |

23 Superior and inferior lingular bronchi
24 Esophageal plexus of left vagus nerve
25 Descending aorta
26 Central tendon of diaphragm covered with pericardium
27 Left phrenic nerve (divided)
28 Costal margin
29 Liver (left lobe)
30 Pharynx
31 Secondary bronchi
32 Esophagus (abdominal part)
33 Diaphragm
34 Abdominal aorta

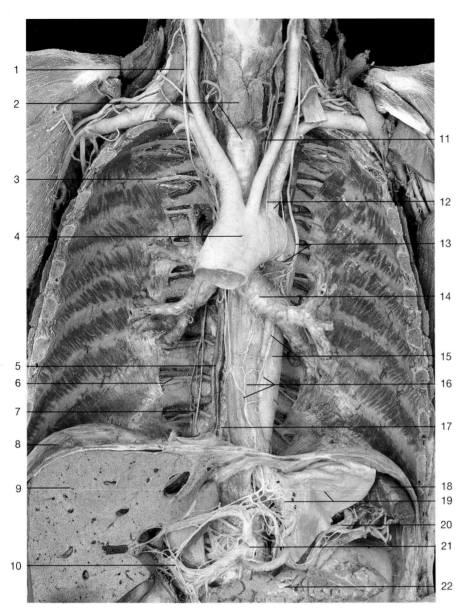

**Posterior mediastinal organs** (anterior aspect).

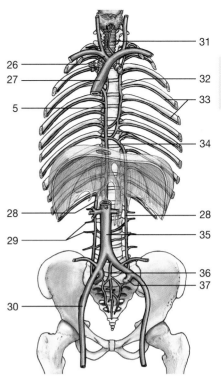

**Veins of the posterior wall of thoracic and abdominal cavities** (anterior aspect).

1   Right vagus nerve
2   Thyroid gland and trachea
3   Intercostal nerve
4   Aortic arch
5   Azygos vein
6   Posterior intercostal artery
7   Greater splanchnic nerve
8   Diaphragm
9   Liver
10  Proper hepatic artery and hepatic plexus
11  Left recurrent laryngeal nerve
12  Inferior cervical cardiac nerves
13  Left vagus nerve and
    left recurrent laryngeal nerve
14  Left primary bronchus
15  Thoracic aorta and left vagus nerve
16  Esophagus and esophageal plexus
17  Thoracic duct
18  Spleen
19  Anterior gastric plexus and stomach (divided)
20  Splenic artery and splenic plexus
21  Celiac trunk and celiac plexus
22  Pancreas
23  Ramus communicans
24  Sympathetic trunk and sympathetic ganglion
25  Posterior intercostal vein and artery
    and intercostal nerve
26  Right brachiocephalic vein
27  Superior vena cava
28  Ascending lumbar vein
29  Lumbar veins
30  Right external iliac vein
31  Trachea
32  Accessory hemiazygos vein
33  Posterior intercostal veins
34  Hemiazygos vein
35  Inferior vena cava
36  Median sacral vein
37  Internal iliac vein

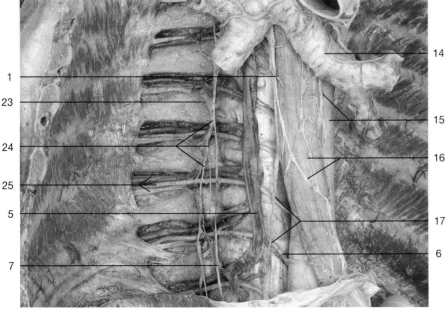

**Inferior segment of posterior mediastinum** (anterior aspect).

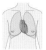

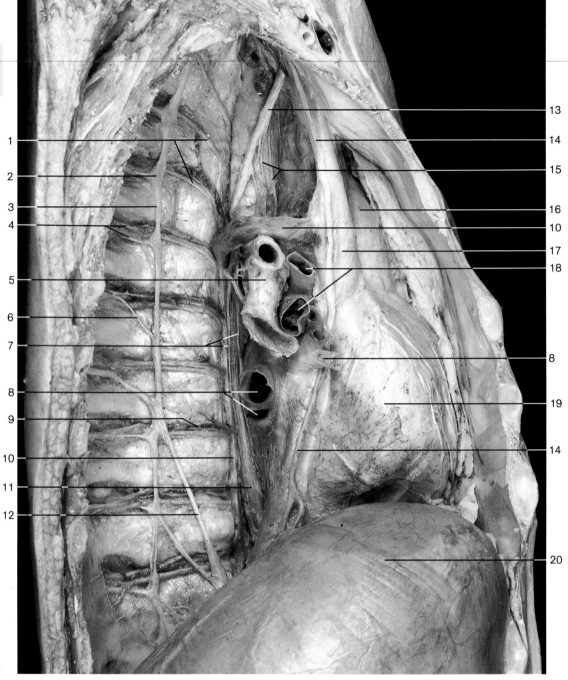

**Mediastinal organs** (right lateral aspect). Right lung and pleura of right half of the thorax have been removed.

| | | |
|---|---|---|
| 1 Posterior intercostal arteries | 7 Esophageal plexus | 14 Right phrenic nerve |
| 2 Ganglion of sympathetic trunk | (branches of right vagus nerve) | 15 Inferior cervical cardiac branches |
| 3 Sympathetic trunk | 8 Pulmonary veins | of vagus nerve |
| 4 Vessels and nerves of the intercostal space | 9 Posterior intercostal vein | 16 Aortic arch |
| (from above: posterior intercostal vein and | 10 Azygos vein | 17 Superior vena cava |
| artery and intercostal nerve) | 11 Esophagus | 18 Right pulmonary artery |
| 5 Right primary bronchus | 12 Greater splanchnic nerve | 19 Heart with pericardium |
| 6 Ramus communicans of sympathetic trunk | 13 Right vagus nerve | 20 Diaphragm |

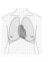

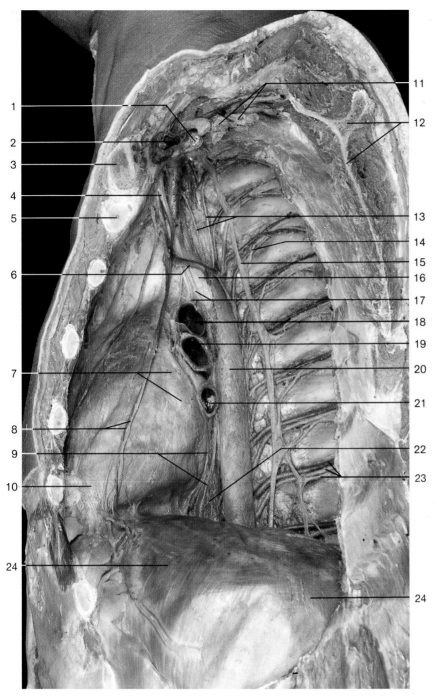

**Mediastinal organs** (left lateral aspect). Posterior and superior mediastinum. The heart with the pericardium is located in situ. Within the posterior mediastinum the descending thoracic aorta and the sympathetic trunk are shown.

**Main branches of descending aorta** (anterior aspect).

| | | |
|---|---|---|
| 1 Subclavian artery | 12 Scapula (divided) | 23 Posterior intercostal artery and vein and intercostal nerve |
| 2 Subclavian vein | 13 Posterior intercostal arteries | 24 Diaphragm |
| 3 Clavicle (divided) | 14 White ramus communicans of sympathetic trunk | 25 Common carotid artery |
| 4 Left vagus nerve | 15 Sympathetic trunk | 26 Subclavian artery |
| 5 First rib (divided) | 16 Aortic arch | 27 Highest intercostal artery |
| 6 Left superior intercostal vein | 17 Left vagus nerve and left recurrent laryngeal nerve | 28 Bifurcation of trachea |
| 7 Left atrium with pericardium | 18 Left pulmonary artery | 29 Celiac trunk |
| 8 Left phrenic nerve and pericardiacophrenic artery and vein | 19 Left primary bronchus | 30 Renal artery |
| 9 Esophageal plexus (branches derived from left vagus nerve) | 20 Thoracic aorta | 31 Superior mesenteric artery |
| 10 Apex of the heart with pericardium | 21 Pulmonary vein | 32 Inferior mesenteric artery |
| 11 Brachial plexus | 22 Esophagus (thoracic part) | 33 Common iliac artery |

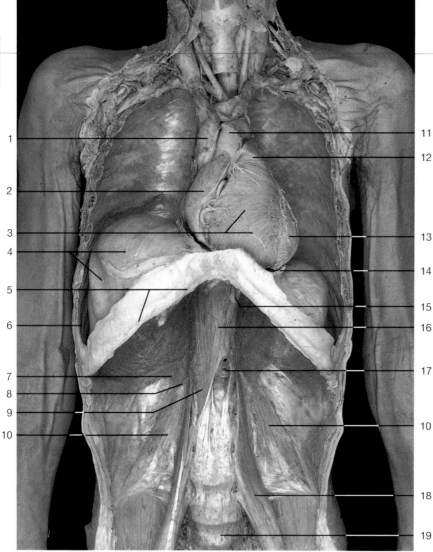

1 Superior vena cava
2 Right atrium
3 Right ventricle
4 Costal part of diaphragm
5 Costal margin
6 Position of costodiaphragmatic recess
7 Lateral arcuate ligament
8 Medial arcuate ligament
9 Right crus of lumbar part of diaphragm
10 Quadratus lumborum muscle
11 Ascending aorta
12 Pulmonary trunk
13 Left ventricle
14 Pericardium and diaphragm
15 Esophageal hiatus and
   abdominal part of esophagus (cut)
16 Lumbar part of diaphragm
17 Aortic hiatus
18 Psoas major muscle
19 Lumbar vertebrae

**Diaphragm in situ** (anterior aspect). Anterior walls of thoracic and abdominal cavities have been removed. Natural position of the heart above the central tendon on the diaphragm is shown.

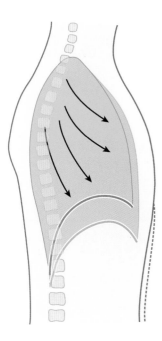

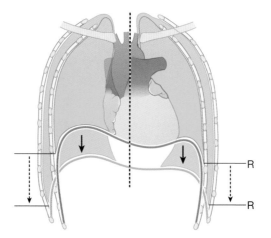

**Changes in the position of the diaphragm and thoracic cage during respiration.** Left: lateral aspect; right: anterior aspect. During inspiration the diaphragm moves downward and the lower part of the thoracic cage expands forward and laterally, causing the costodiaphragmatic recess (R) to enlarge (cf. dotted arrows).

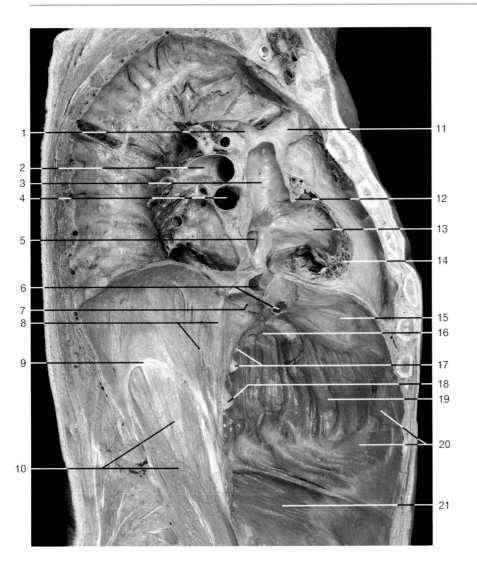

1 Azygos venous arch
2 Right pulmonary artery
3 Superior vena cava
4 Right pulmonary vein
5 Fossa ovalis
6 Hepatic veins
7 Inferior vena cava
8 Right crus of lumbar part
   of diaphragm
9 Medial arcuate ligament
10 Psoas major muscle
11 Left brachiocephalic vein
12 Terminal crista
13 Right atrium
14 Right auricle
15 Central tendon of diaphragm
16 Esophagus
17 Celiac trunk and
   superior mesenteric artery
18 Aorta
19 Costal part of diaphragm
20 Costal margin
21 Transverse abdominal muscle

**Diaphragm and thoracic organs.**
Paramedian section to the right of
the median plane through thoracic
and upper abdominal cavities. The
plane passes through the superior
and inferior vena cava just to the
right of the vertebral bodies. Most
of the heart remains in situ to the
left of this plane (viewed from the
right side).

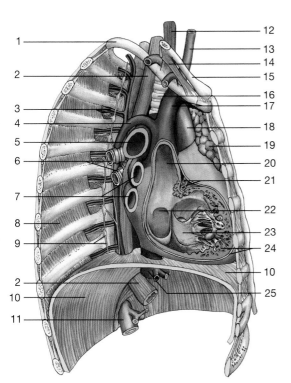

**Diaphragm and thoracic organs** (paramedian section).
The heart is partly dissected.

1 First rib
2 Esophagus
3 Intercostal artery, vein, and nerve
4 Azygos venous arch
5 Pulmonal artery
6 Right bronchi
7 Pulmonary veins
8 Internal intercostal muscle
9 Sympathetic trunk
10 Diaphragm
11 Abdominal aorta
12 Anterior scalene muscle
13 Internal jugular vein
14 Subclavius muscle
15 Clavicle
16 Trachea
17 Junction between superior vena cava
   and left brachiocephalic vein
18 Aorta
19 Remnants of thymus gland
20 Entrance of superior vena cava
   into the right atrium
21 Right coronary artery and vein
22 Fossa ovalis
23 Right atrioventricular valve and
   anterior papillary muscle
24 Right ventricle with pericardium
25 Inferior vena cava

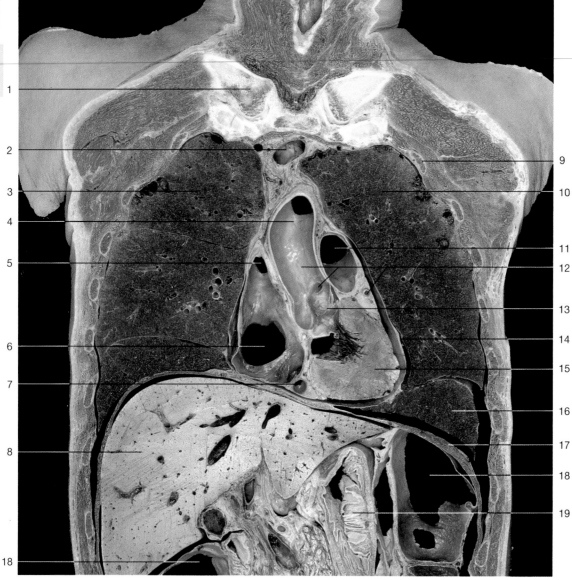

**Coronal section through the thorax** at the level of the ascending aorta (anterior aspect).

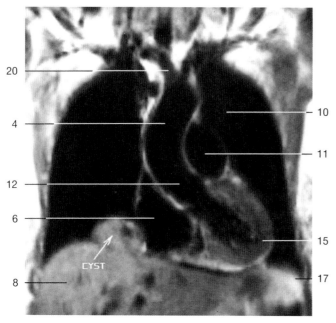

**Coronal section through the thorax** at the level of the ascending aorta (MRI scan).

1  Clavicle
2  Left brachiocephalic vein
3  Upper lobe of right lung
4  Aortic arch
5  Superior vena cava
6  Right atrium
   (entrance of inferior vena cava)
7  Coronary sinus
8  Liver
9  Second rib
10  Upper lobe of left lung
11  Pulmonary trunk
12  Ascending aorta and
   left coronary artery
13  Aortic valve
14  Pericardium
15  Myocardium of left ventricle
16  Lower lobe of left lung
17  Diaphragm
18  Colic flexures
19  Stomach
20  Brachiocephalic trunk

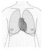

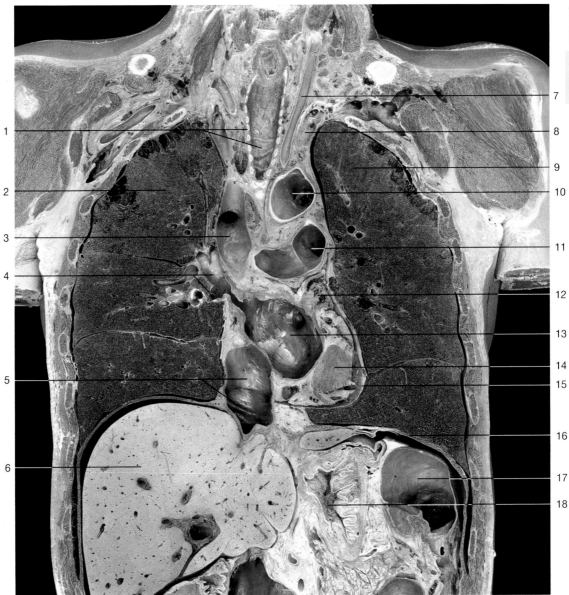

**Coronal section through the thorax** at the level of superior and inferior vena cava (anterior aspect).

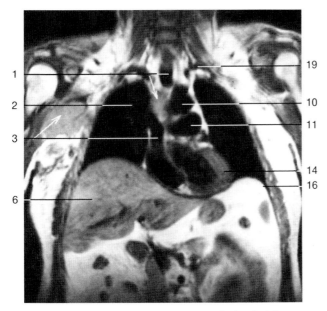

**Coronal section through the thorax** at the level of the superior vena cava (MRI scan). Arrows: metastases of tumor.

1  Trachea
2  Upper lobe of right lung
3  Superior vena cava
4  Right pulmonary veins
5  Inferior vena cava and right atrium
6  Liver
7  Left common carotid artery
8  Left subclavian vein
9  Upper lobe of left lung
10  Aortic arch
11  Left pulmonary artery
12  Left auricle
13  Left atrium with orifices
    of pulmonary veins
14  Left ventricle (myocardium)
15  Pericardium
16  Diaphragm
17  Left colic flexure
18  Stomach
19  Left subclavian artery

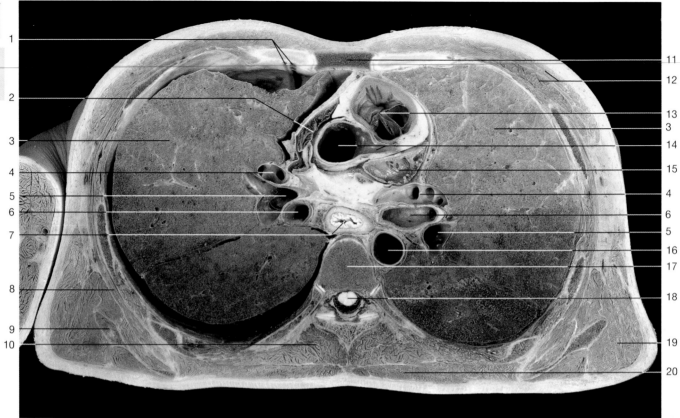

**Horizontal section through the thorax.** Section 1 (from below).

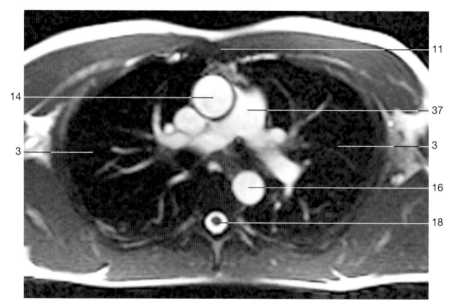

**Horizontal section through the thorax** at the level of section 1 (MRI scan).
(Prof. Bautz and Dr. Janka, Dept. of Radiology, Univ. Erlangen-Nuremberg, Germany.)

| | | | |
|---|---|---|---|
| 1 | Internal thoracic artery and vein | 12 | Pectoralis major and minor muscles |
| 2 | Right atrium | 13 | Conus arteriosus (right ventricle) and |
| 3 | Lung | | pulmonic valve |
| 4 | Pulmonary artery | 14 | Ascending aorta and left coronary artery |
| 5 | Pulmonary vein | | (only in the upper figure) |
| 6 | Primary bronchus | 15 | Left atrium |
| 7 | Esophagus | 16 | Descending aorta |
| 8 | Serratus anterior muscle | 17 | Thoracic vertebra |
| 9 | Scapula | 18 | Spinal cord |
| 10 | Longissimus thoracis muscle | 19 | Latissimus dorsi muscle |
| 11 | Sternum | 20 | Trapezius muscle |

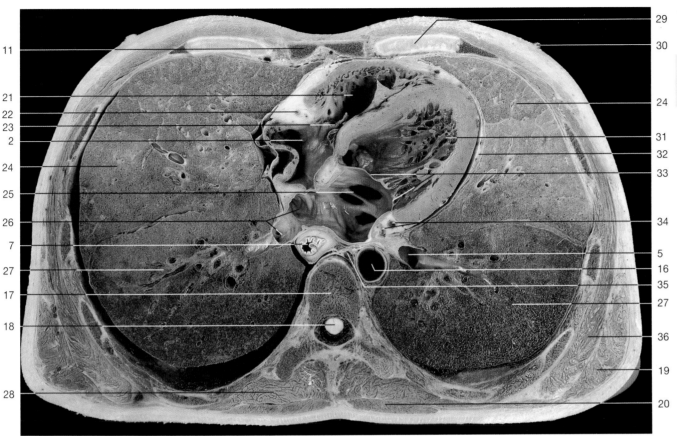

**Horizontal section through the thorax.** Section 2 (from below).

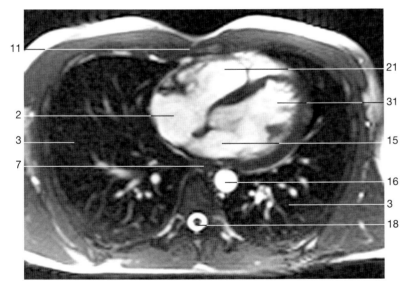

**Horizontal section through the thorax** at the level of section 2 (MRI scan).
(Prof. Bautz and Dr. Janka, Dept. of Radiology, Univ. Erlangen-Nuremberg, Germany.)

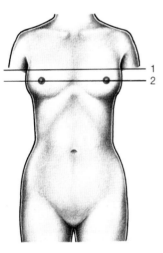

**Horizontal section through the thorax.**
Levels of the sections are indicated.

| 21 | Right ventricle | 30 | Nipple |
|----|----|----|----|
| 22 | Right coronary artery | 31 | Left ventricle |
| 23 | Right atrioventricular valve | 32 | Pericardium |
| 24 | Lung (upper lobe) | 33 | Left atrioventricular valve |
| 25 | Left atrium | 34 | Left coronary artery and coronary sinus |
| 26 | Pulmonary veins | 35 | Accessory hemiazygos vein |
| 27 | Lung (lower lobe) | 36 | Serratus anterior muscle |
| 28 | Erector muscle of spine | 37 | Pulmonary trunk |
| 29 | Third costal cartilage | | |

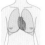

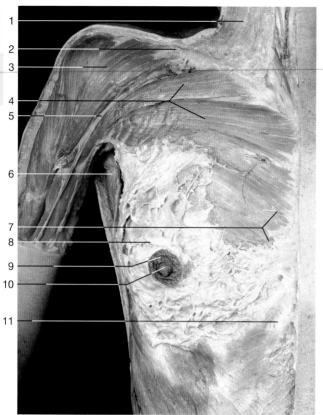

**Dissection of mammary gland** (anterior aspect).

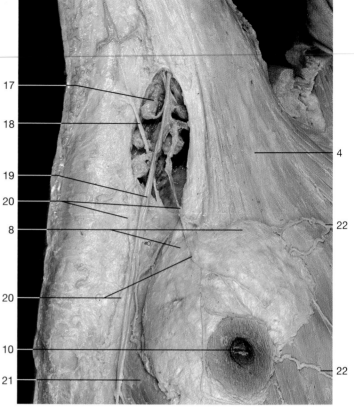

**Dissection of mammary gland and axillary lymph nodes.**

| | | | |
|---|---|---|---|
| 1 | Platysma muscle | 8 | Breast tissue |
| 2 | Clavicle | 9 | Areola |
| 3 | Deltoid muscle | 10 | Nipple (papilla) |
| 4 | Pectoralis major muscle | 11 | Costal margin |
| 5 | Deltopectoral groove and cephalic vein | 12 | Pectoral fascia |
| | | 13 | Mammary gland |
| 6 | Latissimus dorsi muscle | 14 | Serratus anterior muscle (insertion) |
| 7 | Medial mammarian branches of intercostal nerves | 15 | Lactiferous sinus |

| | |
|---|---|
| 16 | Apical lymph nodes |
| 17 | Axillary lymph nodes |
| 18 | Intercostobrachial nerve |
| 19 | Lateral thoracic vein |
| 20 | Lymph vessels |
| 21 | Serratus anterior muscle |
| 22 | Medial branches of intercostal arteries |
| 23 | Pectoralis minor muscle |

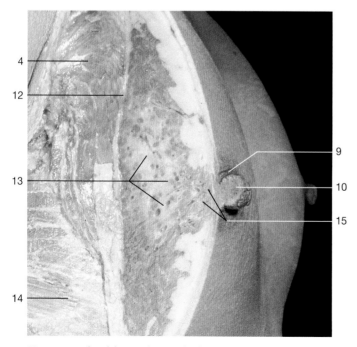

**Mammary gland** (sagittal section) of a pregnant female.

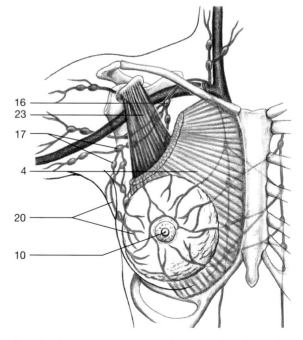

**Lymphatics of the mammary gland.** Most lymph vessels drain into the axillary lymph nodes.

# 5 Abdominal Organs

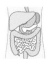

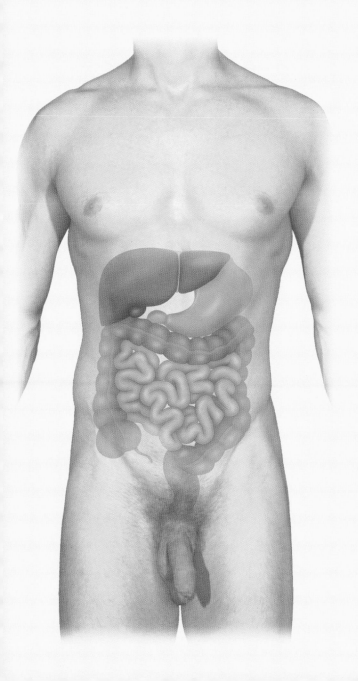

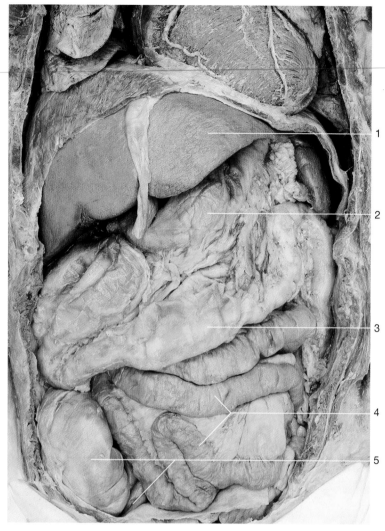

1  Liver (left lobe)
2  Stomach
3  Transverse colon
4  Small intestine
5  Cecum with vermiform appendix
6  Rectus abdominis muscle
7  Small intestine and peritoneum
8  Rib (cut)
9  Bile duct, duodenum, and pancreas
10  Inferior vena cava
11  Body of second lumbar vertebra (L₂)
12  Right kidney
13  Cauda equina and dura mater
14  Linea alba
15  Falciform ligament
16  Stomach and pylorus
17  Superior mesenteric artery and vein
18  Abdominal aorta
19  Pancreas adjacent to lesser sac (omental bursa)
20  Left renal artery and vein
21  Left kidney
22  Psoas major muscle
23  Deep muscles of the back

**Abdominal organs in situ** (anterior aspect). The greater omentum has been partly removed or reflected.

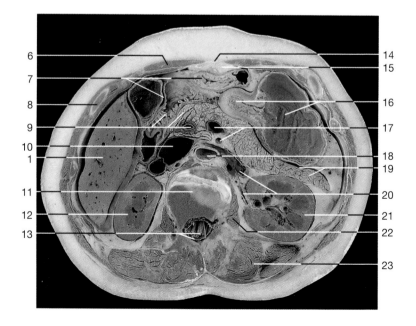

**Horizontal section through the abdominal cavity** at the level of the second lumbar vertebra (from below).

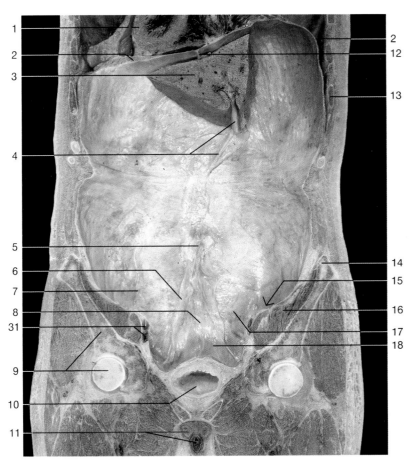

1  Left ventricle with pericardium
2  Diaphragm
3  Remnant of liver
4  Ligamentum teres
   (free margin of falciform ligament)
5  Site of umbilicus
6  Medial umbilical fold
   (containing the obliterated umbilical artery)
7  Lateral umbilical fold
   (containing inferior epigastric artery and vein)
8  Median umbilical fold
   (containing remnant of urachus)
9  Head of femur and pelvic bone
10 Urinary bladder
11 Root of penis
12 Falciform ligament of liver
13 Rib (divided)
14 Iliac crest (divided)
15 Site of deep inguinal ring and
   lateral inguinal fossa
16 Iliopsoas muscle (divided)
17 Medial inguinal fossa
18 Supravesical fossa
19 Posterior layer of rectus sheath
20 Transverse abdominal muscle
21 Umbilicus and arcuate line
22 Inferior epigastric artery
23 Femoral nerve
24 Iliopsoas muscle
25 Remnant of umbilical artery
26 Femoral artery and vein
27 Tendinous intersection
   of rectus abdominis muscle
28 Rectus abdominis muscle
29 Interfoveolar ligament
30 Pubic symphysis (divided)
31 External iliac artery and vein

**Anterior abdominal wall of the male.** Frontal section through pelvic cavity and hip joints (internal aspect).

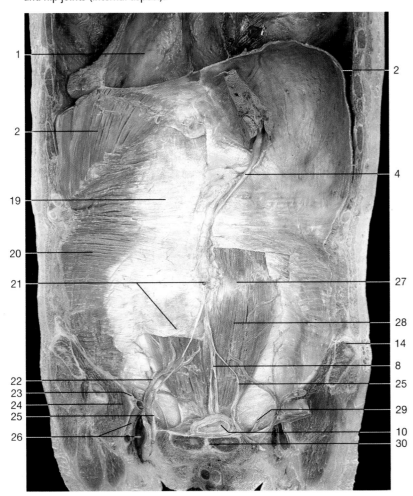

**Anterior abdominal wall of the male**
(internal aspect). The peritoneum and parts of the posterior layer of rectus sheath have been removed. Dissection of inferior epigastric arteries and veins.

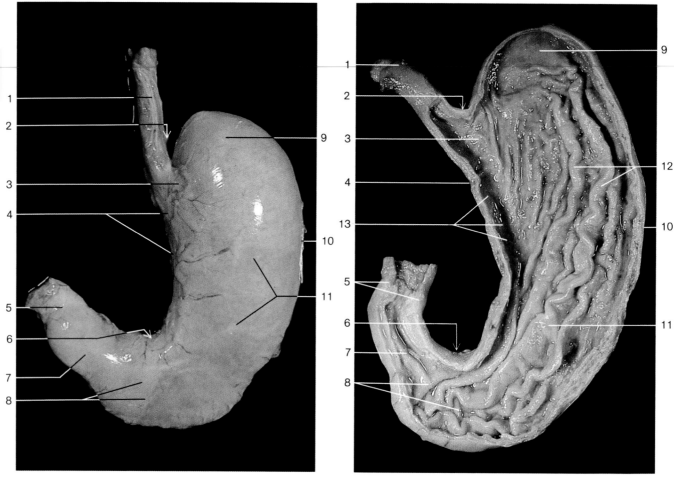

**Stomach** (anterior aspect).

**Mucosa of posterior wall of stomach** (anterior aspect).

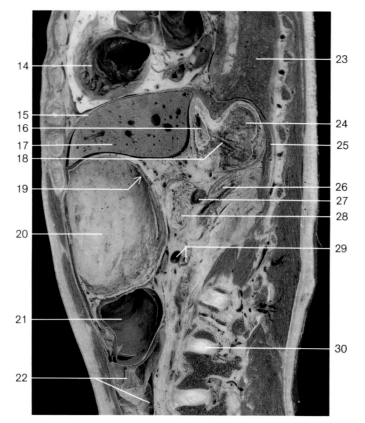

**Position of the stomach** (parasagittal section through upper part of left abdominal cavity 3.5 cm lateral to median plane).

1   Esophagus
2   Cardial notch
3   Cardial part of stomach
4   Lesser curvature of stomach
5   Pyloric sphincter
6   Angular notch (incisura angularis)
7   Pyloric canal
8   Pyloric antrum
9   Fundus of stomach
10  Greater curvature of stomach
11  Body of stomach
12  Folds of mucous membrane (gastric rugae)
13  Gastric canal
14  Right ventricle of heart
15  Diaphragm (cut edge)
16  Abdominal part of esophagus
17  Liver
18  Cardial part of stomach (cut edge)
19  Position of pyloric canal
20  Body of stomach
21  Transverse colon
22  Small intestine
23  Lung (cut edge)
24  Fundus of stomach (section)
25  Lumbar part of diaphragm (cut edge)
26  Suprarenal gland
27  Splenic vein
28  Pancreas
29  Superior mesenteric artery and vein
30  Intervertebral disc

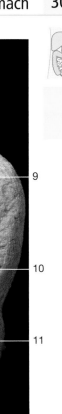

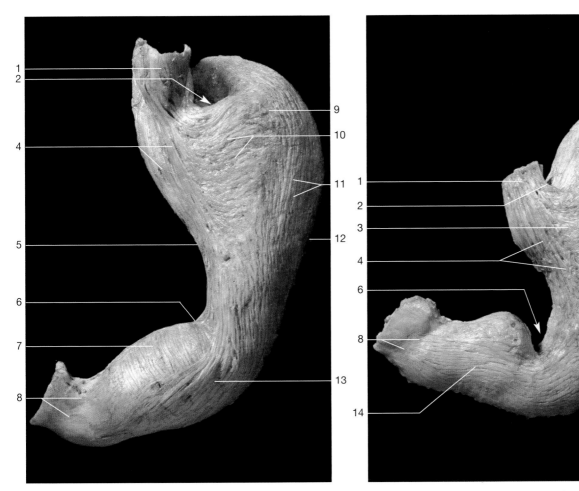

**Muscular coat of stomach,** outer layer (anterior aspect).

**Muscular coat of stomach,** middle layer (anterior aspect).

1   Esophagus (abdominal part)
2   Cardial notch
3   Cardial part of stomach
4   Longitudinal muscle layer at lesser curvature of stomach
5   Lesser curvature
6   Incisura angularis
7   Circular muscle layer of pyloric part of stomach
8   Pyloric sphincter muscle
9   Fundus of stomach
10  Circular muscle layer of fundus of stomach
11  Longitudinal muscle layer of greater curvature of stomach
12  Greater curvature of stomach
13  Longitudinal muscle layer
    (transition from body to pyloric part of stomach)
14  Pyloric part of stomach
15  Oblique muscle fibers

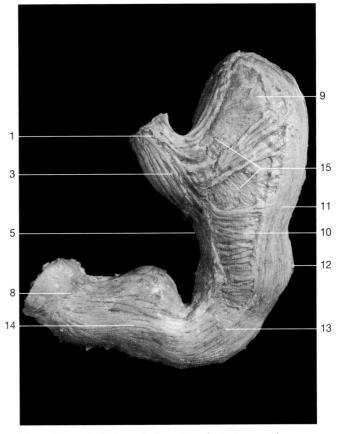

**Muscular coat of stomach,** inner layer (anterior aspect).

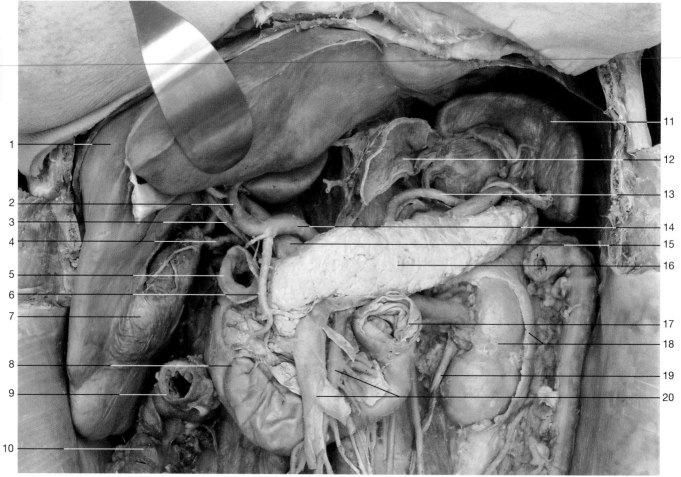

**Upper abdominal region with pancreas, duodenum, spleen, and left kidney** (anterior aspect). Stomach and transverse colon have been removed and the liver elevated; the superior mesenteric vein is slightly enlarged.

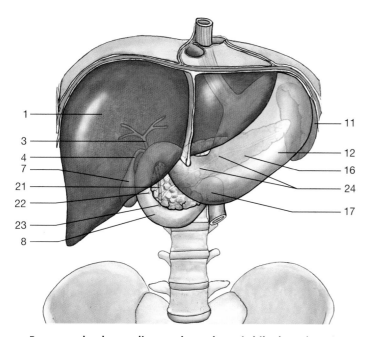

**Pancreas, duodenum, liver, and extrahepatic bile ducts** (anterior aspect).

1   Liver
2   Hepatic artery proper
3   Hepatic duct
4   Cystic duct
5   Pylorus
6   Gastroduodenal artery
7   Gallbladder
8   Duodenum
9   Right colic flexure
10  Ascending colon
11  Spleen
12  Stomach
13  Splenic artery
14  Common hepatic artery
15  Portal vein
16  Pancreas
17  Duodenojejunal flexure
18  Kidney (with capsula adiposa)
19  Ureter
20  Superior mesenteric artery and vein
21  Common bile duct
22  Minor duodenal papilla
23  Major duodenal papilla
24  Pancreatic duct

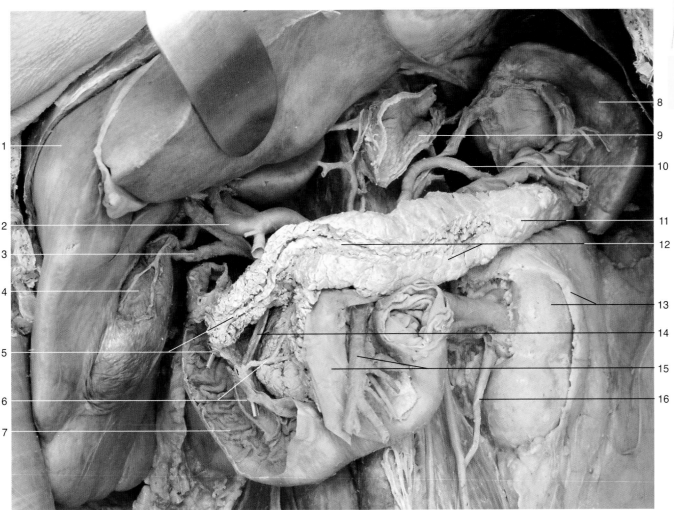

**Upper abdominal region with pancreas, duodenum, spleen, and left kidney** (anterior aspect). Stomach and transverse colon have been removed and the duodenum fenestrated. The liver has been elevated to show the extrahepatic bile ducts. In this case the accessory pancreatic duct represents the main excretory duct of the pancreas.

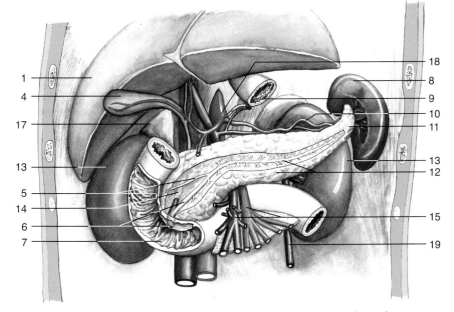

**Upper abdominal organs** (anterior aspect). The schematic drawing shows the most common situation of the pancreatic ducts.

1 Liver
2 Hepatic artery proper
3 Cystic duct
4 Gallbladder
5 Minor duodenal papilla and accessory pancreatic duct
6 Major duodenal papilla and pancreatic duct
7 Duodenum
8 Spleen
9 Stomach
10 Splenic artery
11 Tail of pancreas
12 Pancreas (pancreatic duct and body of pancreas)
13 Kidney (with capsula adiposa in the dissection above)
14 Common bile duct
15 Superior mesenteric artery and vein
16 Ureter
17 Suprarenal gland
18 Aorta with celiac trunk
19 Inferior mesenteric vein

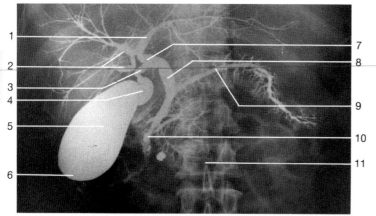

| | |
|---|---|
| 1 | Left hepatic duct |
| 2 | Right hepatic duct |
| 3 | Cystic duct |
| 4 | Neck of gallbladder |
| 5 | Body of gallbladder |
| 6 | Fundus of gallbladder |
| 7 | Common hepatic duct |
| 8 | Common bile duct |
| 9 | Pancreatic duct |
| 10 | Major duodenal papilla |
| 11 | Second lumbar vertebra |
| 12 | Folds of mucous membrane of gallbladder |
| 13 | Muscular coat of gallbladder |
| 14 | Neck of gallbladder (opened) |
| 15 | Cystic duct with spiral fold |
| 16 | Minor duodenal papilla |
| 17 | Accessory pancreatic duct |
| 18 | Uncinate process |
| 19 | Plica circularis of duodenum (Kerckring's fold) |
| 20 | Head of pancreas |
| 21 | Body of pancreas |
| 22 | Tail of pancreas |
| 23 | Descending part of duodenum |
| 24 | Incisure of pancreas |

**Bile ducts, gallbladder, and pancreatic duct** (X-ray, a.-p. direction).

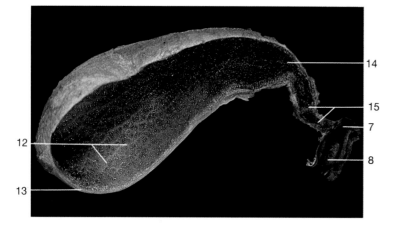

**Isolated gallbladder and cystic duct** (anterior aspect).
The gallbladder has been opened to display the mucous membrane.

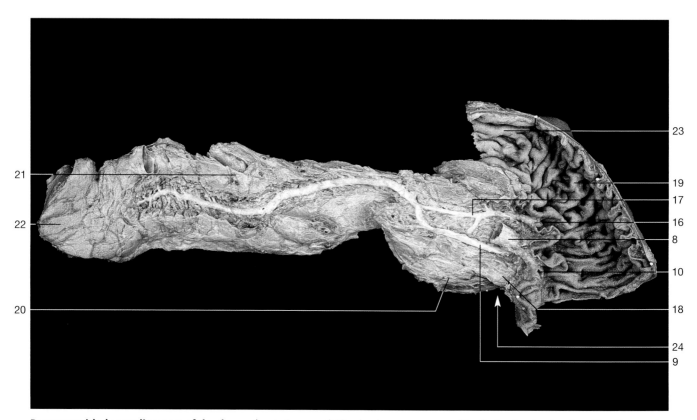

**Pancreas with descending part of duodenum** (posterior aspect). The duodenum was opened to display the duodenal papillae. Pancreatic duct has been dissected, the common bile duct has been divided. The sphincter of Oddi is shown.

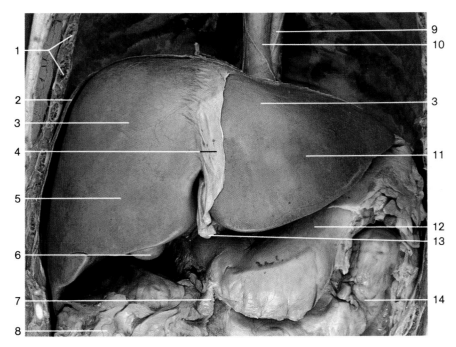

**Liver in situ** (anterior aspect). Part of the diaphragm has been removed.

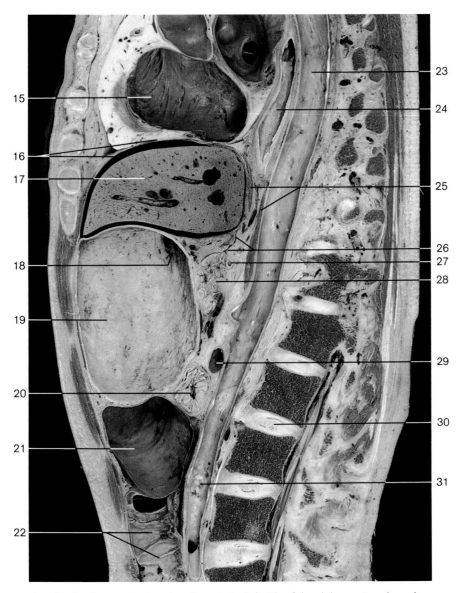

**Liver in situ** (parasagittal section through the left side of the abdomen 2 cm lateral to median plane).

1  Ribs (cut edges)
2  Diaphragm
3  Diaphragmatic surface of liver
4  Falciform ligament of liver
5  Right lobe of liver
6  Fundus of gallbladder
7  Gastrocolic ligament
8  Greater omentum
9  Aorta
10  Esophagus
11  Left lobe of liver
12  Stomach
13  Ligamentum teres
14  Transverse colon
15  Right atrium of heart
16  Central tendon and
    sternal portion of diaphragm
17  Liver (cut edge)
18  Entrance to duodenum (pylorus)
19  Stomach
20  Duodenum
21  Transverse colon
    (divided, dilated)
22  Small intestine
23  Thoracic aorta
    (longitudinally divided)
24  Esophagus
    (longitudinally divided)
25  Esophageal hiatus of diaphragm
26  Omental bursa (lesser sac)
27  Splenic artery
28  Pancreas
29  Left renal vein
30  Intervertebral disc
31  Abdominal aorta
    (longitudinally divided)

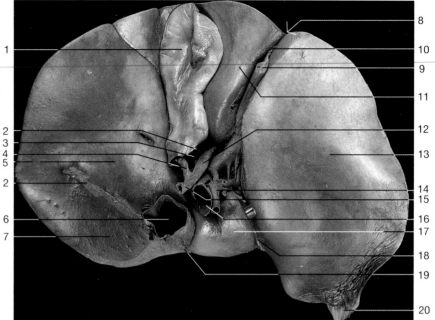

| | |
|---|---|
| 1 | Fundus of gallbladder |
| 2 | Peritoneum (cut edges) |
| 3 | Cystic artery |
| 4 | Cystic duct |
| 5 | Right lobe of liver |
| 6 | Inferior vena cava |
| 7 | Bare area of liver |
| 8 | Notch for ligamentum teres and falciform ligament |
| 9 | Ligamentum teres |
| 10 | Falciform ligament of liver |
| 11 | Quadrate lobe of liver |
| 12 | Common hepatic duct |
| 13 | Left lobe of liver |
| 14 | Hepatic artery proper ⎫ |
| 15 | Common bile duct ⎬ Portal triad |
| 16 | Portal vein ⎭ |
| 17 | Caudate lobe of liver |
| 18 | Ligamentum venosum |
| 19 | Ligament of inferior vena cava |
| 20 | Appendix fibrosa (left triangular ligament) |
| 21 | Coronary ligament of liver |
| 22 | Hepatic veins |
| 23 | Porta hepatis |

**Liver** (inferior aspect). Dissection of porta hepatis. Gallbladder partly collapsed. Ventral margin of liver above.

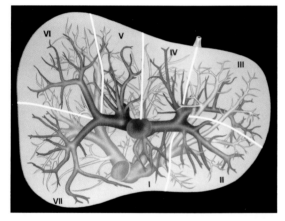

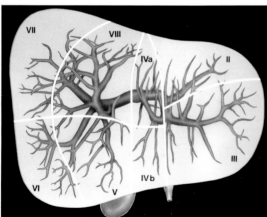

**Segmentation of the liver** (anterior aspect). Liver segments indicated by Roman numerals.

**Liver segments I–VIII.** The three main hepatic veins (blue within both schematic drawings shown on the left) drain the eight segments of the liver that have no visible external markings.
Upper drawing = inferior aspect; lower drawing = superior aspect.

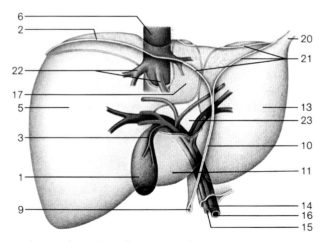

**Liver and margins of peritoneal folds** (anterior aspect).

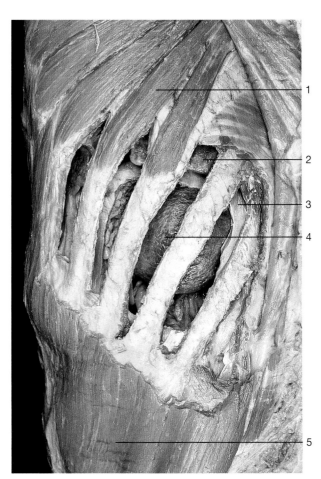

1   Serratus anterior muscle
2   Left lung
3   Diaphragm
4   Spleen
5   External abdominal oblique muscle
6   Gastrosplenic ligament
7   Splenic artery
8   Tail of pancreas
9   Superior border of spleen
10  Anterior border of spleen
11  Border of lung
12  Area of liver
13  Area of stomach
14  Tenth rib
15  Eleventh rib
16  Twelfth rib

**Spleen in situ** (left lateral aspect). Intercostal spaces and diaphragm have been fenestrated.

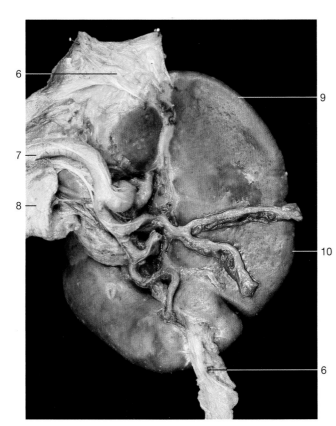

**Spleen** (visceral surface). Hilum of spleen with vessels, nerves, and ligaments.

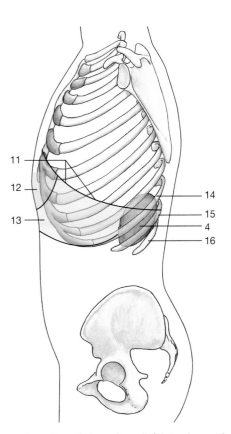

**Location of the spleen** (left lateral aspect).

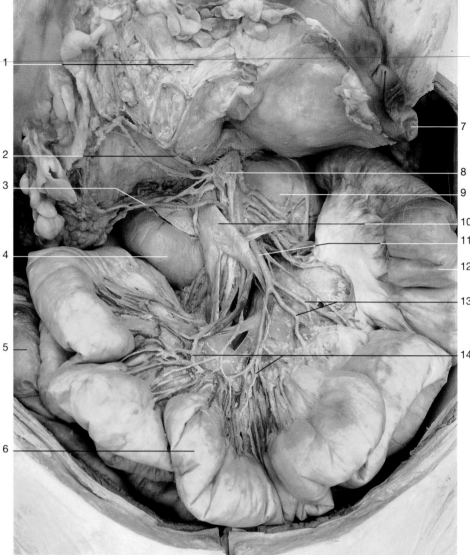

| | |
|---|---|
| 1 | Greater omentum |
| 2 | Middle colic artery |
| 3 | Right colic artery |
| 4 | Duodenum |
| 5 | Ascending colon |
| 6 | Ileum |
| 7 | Transverse colon |
| 8 | Celiac plexus |
| 9 | Duodenojejunal flexure |
| 10 | Superior mesenteric vein |
| 11 | Superior mesenteric artery |
| 12 | Jejunum |
| 13 | Jejunal arteries |
| 14 | Ileal arteries |
| 15 | Liver |
| 16 | Celiac trunk and abdominal aorta |
| 17 | Gallbladder |
| 18 | Pancreas |
| 19 | Ileocolic artery |
| 20 | Stomach |
| 21 | Spleen |
| 22 | Left colic flexure |
| 23 | Appendicular artery |
| 24 | Vermiform appendix |

**Vessels of upper abdominal organs and small intestine** (anterior aspect). Dissection of superior mesenteric artery and vein. Greater omentum and transverse colon are reflected.

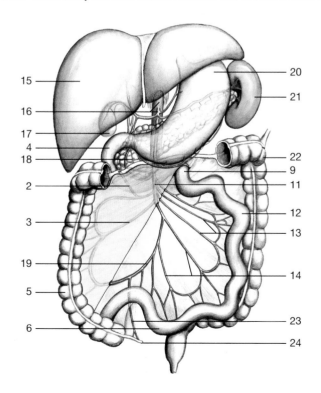

**Arteries of upper abdominal organs and small intestine** (anterior aspect). Main branches of superior mesenteric artery.

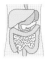

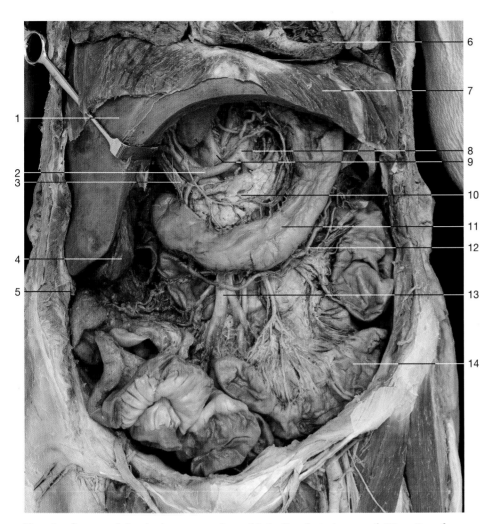

**Vessels of upper abdominal organs and small intestine** (anterior aspect). Dissection of superior mesenteric vein. The liver is dissected and elevated.

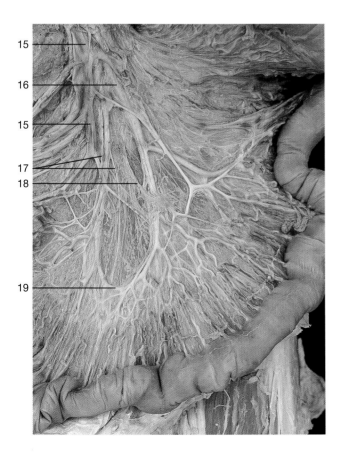

1   Liver
2   Hepatic artery proper
3   Hepatic duct
4   Gallbladder
5   Major duodenal papilla
6   Apex of the heart
7   Diaphragm
8   Common hepatic artery
9   Inferior vena cava
10  Pancreas
11  Stomach
12  Gastro-omental (gastro-epiploic) artery
13  Superior mesenteric vein
14  Small intestine
15  Jejunal vein
16  Superior mesenteric artery
17  Intestinal lymphatic vessels
18  Superior mesenteric plexus
19  Branches of superior mesenteric artery

**Blood and lymphatic vessels of the small intestine** (anterior aspect). Note the arterial arch of the mesenteric artery adjacent the small intestine.

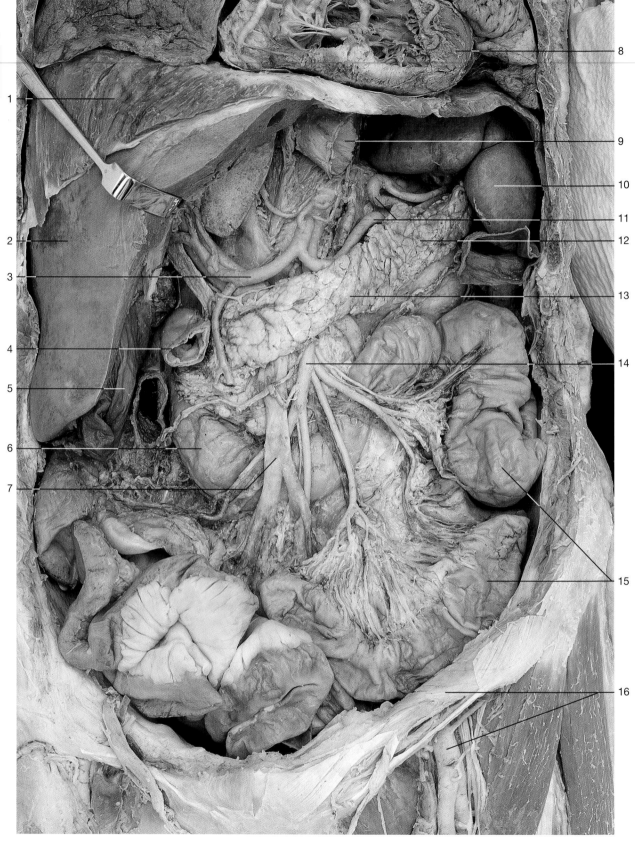

**Vessels of upper abdominal organs and small intestine** (anterior aspect). Stomach and omentum majus have been removed. The liver is elevated.

| | | |
|---|---|---|
| 1 Diaphragm | 7 Superior mesenteric vein | 13 Pancreas |
| 2 Liver | 8 Apex of the heart | 14 Superior mesenteric artery |
| 3 Proper hepatic artery | 9 Esophagus (abdominal part) | 15 Small intestine |
| 4 Duodenum | 10 Spleen | 16 Inguinal ligament and femoral artery |
| 5 Gallbladder | 11 Splenic artery | |
| 6 Inferior duodenal flexure | 12 Tail of pancreas | |

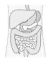

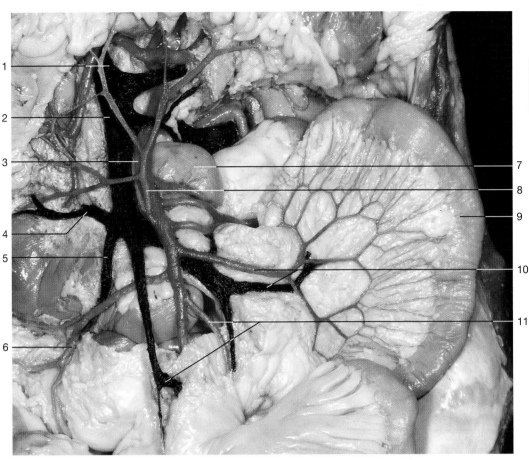

**Dissection of portal venous system** (anterior aspect). Blue = tributaries of portal vein; red = branches of superior mesenteric artery.

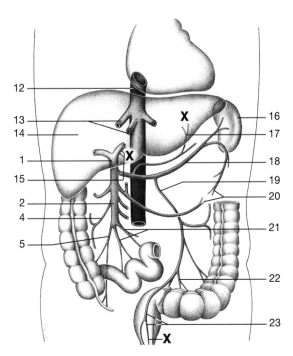

**Main tributaries of portal vein** (anterior aspect). Blue = tributaries of portal vein; violet = inferior vena cava; X = sites of portocaval anastomoses.

1  Portal vein
2  Superior mesenteric vein
3  Superior mesenteric artery
4  Right colic vein
5  Ileocolic vein
6  Ileocolic artery
7  Duodenojejunal flexure
8  Middle colic artery
9  Jejunum
10 Jejunal arteries and veins
11 Ileal arteries and veins
12 Inferior vena cava
13 Hepatic veins
14 Liver
15 Para-umbilical veins
   (located within the
   ligamentum teres)
16 Spleen
17 Left gastric vein
   with esophageal branches
18 Splenic vein
19 Inferior mesenteric vein
20 Gastro-omental veins
21 Ileal veins
22 Sigmoid veins
23 Superior rectal vein

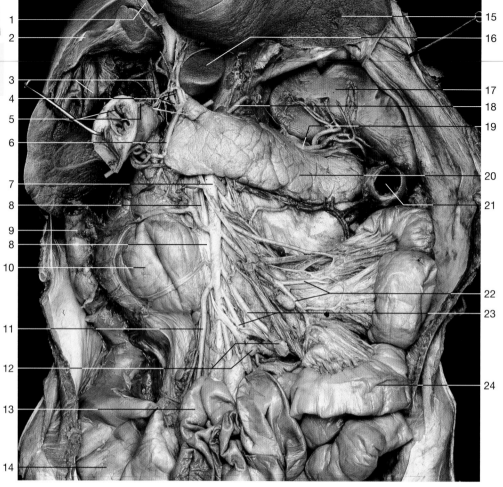

| | |
|---|---|
| 1 | Ligamentum teres |
| 2 | Liver |
| 3 | Gallbladder and common bile duct |
| 4 | Hepatic artery proper and portal vein |
| 5 | Right gastric artery and pylorus |
| 6 | Gastroduodenal artery |
| 7 | Superior mesenteric artery |
| 8 | Superior mesenteric vein |
| 9 | Ascending colon |
| 10 | Duodenum |
| 11 | Ileocolic artery |
| 12 | Lymph nodes |
| 13 | Ileum |
| 14 | Cecum |
| 15 | Left lobe of liver |
| 16 | Caudate lobe of liver |
| 17 | Spleen |
| 18 | Left gastric artery |
| 19 | Splenic artery |
| 20 | Pancreas |
| 21 | Left colic flexure (cut) |
| 22 | Jejunal arteries |
| 23 | Ileal arteries |
| 24 | Jejunum |
| 25 | Middle colic artery |
| 26 | Right colic artery |
| 27 | Appendicular artery |
| 28 | Transverse mesocolon |
| 29 | Duodenojejunal flexure |
| 30 | Inferior mesenteric artery |
| 31 | Left colic artery |
| 32 | Sigmoid arteries |
| 33 | Superior rectal arteries |
| 34 | Inferior vena cava |
| 35 | Abdominal aorta |
| 36 | Descending colon |
| 37 | Ileum |
| 38 | Sigmoid colon |
| 39 | Vermiform appendix |
| 40 | Cecum |

**Superior mesenteric artery and vein in relation to pancreas and duodenum** (anterior aspect). Stomach and transverse colon have been removed and the liver elevated. Note the location of the spleen. A yellow probe is inserted through the omental foramen.

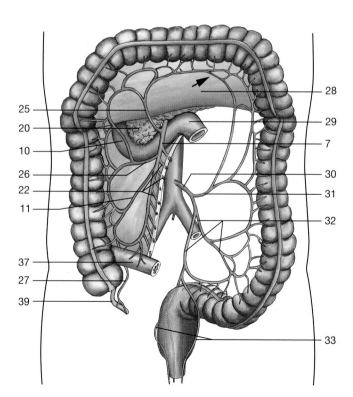

**Main branches of superior and inferior mesenteric arteries** (anterior aspect). Arrow: Riolan's anastomosis.

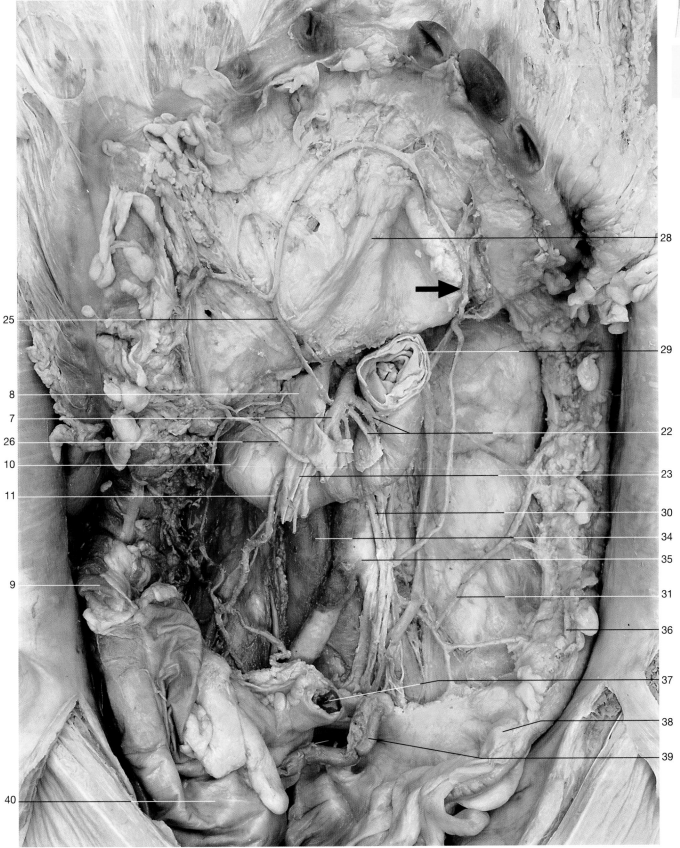

**Vessels of the retroperitoneal organs** (anterior aspect). Dissection of the inferior mesenteric artery and its anastomosis with the middle colic artery (arrow: Riolan's anastomosis). Greater omentum and transverse colon have been reflected and the intestine partly removed. The normally retrocecally located vermiform appendix has been replaced anteriorly. The right common iliac artery is partly obstructed by a blood thrombus.

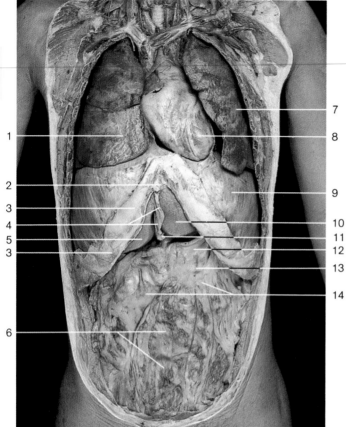

1    Middle lobe of right lung
2    Xiphoid process
3    Costal margin
4    Falciform ligament of liver
5    Quadrate lobe of liver
6    Greater omentum
7    Upper lobe of left lung
8    Heart
9    Diaphragm
10   Left lobe of liver
11   Ligamentum teres
12   Stomach
13   Gastrocolic ligament
14   Transverse colon
15   Taenia coli
16   Appendices epiploicae
17   Cecum
18   Taenia coli
19   Ileum
20   Transverse mesocolon
21   Jejunum
22   Sigmoid colon
23   Position of root of mesentery
24   Vermiform appendix
25   Duodenojejunal flexure
26   Mesentery

**Abdominal organs** (anterior aspect). The anterior thoracic and abdominal walls have been removed.

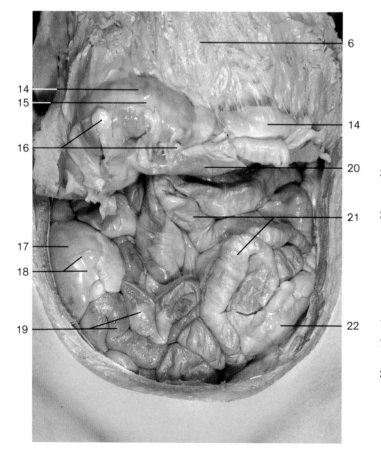

**Abdominal organs** (anterior aspect). The greater omentum, which is fixed to the transverse colon, has been raised.

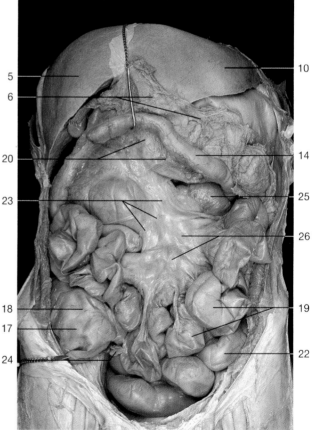

**Abdominal organs** (anterior aspect). The transverse colon has been reflected.

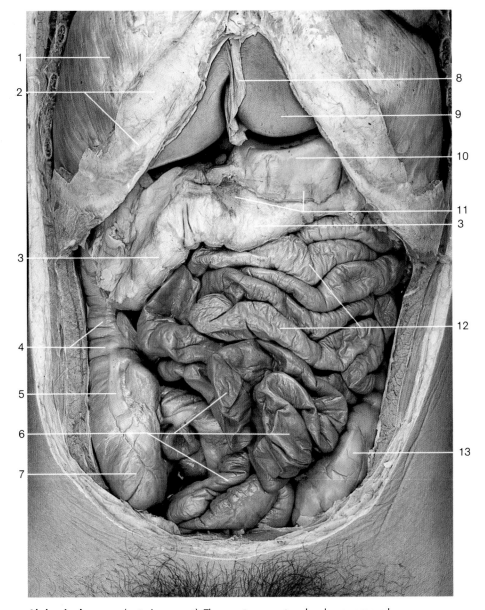

1 Diaphragm
2 Costal margin
3 Transverse colon
4 Ascending colon with haustra
5 Free taenia of cecum
6 Ileum
7 Cecum
8 Falciform ligament of liver
9 Liver
10 Stomach
11 Gastrocolic ligament
12 Jejunum
13 Sigmoid colon
14 Ileocecal valve
15 Ileal ostium
16 Frenulum of ileal opening
17 Ostium of vermiforme appendix
   (probe in the dissection)
18 Ileocolic artery
19 Terminal ileum
20 Appendicular artery
21 Vermiform appendix
22 Meso-appendix
23 Mesentery

**Abdominal organs** (anterior aspect). The greater omentum has been removed.

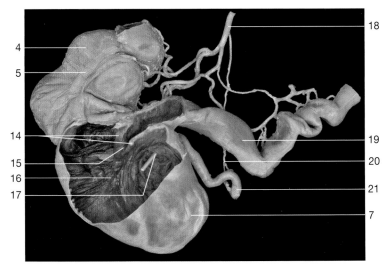

**Ascending colon, cecum, and vermiform appendix.** The cecum has been opened. Note the probe in the entrance of the vermiform appendix.

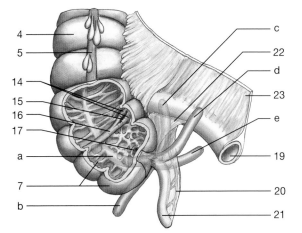

**Variations in the position of the vermiform appendix.** The cecum has been opened to show the ileal opening. a = retrocecal; b = paracolic; c = retro-ileal; d = pre-ileal; e = subcecal.

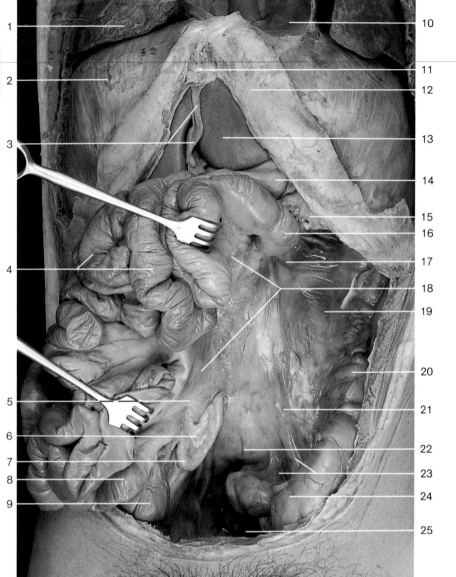

1   Lung
2   Diaphragm
3   Falciform ligament of liver
4   Jejunum
5   Ileocecal fold
6   Meso-appendix
7   Vermiform appendix
8   Terminal ileum
9   Cecum
10  Pericardial sac
11  Xiphoid process
12  Costal margin
13  Liver
14  Stomach
15  Transverse colon
16  Duodenojejunal flexure
17  Inferior duodenal fold
18  Mesentery
19  Position of left kidney
20  Descending colon
21  Position of left common iliac artery
22  Sacral promontory
23  Sigmoid mesocolon
24  Sigmoid colon
25  Rectum
26  Beginning of jejunum
27  Peritoneum
    of posterior abdominal wall
28  Transverse mesocolon
29  Superior duodenal fold
30  Superior duodenal recess
31  Retroduodenal recess
32  Free taenia of ascending colon
33  Ileocecal valve
34  Frenulum of ileocecal valve
35  Orifice of vermiform appendix
    (probe)
36  Ileocolic artery
37  Vermiform appendix
    with appendicular artery
38  Ascending colon

**Abdominal organs with mesenteries** (anterior aspect). The small intestine has been reflected laterally to demonstrate the mesentery.

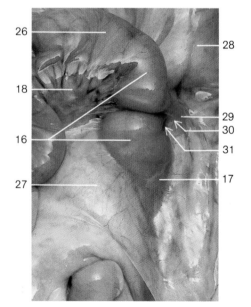

**Duodenojejunal flexure**
(enlargement of preceding figure).

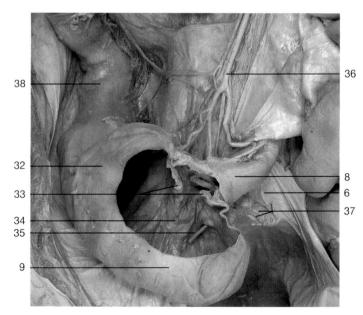

**Ileocecal valve** (anterior aspect). Cecum and terminal part of the ileum have been opened.

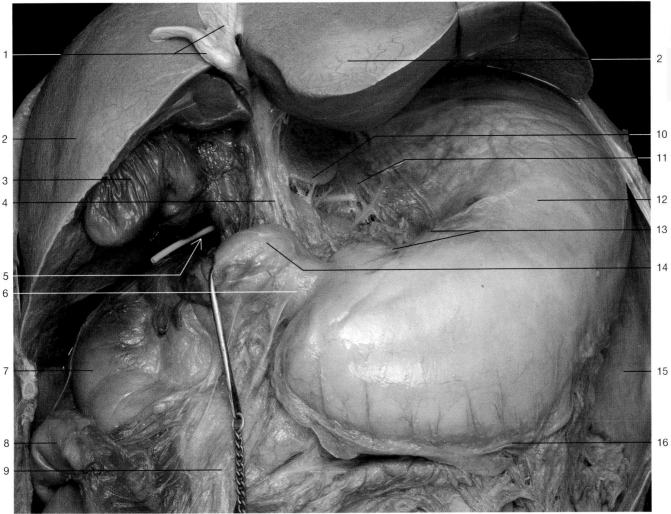

**Upper abdominal organs** (anterior aspect). Thorax and anterior part of diaphragm have been removed and the liver raised to display the **lesser omentum.** A probe has been inserted into the epiploic foramen and lesser sac.

1 Falciform ligament and ligamentum teres
2 Liver
3 Gallbladder (fundus)
4 Hepatoduodenal ligament
5 Epiploic foramen (probe)
6 Pylorus
7 Descending part of duodenum
8 Right colic flexure
9 Gastrocolic ligament
10 Caudate lobe of liver (behind lesser omentum)
11 Lesser omentum
12 Stomach
13 Lesser curvature of stomach
14 Superior part of duodenum
15 Diaphragm
16 Greater curvature of stomach
   with gastro-omental vessels
17 Twelfth thoracic vertebra
18 Right kidney
19 Right suprarenal gland
20 Inferior vena cava
21 Falciform ligament of liver
22 Abdominal aorta
23 Spleen
24 Lienorenal ligament
25 Gastrosplenic ligament
26 Pancreas
27 Lesser sac (omental bursa)

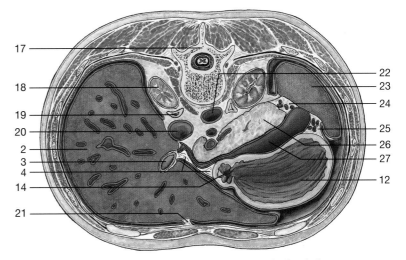

**Horizontal section through the lesser sac** above the level of epiploic foramen (superior aspect).

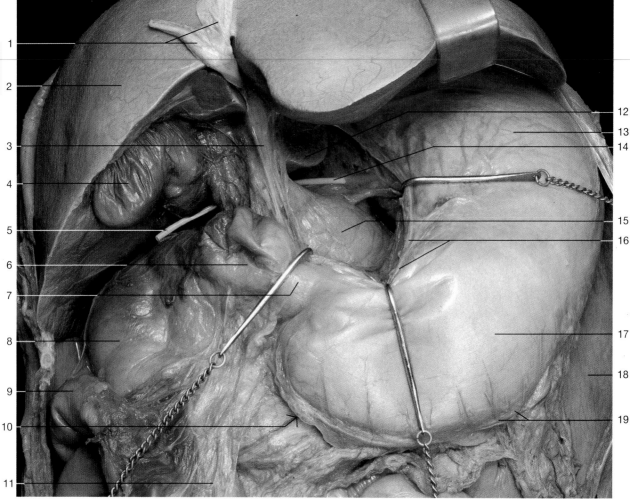

**Upper abdominal organs** (anterior aspect). **Lesser sac.** The lesser omentum has been partly removed and the liver and stomach have been slightly reflected.

| | | | |
|---|---|---|---|
| 1 | Falciform ligament and ligamentum teres | 18 | Diaphragm |
| 2 | Liver | 19 | Greater curvature with gastro-omental vessels |
| 3 | Hepatoduodenal ligament | 20 | Head of pancreas and gastropancreatic fold |
| 4 | Gallbladder | 21 | Spleen |
| 5 | Probe within the epiploic foramen | 22 | Tail of pancreas |
| 6 | Superior part of duodenum | 23 | Left colic flexure |
| 7 | Pylorus | 24 | Root of transverse mesocolon |
| 8 | Descending part of duodenum | 25 | Transverse mesocolon |
| 9 | Right colic flexure | 26 | Gastrocolic ligament (cut edge) |
| 10 | Gastrocolic ligament | 27 | Transverse colon |
| 11 | Greater omentum | 28 | Umbilicus |
| 12 | Caudate lobe of liver | 29 | Small intestine |
| 13 | Fundus of stomach | 30 | Lesser omentum |
| 14 | Probe at the level of the vestibule of lesser sac (through epiploic foramen) | 31 | Lesser sac (omental bursa) |
| | | 32 | Duodenum |
| 15 | Head of pancreas | 33 | Mesentery |
| 16 | Lesser curvature of stomach | 34 | Sigmoid colon |
| 17 | Body of stomach | | |

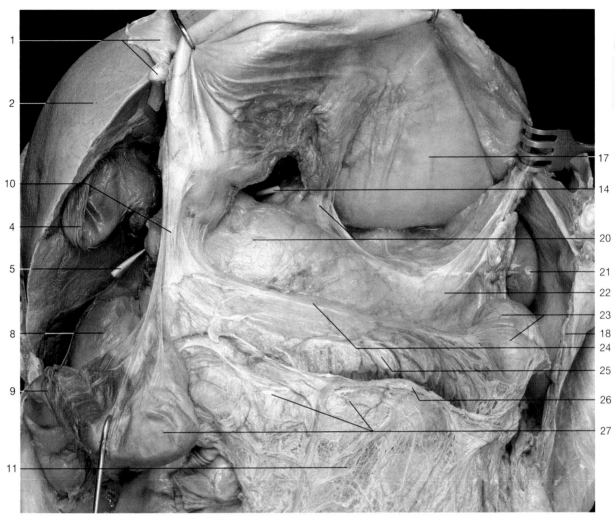

**Upper abdominal organs** (anterior aspect). **Lesser sac.** The gastrocolic ligament has been divided and the whole stomach raised to display the posterior wall of the lesser sac.

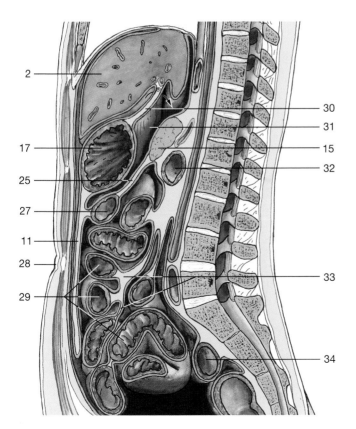

**Midsagittal section through the abdominal cavity,** demonstrating the site of lesser sac.
Blue = lesser sac (omental bursa); green = peritoneum; arrow: entrance to the lesser sac (epiploic foramen).

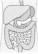

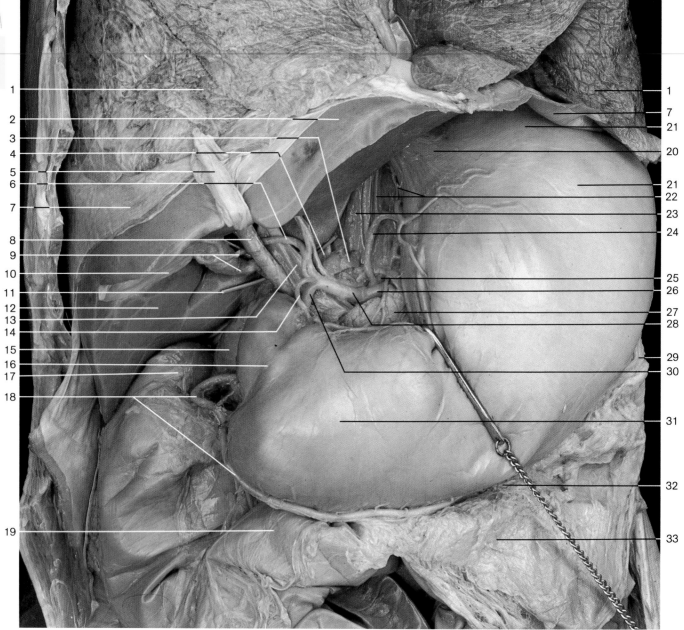

**Upper abdominal organs** (anterior aspect). **Celiac trunk.** The lesser omentum has been removed and the lesser curvature of the stomach reflected to display the branches of the celiac trunk. The probe is situated within the epiploic foramen.

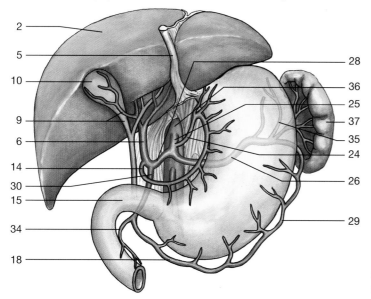

**Arteries of upper abdominal organs and branches of celiac trunk.**

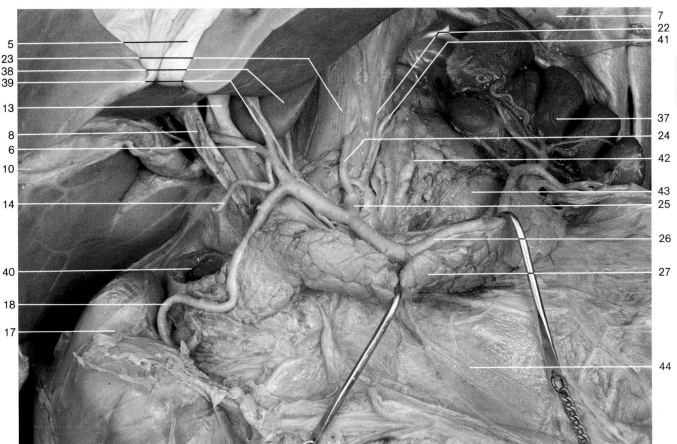

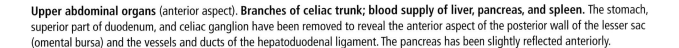

**Upper abdominal organs** (anterior aspect). **Branches of celiac trunk; blood supply of liver, pancreas, and spleen.** The stomach, superior part of duodenum, and celiac ganglion have been removed to reveal the anterior aspect of the posterior wall of the lesser sac (omental bursa) and the vessels and ducts of the hepatoduodenal ligament. The pancreas has been slightly reflected anteriorly.

| | |
|---|---|
| 1   Lung | 23   Lumbar part of diaphragm |
| 2   Liver (visceral surface) | 24   Left gastric artery |
| 3   Lymph node | 25   Celiac trunk |
| 4   Inferior vena cava | 26   Splenic artery |
| 5   Ligamentum teres (reflected) | 27   Pancreas |
| 6   Right branch of hepatic artery proper | 28   Common hepatic artery |
| 7   Diaphragm | 29   Left gastro-omental (gastro-epiploic) artery |
| 8   Common hepatic duct (dilated) | 30   Gastroduodenal artery |
| 9   Cystic duct and artery | 31   Pyloric part of stomach |
| 10   Gallbladder | 32   Greater curvature of stomach |
| 11   Probe within the epiploic foramen | 33   Gastrocolic ligament |
| 12   Right lobe of liver | 34   Supraduodenal artery |
| 13   Portal vein | 35   Short gastric arteries |
| 14   Right gastric artery | 36   Aorta |
| 15   Duodenum | 37   Spleen |
| 16   Pylorus | 38   Caudate lobe of liver |
| 17   Right colic flexure | 39   Left branch of hepatic artery proper |
| 18   Right gastro-omental (gastro-epiploic) artery | 40   Descending part of duodenum (cut) |
| 19   Transverse colon | 41   Left inferior phrenic artery |
| 20   Abdominal part of esophagus (cardiac part of stomach) | 42   Suprarenal gland |
| 21   Fundus of stomach | 43   Kidney |
| 22   Esophageal branches of left gastric artery | 44   Transverse mesocolon |

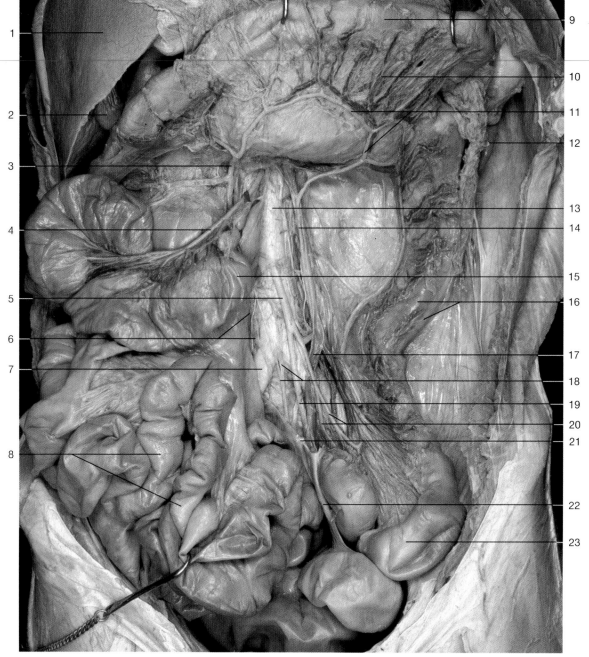

**Lower abdominal organs** (anterior aspect). **Inferior mesenteric artery and autonomic plexus.** The transverse colon with the mesocolon has been raised and the small intestine reflected.

| | | | |
|---|---|---|---|
| 1 | Liver | 12 | Spleen |
| 2 | Gallbladder | 13 | Abdominal aorta |
| 3 | Middle colic artery | 14 | Left colic artery |
| 4 | Jejunal artery | 15 | Duodenojejunal flexure |
| 5 | Inferior mesenteric artery | 16 | Descending colon (free taenia of colon) |
| 6 | Sympathetic nerves and ganglia | 17 | Inferior mesenteric vein |
| 7 | Right common iliac artery | 18 | Superior hypogastric plexus |
| 8 | Small intestine (ileum) | 19 | Superior rectal artery |
| 9 | Transverse colon (reflected) | 20 | Sigmoid arteries |
| 10 | Transverse mesocolon | 21 | Peritoneum (cut edge) |
| 11 | Anastomosis between middle and left colic artery | 22 | Sigmoid mesocolon |
| | | 23 | Sigmoid colon |

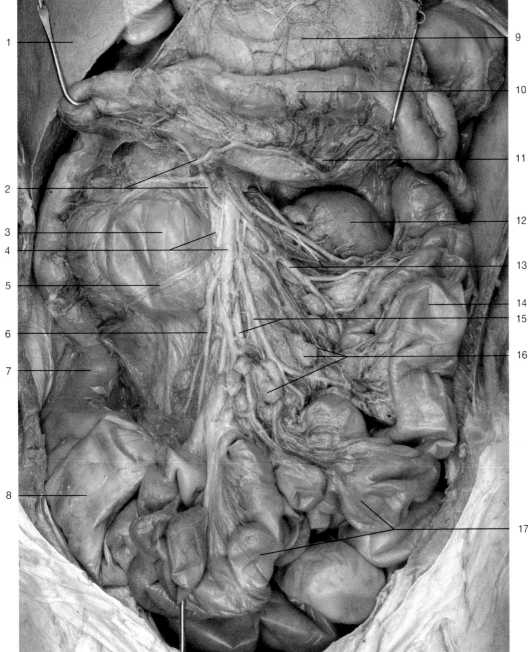

| | |
|---|---|
| 1 | Liver |
| 2 | Middle colic artery |
| 3 | Horizontal part of duodenum (extended) |
| 4 | Superior mesenteric artery and vein |
| 5 | Right colic artery |
| 6 | Ileocolic artery |
| 7 | Ascending colon |
| 8 | Cecum |
| 9 | Greater omentum (reflected) |
| 10 | Transverse colon |
| 11 | Transverse mesocolon |
| 12 | Duodenojejunal flexure |
| 13 | Jejunal arteries |
| 14 | Jejunum |
| 15 | Ileal arteries |
| 16 | Mesenteric lymph nodes and lymph vessels |
| 17 | Ileum |
| 18 | Abdominal aorta |
| 19 | Inferior vena cava |
| 20 | Stomach |
| 21 | Spleen |
| 22 | Splenic artery |
| 23 | Head of pancreas |
| 24 | Superior mesenteric artery |

**Lower abdominal organs** (anterior aspect). **Superior mesenteric artery and mesenteric lymph nodes.**
The transverse colon has been reflected.

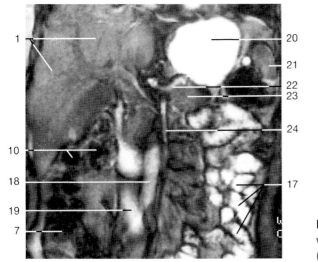

**Frontal section through the abdominal cavity.** The intestinal tract and
vessels are filled with a paramagnetic substance (Gadolinium; MRI scan).
(Prof. Rödl, Univ. Erlangen-Nuremberg, Germany.)

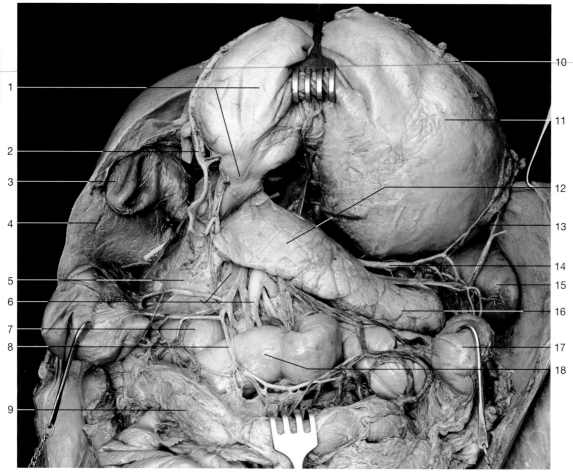

**Posterior abdominal wall with pancreas and extrahepatic bile ducts in situ** (anterior aspect).
The gastrocolic ligament has been divided and the transverse colon and the stomach
replaced to display the pancreas and superior mesenteric vessels.

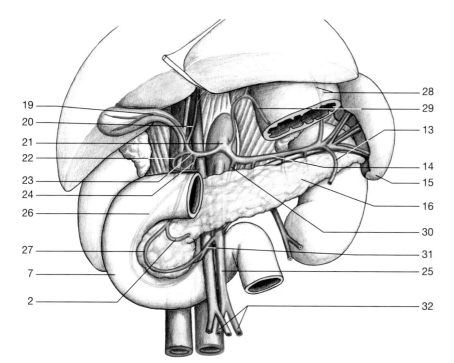

**Blood supply of upper abdominal organs** (compare with dissection depicted on
following page). Note the branching of the celiac trunk not visible behind the body of
pancreas, the main arterial supply of liver, spleen, pancreas, stomach, and duodenum.

1  Stomach (pyloric part) and pylorus
2  Right gastro-omental (gastro-epiploic) artery
3  Fundus of gallbladder
4  Liver (right lobe)
5  Head of pancreas
6  Superior mesenteric artery and vein
7  Duodenum
8  Middle colic artery
9  Transverse colon
10  Greater curvature of stomach
    (remnants of gastrocolic ligament)
11  Body of stomach
12  Body of pancreas
13  Left gastro-omental (gastro-epiploic) artery
14  Splenic artery
15  Spleen
16  Tail of pancreas
17  Left colic flexure
18  Jejunum
19  Cystic artery
20  Hepatic artery proper
21  Celiac trunk
22  Right gastric artery
23  Common hepatic artery
24  Gastroduodenal artery
25  Superior mesenteric artery
26  Superior posterior pancreaticoduodenal artery
27  Superior anterior pancreaticoduodenal artery
28  Short gastric arteries
29  Left gastric artery
30  Posterior pancreatic branch of splenic artery
31  Inferior pancreaticoduodenal artery
32  Jejunal arteries

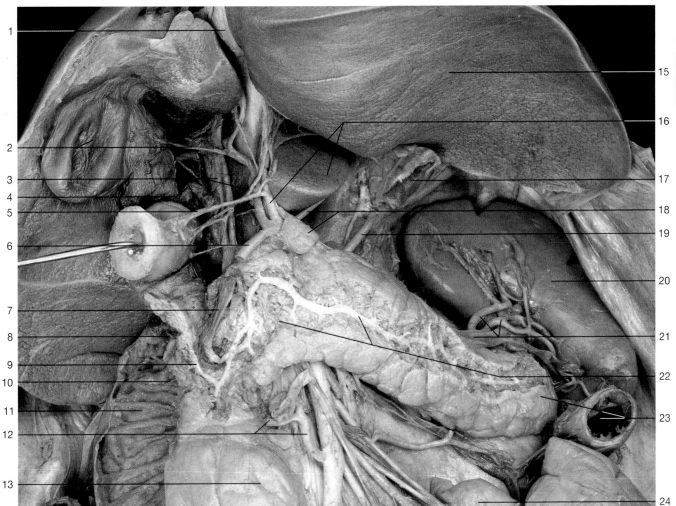

**Posterior abdominal wall with pancreas, extrahepatic bile ducts, spleen, and liver with their vessels in situ** (anterior aspect). The stomach has been removed, the liver elevated, and the descending part of duodenum fenestrated to display the openings of the pancreatic ducts. The pancreatic ducts were dissected. Note the location of superior mesenteric artery and vein between duodenum and pancreas.

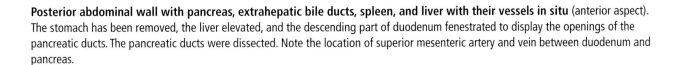

1  Ligamentum teres
2  Gallbladder and cystic artery
3  Common hepatic duct and portal vein
4  Cystic duct
5  Right gastric artery (pylorus with superior part of duodenum, cut and reflected)
6  Gastroduodenal artery
7  Common bile duct
8  Probe within the minor duodenal papilla
9  Accessory pancreatic duct
10  Probe within the major duodenal papilla
11  Descending part of duodenum (opened)
12  Middle colic artery and inferior pancreaticoduodenal artery

13  Horizontal part of duodenum (distended)
14  Superior mesenteric artery
15  Liver (left lobe)
16  Caudate lobe of liver and hepatic artery proper
17  Abdominal part of esophagus (cut)
18  Probe in epiploic foramen and lymph node
19  Left gastric artery
20  Spleen
21  Splenic vein and branches of splenic artery
22  Main pancreatic duct and head of pancreas
23  Left colic flexure and tail of pancreas
24  Duodenojejunal flexure

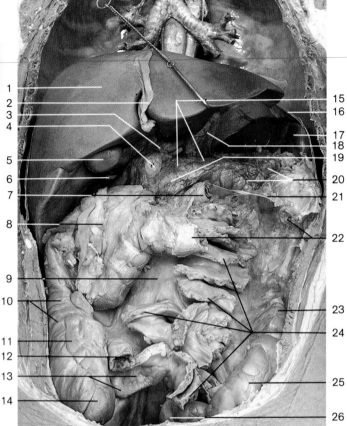

1  Liver
2  Falciform ligament
3  Hepatoduodenal ligament
4  Pylorus (divided)
5  Gallbladder
6  Probe within the epiploic foramen
7  Duodenojejunal flexure (divided)
8  Greater omentum
9  Root of mesentery
10  Ascending colon
11  Free colic taenia
12  End of ileum (divided)
13  Vermiform appendix with meso-appendix
14  Cecum
15  Pancreas and site of lesser sac
16  Diaphragm
17  Spleen
18  Cardia (part of stomach, divided)
19  Head of pancreas
20  Body and tail of pancreas
21  Transverse mesocolon
22  Transverse colon (divided)
23  Descending colon
24  Cut edge of mesentery
25  Sigmoid colon
26  Rectum
27  Attachment of bare area of liver
28  Inferior vena cava
29  Kidney
30  Attachment of right colic flexure
31  Root of transverse mesocolon
32  Junction between descending and horizontal parts of duodenum
33  Bare surface for ascending colon
34  Ileocecal recess
35  Retrocecal recess
36  Root of meso-appendix
37  Superior recess  ⎫
38  Isthmus (opening)  ⎬ of lesser sac (omental bursa)
39  Splenic recess  ⎭
40  Superior duodenal recess
41  Inferior duodenal recess
42  Bare surface for descending colon
43  Paracolic recesses
44  Root of mesentery
45  Root of mesosigmoid
46  Intersigmoid recess
47  Hepatic veins
48  Duodenojejunal flexure
49  Attachment of left colic flexure
50  Esophagus
51  Entrance to lesser sac through the epiploic foramen (arrow)

**Abdominal cavity** after removal of stomach, jejunum, ileum, and part of the transverse colon. The liver has been slightly raised.

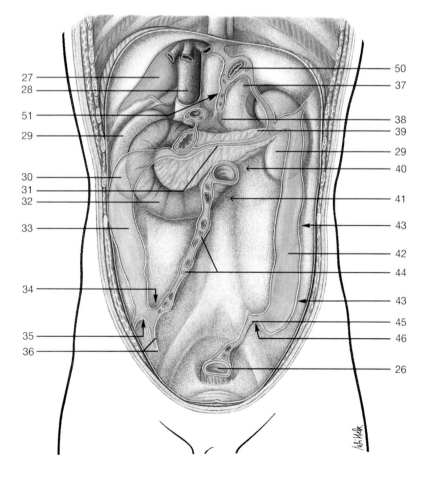

**Peritoneal reflections from organs and the position of root of mesentery and peritoneal recesses on the posterior abdominal wall.**
Arrows: position of peritoneal recesses.

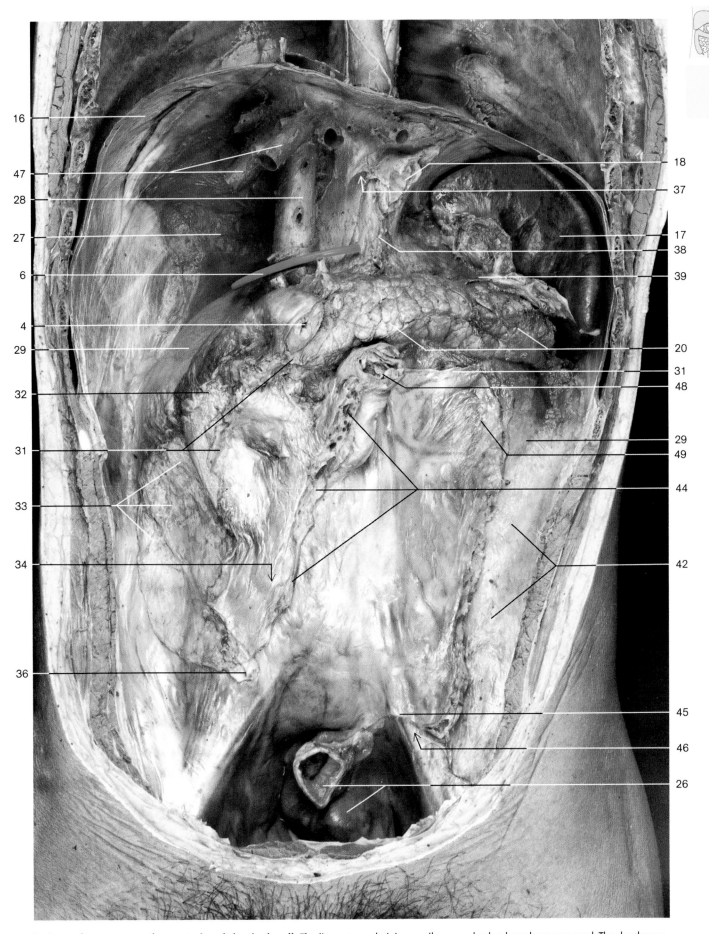

**Peritoneal recesses on the posterior abdominal wall.** The liver, stomach, jejunum, ileum, and colon have been removed. The duodenum, pancreas, and spleen have been left in place. Arrows: position of peritoneal recesses.

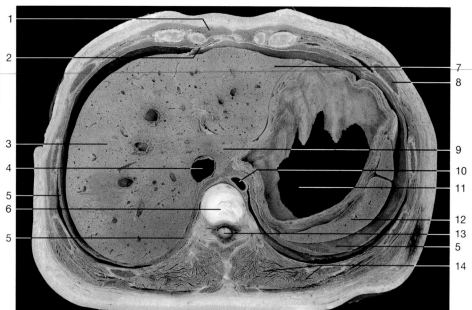

**Horizontal section through the abdominal cavity.**
Section 1 (from below).

1   Rectus abdominis muscle
2   Falciform ligament
3   Liver (right lobe)
4   Inferior vena cava
5   Diaphragm
6   Intervertebral disc
7   Liver (left lobe)
8   Rib
9   Liver (caudate lobe)
10  Abdominal (descending) aorta
11  Stomach
12  Spleen
13  Spinal cord
14  Longissimus thoracis and
     iliocostalis muscles
15  Rectus abdominis muscle
16  External abdominal oblique
     muscle
17  Transverse colon
18  Head of pancreas
19  Major duodenal papilla
20  Duodenum
21  Suprarenal gland and ureter
22  Kidney
23  Body of vertebra
24  Round ligament of liver
25  Small intestine
26  Superior mesenteric artery and
     vein
27  Psoas major muscle
28  Descending colon
29  Quadratus lumborum muscle
30  Cauda equina

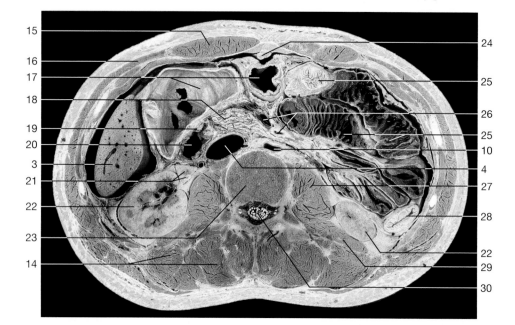

**Horizontal section through the abdominal cavity** at the level of major duodenal papilla.
Section 2 (from below).

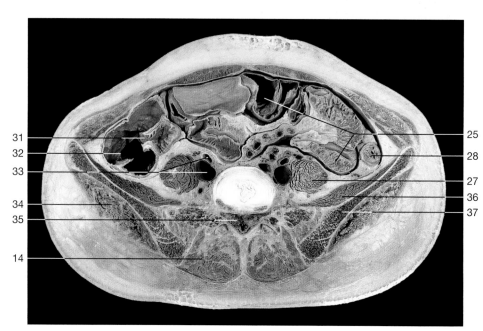

**Horizontal section through the abdominal cavity.**
Section 3 (from below).

31  Ileocecal valve
32  Cecum
33  Common iliac artery and vein
34  Gluteus medius muscle
35  Vertebral canal and dura mater
36  Iliacus muscle
37  Ilium
38  Right renal vein
39  Common iliac arteries
40  Spinous process
41  Internal abdominal oblique muscle
42  Transverse abdominal muscle
43  Longissimus muscle

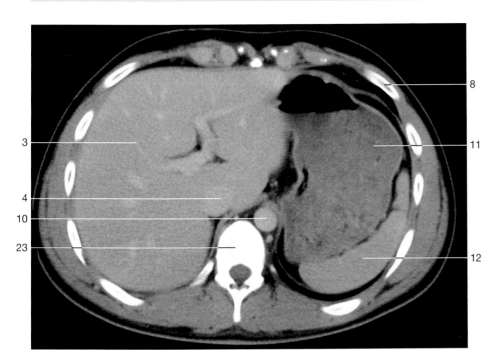

**Horizontal section through the abdominal cavity** at the level of section 1 (MRI scan). (Prof. Uder, Dept. of Radiology, Univ. Erlangen-Nuremberg, Germany.)

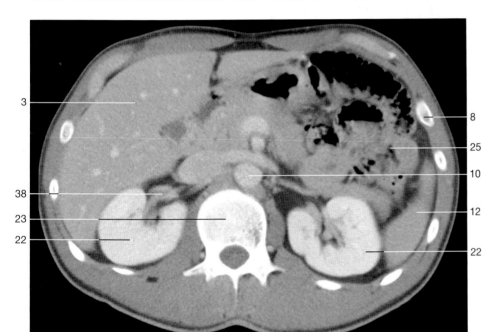

**Horizontal section through the abdominal cavity** at the level of section 2 (MRI scan). (Prof. Uder, Dept. of Radiology, Univ. Erlangen-Nuremberg, Germany.)

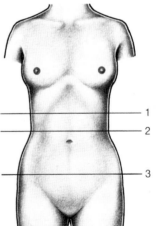

**Horizontal section through the abdominal cavity.** Levels of the sections are indicated.

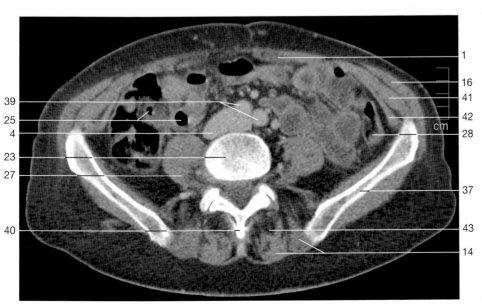

**Horizontal section through the abdominal cavity** at the level of section 3 (MRI scan). (Prof. Uder, Dept. of Radiology, Univ. Erlangen-Nuremberg, Germany.)

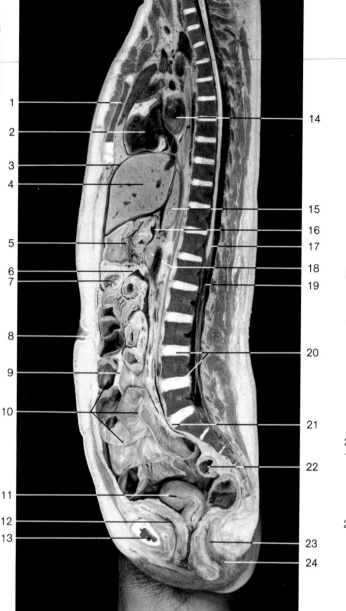

**Midsagittal section through the female trunk.**

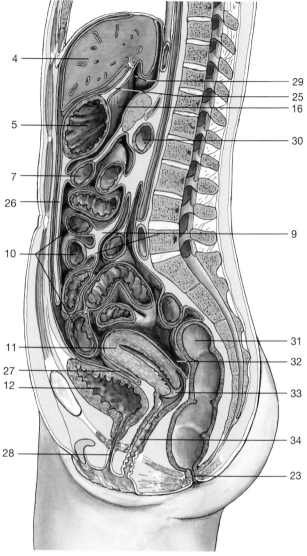

**Midsagittal section through the female trunk.**
Blue = lesser sac (omental bursa); green = peritoneum.

| | | | | |
|---|---|---|---|---|
| 1 | Sternum | 13 | Pubic symphysis | 24 Anus |
| 2 | Right ventricle of heart | 14 | Left atrium of heart | 25 Lesser omentum |
| 3 | Diaphragm | 15 | Caudate lobe of liver | 26 Greater omentum |
| 4 | Liver | 16 | Lesser sac (omental bursa) | 27 Vesico-uterine pouch |
| 5 | Stomach | 17 | Conus medullaris | 28 Urethra |
| 6 | Transverse mesocolon | 18 | Pancreas | 29 Epiploic (omental) foramen |
| 7 | Transverse colon | 19 | Cauda equina | 30 Duodenum |
| 8 | Umbilicus | 20 | Intervertebral discs | 31 Rectum |
| 9 | Mesentery | | (lumbar vertebral column) | 32 Recto-uterine pouch |
| 10 | Small intestine | 21 | Sacral promontory | 33 Vaginal part of cervix of uterus |
| 11 | Uterus | 22 | Sigmoid colon | 34 Vagina |
| 12 | Urinary bladder | 23 | Anal canal | |

# 6 Retroperitoneal Organs

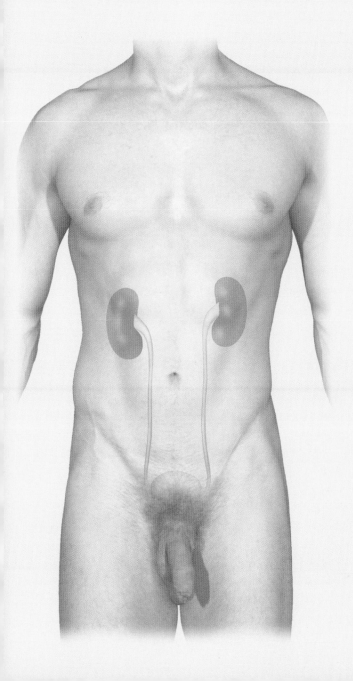

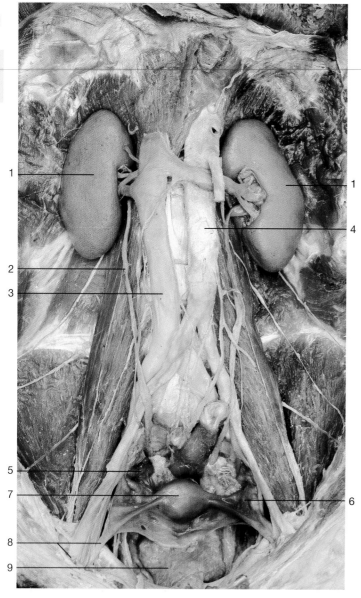

1  Kidney
2  Ureter
3  Inferior vena cava
4  Abdominal aorta
5  Ovary
6  Uterine tube
7  Uterus
8  Round ligament of uterus and inguinal canal
9  Urinary bladder

**Retroperitoneal organs of the female in situ**
(anterior aspect). View of the female pelvis showing uterus
with uterine ligaments, ovary, and urinary bladder.

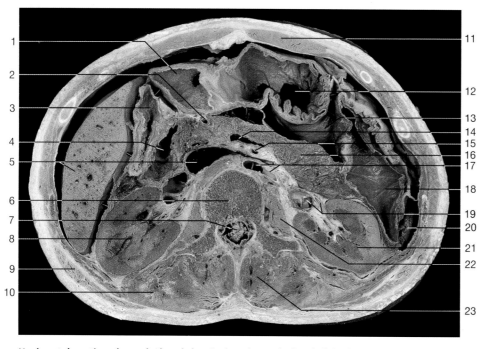

1  Pyloric antrum
2  Gastroduodenal artery
3  Descending part of duodenum
4  Vestibule of lesser sac
5  Inferior vena cava and liver
6  Body of first lumbar vertebra
7  Cauda equina
8  Right kidney
9  Latissimus dorsi muscle
10  Iliocostalis muscle
11  Rectus abdominis muscle
12  Stomach
13  Lesser sac
14  Splenic vein
15  Superior mesenteric artery
16  Pancreas
17  Aorta and left renal artery
18  Transverse colon
19  Renal artery and vein
20  Spleen
21  Left kidney
22  Psoas major muscle
23  Multifidus muscle

**Horizontal section through the abdominal cavity** at the level of the first lumbar vertebra
(from below).

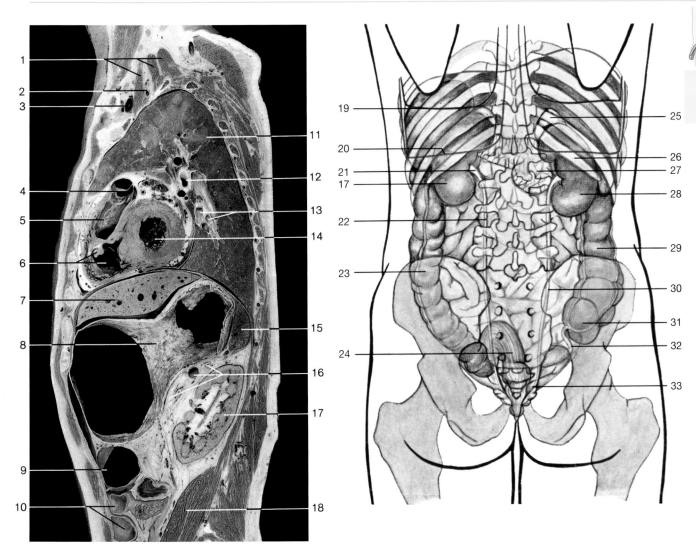

**Parasagittal section through thoracic and abdominal cavities** at the level of the left kidney 5.5 cm left to median plane.

**Positions of urinary organs** (posterior aspect). Notice that the upper part of the kidney reaches the level of the margin of pleura and lung.

| | |
|---|---|
| 1 Anterior, middle, and posterior scalene muscles | 19 Margin of lung |
| 2 Left subclavian artery | 20 Margin of pleura |
| 3 Left subclavian vein | 21 Renal pelvis |
| 4 Pulmonic valve | 22 Left ureter |
| 5 Arterial cone | 23 Descending colon |
| 6 Right ventricle of heart | 24 Rectum |
| 7 Liver | 25 Suprarenal gland |
| 8 Stomach | 26 Twelfth rib |
| 9 Transverse colon | 27 Pancreas |
| 10 Small intestine | 28 Right kidney |
| 11 Left lung | 29 Ascending colon |
| 12 Left main bronchus | 30 Right ureter |
| 13 Branches of pulmonary vein | 31 Cecum |
| 14 Left ventricle of heart | 32 Vermiform appendix |
| 15 Spleen | 33 Urinary bladder |
| 16 Splenic artery and vein, and pancreas | 34 Inferior vena cava |
| 17 Left kidney | 35 Body of lumbar vertebra (L$_1$) |
| 18 Psoas major muscle | 36 Iliocostal muscle |
| | 37 Superior mesenteric artery |
| | 38 Abdominal aorta |

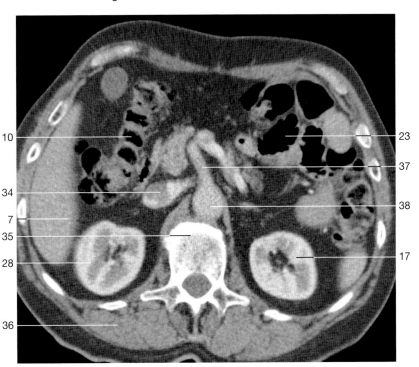

**Horizontal section through the abdominal cavity** (MRI scan). (Prof. Uder, Dept. of Radiology, Univ. Erlangen-Nuremberg, Germany.)

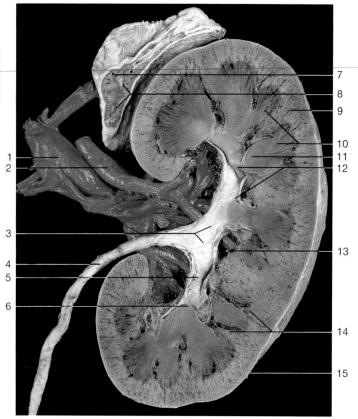

1 Renal vein
2 Renal artery
3 Renal pelvis
4 Abdominal part of ureter
5 Major renal calyx
6 Cribriform area of renal papilla
7 Cortex of suprarenal gland
8 Medulla of suprarenal gland
9 Cortex of kidney
10 Medulla of kidney
11 Renal papilla
12 Minor renal calyx
13 Renal sinus
14 Renal columns
15 Fibrous capsule of kidney

**Coronal section through right kidney and suprarenal gland** (posterior aspect). The renal pelvis has been opened and the fatty tissue removed to display the renal vessels.

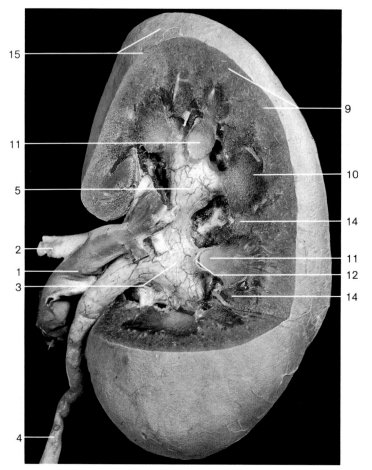

**Right kidney** (posterior aspect). Partial coronal section to expose internal aspect of the kidney.

Each kidney can be divided into five segments supplied by individual interlobar arteries known as end arteries. Thus, obstruction leads to infarcts marking the trace of segment borders. The anterior kidney surface reveals four segments; the posterior, only three (1, 4, and 5).

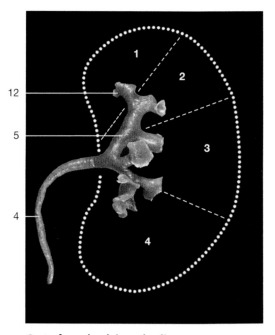

**Cast of renal pelvis and calices.**
1–4 = Renal segments on anterior surface.

1  Hepatic vein
2  Anterior and posterior vagal trunk
3  Inferior vena cava
4  Lumbar part of diaphragm
5  Right greater and lesser splanchnic nerves
6  Celiac trunk
7  Celiac ganglion and plexus
8  Superior mesenteric artery
9  Left renal vein
10  Right sympathetic trunk and ganglion
11  Abdominal aorta
12  Left sympathetic trunk
13  Esophagus (cut) and
     left greater splanchnic nerve
14  Left suprarenal gland
15  Left renal artery
16  Renal pelvis
17  Renal papilla with minor calyx
18  Left testicular vein
19  Ureter
20  Psoas major muscle
21  Quadratus lumborum muscle
22  Lumbar vertebra (L$_2$)
23  Renal calyx
24  Catheter

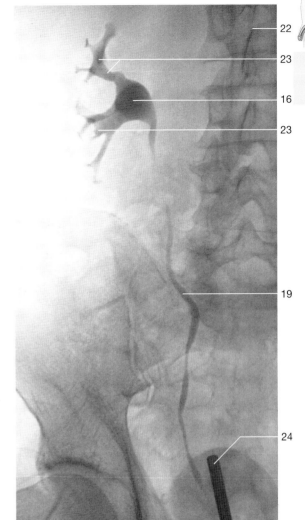

**Renal pelvis with calices and ureter** (X-ray, retrograde injection). (Courtesy of Prof. Herrlinger, Fürth, Germany.)

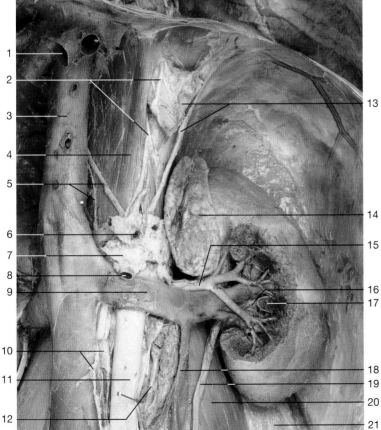

**Left kidney and suprarenal gland in situ.** The anterior cortical layer of the kidney has been removed to display the renal pelvis and papillae.

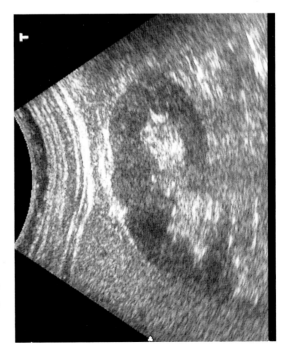

**Right kidney** (ultrasound image).
(Courtesy of Prof. Herrlinger, Fürth, Germany.)

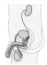

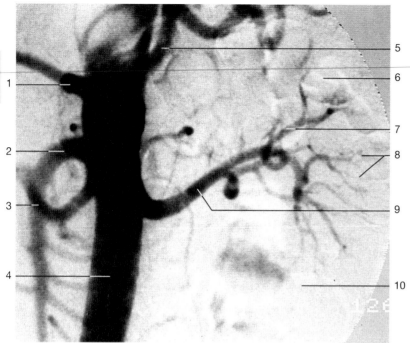

**Subtraction angiography of the abdominal aorta with renal artery and renal vessels.**

1 Celiac trunk
2 Superior mesenteric artery
3 Middle colic artery
4 Abdominal aorta (with catheter in the figure below)
5 Splenic artery
6 Upper pole of kidney
7 Anterior branch of renal artery
8 Interlobular arteries
9 Renal artery
10 Lower pole of kidney
11 Common iliac artery
12 Posterior branch of renal artery
13 Anterior superior segmental artery of renal artery
14 Superior suprarenal artery
15 Upper capsular artery
16 Perforating artery
17 Lower capsular artery
18 Ureter
19 Right inferior phrenic artery
20 Left inferior phrenic artery
21 Middle suprarenal artery
22 Inferior suprarenal artery
23 Anterior segmental artery of renal artery
24 Left testicular (or ovarian) artery
25 Inferior mesenteric artery

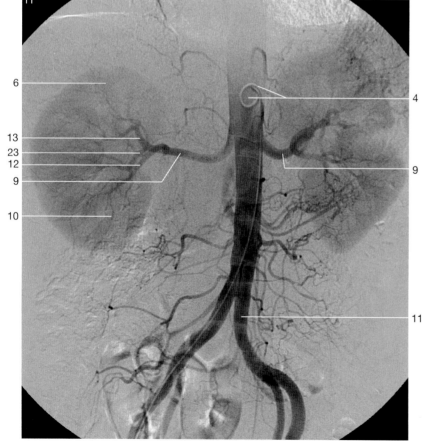

**Arteriography of the abdominal aorta with renal arteries and renal vessels.**
(Courtesy of Dr. Wieners, Dept. of Radiology, Berlin, Germany.)

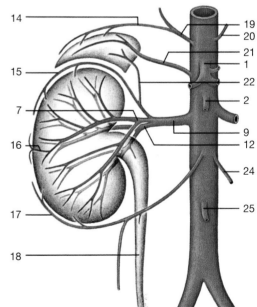

**Arteries of kidney and suprarenal gland.**

1   Diaphragm
2   Hepatic veins
3   Inferior vena cava
4   Common hepatic artery
5   Suprarenal gland
6   Celiac trunk
7   Right renal vein
8   Kidney
9   Abdominal aorta
10  Subcostal nerve
11  Iliohypogastric nerve
12  Central tendon
    of diaphragm
13  Inferior phrenic artery
14  Cardic part of stomach
15  Spleen
16  Splenic artery
17  Superior renal artery
18  Superior mesenteric artery
19  Psoas major muscle
20  Inferior mesenteric artery
21  Ureter
22  Glomerulus
23  Afferent arteriole of glomerulus
24  Glomeruli
25  Radiating cortical artery
26  Subcortical or arcuate artery
27  Subcortical or arcuate vein
28  Interlobular vein
29  Interlobular artery
30  Interlobar artery and vein
31  Vessels of renal capsule
32  Efferent arteriole of glomerulus
33  Vasa recta of renal medulla
34  Spiral arteries of renal pelvis

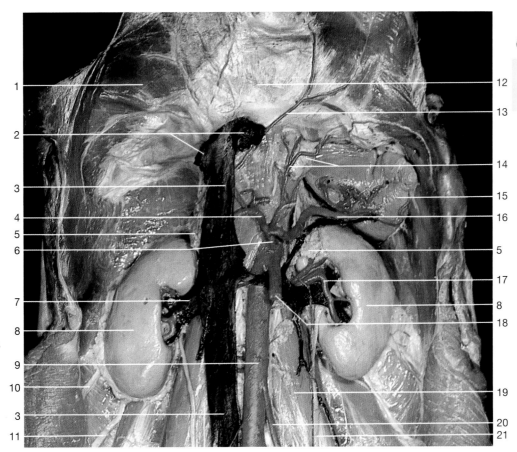

**Retroperitoneal organs, kidneys, and suprarenal glands in situ** (anterior aspect).
Red = arteries; blue = veins.

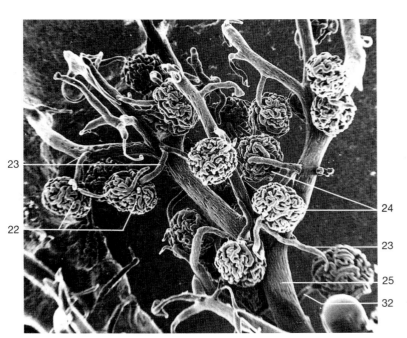

**Scanning electron micrograph showing glomeruli and associated arteries** (magn. 210 ×).

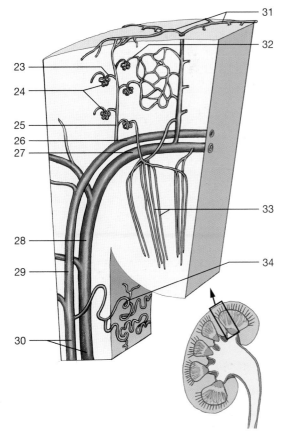

**Architecture of the vascular system of the kidney.**

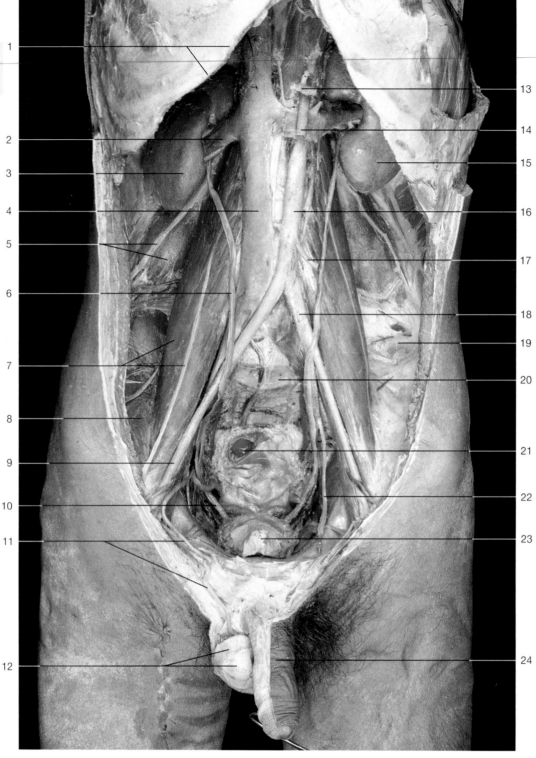

**Retroperitoneal organs, urinary system in the male** (anterior aspect). The peritoneum has been removed.

| | | |
|---|---|---|
| 1 Costal arch | 8 Iliacus muscle | 17 Inferior mesenteric artery |
| 2 Right renal vein | 9 External iliac artery | 18 Common iliac artery |
| 3 Right kidney | 10 Ureter (pelvic part) | 19 Iliac crest |
| 4 Inferior vena cava | 11 Ductus deferens | 20 Sacral promontory |
| 5 Iliohypogastric nerve and quadratus lumborum muscle | 12 Testis and epididymis | 21 Rectum (cut) |
| 6 Ureter (abdominal part) | 13 Celiac trunk | 22 Medial umbilical ligament |
| 7 Psoas major muscle and genitofemoral nerve | 14 Superior mesenteric artery | 23 Urinary bladder |
| | 15 Left kidney | 24 Penis |
| | 16 Abdominal aorta | |

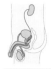

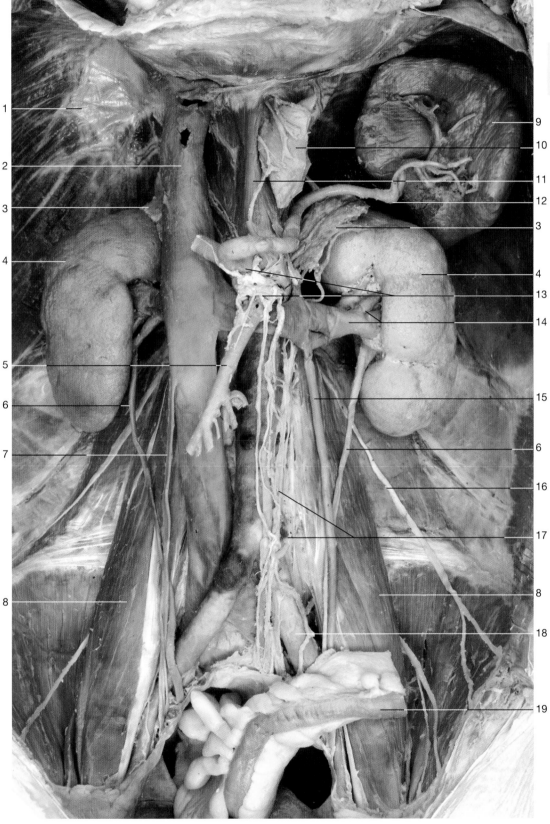

**Retroperitoneal organs, urinary system in the male** (anterior aspect). The peritoneum has been removed. Note the autonomic plexus and ganglia at the abdominal aorta.

| | | | |
|---|---|---|---|
| 1 Diaphragm | 7 Right spermatic vein | 12 Splenic artery | 17 Superior hypogastric plexus and ganglion |
| 2 Inferior vena cava | 8 Psoas major muscle | 13 Celiac trunk and celiac ganglion | 18 Left common iliac artery |
| 3 Suprarenal gland | 9 Spleen | 14 Renal artery and vein | 19 Sigmoid colon |
| 4 Kidney | 10 Cardiac part of stomach | 15 Left spermatic vein | |
| 5 Superior mesenteric artery | 11 Abdominal aorta | 16 Ilio-inguinal nerve | |
| 6 Ureter | | | |

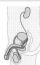

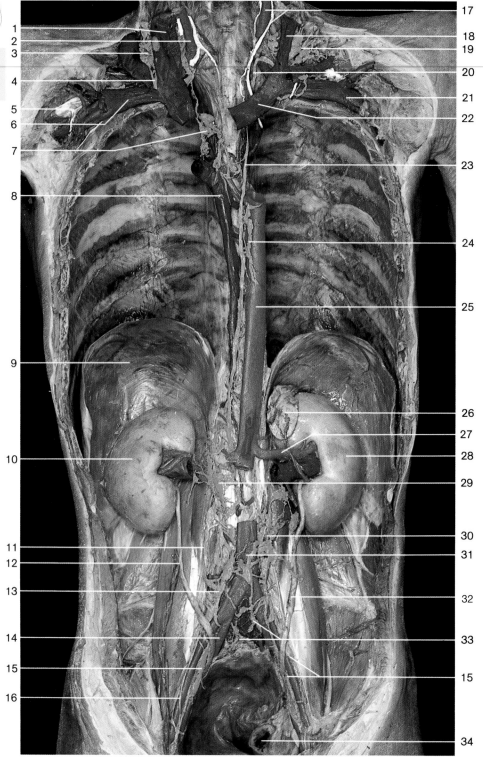

**Lymph vessels and lymph nodes of the posterior wall of thoracic and abdominal cavities**
(anterior aspect). Green = lymph vessels and nodes; blue = veins; red = arteries; white = nerves.

| | | | |
|---|---|---|---|
| 1 | Internal jugular vein | 10 | Right kidney |
| 2 | Right common carotid artery and right vagus nerve | 11 | Right lumbar trunk |
| | | 12 | Right ureter |
| 3 | Jugulo-omohyoid lymph node | 13 | Common iliac lymph nodes |
| 4 | Right lymphatic duct | 14 | Right internal iliac artery |
| 5 | Subclavian trunk | 15 | External iliac lymph nodes |
| 6 | Right subclavian vein | 16 | Right external iliac artery |
| 7 | Bronchomediastinal trunk | 17 | Left common carotid artery and left vagus nerve |
| 8 | Azygos vein | | |
| 9 | Diaphragm | 18 | Internal jugular vein |

| | |
|---|---|
| 19 | Deep cervical lymph nodes |
| 20 | Thoracic duct entering left jugular angle |
| 21 | Left subclavian vein |
| 22 | Left brachiocephalic vein |
| 23 | Thoracic duct |
| 24 | Mediastinal lymph nodes |
| 25 | Thoracic aorta |
| 26 | Left suprarenal gland |
| 27 | Left renal artery |

| | |
|---|---|
| 28 | Left kidney |
| 29 | Cisterna chyli |
| 30 | Lumbar lymph nodes |
| 31 | Abdominal aorta |
| 32 | Left ureter |
| 33 | Sacral lymph nodes |
| 34 | Rectum (cut edge) |
| 35 | Aortic arch |
| 36 | Superior vena cava |
| 37 | Intercostal vein |
| 38 | Left jugular trunk |
| 39 | Left subclavian artery |
| 40 | Quadratus lumborum muscle |
| 41 | Psoas major muscle |
| 42 | Parotid lymph nodes |
| 43 | Axillary lymph nodes |

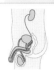

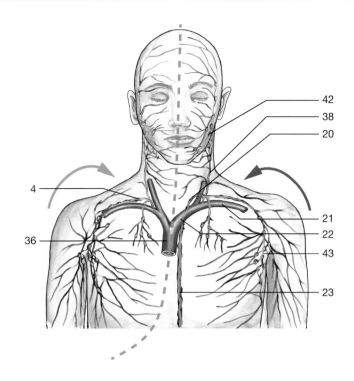

**Lymph vessels and lymph nodes of the upper part of the body.** Dotted red line = border between irrigation areas of the right and left part of the body.

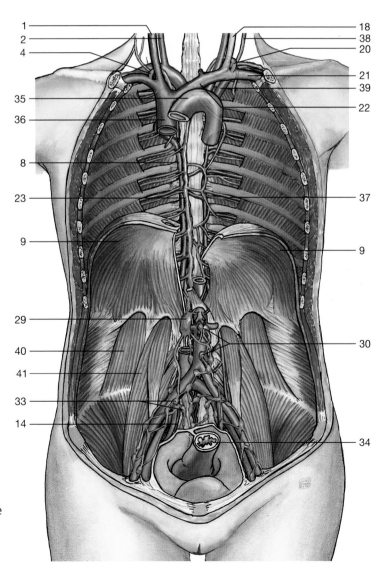

**Lymph vessels and lymph nodes of the posterior wall of thoracic and abdominal cavities** (anterior aspect). Note the course of the thoracic duct from the cisterna chyli to the left venous angle. The lymph vessels of the intercostal spaces communicate mainly with the thoracic duct.

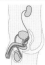

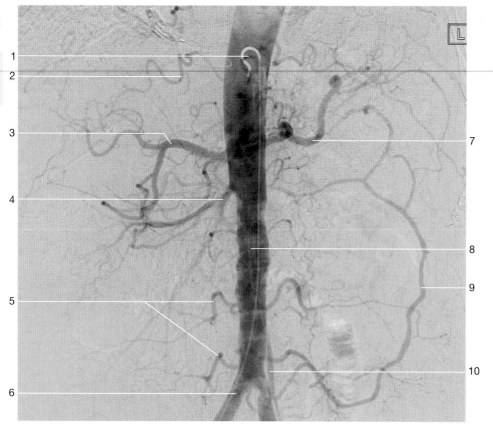

1   Abdominal aorta
    (containing partly the
    catheter)
2   Superior suprarenal artery
3   Hepatic artery
4   Superior mesenteric artery
5   Lumbal arteries
6   Common iliac artery
    (with catheter)
7   Splenic artery
8   Abdominal aorta
    (partly sclerotized)
9   Left colic artery
10  Inferior mesenteric artery
11  Inferior phrenic arteries
12  Middle suprarenal artery
13  Right colic artery
14  Ileocolic artery
15  Sigmoid arteries
16  Superior rectal artery

**Arteriography of the abdominal aorta.** The distal portion of the aorta reveals sclerotic changes.
(Courtesy of Dr. Wieners, Dept. of Radiology, Berlin, Germany.)

**Course of the superior and inferior mesenteric arteries within the retroperitoneal
space** supplying the ascending and descending parts of the colon (anterior aspect).

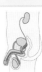

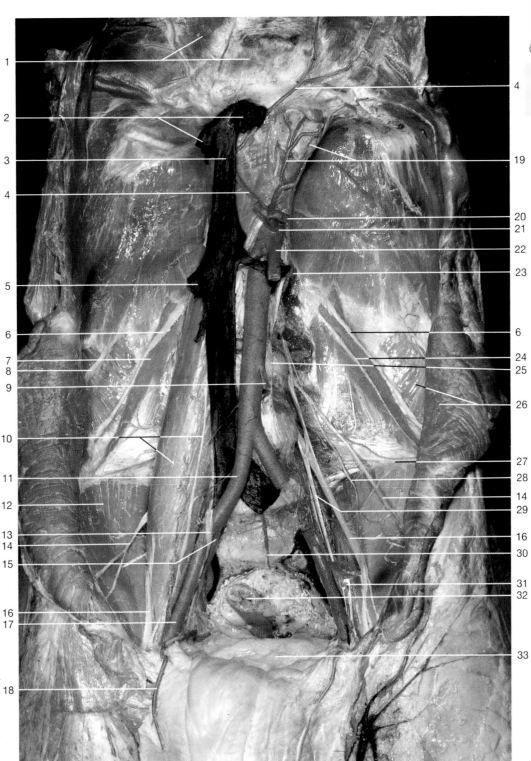

**Vessels and nerves within the retroperitoneal space** (anterior aspect). Part of the left psoas major muscle has been removed to display the lumbar plexus. Red = arteries; blue = veins.

| | | | |
|---|---|---|---|
| 1 | Diaphragm | 10 | Right genitofemoral nerve and psoas major muscle |
| 2 | Hepatic veins | 11 | Common iliac artery |
| 3 | Inferior vena cava | 12 | Iliacus muscle |
| 4 | Inferior phrenic artery | 13 | Right ureter (divided) |
| 5 | Right renal vein | 14 | Lateral femoral cutaneous nerve |
| 6 | Iliohypogastric nerve | 15 | Internal iliac artery |
| 7 | Quadratus lumborum muscle | 16 | Femoral nerve |
| 8 | Subcostal nerve | 17 | External iliac artery |
| 9 | Inferior mesenteric artery | 18 | Inferior epigastric artery |

| | |
|---|---|
| 19 | Cardiac part of stomach and esophageal branches of left gastric artery |
| 20 | Splenic artery |
| 21 | Celiac trunk |
| 22 | Superior mesenteric artery |
| 23 | Left renal artery |
| 24 | Ilio-inguinal nerve |
| 25 | Sympathetic trunk |
| 26 | Transverse abdominal muscle |

| | |
|---|---|
| 27 | Iliac crest |
| 28 | Left genitofemoral nerve |
| 29 | Left obturator nerve |
| 30 | Median sacral artery |
| 31 | Psoas major muscle (divided) with supplying artery |
| 32 | Rectum (cut) |
| 33 | Urinary bladder |

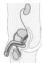

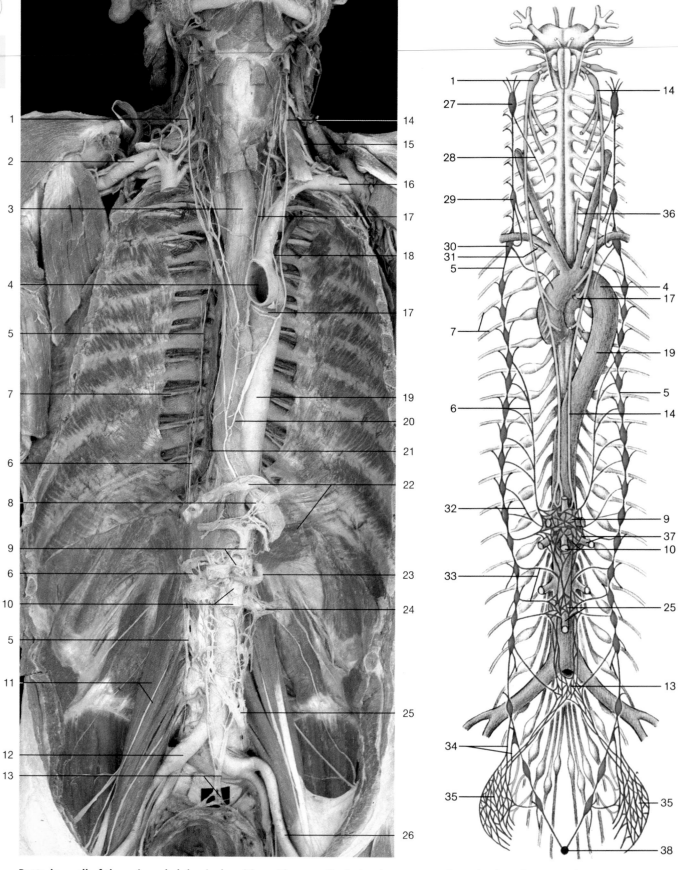

**Posterior wall of thoracic and abdominal cavities with sympathetic trunk, vagus nerve, and autonomic ganglia** (anterior aspect). Thoracic and abdominal organs removed, except for the esophagus and aorta.

**Organization of autonomic nervous system.**
Yellow = parasympathetic nerves;
green = sympathetic nerves.

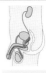

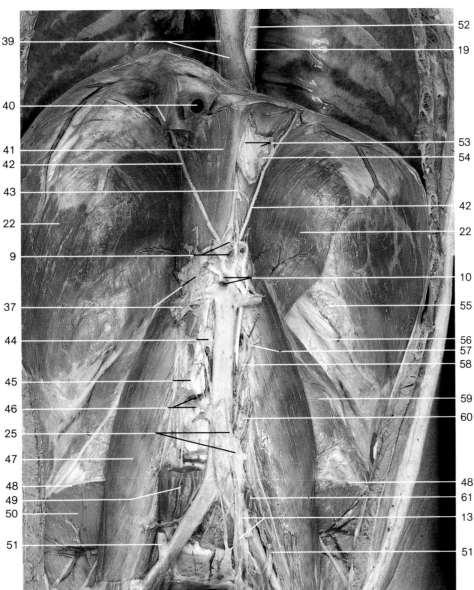

**Ganglia and plexus of the autonomic nervous system within the retroperitoneal space** (anterior aspect). The kidneys and the inferior vena cava with its tributaries have been removed.

| | | | |
|---|---|---|---|
| 1 | Right vagus nerve | 16 | Left subclavian artery |
| 2 | Right subclavian artery | 17 | Left recurrent laryngeal nerve |
| 3 | Esophagus | 18 | Inferior cervical cardiac nerve |
| 4 | Aortic arch | 19 | Thoracic aorta |
| 5 | Sympathetic trunk | 20 | Esophageal plexus |
| 6 | Greater splanchnic nerve | 21 | Azygos vein |
| 7 | Intercostal nerve | 22 | Diaphragm |
| 8 | Abdominal part of esophagus and vagal trunk | 23 | Splenic artery |
| | | 24 | Left renal artery and plexus |
| 9 | Celiac trunk with celiac ganglion | 25 | Inferior mesenteric ganglion and artery |
| 10 | Superior mesenteric artery and ganglion | 26 | Left external iliac artery |
| | | 27 | Superior cervical ganglion of sympathetic trunk |
| 11 | Psoas major muscle and genitofemoral nerve | 28 | Superior cardiac branch of sympathetic trunk |
| 12 | Common iliac artery | 29 | Middle cervical ganglion of sympathetic trunk |
| 13 | Superior hypogastric plexus and ganglion | 30 | Inferior cervical ganglion of sympathetic trunk |
| 14 | Left vagus nerve | | |
| 15 | Brachial plexus | | |

| | | | |
|---|---|---|---|
| 31 | Right recurrent laryngeal nerve | 46 | Lumbar artery and vein |
| 32 | Lesser splanchnic nerve | 47 | Psoas major muscle |
| 33 | Lumbar splanchnic nerves | 48 | Iliac crest |
| 34 | Sacral splanchnic nerves | 49 | Inferior vena cava |
| 35 | Inferior hypogastric ganglion and plexus | 50 | Iliacus muscle |
| | | 51 | Ureter |
| 36 | Left recurrent laryngeal nerve | 52 | Left vagus nerve forming the esophageal plexus |
| 37 | Aorticorenal plexus and renal artery | 53 | Left vagus nerve forming the gastric plexus |
| 38 | Ganglion impar | 54 | Esophagus continuing into the cardiac part of stomach |
| 39 | Esophagus with branches of vagus nerve | 55 | Lumbocostal triangle |
| 40 | Hepatic veins | 56 | Position of twelfth rib |
| 41 | Right crus of diaphragm | 57 | Left lumbar lymph trunk |
| 42 | Inferior phrenic artery | 58 | Ganglion of sympathetic trunk |
| 43 | Right vagus nerve entering the celiac ganglion | 59 | Quadratus lumborum muscle |
| 44 | Right lumbar lymph trunk | 60 | Lumbar part of left sympathetic trunk |
| 45 | Lumbar part of right sympathetic trunk | 61 | Iliac lymph vessels |

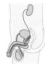

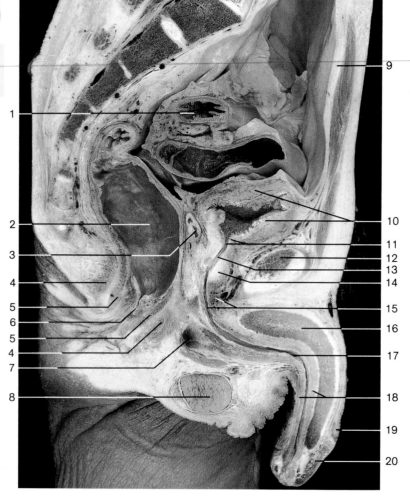

1    Sigmoid colon
2    Ampulla of rectum
3    Ampulla of ductus deferens
4    External anal sphincter muscle
5    Internal anal sphincter muscle
6    Anal canal
7    Bulb of penis
8    Testis (cut surface)
9    Median umbilical ligament
10   Urinary bladder
11   Internal urethral orifice and sphincter
12   Pubic symphysis
13   Prostatic part of urethra
14   Prostate gland
15   Membranous part of urethra and
     external urethral sphincter
16   Corpus cavernosum of penis
17   Spongy urethra
18   Corpus spongiosum of penis
19   Foreskin or prepuce
20   Glans penis
21   Kidney
22   Renal pelvis
23   Abdominal part of ureter
24   Pelvic part of ureter
25   Seminal vesicle
26   Ejaculatory duct
27   Bulbo-urethral gland (Cowper's gland)
28   Ductus deferens
29   Epididymis
30   Umbilicus
31   Trigone of urinary bladder and
     ureteric orifice
32   Navicular fossa of urethra
33   External urethral orifice
34   Testis
35   Sacrum

**Male urogenital system** (midsagittal section through the pelvic cavity).

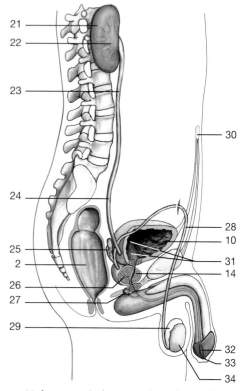

**Male urogenital system** (lateral aspect).

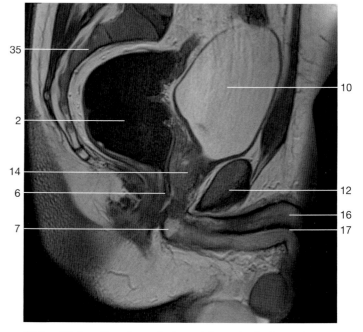

**Midsagittal section through the pelvic cavity in the male**
(MRI scan). (Prof. Uder, Dept. of Radiology, Univ. Erlangen-
Nuremberg, Germany.)

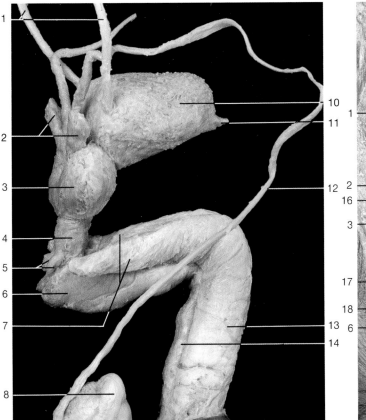

**Male genital organs, isolated** (right lateral aspect).

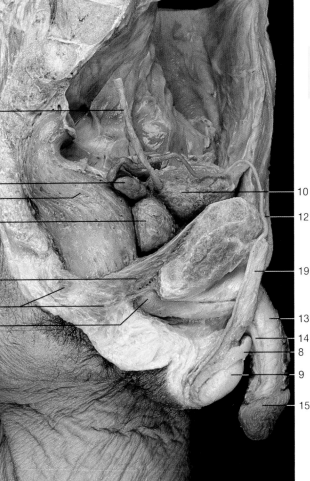

**Male genital organs in situ** (right lateral aspect).

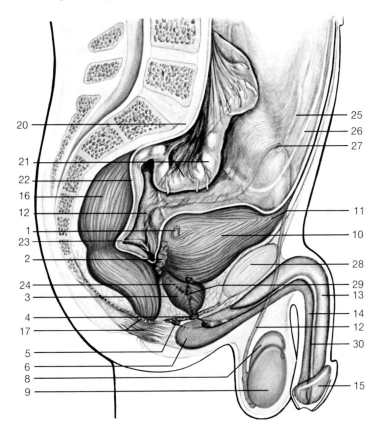

**Positions of male genital organs** (right lateral aspect).

1 Ureter
2 Seminal vesicle
3 Prostate gland
4 Urogenital diaphragm and membranous part of urethra
5 Bulbo-urethral gland (Cowper's gland)
6 Bulb of penis
7 Left and right crus penis
8 Epididymis
9 Testis
10 Urinary bladder
11 Apex of urinary bladder
12 Ductus deferens
13 Corpus cavernosum of penis
14 Corpus spongiosum of penis
15 Glans penis
16 Ampulla of rectum
17 Levator ani muscle
18 Anal canal and external anal sphincter muscle
19 Spermatic cord (cut)
20 Sacral promontory
21 Sigmoid colon
22 Peritoneum (cut edge)
23 Rectovesical pouch
24 Ejaculatory duct
25 Lateral umbilical fold
26 Medial umbilical fold
27 Deep inguinal ring and ductus deferens
28 Pubic symphysis
29 Prostatic part of urethra
30 Spongy urethra

| | |
|---|---|
| 1 | Ureter |
| 2 | Ductus deferens |
| 3 | Interureteric fold |
| 4 | Ureteric orifice |
| 5 | Seminal vesicle |
| 6 | Trigone of urinary bladder |
| 7 | Prostatic urethra with seminal colliculus and urethral crest |
| 8 | Deep transverse perineal muscle |
| 9 | Membranous urethra |
| 10 | Spongy urethra |
| 11 | Mucous membrane of urinary bladder |
| 12 | Internal urethral orifice and uvula of urinary bladder |
| 13 | Prostate |
| 14 | Prostatic utricle |
| 15 | Right and left corpus cavernosum of penis |
| 16 | Ejaculatory duct |
| 17 | Sphincter urethrae muscle |
| 18 | Sphincter muscle of urinary bladder |
| 19 | Bulbo-urethral gland (Cowper's gland) |
| 20 | Crus penis |
| 21 | Orifices of bulbo-urethral glands |
| 22 | Glans penis |
| 23 | Ureteric orifices |

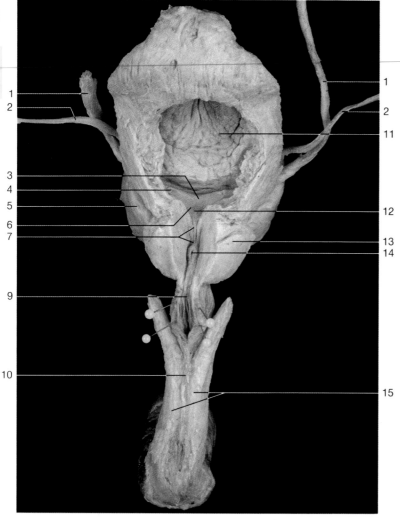

**Male genital organs and urinary bladder, isolated** (anterior aspect). Urinary bladder, prostate, and urethra have been opened. The urinary bladder is contracted.

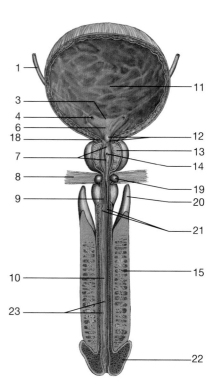

**Posterior half of male urethra and prostate** in continuity with the neck of urinary bladder (anterior aspect).

**Male genital organs and urinary bladder** (anterior aspect). Urinary bladder, urethra, and penis have been dissected.

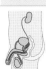

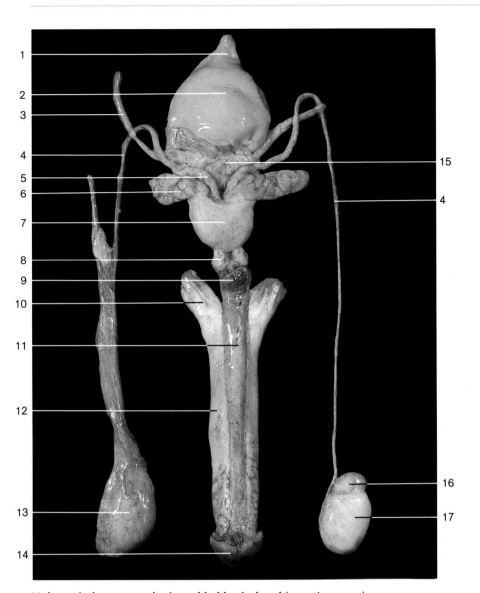

1 Apex of urinary bladder
   with urachus
2 Urinary bladder
3 Ureter
4 Ductus deferens
5 Ampulla of ductus deferens
6 Seminal vesicle
7 Prostate
8 Bulbo-urethral gland (Cowper's gland)
9 Bulb of penis
10 Crus penis
11 Corpus spongiosum of penis
12 Corpus cavernosum of penis
13 Testis and epididymis with coverings
14 Glans penis
15 Fundus of urinary bladder
16 Head of epididymis
17 Testis
18 Mucous membrane of bladder
19 Trigone of bladder
20 Ureteric orifice
21 Internal urethral orifice
22 Seminal colliculus
23 Prostate
24 Prostatic urethra
25 Membranous urethra
26 Spongy (penile) urethra
27 Skin of penis
28 Deep dorsal vein of penis (unpaired)
29 Dorsal artery of penis (paired)
30 Tunica albuginea
   of corpora cavernosa
31 Septum of penis
32 Deep artery of penis
33 Tunica albuginea
   of corpus spongiosum
34 Deep fascia of penis

**Male genital organs and urinary bladder, isolated** (posterior aspect).

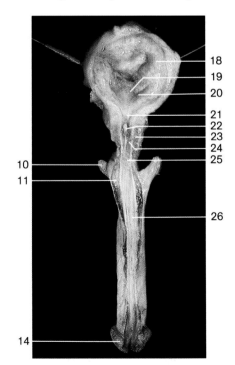

**Urinary bladder, urethra, and penis**
(anterior aspect, opened longitudinally).

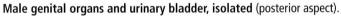

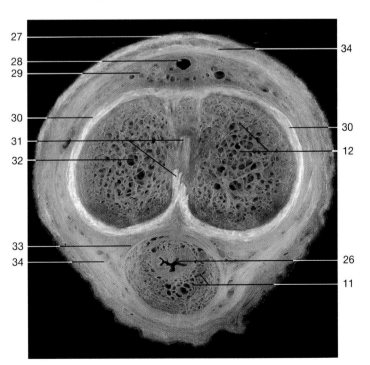

**Cross section through the penis** (inferior aspect).

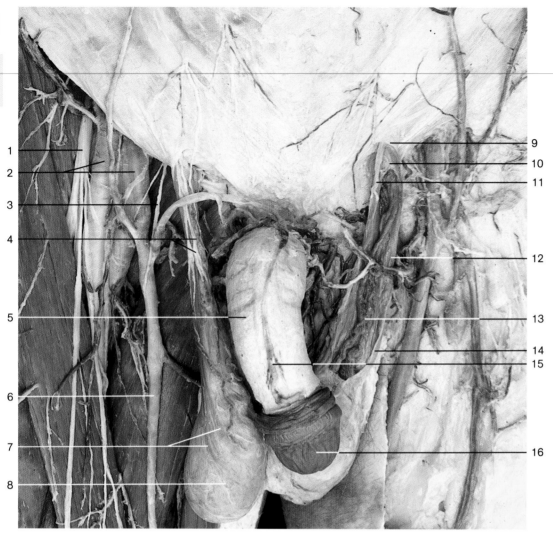

**Male external genital organs with penis, testis, and spermatic cord,** superficial layer (anterior aspect).

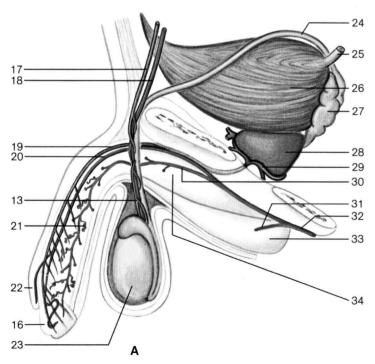

**Vessels of male genital organs.**
A = lateral aspect; B = cross section through the penis.

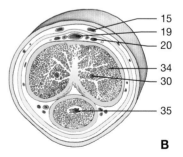

**B**

1   Femoral nerve
2   Femoral artery and vein
3   Femoral branch of genitofemoral nerve
4   Spermatic cord with genital branch
    of genitofemoral nerve
5   Penis with deep fascia
6   Great saphenous vein
7   Cremaster muscle
8   Testis with cremaster muscle
9   Superficial inguinal ring
10  Internal spermatic fascia (cut edge)
11  Ilio-inguinal nerve
12  Left spermatic cord
13  Pampiniform venous plexus
14  External spermatic fascia
15  Superficial dorsal vein of penis

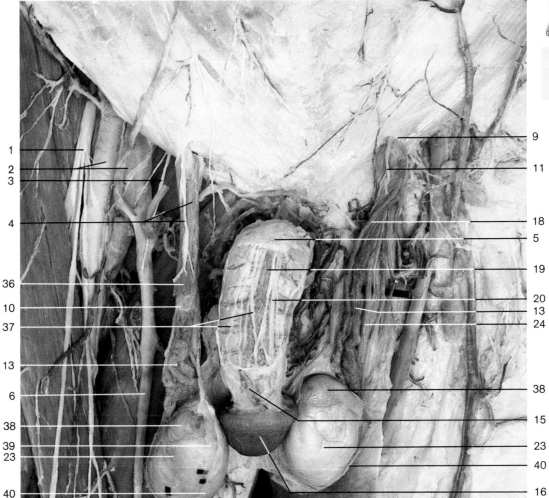

1
2
3

4

36
10
37

13

6

38
39
23

40

9
11

18
5

19

20
13
24

38

15

23
40
16

| 16 | Glans penis |
| 17 | Testicular vein |
| 18 | Testicular artery |
| 19 | Deep dorsal vein of penis |
| 20 | Dorsal artery of penis |
| 21 | Helicine arteries |
| 22 | Prepuce |
| 23 | Testis with tunica albuginea |
| 24 | Ductus deferens |
| 25 | Ureter |
| 26 | Urinary bladder |
| 27 | Seminal vesicle |
| 28 | Prostate |
| 29 | Vesicoprostatic venous plexus |
| 30 | Deep artery of penis |
| 31 | Artery of bulb of penis |
| 32 | Internal pudendal artery |
| 33 | Corpus spongiosum of penis |
| 34 | Corpus cavernosum of penis |
| 35 | Urethra |
| 36 | Cremasteric fascia with cremaster muscle |
| 37 | Dorsal nerve of penis |
| 38 | Epididymis |
| 39 | Tunica vaginalis (visceral layer) |
| 40 | Tunica vaginalis (parietal layer) |
| 41 | Inguinal ligament |
| 42 | Femoral cutaneous nerve |
| 43 | Deep inguinal ring |
| 44 | Ductus deferens and testicular artery |
| 45 | Hiatus saphenous |
| 46 | Epididymis |

**Male external genital organs with penis, testis, and spermatic cord,** deeper layer (anterior aspect).
The deep fascia of the penis has been opened to display the dorsal nerves and vessels.

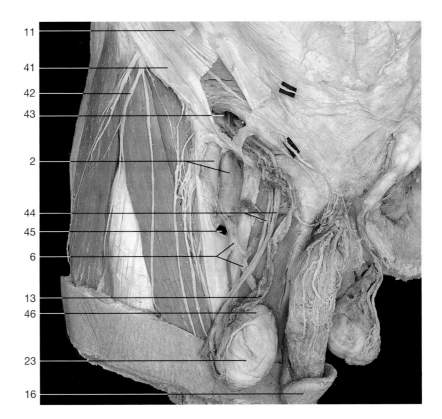

11

41

42
43

2

44
45

6

13
46

23

16

**Male external genital organs and
inguinal region** (anterior aspect).
Dissection of the inguinal channel.

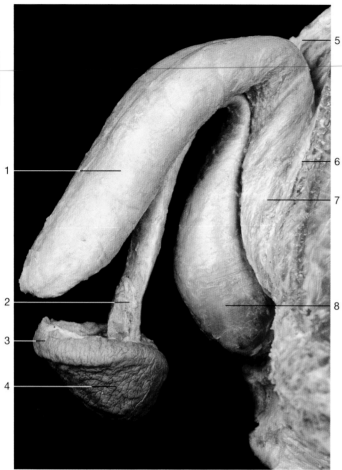

**Male external genital organs** (oblique-lateral aspect). The corpus spongiosum of the penis with the glans penis has been isolated and reflected.

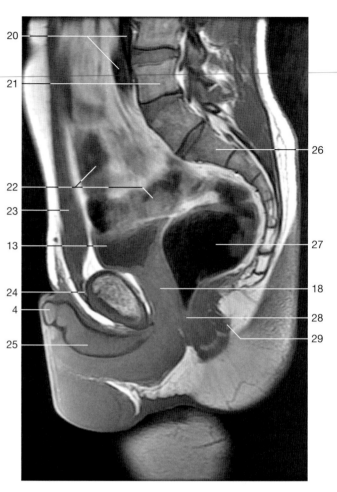

**Sagittal section through the pelvic cavity with the male genital organs** (MRI scan). (From Heuck et al., MRT-Atlas, 2009.)

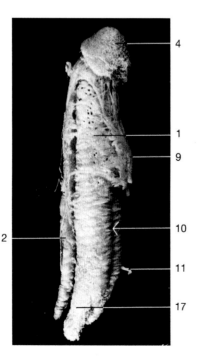

**Resin cast of an erected penis.**

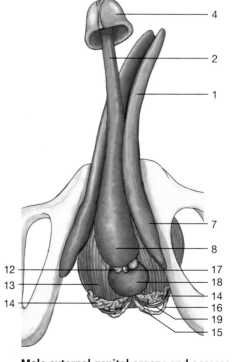

**Male external genital organs and accessory glands.**

| | |
|---|---|
| 1 | Corpus cavernosum of penis |
| 2 | Corpus spongiosum of penis |
| 3 | Corona of glans penis |
| 4 | Glans penis |
| 5 | Suspensory ligament of penis |
| 6 | Pubis (inferior pubic ramus, dissected) |
| 7 | Crus penis |
| 8 | Bulb of penis |
| 9 | Dorsal vein of penis |
| 10 | Septum pectiniforme |
| 11 | Dorsal artery of penis |
| 12 | Bulbo-urethral gland (Cowper's gland) |
| 13 | Urinary bladder |
| 14 | Seminal vesicle |
| 15 | Ampulla of ductus deferens |
| 16 | Ductus deferens |
| 17 | Membranous urethra |
| 18 | Prostate |
| 19 | Ureter |
| 20 | Common iliac artery and vein |
| 21 | Fifth lumbar vertebral body |
| 22 | Intestinal loops |
| 23 | Rectus abdominis muscle |
| 24 | Pubic symphysis |
| 25 | Root of penis |
| 26 | Sacrum |
| 27 | Ampulla of rectum |
| 28 | Anal canal |
| 29 | External anal sphincter muscle |

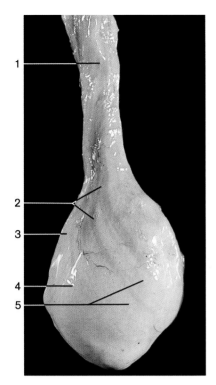

**Testis and epididymis** with investing layers (lateral aspect).

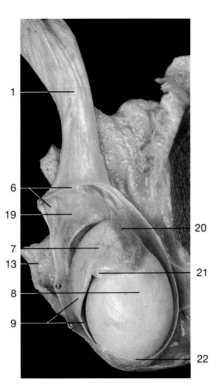

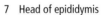

**Testis and epididymis** (lateral aspect). The tunica vaginalis has been opened.

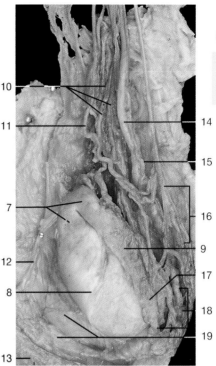

**Testis, epididymis, and spermatic cord** (left side, postero-lateral aspect). Dissection of spermatic cord and ductus deferens.

| | |
|---|---|
| 1 | Spermatic cord covered with cremasteric fascia |
| 2 | Cremaster muscle |
| 3 | Position of epididymis |
| 4 | Internal spermatic fascia |
| 5 | Position of testis |
| 6 | Internal spermatic fascia with adjacent investing layers of testis (cut surface) |

| | |
|---|---|
| 7 | Head of epididymis |
| 8 | Testis with tunica vaginalis (visceral layer) |
| 9 | Body of epididymis |
| 10 | Pampiniform venous plexus (anterior veins) |
| 11 | Testicular artery |
| 12 | Tunica vaginalis (parietal layer, cut edge) |
| 13 | Skin and dartos muscle (reflected) |
| 14 | Ductus deferens |

| | |
|---|---|
| 15 | Artery of ductus deferens |
| 16 | Posterior veins of pampiniform plexus |
| 17 | Tail of epididymis |
| 18 | Transition of epididymal duct to ductus deferens and venous plexus |
| 19 | Parietal layer of tunica vaginalis |
| 20 | Appendix of epididymis |
| 21 | Appendix of testis |
| 22 | Gubernaculum testis |

**Longitudinal section through testis and epididymis.** The left figure shows the testicular septa after removal of the seminiferous tubules.

| | |
|---|---|
| 1 | Spermatic cord (cut surface) |
| 2 | Head of epididymis (cut surface) |
| 3 | Septa of testis |
| 4 | Mediastinum testis |
| 5 | Tunica albuginea |
| 6 | Superior pole of testis |
| 7 | Convoluted seminiferous tubules |
| 8 | Inferior pole of testis |

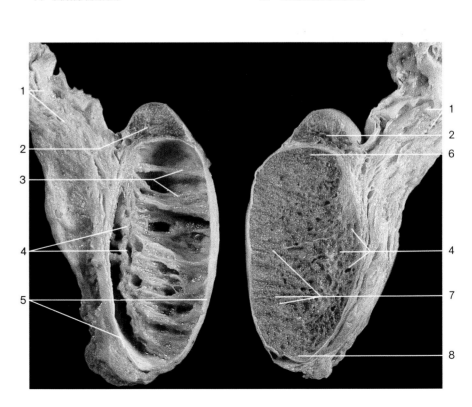

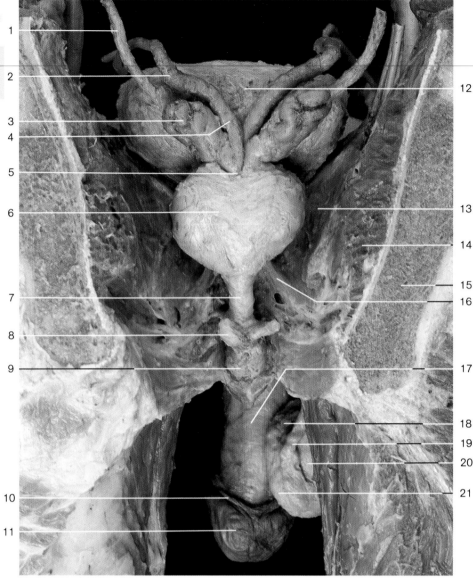

| | |
|---|---|
| 1 | Ureter |
| 2 | Ductus deferens |
| 3 | Seminal vesicle |
| 4 | Ampulla of ductus deferens |
| 5 | Ejaculatory duct (proximal portion) |
| 6 | Prostate |
| 7 | Membranous urethra |
| 8 | Bulbo-urethral gland (Cowper's gland) |
| 9 | Bulb of penis |
| 10 | Penis |
| 11 | Glans penis |
| 12 | Urinary bladder |
| 13 | Levator ani muscle |
| 14 | Obturator internus muscle |
| 15 | Pelvic bone (cut edge) |
| 16 | Puboprostatic ligament |
| 17 | Corpus spongiosum of penis |
| 18 | Head of epididymis |
| 19 | Beginning of ductus deferens |
| 20 | Testis |
| 21 | Tail of epididymis |
| 22 | Corpus cavernosum of penis |
| 23 | Spermatic cord |
| 24 | Pectineus and adductor muscles |
| 25 | Pubis |
| 26 | Prostatic part of urethra (seminal colliculus) |
| 27 | Rectum |
| 28 | Sciatic nerve |
| 29 | Great saphenous vein |
| 30 | Sartorius muscle |
| 31 | Femoral artery and vein |
| 32 | Rectus femoris muscle |
| 33 | Tensor fasciae latae muscle |
| 34 | Pectineus muscle |
| 35 | Iliopsoas muscle |
| 36 | Vastus lateralis muscle |
| 37 | Obturator externus muscle |
| 38 | Femur |
| 39 | Ischial tuberosity |
| 40 | Gluteus maximus muscle |

**Accessory glands of male genital organs.** Coronal section through the pelvic cavity. Posterior aspect of urinary bladder, prostate, and seminal vesicles.

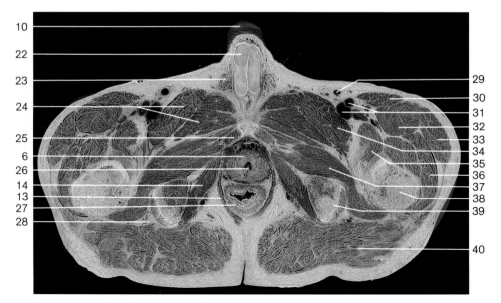

**Horizontal section through the pelvic cavity in the male** at the level of prostate.

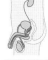

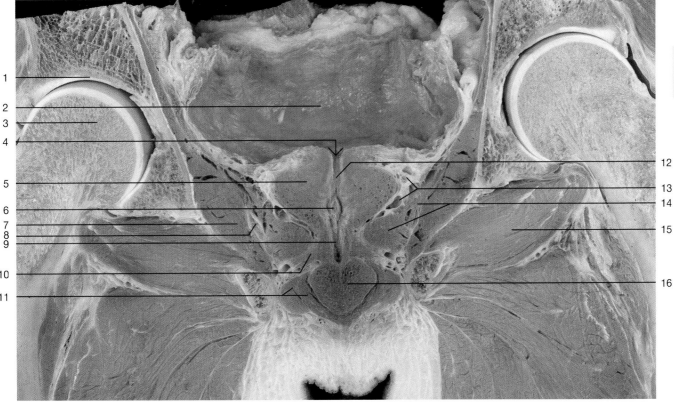

**Coronal section through the pelvic cavity in the male** at the level of prostate and hip joint (anterior aspect).

| | | | |
|---|---|---|---|
| 1 | Acetabulum of hip joint | 12 | Prostatic part of urethra |
| 2 | Urinary bladder | 13 | Prostatic plexus |
| 3 | Head of femur | 14 | Levator ani muscle |
| 4 | Internal urethral orifice | 15 | Obturator externus muscle |
| 5 | Prostate | 16 | Bulb of penis |
| 6 | Seminal colliculus | 17 | Median umbilical fold with remnant of urachus |
| 7 | Obturator internus muscle | 18 | Rectovesical pouch |
| 8 | Ischiorectal fossa | 19 | Rectum |
| 9 | Membranous urethra | 20 | Sacrum |
| 10 | Deep transverse perineal muscle | 21 | Inferior epigastric artery |
| 11 | Crus penis and ischiocavernosus muscle | | |

| | |
|---|---|
| 22 | Medial umbilical fold with remnant of umbilical artery |
| 23 | Deep inguinal ring and ductus deferens |
| 24 | Deep iliac circumflex artery |
| 25 | External iliac artery and vein |
| 26 | Femoral nerve |
| 27 | Iliopsoas muscle |
| 28 | Ureter |
| 29 | Obturator nerve and internal iliac artery |
| 30 | Ilium and sacrum |

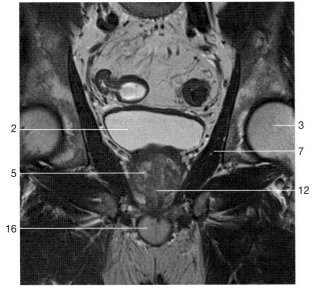

**Coronal section through the pelvic cavity in the male** (MRI scan). (Prof. Uder, Dept. of Radiology, Univ. Erlangen-Nuremberg, Germany.)

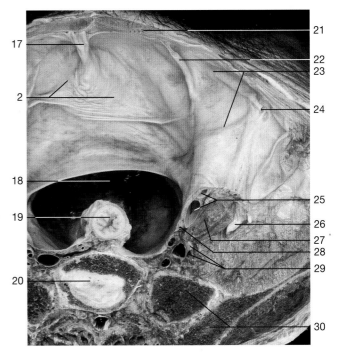

**Pelvic cavity in the male** (from above).

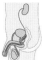

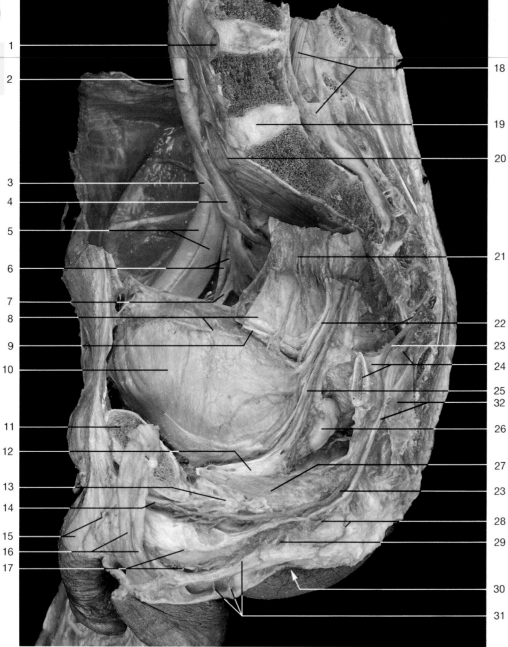

**Vessels of the pelvic cavity in the male** (right half, parasagittal section). The arteries have been injected with red resin. The parietal layer of peritoneum has been removed. The urinary bladder is filled to a great extent.

| | |
|---|---|
| 1 Left common iliac artery | 18 Cauda equina and dura mater (divided) |
| 2 Right common iliac artery | 19 Intervertebral disc |
| 3 Right ureter | between fifth lumbar vertebra and sacrum |
| 4 Right internal iliac artery | 20 Sacral promontory |
| 5 Right external iliac artery and vein | 21 Mesosigmoid |
| 6 Right obturator artery and nerve | 22 Left ureter |
| 7 Umbilical artery | 23 Left internal pudendal artery |
| 8 Sigmoid and superior vesical artery | 24 Ischial spine (cut), sacrospinal ligament, and |
| 9 Left ductus deferens | inferior gluteal artery |
| 10 Urinary bladder | 25 Left inferior vesical artery |
| 11 Pubis (cut) | 26 Seminal vesicle |
| 12 Prostate | 27 Levator ani muscle |
| 13 Vesicoprostatic venous plexus | 28 Branches of inferior rectal artery |
| 14 Deep dorsal vein of penis and | 29 Perineal artery |
| dorsal artery of penis | 30 Anus |
| 15 Penis and superficial dorsal vein | 31 Posterior scrotal branches |
| 16 Spermatic cord and testicular artery | 32 Pudendal nerve and sacrotuberal ligament |
| 17 Bulb of penis and deep artery of penis | |

1   Internal iliac artery
2   External iliac artery
3   Ureter
4   Obturator nerve
5   Umbilical artery
6   Deep inguinal ring
7   Urinary bladder (vesica urinaria)
8   Symphysis
9   Prostatic part of urethra
10  Sphincter muscle of urethra
11  Urethra (spongy part)
12  Cavernous body of penis
13  Glans penis
14  Sacrum
15  Promontory
16  Lateral sacral artery
17  Plexus sacralis
18  Inferior gluteal artery
19  Internal pudendal artery
20  Obturator artery
21  Inferior hypogastric plexus
22  Ductus deferens
23  Seminal vesicle (vesicula seminalis)
24  Rectum
25  Prostatic venous plexus
26  Prostate
27  Anal canal
28  Spongy part of penis
29  Pampiniform plexus
30  Testis and epididymis
31  Common iliac artery
32  Umbilical artery
33  Medial umbilical ligament
34  Branches of superior vesical artery
35  Urogenital diaphragm
36  Deep artery of penis
37  Dorsal artery of penis
38  Penis
39  Iliolumbar artery
40  Superior gluteal artery
41  Middle rectal artery
42  Levator ani muscle
43  Inferior rectal artery
44  Inferior vesical artery
45  Testicular artery
46  Artery of bulb of penis
47  Septum of penis

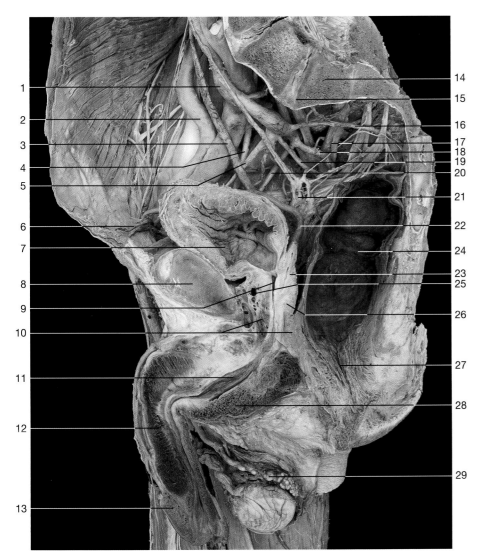

**Vessels of the pelvic cavity in the male** (medial aspect, midsagittal section). The gluteus maximus muscle has been removed.

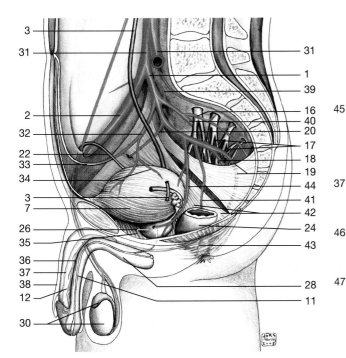

**Main branches of internal iliac artery in the male** (lateral aspect).

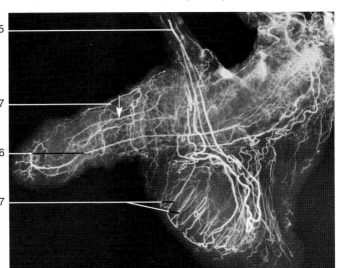

**Arteriography of male genital organs** (lateral aspect). Arrow: helicine artery.

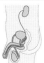

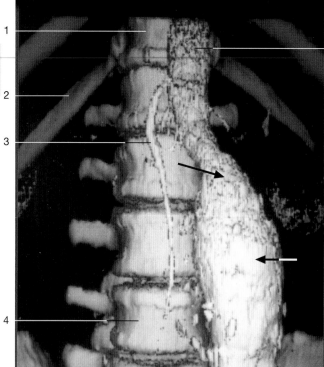

1 Twelfth thoracic vertebra (Th$_{12}$)
2 Twelfth rib (rib XII)
3 Inferior mesenteric artery
4 Fourth lumbar vertebra (L$_4$)
5 Sacrum
6 Sacro-iliac articulation
7 Aorta (abdominal part)
8 Left common iliac artery (included into the aneurysm)
9 Aorta with aneurysm
10 Body of lumbar vertebra
11 Intrinsic muscles of the back
12 Thrombotic part of the aneurysm (green)
13 Inferior vena cava (compressed, blue)
14 Iliopsoas muscle
15 Vertebral canal
16 Aneurysm of the aorta (red)

**Abdominal part of the aorta showing an infrarenal aneurysm** with involvement of both iliac arteries (arrows; 3-D reconstruction). (Courtesy of Prof. Rupprecht and Dr. Rexer, Klinikum Fürth, Germany.)

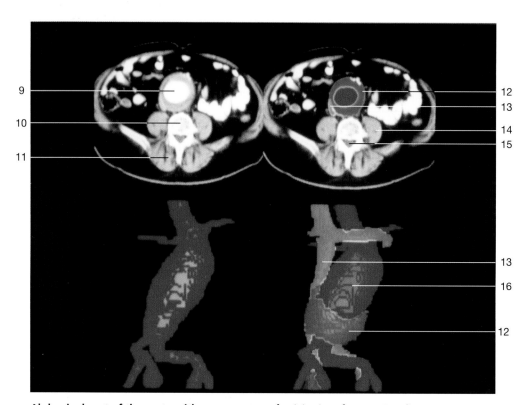

**Abdominal part of the aorta with an aneurysm,** after injection of contrast medium.
Above = horizontal sections through the abdominal cavity, showing different contrast medium concentrations within the aorta and the aneurysm; below = 3-D reconstruction of the aneurysm; red = aorta; green = thrombotic areas; blue = inferior vena cava (partly compressed).

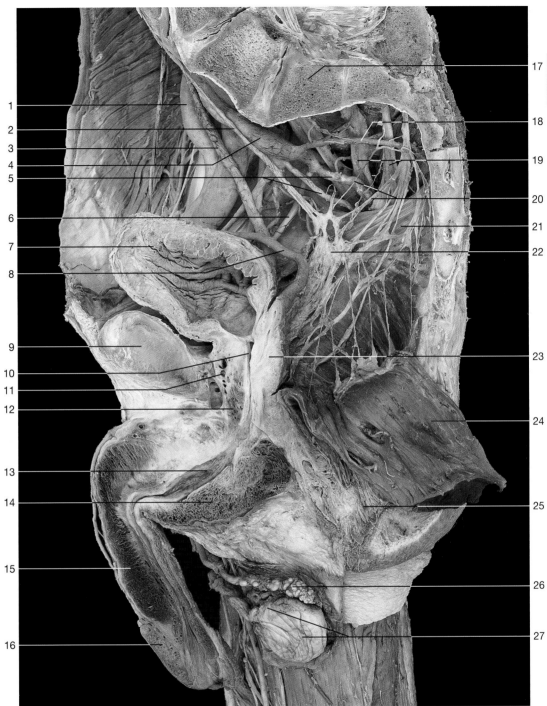

**Vessels and nerves of the pelvic cavity in the male** (medial aspect, midsagittal section). The rectum was reflected to display the inferior hypogastric plexus.

| | | | |
|---|---|---|---|
| 1 | External iliac artery | 10 | Prostatic part of urethra |
| 2 | Right hypogastric nerve | 11 | Prostatic venous plexus |
| 3 | Ureter | 12 | Sphincter urethrae muscle |
| 4 | Internal iliac artery | 13 | Spongy part of urethra |
| 5 | Inferior gluteal artery and | 14 | Corpus spongiosum penis |
| | internal pudendal artery | 15 | Corpus cavernosum penis |
| 6 | Obturator artery | 16 | Glans penis |
| 7 | Urinary bladder | 17 | Sacrum |
| 8 | Ductus deferens | 18 | Lateral sacral artery |
| 9 | Symphysis pubica | 19 | Sacral plexus |

| | |
|---|---|
| 20 | Pelvic splanchnic nerves (nervi erigentes) |
| 21 | Levator ani muscle |
| 22 | Inferior hypogastric plexus (pelvic plexus) |
| 23 | Prostate |
| 24 | Rectum (reflected) |
| 25 | Anal canal and external anal sphincter muscle |
| 26 | Pampiniform plexus continuous with testicular vein |
| 27 | Testis and epididymis |

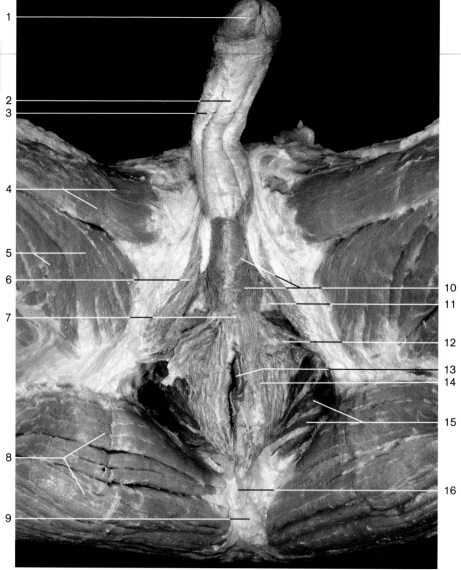

1 Glans penis
2 Corpus spongiosum of penis
3 Corpus cavernosum of penis
4 Gracilis muscle
5 Adductor muscles
6 Ischiocavernosus muscle
   overlying crus of penis
7 Perineal body
8 Gluteus maximus muscle
9 Coccyx
10 Bulbospongiosus muscle
11 Deep transverse perineus muscle
   covered by inferior fascia
   of urogenital diaphragm
12 Superficial transverse
   perineus muscle
13 Anus
14 External anal sphincter muscle
15 Levator ani muscle
16 Anococcygeal ligament
17 Testis
18 Urethra
19 Deep dorsal vein of penis
20 Dorsal artery of penis
21 Deep transverse perineal muscle
22 Obturator internus muscle
23 Sacrotuberal ligament

**Urogenital diaphragm and external genital organs in the male** with muscles of the pelvic floor (from below).

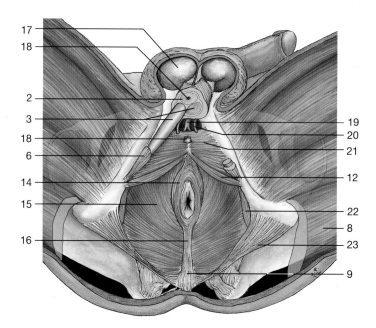

**Urogenital and anal regions in the male** (from below). Muscles of urogenital and pelvic diaphragms.

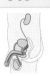

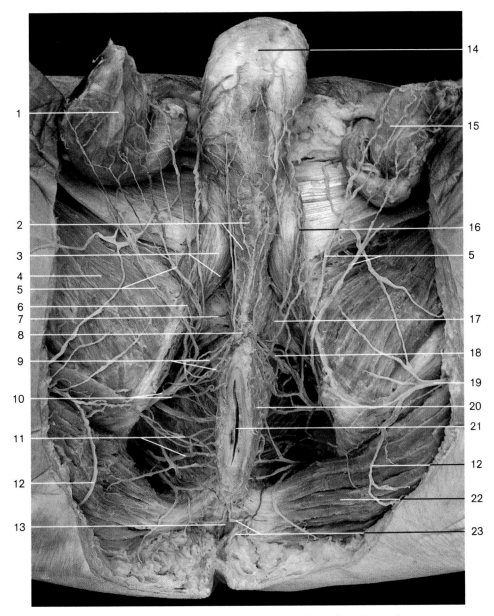

1  Right testis
   (reflected laterally and upward)
2  Bulbospongiosus muscle
3  Ischiocavernosus muscle
4  Adductor magnus muscle
5  Posterior scrotal nerves and
   superficial perineal arteries
6  Posterior scrotal artery and vein
7  Right artery of bulb of penis
8  Perineal body
9  Perineal branches
   of pudendal nerve
10 Pudendal nerve and
   internal pudendal artery
11 Inferior rectal arteries and nerves
12 Inferior cluneal nerves
13 Coccyx (location)
14 Penis
15 Left testis (reflected laterally)
16 Left posterior scrotal artery
17 Deep transverse perineal muscle
18 Left artery of bulb of penis
19 Branch of posterior femoral
   cutaneous nerve
20 External anal sphincter muscle
21 Anus
22 Gluteus maximus muscle
23 Anococcygeal nerves
24 Acetabulum (femur removed)
25 Ligament of femoral head
26 Body of ischium (cut)
27 Sciatic nerve
28 Coccygeus muscle
29 Levator ani muscle
   a  Iliococcygeus muscle
   b  Pubococcygeus muscle
   c  Puborectalis muscle
30 Prostatic venous plexus
31 Pubis
32 Testis

**Urogenital diaphragm and external genital organs in the male** with vessels and nerves (from below). The testes have been reflected laterally.

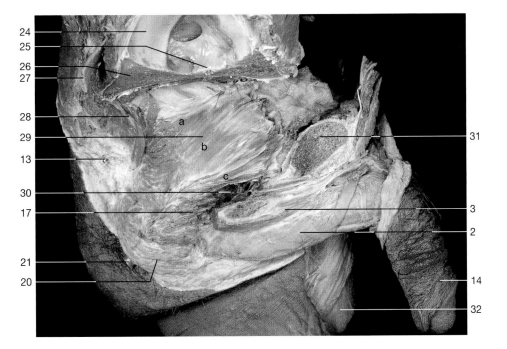

**Pelvic diaphragm and external genital organs in the male** (lateral aspect). The right half of the pelvis including the obturator internus muscle and femur have been removed to display the right half of the levator ani muscle.

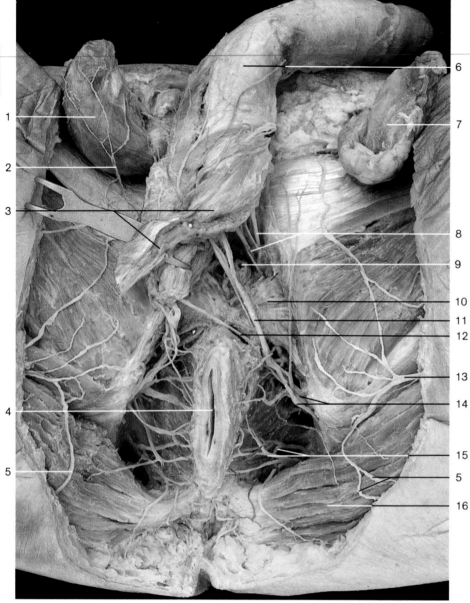

| | |
|---|---|
| 1 | Right testis (reflected) |
| 2 | Posterior scrotal nerves |
| 3 | Left crus penis with ischiocavernosus muscle |
| 4 | Anus |
| 5 | Inferior cluneal nerves |
| 6 | Penis |
| 7 | Left testis (reflected) |
| 8 | Dorsal artery and nerve of penis |
| 9 | Urethra |
| 10 | Deep transverse perineus muscle |
| 11 | Perineal branches of pudendal nerve |
| 12 | Artery of bulb of penis (reflected) |
| 13 | Branch of posterior femoral cutaneous nerve |
| 14 | Internal pudendal artery and pudendal nerve |
| 15 | Inferior rectal arteries and nerves |
| 16 | Gluteus maximus muscle |
| 17 | Dorsal nerve of penis |
| 18 | Posterior femoral cutaneous nerve |
| 19 | Perineal and anal branches of pudendal nerve |
| 20 | Pudendal nerve |
| 21 | Inferior rectal nerves |
| 22 | Bulbospongiosus muscle |
| 23 | Ischiocavernosus muscle |
| 24 | Dorsal artery of penis |
| 25 | Perineal artery |
| 26 | External anal sphincter muscle |
| 27 | Internal pudendal artery and vein |
| 28 | Inferior rectal arteries |

**Urogenital diaphragm and external genital organs in the male** (from below). The left crus penis has been isolated and reflected laterally together with the bulb of the penis. The urethra has been cut.

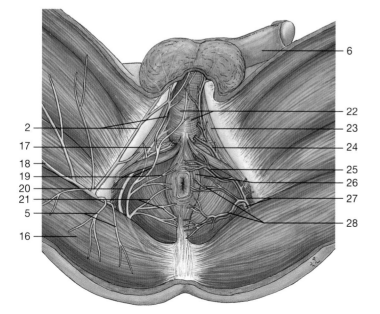

**Urogenital and anal regions in the male** (from below). Right side: nerves; left side: arteries and veins.

1   Right testis (reflected)
2   Corpus spongiosum of penis
3   Corpus cavernosum of penis
4   Perineal branch
    of posterior femoral cutaneous nerve
5   Posterior scrotal arteries and nerves
6   Deep artery of penis
7   Deep transverse perineal muscle
8   Right perineal nerves
9   Inferior rectal nerves
10  Inferior cluneal nerve
11  Anococcygeal nerves
12  Left spermatic cord
13  Left testis (cut surface)
14  Dorsal artery and nerve of penis
15  Deep dorsal vein of penis
16  Urethra (cut)
17  Artery of bulb of penis
18  Superficial transverse perineus
    muscle
19  Left artery of bulb of penis
20  Perineal branch of pudendal nerve
21  Anus
22  External anal sphincter muscle
23  Gluteus maximus muscle
24  Obturator fascia with Alcock's canal
    for pudendal nerve, and
    internal pudendal artery and vein
25  Sacrotuberous ligament
26  Coccyx
27  Urogenital diaphragm
    with superficial investing fascia
    of perineum (perineal fascia)

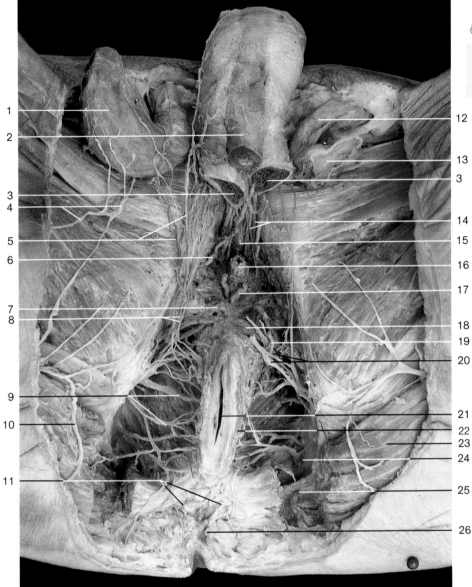

**Urogenital diaphragm and
external genital organs in the
male** (from below). The root of the
penis has been cut. Dissection of the
urogenital diaphragm.

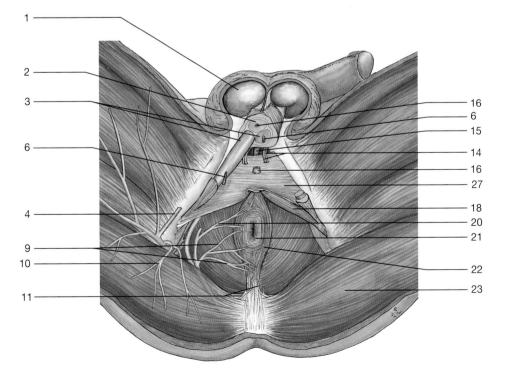

**Urogenital and anal regions in
the male** (from below). Muscles of
urogenital and pelvic diaphragms.
Light blue = perineal fascia.

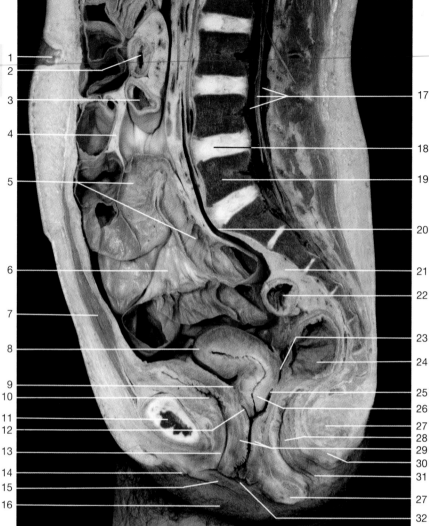

1 Umbilicus
2 Duodenum
3 Ascending part of duodenum
4 Root of mesentery
5 Small intestine
6 Mesentery
7 Rectus abdominis muscle
8 Uterus
9 Vesico-uterine pouch
10 Urinary bladder (collapsed)
11 Pubic symphysis
12 Anterior fornix of vagina
13 Urethra
14 Clitoris
15 Labium minus
16 Labium majus
17 Vertebral canal with cauda equina
18 Intervertebral disc
19 Body of fifth lumbar vertebra ($L_5$)
20 Sacral promontory
21 Mesosigmoid
22 Sigmoid colon
23 Recto-uterine pouch
   (of Douglas)
24 Ampulla of rectum
25 Posterior fornix of vagina
26 Cervix of uterus
27 External anal sphincter muscle
28 Anal canal
29 Vagina
30 Internal anal sphincter muscle
31 Anus
32 Hymen
33 Abdominal aorta
34 Discus intervertebralis, promontory
35 Sacrum
36 Rectum

**Female urogenital system** (midsagittal section through the pelvic cavity). The urinary bladder is empty; the position and shape of the uterus are normal.

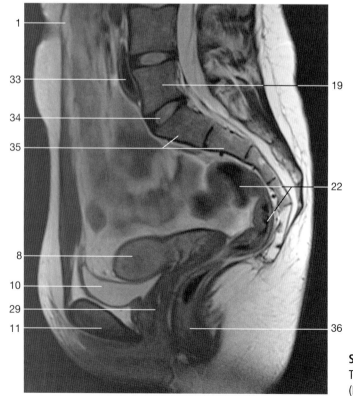

**Sagittal section through the pelvic cavity of a young female.**
The uterus reveals an extreme anteflexion (MRI scan).
(Prof. Uder, Dept. of Radiology, Univ. Erlangen-Nuremberg, Germany.)

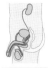

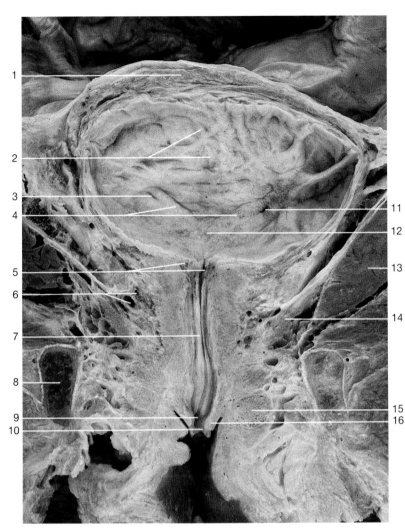

**Coronal section through the urinary bladder and urethra in the female** (anterior aspect).

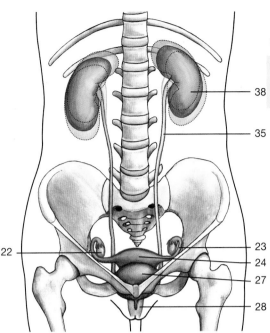

**Position of kidneys, urinary, and genital organs in the female** (anterior aspect). The excursions of the kidneys are indicated.

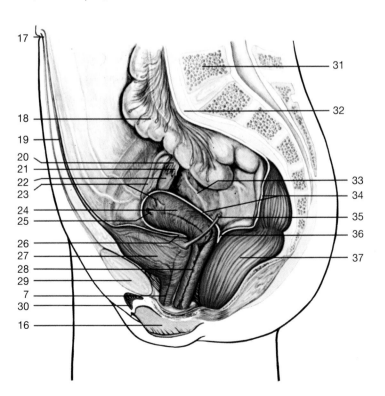

**Position of female genital organs** (medial aspect).

1   Muscular coat of urinary bladder
2   Folds of mucous membrane of urinary bladder
3   Right ureteric orifice
4   Interureteric fold
5   Internal urethral orifice
6   Vesico-uterine venous plexus
7   Urethra
8   Pubis (cut edge)
9   External urethral orifice
10  Vestibule of vagina
11  Left ureteric orifice
12  Trigone of bladder
13  Obturator internus muscle
14  Levator ani muscle
15  Bulb of vestibule
16  Left labium minus
17  Umbilicus
18  Sigmoid colon
19  Median umbilical fold with urachus
20  Infundibulum of uterine tube
21  Fimbriae of uterine tube
22  Ovary
23  Uterine tube (isthmus)
24  Uterus
25  Round ligament of uterus
26  Vesico-uterine pouch
27  Urinary bladder
28  Vagina
29  Pubic symphysis
30  Clitoris
31  Body of fifth lumbar vertebra (L$_5$)
32  Sacral promontory
33  Right ureter
34  Peritoneum (cut edge)
35  Left ureter
36  Recto-uterine pouch (of Douglas)
37  Rectal ampulla
38  Kidney

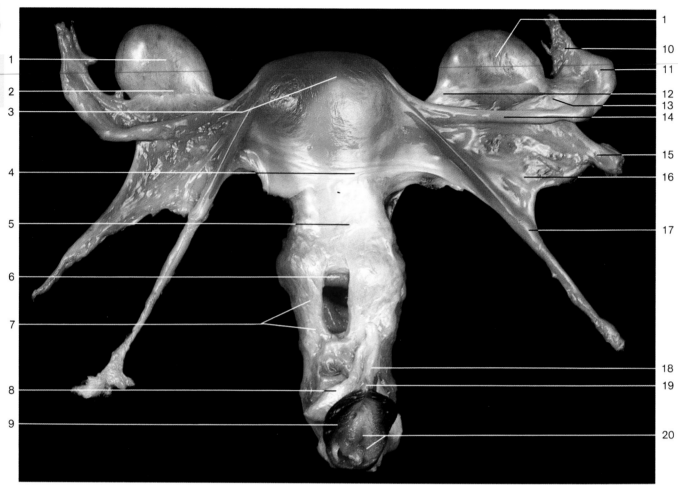

**Female genital organs, isolated** (anterior aspect). The anterior wall of the vagina has been opened to display the vaginal portion of the cervix.

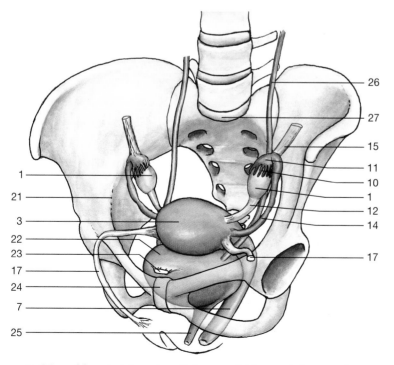

**Position of female internal genital organs** (oblique-anterior aspect).

1   Ovary
2   Mesovarium
3   Fundus of uterus
4   Vesico-uterine pouch
5   Cervix of uterus
6   Vaginal portion of cervix
7   Vagina
8   Crus of clitoris
9   Labium minus
10  Fimbriae of uterine tube
11  Infundibulum of uterine tube
12  Ligament of the ovary
13  Mesosalpinx
14  Uterine tube
15  Suspensory ligament of ovary
    (caudally displaced)
16  Broad ligament of uterus
17  Round ligament of uterus
18  Corpus cavernosum of clitoris
19  Glans of clitoris
20  Hymen and vaginal orifice
21  Linea terminalis
22  Urinary bladder
23  Medial umbilical ligament
24  Pubic symphysis
25  Urethra
26  Ureter
27  Promontory

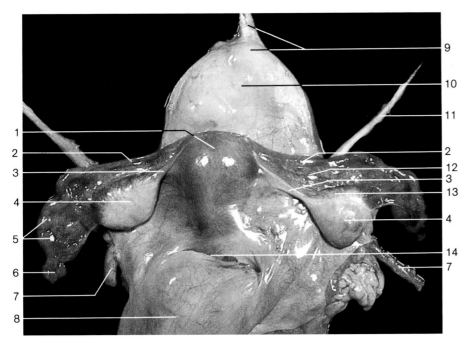

1   Fundus of uterus
2   Uterine tube
3   Ligament of the ovary
4   Ovary
5   Infundibulum of uterine tube
6   Fimbriae of uterine tube
7   Ureter
8   Rectum
9   Apex of urinary bladder and
    median umbilical ligament
10  Urinary bladder (fenestrated
    in the dissection in the middle)
11  Round ligament of uterus
12  Mesosalpinx
13  Mesovarium
14  Recto-uterine pouch (of Douglas)
15  Vesico-uterine pouch
16  Body of uterus
17  Cervix of uterus
18  Vaginal portion of cervix of uterus
19  Vagina
20  Mucous membrane
    of uterus congestion
21  Anterior fornix of vagina

**Female genital organs, isolated** (supero-posterior aspect).

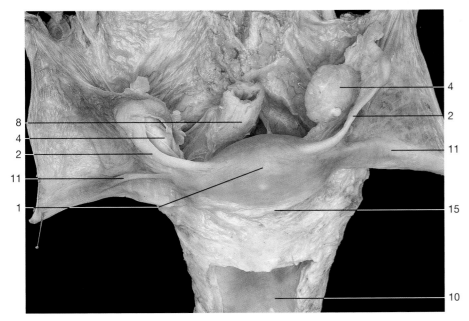

**Uterus and related organs, isolated** (superior aspect). The left ovary is enlarged.

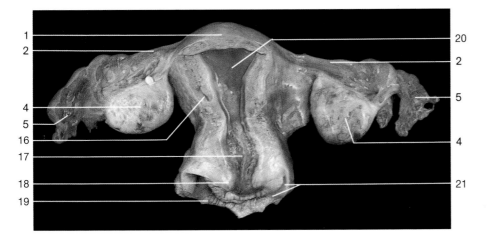

**Uterus and related organs, isolated** (posterior aspect). The posterior wall of the uterus
has been opened.

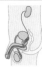

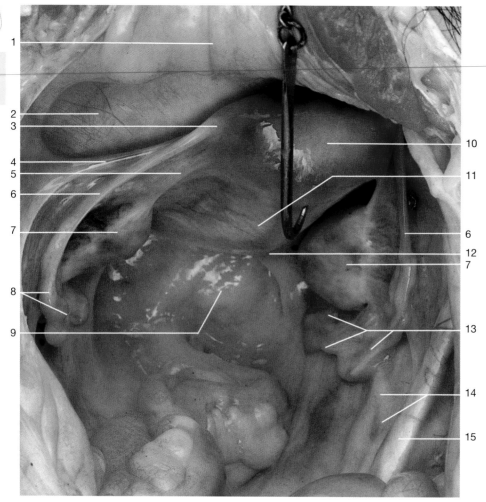

**Female internal genital organs.** View of the pelvic cavity (superior aspect). The uterus has been reflected to the right.

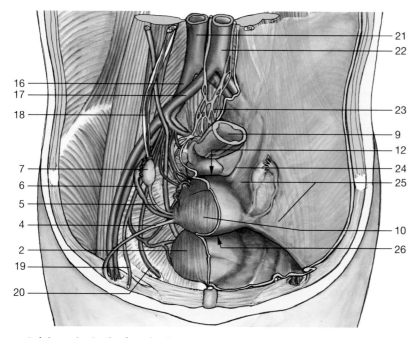

**Pelvic cavity in the female showing uterus and related organs** (antero-superior aspect). The peritoneal cover removed on the right side. Arrows: vesico-uterine and recto-uterine pouches.

1 Median umbilical fold with urachus
2 Urinary bladder
3 Insertion of uterine tube at fundus of uterus
4 Round ligament of uterus
5 Ligament of ovary
6 Uterine tube (isthmus)
7 Ovary
8 Ampulla of uterine tube
9 Rectum
10 Uterus
11 Vagina
12 Recto-uterine pouch (of Douglas)
13 Fimbriae of uterine tube
14 Suspensory ligament of ovary
15 Right common iliac artery (covered by peritoneum)
16 Common iliac vein
17 Common iliac artery
18 Ovarian artery and vein
19 Umbilical fold
20 Obturator artery
21 Inferior vena cava
22 Abdominal aorta
23 Superior hypogastric plexus
24 Recto-uterine fold
25 Broad ligament of uterus
26 Vesico-uterine pouch

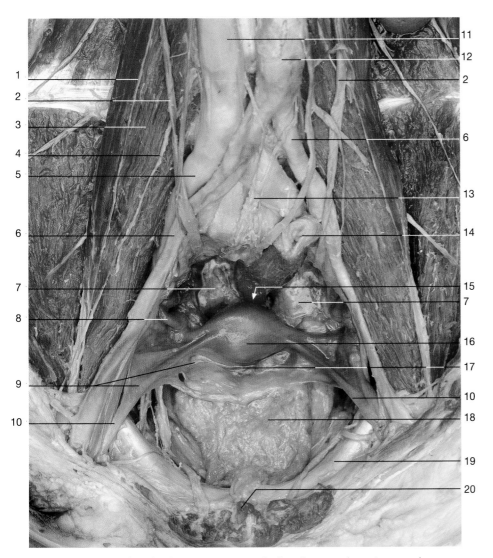

1 Ilio-inguinal nerve
2 Ureter
3 Psoas major muscle
4 Genitofemoral nerve
5 Common iliac vein
6 Common iliac artery
7 Ovary
8 Uterine tube
9 Peritoneum
10 Round ligament of uterus
11 Inferior vena cava
12 Abdominal aorta
13 Superior hypogastric plexus
14 Rectum
15 Recto-uterine pouch (of Douglas)
16 Uterus
17 Vesico-uterine pouch
18 Urinary bladder
19 Iliac crest
20 Pubic symphysis
21 Rectal ampulla
22 Obturator internus muscle
23 Promontorium
24 Sigmoid colon
25 Head of femur
26 Urethra
27 Vagina
28 Labium minus

**Pelvic cavity in the female showing uterus and related organs** (superior aspect).
The peritoneum has been mostly removed.

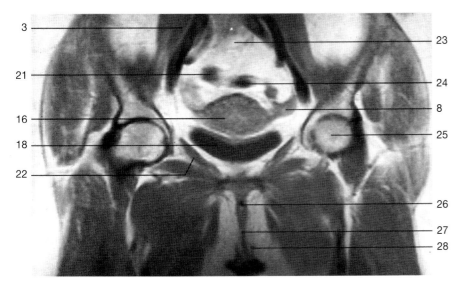

**Horizontal section through the pelvic cavity in the female** (MRI scan).
(Prof. Uder, Dept. of Radiology, Univ. Erlangen-Nuremberg, Germany.)

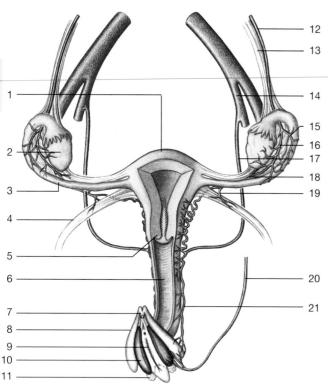

**Arteries of female genital organs.**

**Main drainage routes of lymph vessels of uterus and related organs** (indicated by arrows).

| | | | |
|---|---|---|---|
| 1 Uterus | 10 Bulb of vestibule | 19 Artery of round ligament | 28 Internal iliac lymph nodes |
| 2 Ovary | 11 Greater vestibular gland | 20 Internal pudendal artery | 29 Superior gluteal artery |
| 3 Uterine tube | 12 Ovarian artery | 21 Vaginal artery | 30 Obturator artery |
| 4 Round ligament of uterus | 13 Suspensory ligament of ovary | 22 Lumbar lymph nodes | 31 Inferior gluteal artery |
| 5 Vaginal portion of cervix of uterus | 14 Internal iliac artery | 23 External iliac lymph nodes | 32 Middle sacral artery |
| 6 Vagina | 15 Tubal branch of ovarian artery | 24 Inguinal lymph nodes | 33 Femoral artery |
| 7 Clitoris | 16 Ovarian branch of ovarian artery | 25 Abdominal aorta | 34 Vessels of labium majus |
| 8 Corpus cavernosum of clitoris | 17 Uterine artery | 26 External iliac artery | 35 Femur |
| 9 Vaginal orifice | 18 Ovarian branch of uterine artery | 27 Sacral lymph nodes | |

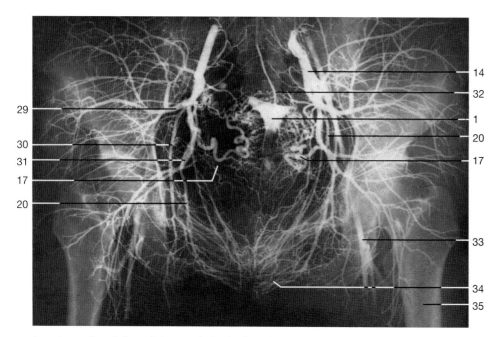

**Arteriography of the pelvic vessels in the female** (a.-p. direction).

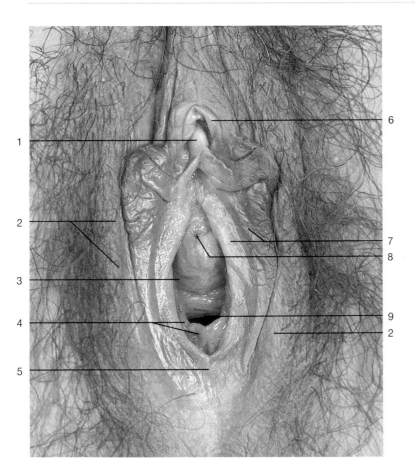

1  Glans of clitoris
2  Labium majus
3  Vestibule of vagina
4  Hymen
5  Posterior labial commissure
6  Prepuce of clitoris
7  Labium minus
8  External urethral orifice
9  Vaginal orifice
10 Body of clitoris
11 Crus of clitoris
12 Bulb of vestibule with bulbospongiosus muscle
13 Frenulum of clitoris
14 Greater vestibular gland
15 Ureter
16 Adnexa of uterus
17 Cavernous body of clitoris
18 Anus and internal anal sphincter
19 Urachus
20 Urinary bladder
21 Infundibulum of uterine tube
22 Ovary
23 Uterine tube
24 Suspensory ligament of ovary
25 Perineal body
26 External anal sphincter

**Female external genital organs in situ** (anterior aspect). Labia reflected.

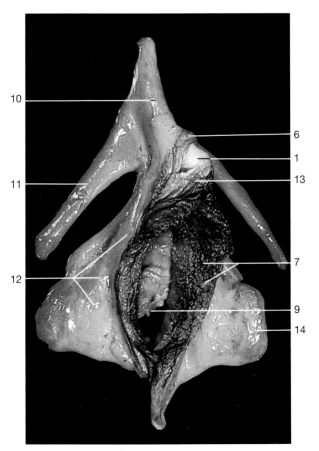

**Cavernous tissue of female external genital organs,** isolated (anterior aspect).

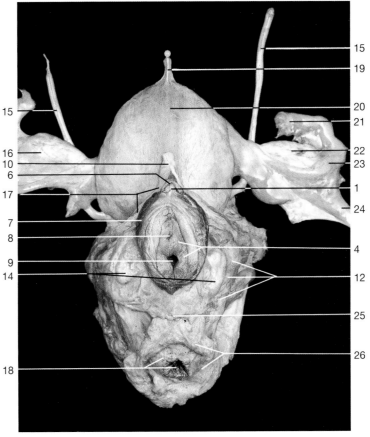

**Female external genital organs** in relation to internal genital organs and urinary system, isolated (anterior aspect).

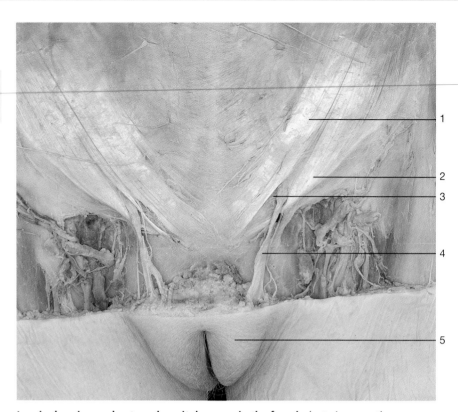

1   Medial crus of superficial inguinal ring
2   Lateral crus of superficial inguinal ring
3   Superficial inguinal ring
4   Round ligament of uterus
5   Outer labia (labium majus)
6   Rectus abdominis muscle and
    inferior epigastric artery
7   Deep inguinal ring with ilio-inguinal nerve
8   Inguinal ligament
9   Femoral nerve
10  Femoral artery

**Inguinal region and external genital organs in the female** (anterior aspect).
Dissection of the inguinal canal and round ligament of uterus of a child.

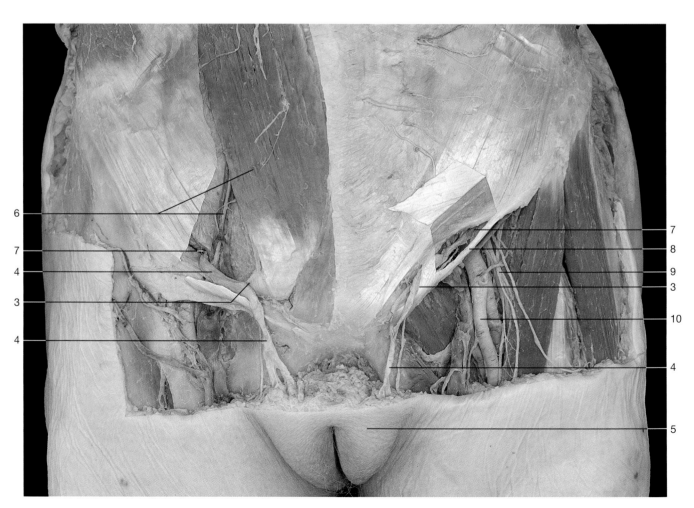

**Inguinal region and external genital organs in the female** (anterior aspect). The inguinal canal has been opened. The round ligament of uterus and the ilio-inguinal nerve have been dissected.

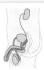

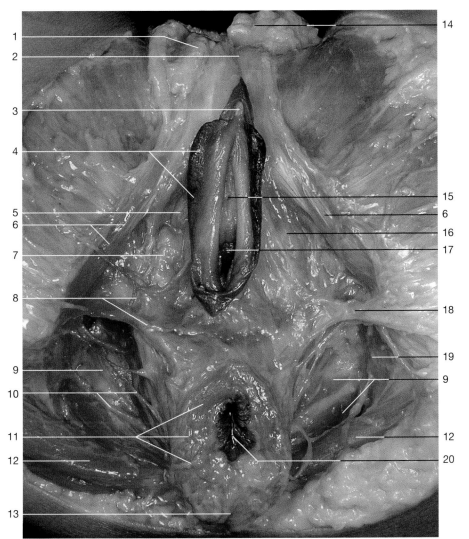

1    Fatty tissue
      encasing round ligament of uterus
2    Position of pubic symphysis
3    Clitoris
4    Labium minus
5    Bulb of vestibule
6    Ischiocavernosus muscle
7    Greater vestibular gland
8    Perineal branches of pudendal nerve
9    Levator ani muscle
10   Inferior rectal nerves
11   External anal sphincter muscle
12   Gluteus maximus muscle
13   Coccyx
14   Fatty tissue of mons pubis
15   External orifice of urethra
16   Urogenital diaphragm with fascia
      of deep transverse perineal muscle
17   Vaginal orifice
18   Superficial transverse perineal muscle
19   Obturator internus muscle
20   Anus
21   Suspensory ligament of clitoris
22   Glans of clitoris
23   Crus of clitoris
24   Perineal body
25   Prepuce of clitoris
26   Frenulum of clitoris
27   Posterior commissure of labia

**External genital organs and urogenital diaphragm in the female,** superficial layer
(inferior aspect).

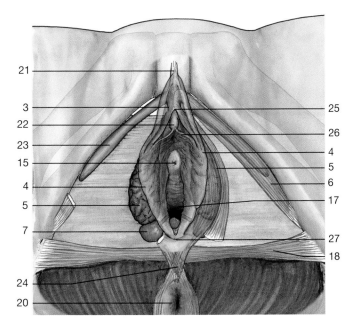

**External genital organs with cavernous tissue in the female**
(inferior aspect). Blue = cavernous tissue of clitoris and bulb of vestibule.

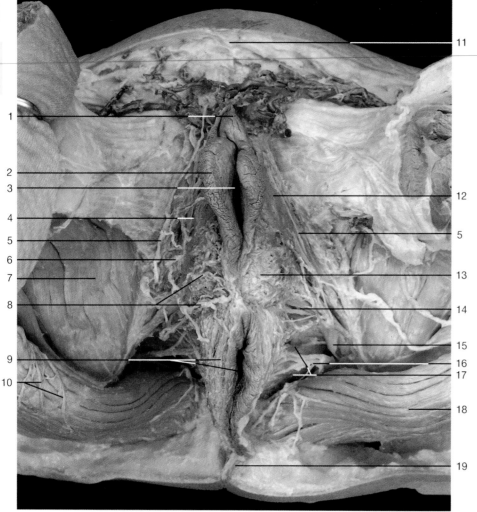

1   Prepuce of clitoris
2   Labium minus
3   Vaginal orifice
4   Deep transverse perineal muscle
5   Dorsal nerve of clitoris
6   Posterior labial nerves
7   Great adductor muscle
8   Perineal branch of pudendal nerve
9   Anus and
    external anal sphincter muscle
10  Inferior cluneal nerves
11  Mons pubis
12  Crus of clitoris
    with ischiocavernosus muscle
13  Bulb of vestibule
14  Superficial transverse perineal muscle
15  Pudendal nerve and
    internal pudendal artery
16  Inferior rectal nerves
17  Levator ani muscle
18  Gluteus maximus muscle
19  Anococcygeal ligament
20  External urethral orifice

**External genital organs and urogenital diaphragm in the female,** superficial layer (inferior aspect). On the right side the bulb of vestibule has been removed.

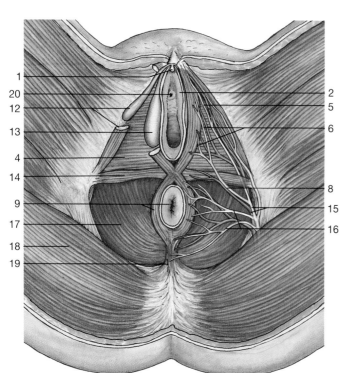

**Urogenital and pelvic diaphragms in the female** (inferior aspect). Muscles, nerves, and arteries have been displayed. The bulb of vestibule has been partly removed.

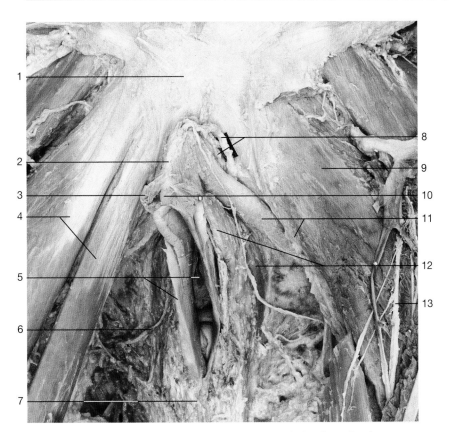

1   Position of pubic symphysis
2   Body of clitoris
3   Prepuce of clitoris
4   Adductor longus and gracilis muscles
5   External orifice of vagina and
    labium minus
6   Posterior labial nerve
7   Perineal body
8   Deep artery of clitoris and
    dorsal nerve of clitoris
9   Adductor brevis muscle
10  Glans of clitoris
11  Crus of clitoris and
    ischiocavernosus muscle
12  Bulb of vestibule and
    bulbospongiosus muscle
13  Anterior branch of obturator nerve

**External genital organs in the female** (anterior aspect). The clitoris has been dissected and slightly reflected to the right. The prepuce of clitoris has been divided to display the glans.

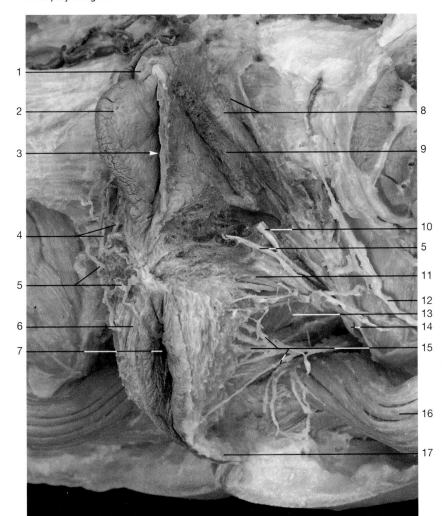

1   Clitoris
2   Labium minus
3   Vaginal orifice
4   Posterior labial nerves
5   Perineal branches of pudendal nerve
6   External anal sphincter muscle
7   Anus
8   Crus of clitoris and ischiocavernosus muscle
9   Bulb of vestibule
10  Dorsal artery of clitoris
11  Superficial transverse perineal muscle
12  Perineal branch
    of posterior femoral cutaneous nerve
13  Levator ani muscle
14  Internal pudendal artery
15  Inferior rectal nerves
16  Gluteus maximus muscle
17  Anococcygeal ligament

**External genital organs and urogenital diaphragm in the female** (latero-inferior aspect). The bulb of vestibule has been partly removed. The left labium minus was cut away.

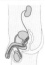

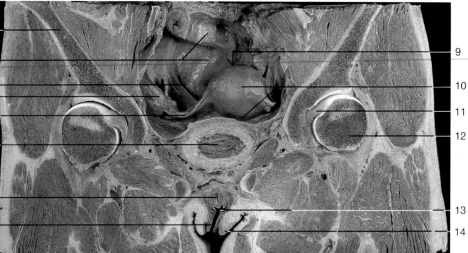

1 Ilium
2 Rectum
3 Recto-uterine fold
4 Ovary
5 Uterine tube
6 Urinary bladder
7 Urethra
8 Labium minus
9 Recto-uterine pouch
10 Uterus and
   vesico-uterine pouch
11 Ligament
   of the head of femur
12 Head of femur
13 Vestibule of vagina
14 Labium majus
15 Pyramidalis muscle
16 Femoral nerve
17 Femoral artery and vein
18 Small intestine
19 Broad ligament of uterus

**Coronal section through the pelvic cavity of the female** at the level of the hip joints.

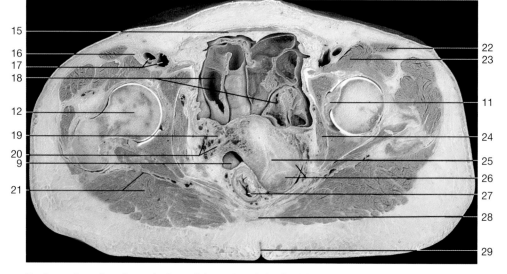

**Horizontal section through the pelvic cavity of the female** at the level of the uterus (inferior aspect). The uterus is retroverted to the left.

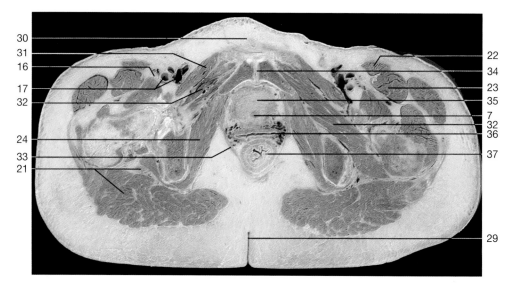

**Horizontal section through the pelvic cavity of the female** at the level of the urethral sphincter muscle and vagina (inferior aspect).

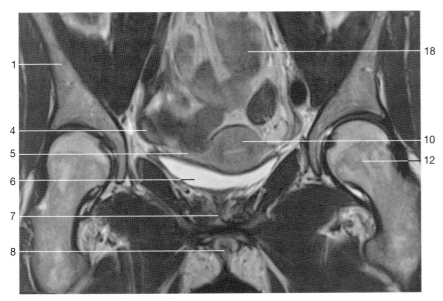

20 Uterine venous plexus
21 Sciatic nerve and
   gluteus maximus muscle
22 Sartorius muscle
23 Iliopsoas muscle
24 Obturator internus muscle
25 Endometrium
26 Myometrium
27 Rectal ampulla
28 Coccyx
29 Anal cleft
30 Mons pubis
31 Pectineus muscle
32 Obturator externus muscle
33 Levator ani muscle
34 Pubic symphysis
35 Urethral sphincter muscle
   (base of urinary bladder)
36 Vagina
37 Rectum (anal canal)

**Coronal section through the pelvic cavity of the female** at the level of the hip joints (MRI scan). (Prof. Uder, Dept. of Radiology, Univ. Erlangen-Nuremberg, Germany.)

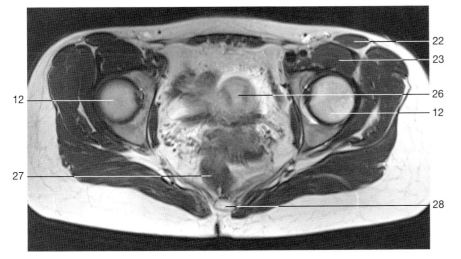

**Horizontal section through the pelvic cavity of the female** at the level of the uterus (MRI scan). (Prof. Uder, Dept. of Radiology, Univ. Erlangen-Nuremberg, Germany.)

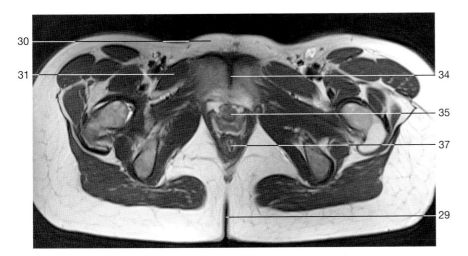

**Horizontal section through the pelvic cavity of the female** at the level of urethral sphincter muscle and vagina (MRI scan). (Prof. Uder, Dept. of Radiology, Univ. Erlangen-Nuremberg, Germany.)

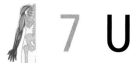

# 7 Upper Limb

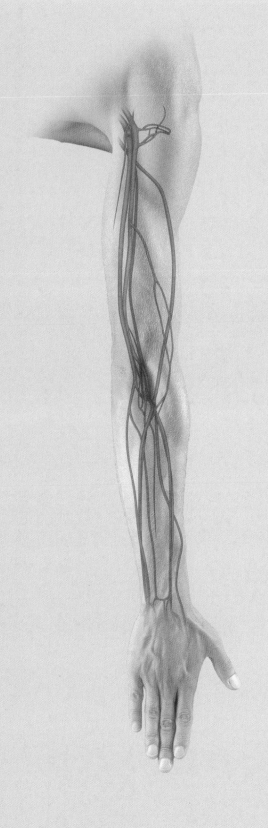

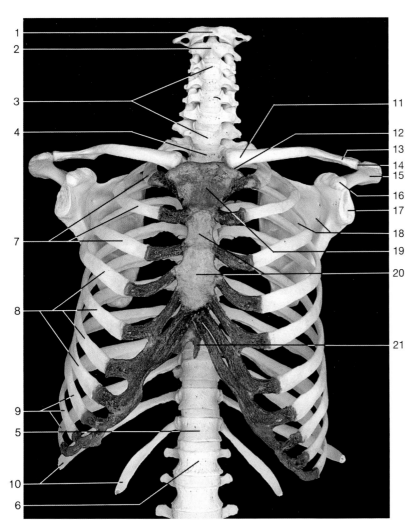

**Vertebral column**
1   Atlas (C$_1$)
2   Axis (C$_2$)
3   Third to seventh cervical vertebrae (C$_3$–C$_7$)
4   First thoracic vertebra (Th$_1$)
5   Twelfth thoracic vertebra (Th$_{12}$)
6   First lumbar vertebra (L$_1$)

**Ribs**
7   First to third ribs        } True ribs
8   Fourth to seventh ribs
9   Eighth to tenth ribs       } False ribs
10  Eleventh and twelfth ribs
    (floating ribs)

**Clavicle (A)**
11  Sternal end
12  Sternoclavicular joint
13  Acromial end
14  Acromioclavicular joint

**Scapula (B)**
15  Acromion
16  Coracoid process
17  Glenoid cavity
18  Costal surface

**Sternum (C)**
19  Manubrium
20  Body
21  Xiphoid process

**Skeleton of shoulder girdle and thorax** (anterior aspect).
The cartilaginous parts of the ribs appear dark brown.

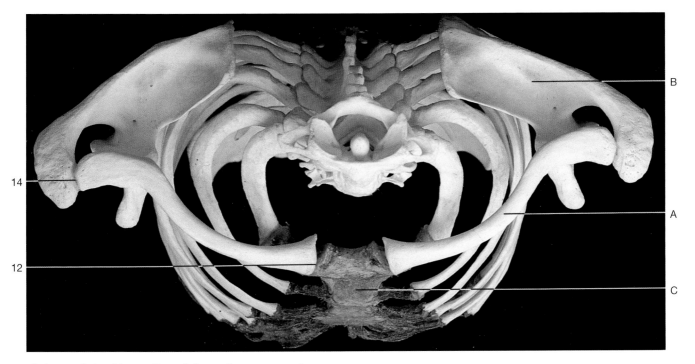

**Skeleton of shoulder girdle and thorax** (superior aspect).

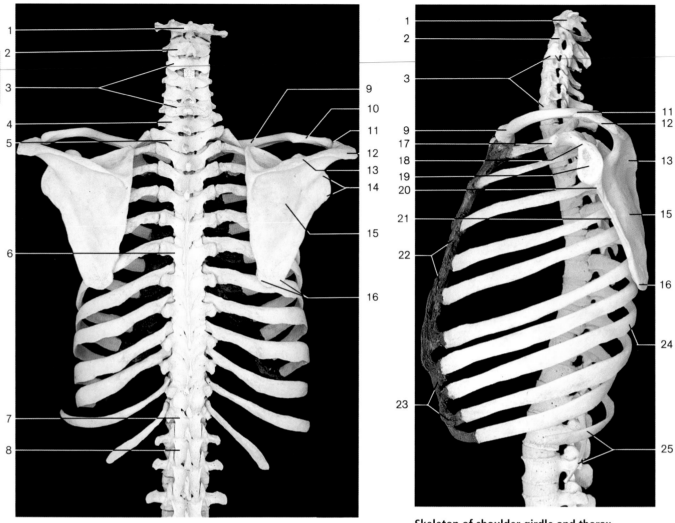

**Skeleton of shoulder girdle and thorax** (posterior aspect).

**Skeleton of shoulder girdle and thorax** (lateral aspect).

**Vertebral column**
1   Atlas
2   Axis
3   Third to sixth cervical vertebrae
4   Seventh vertebra (vertebra prominens)
5   First thoracic vertebra
6   Sixth thoracic vertebra
7   Twelfth thoracic vertebra
8   First lumbar vertebra

**Clavicle**
9   Sternal end
10  Acromial end
11  Acromioclavicular joint

**Scapula**
12  Acromion
13  Spine of scapula
14  Lateral angle
15  Posterior surface
16  Inferior angle
17  Coracoid process
18  Supraglenoid tubercle
19  Glenoid cavity
20  Infraglenoid tubercle
21  Lateral margin

**Thorax**
22  Body of sternum
23  Subcostal angle
24  Angle of rib
25  Floating ribs

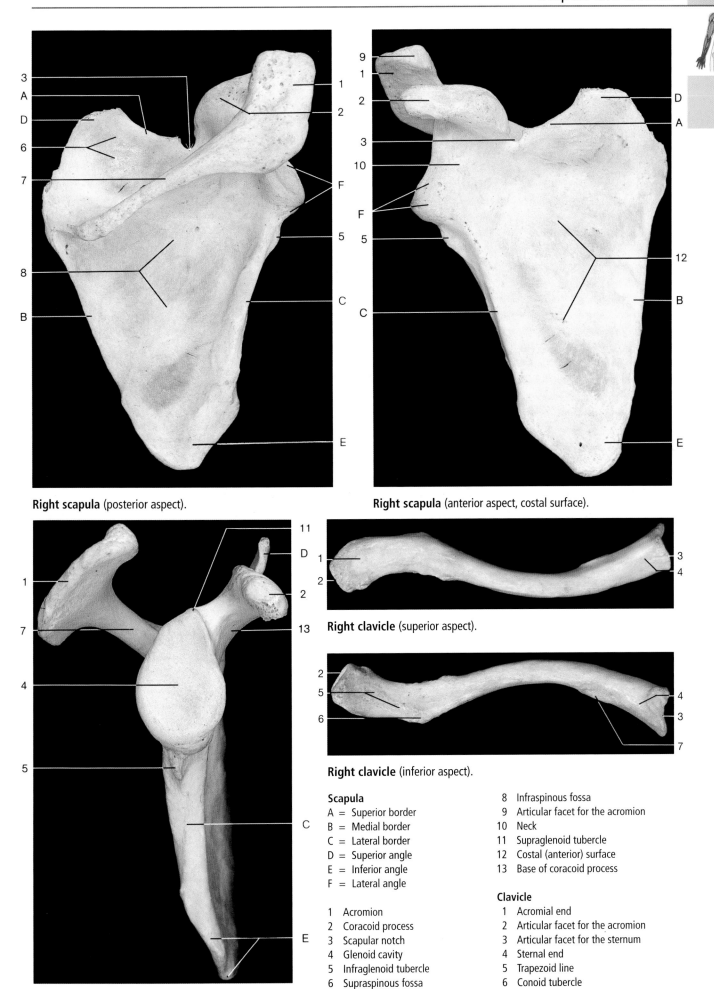

**Right scapula** (posterior aspect).

**Right scapula** (anterior aspect, costal surface).

**Right scapula** (lateral aspect).

**Right clavicle** (superior aspect).

**Right clavicle** (inferior aspect).

**Scapula**
A = Superior border
B = Medial border
C = Lateral border
D = Superior angle
E = Inferior angle
F = Lateral angle

1  Acromion
2  Coracoid process
3  Scapular notch
4  Glenoid cavity
5  Infraglenoid tubercle
6  Supraspinous fossa
7  Spine
8  Infraspinous fossa
9  Articular facet for the acromion
10  Neck
11  Supraglenoid tubercle
12  Costal (anterior) surface
13  Base of coracoid process

**Clavicle**
1  Acromial end
2  Articular facet for the acromion
3  Articular facet for the sternum
4  Sternal end
5  Trapezoid line
6  Conoid tubercle
7  Impression of costoclavicular ligament

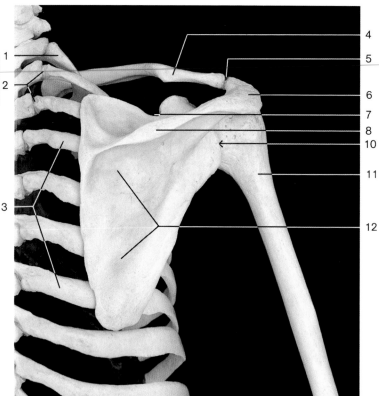

| | |
|---|---|
| 1 | First rib |
| 2 | Position of costotransverse joints |
| 3 | Fourth to seventh ribs |
| 4 | Clavicle |
| 5 | Position of acromioclavicular joint |
| 6 | Acromion |
| 7 | Scapular notch |
| 8 | Spine of scapula |
| 9 | Head of humerus |
| 10 | Glenoid cavity |
| 11 | Surgical neck of humerus |
| 12 | Posterior surface of scapula |
| 13 | Coracoid process |
| 14 | Infraglenoid tubercle |
| 15 | Greater tubercle of humerus |
| 16 | Anatomical neck of humerus |

**Bones of shoulder joint** (posterior aspect).

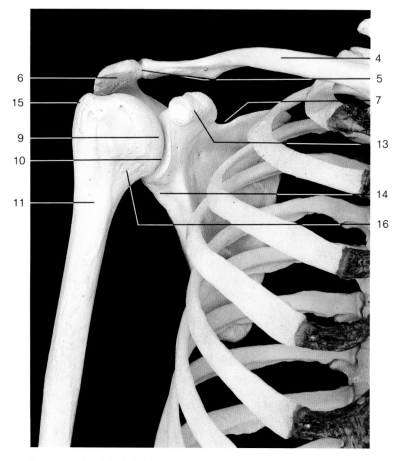

**Bones of shoulder joint** (anterior aspect).

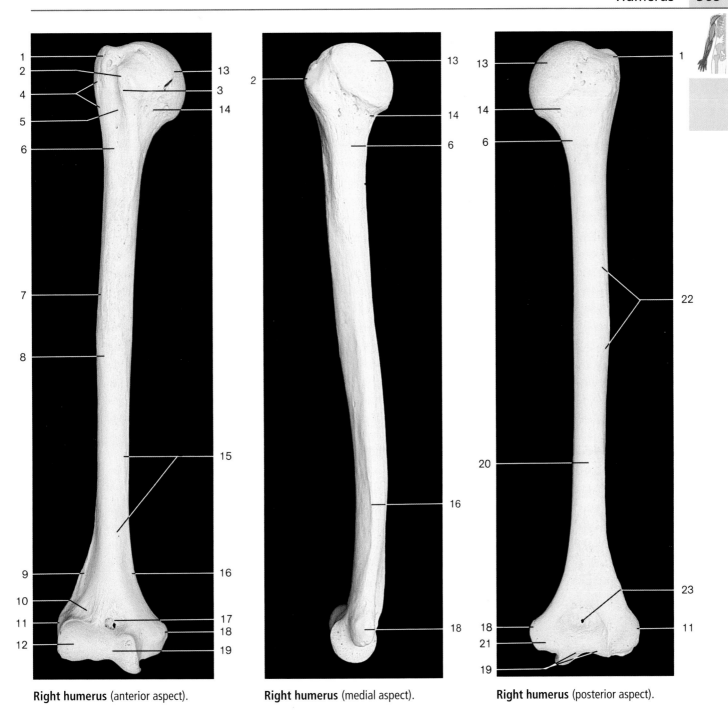

**Right humerus** (anterior aspect).

**Right humerus** (medial aspect).

**Right humerus** (posterior aspect).

**Humerus**

| | | | | | | |
|---|---|---|---|---|---|---|
| 1 | Greater tubercle | 7 | Deltoid tuberosity | 13 | Head | 19 | Trochlea |
| 2 | Lesser tubercle | 8 | Antero-lateral surface | 14 | Anatomical neck | 20 | Posterior surface |
| 3 | Crest of lesser tubercle | 9 | Lateral supracondylar ridge | 15 | Antero-medial surface | 21 | Groove for ulnar nerve |
| 4 | Crest of greater tubercle | 10 | Radial fossa | 16 | Medial supracondylar ridge | 22 | Groove for radial nerve |
| 5 | Intertubercular sulcus | 11 | Lateral epicondyle | 17 | Coronoid fossa | 23 | Olecranon fossa |
| 6 | Surgical neck | 12 | Capitulum | 18 | Medial epicondyle | | |

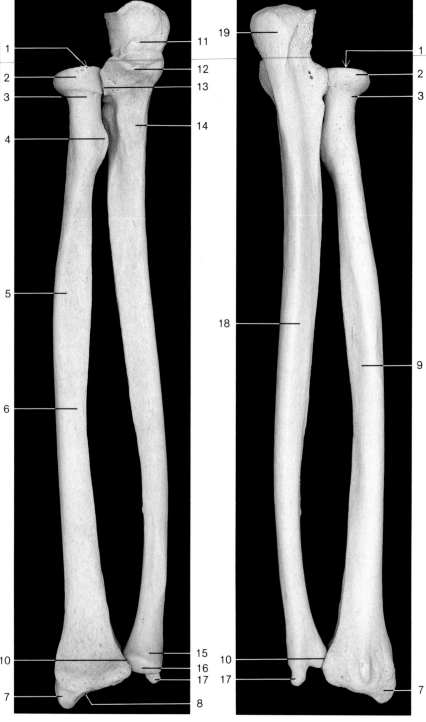

**Radius**
1   Head
2   Articular circumference
3   Neck
4   Radial tuberosity
5   Shaft
6   Anterior surface
7   Styloid process
8   Articular surface
9   Posterior surface
10   Ulnar notch

**Ulna**
11   Trochlear notch
12   Coronoid process
13   Radial notch
14   Ulnar tuberosity
15   Head
16   Articular circumference
17   Styloid process
18   Posterior surface
19   Olecranon

**Bones of right forearm, radius, and ulna** (anterior aspect).

**Bones of right forearm, radius, and ulna** (posterior aspect).

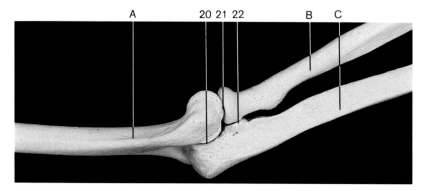

**Articulations at the right elbow**
20   Site of humero-ulnar joint
21   Site of humeroradial joint
22   Site of proximal radio-ulnar joint

A = Humerus
B = Radius
C = Ulna

**Bones of the right elbow joint** (lateral aspect).

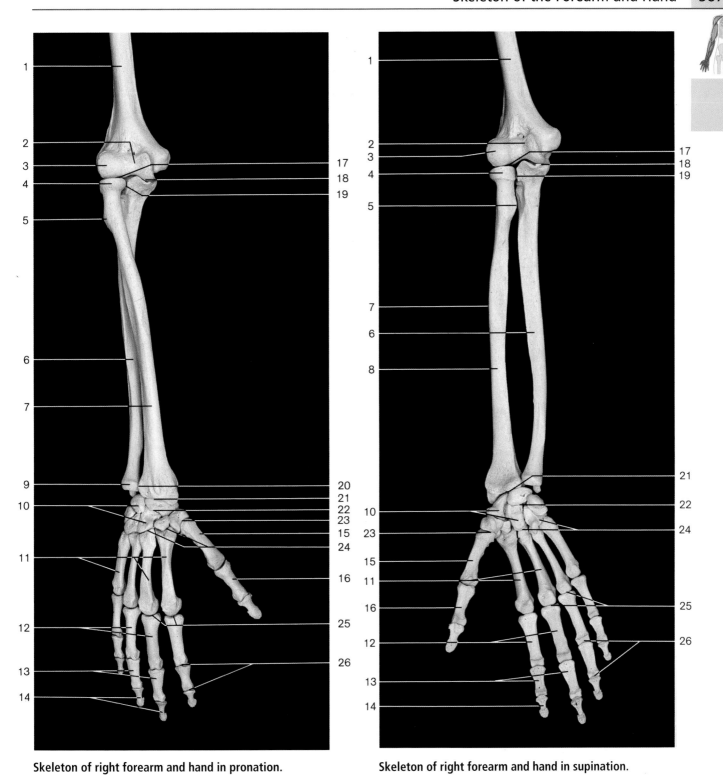

**Skeleton of right forearm and hand in pronation.**

**Skeleton of right forearm and hand in supination.**

| | | | |
|---|---|---|---|
| 1 | Humerus | 9 | Articular circumference of ulna |
| 2 | Trochlea of humerus | 10 | Carpal bones |
| 3 | Capitulum of humerus | 11 | Metacarpal bones |
| 4 | Articular circumference of radius | 12 | Proximal phalanges |
| 5 | Radial tuberosity | 13 | Middle phalanges |
| 6 | Anterior surface of ulna | 14 | Distal phalanges |
| 7 | Posterior surface of radius | 15 | Metacarpal bone of thumb |
| 8 | Anterior surface of radius | 16 | Proximal phalanx of thumb |

**Sites of joints**

17 Humeroradial joint
18 Humero-ulnar joint
19 Proximal radio-ulnar joint
20 Distal radio-ulnar joint
21 Wrist joint
22 Midcarpal joint
23 Carpometacarpal joint of thumb
24 Carpometacarpal joints
25 Metacarpophalangeal joints
26 Interphalangeal joints of the hand

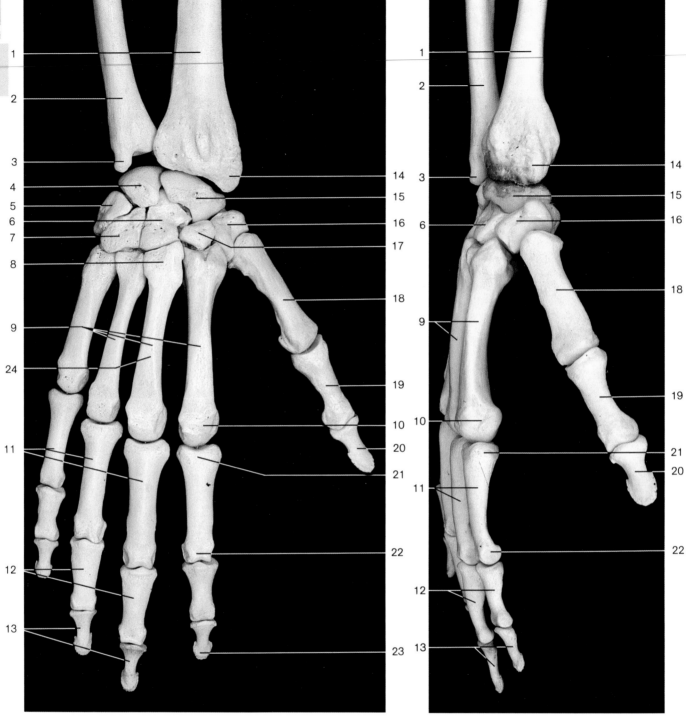

**Skeleton of right wrist and hand** (dorsal aspect).

**Skeleton of right wrist and hand** (medial aspect).

| | | | |
|---|---|---|---|
| 1 | Radius | 8 | Base of third metacarpal bone |
| 2 | Ulna | 9 | Metacarpal bones |
| 3 | Styloid process of ulna | 10 | Head of metacarpal bone |
| 4 | Lunate bone ⎤ | 11 | Proximal phalanges of the hand |
| 5 | Triquetral bone ⎟ Carpal bones | 12 | Middle phalanges of the hand |
| 6 | Capitate bone ⎟ | 13 | Distal phalanges of the hand |
| 7 | Hamate bone ⎦ | 14 | Styloid process of radius |

| | | | |
|---|---|---|---|
| 15 | Scaphoid bone ⎤ | 22 | Head of second |
| 16 | Trapezium bone ⎟ Carpal bones | | proximal phalanx |
| 17 | Trapezoid bone ⎦ | 23 | Tuberosity |
| 18 | Metacarpal bone of thumb | | of distal phalanx |
| 19 | Proximal phalanx of thumb | 24 | Body of third |
| 20 | Distal phalanx of thumb | | metacarpal bone |
| 21 | Base of second proximal phalanx | | |

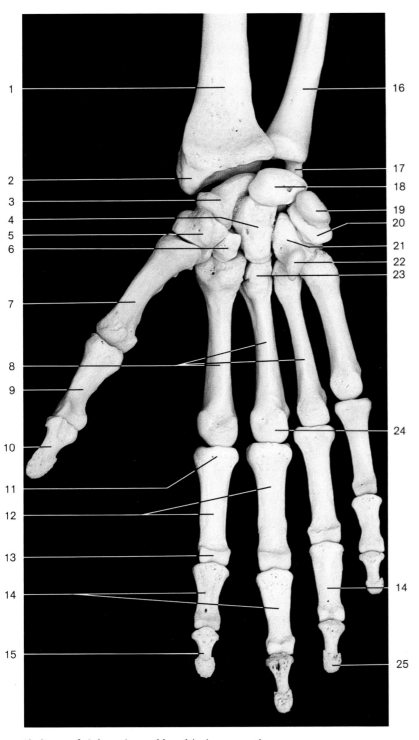

1   Radius
2   Styloid process of radius
3   Scaphoid bone ⎤
4   Capitate bone ⎥
5   Trapezium      ⎬ Carpal bones
6   Trapezoid bone ⎦
7   First metacarpal bone
8   Second to fourth metacarpal bones
9   Proximal phalanx of thumb
10  Distal phalanx of thumb
11  Base of second proximal phalanx
12  Proximal phalanges
13  Head of second proximal phalanx
14  Middle phalanges
15  Distal phalanx
16  Ulna
17  Styloid process of ulna
18  Lunate bone      ⎤
19  Pisiform bone    ⎥
20  Triquetral bone  ⎬ Carpal bones
21  Hamate bone      ⎦
22  Hamulus or hook
    of hamate bone
23  Base of third metacarpal bone
24  Head of metacarpal bone
25  Tuberosity of distal phalanx

**Skeleton of right wrist and hand** (palmar aspect).

The human hand is one of the most admirable structures of the human body. The carpometacarpal joint of the thumb, a saddle joint, enjoys wide mobility so that the thumb can come into contact with all other fingers, thus enabling the hand to become an instrument for grasping and psychologic expression. During evolution, these newly developed functions appeared after the erect posture of the human body was achieved. An inevitable prerequisite for the development of human cultures is not only the differentiation of the brain but also the development of an organ capable of realizing its ideas: the human hand.

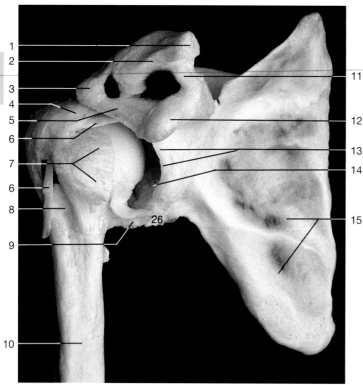

**Right shoulder joint.** The anterior part of the articular capsule has been removed and the head of the humerus has been slightly rotated outward to show the cavity of the joint.

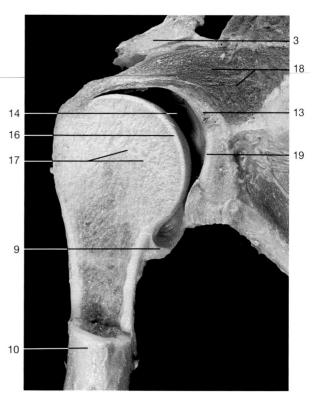

**Coronal section through the right shoulder joint** (anterior aspect).

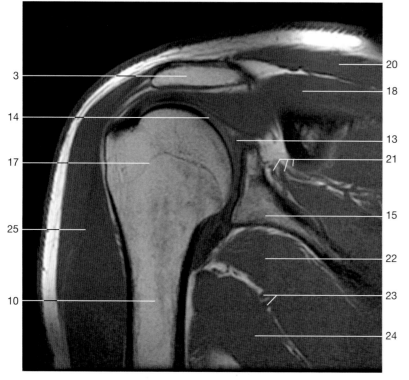

**Coronal section through the right shoulder joint** (MRI scan). (Courtesy of Prof. Heuck, Munich, Germany.)

1  Acromial end of clavicle
2  Acromioclavicular joint
3  Acromion
4  Tendon of supraspinatus muscle (attached to the articular capsule)
5  Coraco-acromial ligament
6  Tendon of long head of biceps brachii muscle
7  Tendon of subscapularis muscle (attached to the articular capsule)
8  Intertubercular sulcus
9  Articular capsule of shoulder joint
10  Humerus
11  Trapezoid ligament
12  Coracoid process
13  Glenoid labrum
14  Shoulder joint (joint cavity)
15  Scapula
16  Head of humerus
17  Epiphysial line
18  Supraspinatus muscle
19  Glenoid cavity
20  Trapezius muscle
21  Suprascapular artery, vein, and nerve
22  Teres major muscle
23  Circumflexa scapular artery and vein
24  Latissimus dorsi muscle
25  Deltoid muscle
26  Tendon of long head of triceps brachii muscle

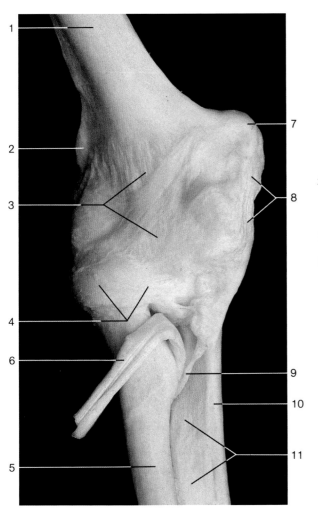

**Ligaments of the elbow joint** (anterior aspect).

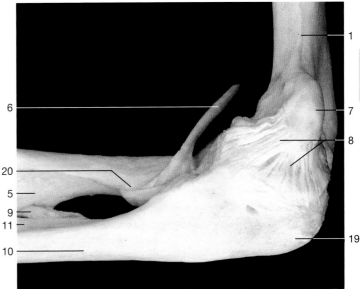

**Ligaments of the elbow joint** (medial aspect).

| | | | |
|---|---|---|---|
| 1 | Humerus | 11 | Interosseous membrane |
| 2 | Lateral epicondyle of humerus | 12 | Radial fossa |
| 3 | Articular capsule | 13 | Capitulum of humerus |
| 4 | Anular ligament | 14 | Head of radius |
| | of proximal radio-ulnar joint | 15 | Radial collateral ligament |
| 5 | Radius | 16 | Coronoid fossa |
| 6 | Tendon of biceps brachii muscle | 17 | Trochlea of humerus |
| 7 | Medial epicondyle of humerus | 18 | Coronoid process of ulna |
| 8 | Ulnar collateral ligament | 19 | Olecranon |
| 9 | Oblique chord | 20 | Radial tuberosity |
| 10 | Ulna | | |

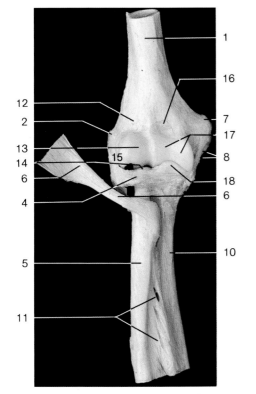

**Elbow joint with ligaments** (anterior aspect). Articular capsule has been removed to show the anular ligament.

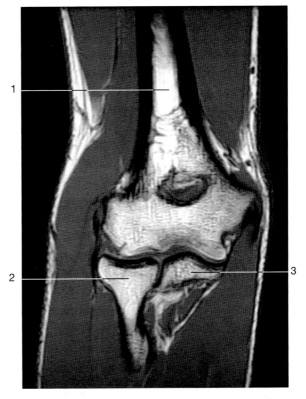

**Coronal section through the elbow joint** (MRI scan). (Courtesy of Prof. Heuck, Munich, Germany.)

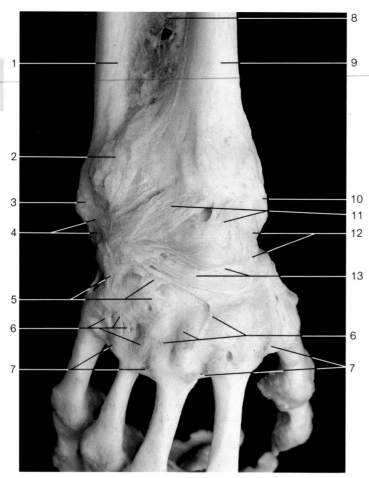

1  Ulna
2  Exostosis (pathological)
3  Head of ulna
4  Ulnar carpal collateral ligament
5  Deep intercarpal ligaments
6  Dorsal carpometacarpal ligaments
7  Dorsal metacarpal ligaments
8  Interosseous membrane
9  Radius
10  Styloid process of radius
11  Dorsal radiocarpal ligament
12  Radial collateral ligament
13  Articular capsule and dorsal intercarpal ligaments
14  Palmar radiocarpal ligament
15  Tendon of flexor carpi radialis muscle (cut)
16  Radiating carpal ligament
17  Palmar carpometacarpal ligaments
18  First metacarpal bone
19  Palmar ulnocarpal ligament
20  Tendon of flexor carpi ulnaris muscle (cut)
21  Pisohamate ligament
22  Pisometacarpal ligament
23  Palmar metacarpal ligaments
24  Fifth metacarpal bone
25  Articular disc (ulnocarpal)
26  Lunate bone
27  Triquetral bone
28  Hamate bone
29  Scaphoid (navicular) bone
30  Capitate bone
31  Trapezoid bone
32  Second and third metacarpal bones
33  Dorsal interossei muscles

**Ligaments of hand and wrist** (dorsal aspect).

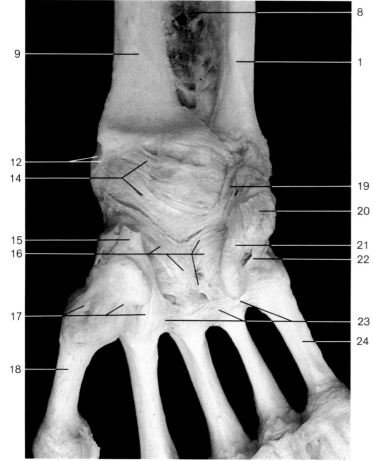

**Ligaments of hand and wrist** (palmar aspect).

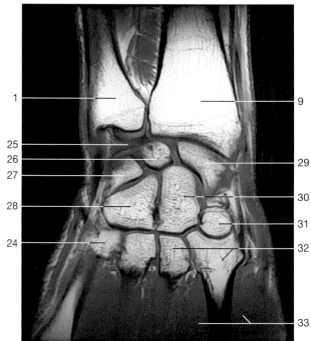

**Coronal section through the hand and wrist** (MRI scan).
(Courtesy of Prof. Heuck, Munich, Germany.) Note the location
of the wrist joint.

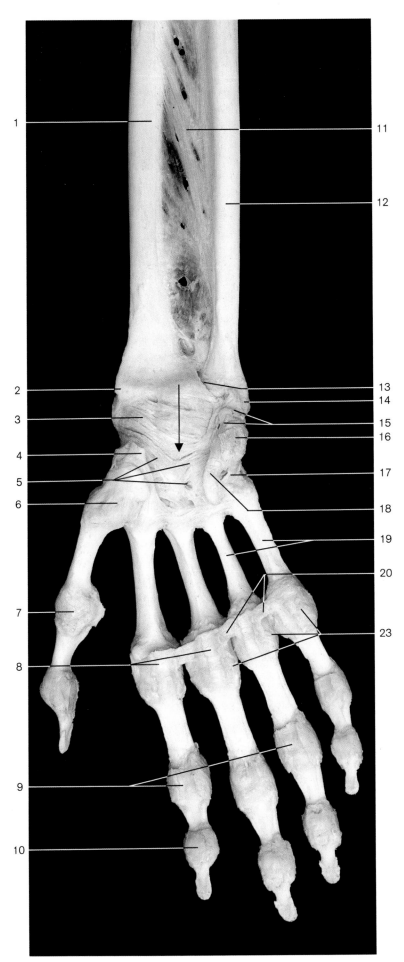

1   Radius
2   Styloid process of radius
3   Palmar radiocarpal ligament
4   Tendon of flexor carpi radialis muscle (cut)
5   Radiating carpal ligament
6   Articular capsule of carpometacarpal joint
    of thumb
7   Articular capsule of metacarpophalangeal joint
    of thumb
8   Palmar ligaments and articular capsule
    of metacarpophalangeal joints
9   Palmar ligaments and articular capsule
    of interphalangeal joints
10  Articular capsule
11  Interosseous membrane
12  Ulna
13  Distal radio-ulnar joint
14  Styloid process of ulna
15  Palmar ulnocarpal ligament
16  Pisiform bone
    with tendon of flexor carpi ulnaris muscle
17  Pisometacarpal ligament
18  Pisohamate ligament
19  Metacarpal bones
20  Deep transverse metacarpal ligaments
21  Tendons of extensor muscles and
    articular capsule
22  Collateral ligament of interphalangeal joint
23  Collateral ligaments
    of metacarpophalangeal joints
24  Second metacarpal bone

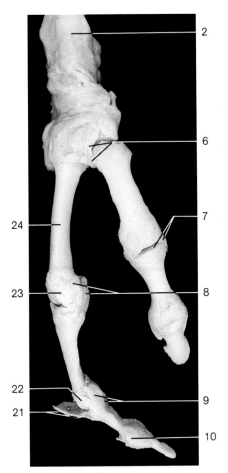

**Ligaments of forearm, hand, and fingers** (palmar aspect). The arrow indicates the location of the carpal tunnel.

**Ligaments of fingers** (lateral aspect).

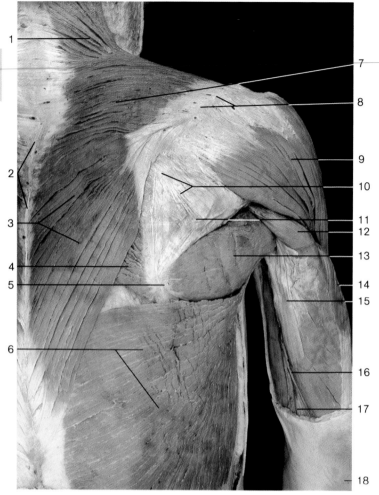

1   Descending fibers of trapezius muscle
2   Spinous processes of thoracic vertebrae
3   Ascending fibers of trapezius muscle
4   Rhomboid major muscle
5   Inferior angle of scapula
6   Latissimus dorsi muscle
7   Transverse fibers of trapezius muscle
8   Spine of scapula
9   Posterior fibers of deltoid muscle
10  Infraspinatus muscle and infraspinous fascia
11  Teres minor muscle and fascia
12  Long head of triceps brachii muscle
13  Teres major muscle
14  Lateral head of triceps brachii muscle
15  Tendon of triceps brachii muscle
16  Medial intermuscular septum
17  Ulnar nerve
18  Olecranon

**Muscles of shoulder and arm,** superficial layer (right side, posterior aspect).

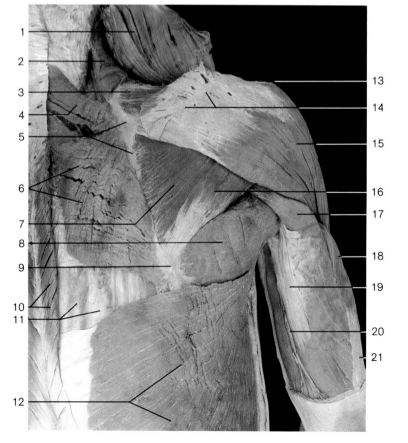

1   Trapezius muscle (reflected)
2   Levator scapulae muscle
3   Supraspinatus muscle
4   Rhomboid minor muscle
5   Medial border of scapula
6   Rhomboid major muscle
7   Infraspinatus muscle
8   Teres major muscle
9   Inferior angle of scapula
10  Cut edge of trapezius muscle
11  Intrinsic muscles of back with fascia
12  Latissimus dorsi muscle
13  Acromion
14  Spine of scapula
15  Deltoid muscle
16  Teres minor muscle
17  Long head of triceps brachii muscle
18  Lateral head of triceps brachii muscle
19  Medial head of triceps brachii muscle
20  Medial intermuscular septum
21  Tendon of triceps brachii muscle

**Muscles of shoulder and arm,** deeper layer (right side, posterior aspect). The trapezius muscle has been cut near its origin at the vertebral column and reflected upward.

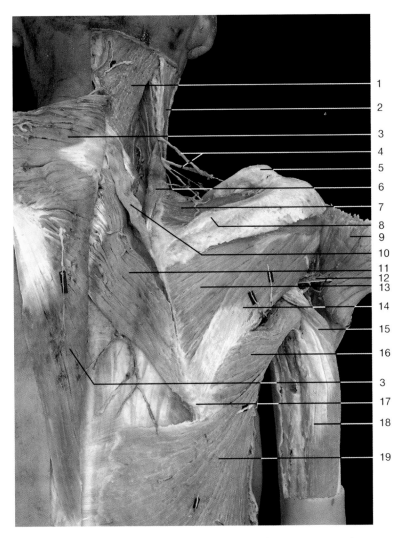

1   Splenius capitis muscle
2   Sternocleidomastoid muscle
3   Trapezius muscle (reflected)
4   Lateral supraclavicular nerves
5   Clavicle
6   Levator scapulae muscle
7   Supraspinatus muscle
8   Spine of scapula
9   Deltoid muscle (reflected)
10  Rhomboid minor muscle
11  Rhomboid major muscle
12  Axillary nerve and
    posterior circumflex humeral artery
13  Infraspinatus muscle
14  Teres minor muscle
15  Long head of triceps brachii muscle
16  Teres major muscle
17  Inferior angle of scapula
18  Triceps brachii muscle
19  Latissimus dorsi muscle

**Muscles of shoulder and arm,** deeper layer (right side, posterior aspect).
The trapezius and deltoid muscles have been divided and reflected.

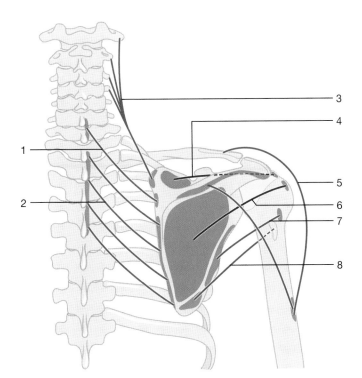

**Position and course of the main shoulder muscles**
(posterior aspect).

◁

1   Rhomboid minor muscle (red)
2   Rhomboid major muscle (red)
3   Levator scapulae muscle (red)
4   Supraspinatus muscle (blue)
5   Deltoid muscle (red)
6   Infraspinatus muscle (blue)
7   Teres minor muscle (red)
8   Teres major muscle (red)

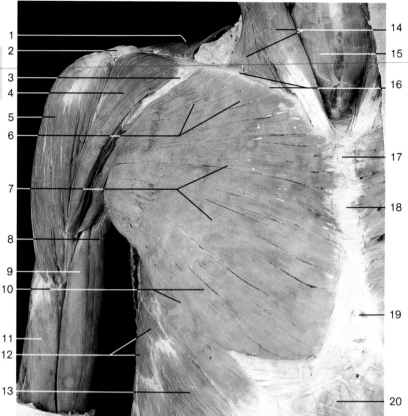

1   Trapezius muscle
2   Acromion
3   Deltopectoral triangle
4   Clavicular part of deltoid muscle
    (anterior fibers)
5   Acromial part of deltoid muscle
    (central fibers)
6   Clavicular part of pectoralis major muscle
7   Sternocostal part of pectoralis major muscle
8   Short head of biceps brachii muscle
9   Long head of biceps brachii muscle
10  Abdominal part of pectoralis major muscle
11  Brachialis muscle
12  Serratus anterior muscle
13  External abdominal oblique muscle
14  Sternocleidomastoid muscle
15  Infrahyoid muscles
16  Clavicle
17  Manubrium sterni
18  Body of sternum
19  Xiphoid process
20  Anterior layer of sheath
    of rectus abdominis muscle

**Shoulder, arm, and pectoral muscles,** superficial layer (right side, anterior aspect).

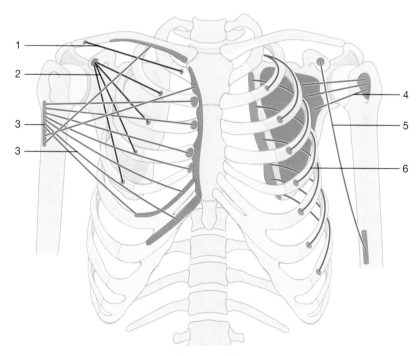

**Position and course of pectoral and shoulder muscles** (anterior aspect).

1   Subclavius muscle (blue)
2   Pectoralis minor muscle (blue)
3   Pectoralis major muscle (red)
4   Subscapularis muscle (red)
5   Coracobrachialis muscle (red)
6   Serratus anterior muscle (green)

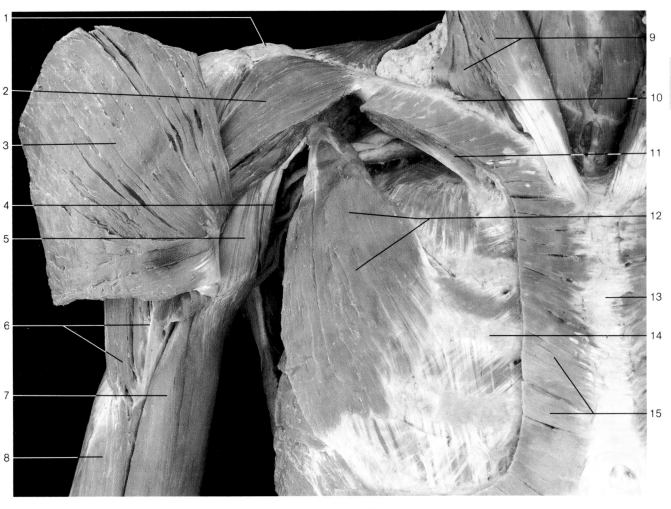

**Shoulder, arm, and pectoral muscles,** deep layer (right side, anterior aspect).

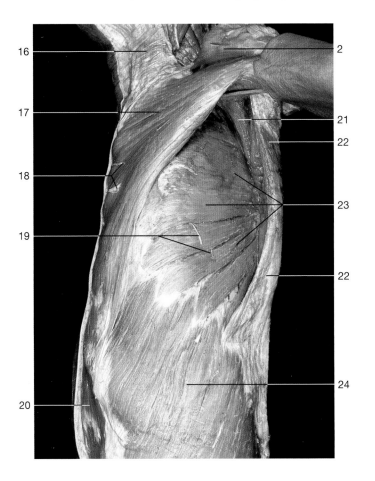

1   Acromion
2   Clavicular part of deltoid muscle
3   Pectoralis major muscle (reflected)
4   Coracobrachialis muscle
5   Short head of biceps brachii muscle
6   Deltoid muscle (insertion on humerus)
7   Long head of biceps brachii muscle
8   Brachialis muscle
9   Sternocleidomastoid muscle
10  Clavicle
11  Subclavius muscle
12  Pectoralis minor muscle
13  Sternum
14  Third rib
15  Pectoralis major muscle (cut)
16  Platysma muscle
17  Pectoralis major muscle forming the anterior axillary fold
18  Anterior cutaneous branches of intercostal nerves
19  Lateral cutaneous branches of intercostal nerves
20  Rectus abdominis muscle
21  Subscapularis muscle
22  Latissimus dorsi muscle forming the posterior axillary fold
23  Serratus anterior muscle forming the medial wall of the axilla
24  External abdominal oblique muscle

**Axillary fossa and serratus anterior muscle**
(left side, lateral aspect).

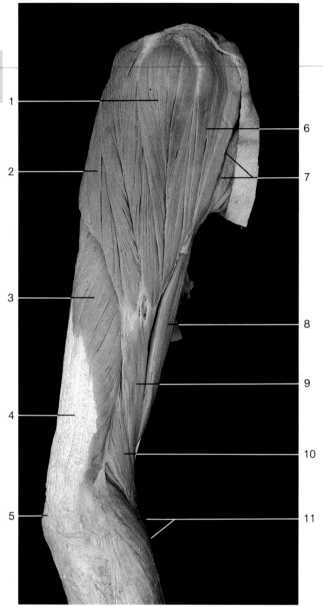

**Muscles of the arm** (right side, lateral aspect).

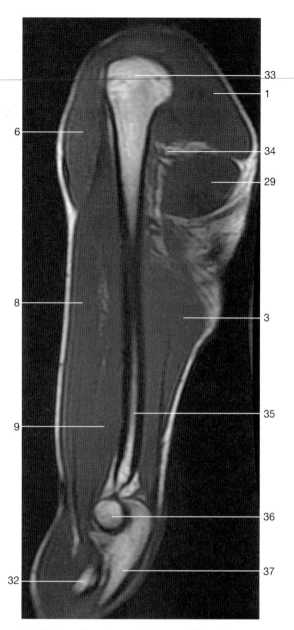

**Sagittal section through the arm** (right side; MRI scan). (From Heuck et al., MRT-Atlas, 2009.)

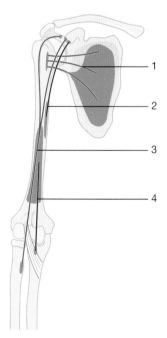

**Position and course of flexors of the arm** (anterior aspect).

1   Subscapularis muscle (red)
2   Coracobrachialis muscle (blue)
3   Biceps brachii muscle (red)
4   Brachialis muscle (blue)

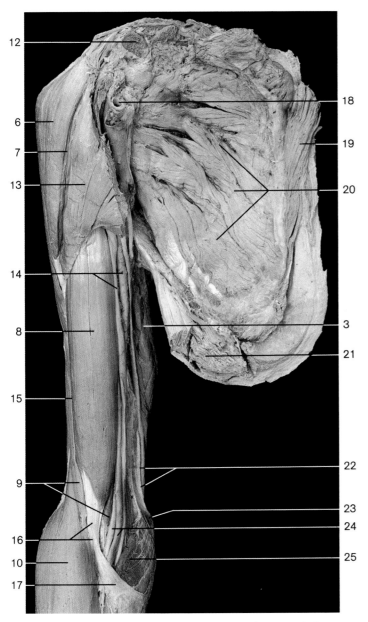

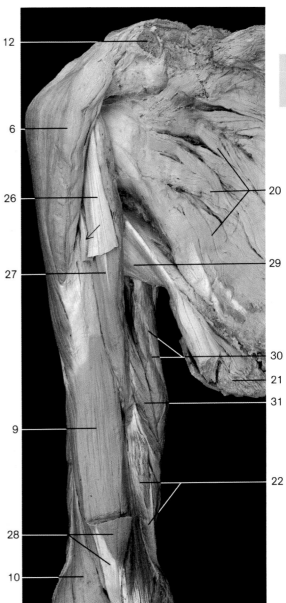

**Muscles of the arm** (right side, anterior aspect). The arm with the scapula and attached muscles has been removed from the trunk.

**Muscles of the arm** (right side, anterior aspect). Part of the biceps brachii muscle has been removed.
Arrow: tendon of long head of biceps brachii muscle.

| | |
|---|---|
| 1 Acromial part of deltoid muscle (central fibers) | 20 Subscapularis muscle |
| 2 Scapular part of deltoid muscle (posterior fibers) | 21 Latissimus dorsi muscle (divided) |
| 3 Triceps brachii muscle | 22 Medial intermuscular septum |
| 4 Tendon of triceps brachii muscle | 23 Medial epicondyle of humerus |
| 5 Olecranon | 24 Brachial artery and median nerve |
| 6 Clavicular part of deltoid muscle (anterior fibers) | 25 Pronator teres muscle |
| 7 Deltopectoral groove | 26 Tendon of short head of biceps brachii muscle |
| 8 Biceps brachii muscle | 27 Coracobrachialis muscle |
| 9 Brachialis muscle | 28 Distal part of biceps brachii muscle |
| 10 Brachioradialis muscle | 29 Teres major muscle |
| 11 Extensor carpi radialis longus muscle | 30 Long head of triceps brachii muscle |
| 12 Clavicle (divided) | 31 Medial head of triceps brachii muscle |
| 13 Pectoralis major muscle | 32 Radius |
| 14 Medial intermuscular septum with vessels and nerves | 33 Head of humerus |
| 15 Lateral intermuscular septum | 34 Axillary nerve |
| 16 Tendon of biceps brachii muscle | 35 Humerus |
| 17 Bicipital aponeurosis | 36 Trochlea |
| 18 Axillary artery | 37 Ulna |
| 19 Rhomboid major muscle | |

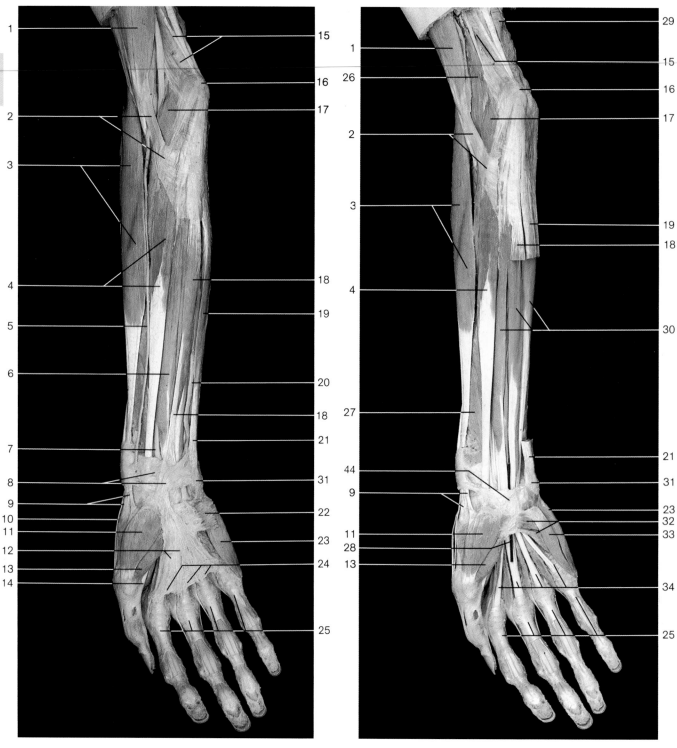

**Flexor muscles of forearm and hand,** superficial layer (right side, anterior aspect).

**Flexor muscles of forearm and hand,** superficial layer (right side, anterior aspect). The palmaris longus and flexor carpi ulnaris muscles have been removed.

  1　Biceps brachii muscle
  2　Bicipital aponeurosis
  3　Brachioradialis muscle
  4　Flexor carpi radialis muscle
  5　Radial artery
  6　Flexor digitorum superficialis muscle
  7　Median nerve
  8　Antebrachial fascia and tendon of palmaris longus muscle
  9　Tendon of abductor pollicis longus muscle
10　Tendon of extensor pollicis brevis muscle
11　Abductor pollicis brevis muscle

12　Palmar aponeurosis
13　Superficial head of flexor pollicis brevis muscle
14　Tendon of flexor pollicis longus muscle
15　Medial intermuscular septum
16　Medial epicondyle of humerus
17　Humeral head of pronator teres muscle
18　Palmaris longus muscle
19　Flexor carpi ulnaris muscle
20　Ulnar artery
21　Tendon of flexor carpi ulnaris muscle
22　Palmaris brevis muscle

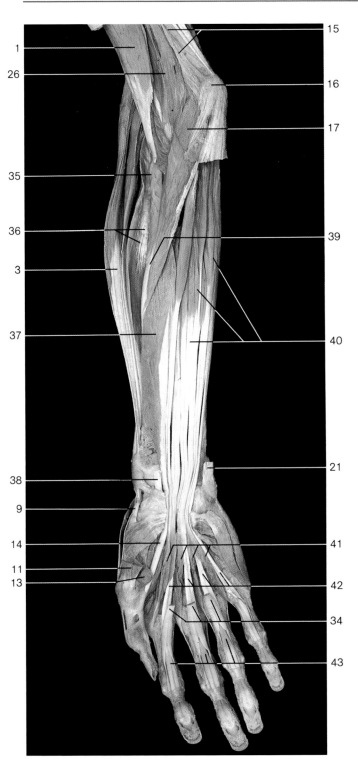

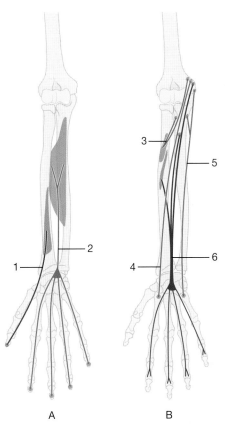

A          B

**Position and course of flexors of forearm and hand**
(anterior aspect).

| **A  Deep flexors** | **B  Superficial flexors** |
|---|---|
| 1  Flexor pollicis<br>   longus muscle (blue) | 3  Pronator teres muscle (red) |
| 2  Flexor digitorum<br>   profundus muscle (red) | 4  Flexor carpi radialis muscle<br>   (red) |
| | 5  Flexor carpi ulnaris muscle<br>   (red) |
| | 6  Flexor digitorum superficialis muscle<br>   (blue) |

**Flexor muscles of forearm and hand,** middle layer (right side,
anterior aspect). The palmaris longus, flexor carpi radialis, and ulnaris
muscles have been removed. The flexor retinaculum has been divided.

23  Abductor digiti minimi muscle
24  Transverse fasciculi of palmar aponeurosis
25  Digital fibrous sheaths of tendons of flexor digitorum muscle
26  Brachialis muscle
27  Flexor pollicis longus muscle
28  Carpal tunnel (canalis carpi, probe)
29  Triceps brachii muscle
30  Flexor digitorum superficialis muscle
31  Pisiform bone
32  Opponens digiti minimi muscle
33  Flexor digiti minimi brevis muscle
34  Tendons of flexor digitorum superficialis muscle

35  Supinator muscle
36  Radius and extensor carpi radialis brevis muscle
37  Flexor pollicis longus muscle
38  Tendon of flexor carpi radialis muscle
39  Pronator teres muscle (insertion of radius)
40  Flexor digitorum profundus muscle
41  Lumbrical muscles
42  Tendons of flexor digitorum profundus muscle
43  Tendons of flexor digitorum profundus muscle
    having passed through the divided tendons
    of the flexor digitorum superficialis muscle
44  Flexor retinaculum

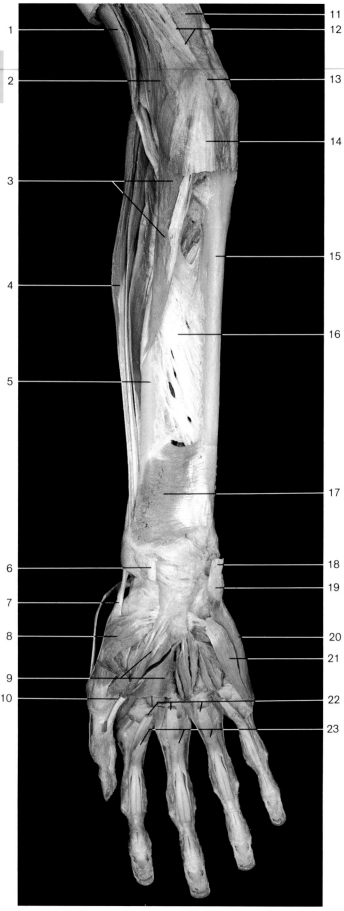

1
2
3
4
5
6
7
8
9
10

11
12

13

14

15

16

17

18
19

20
21

22
23

1 Biceps brachii muscle
2 Brachialis muscle
3 Pronator teres muscle
4 Brachioradialis muscle
5 Radius
6 Tendon of flexor carpi radialis muscle
7 Tendon of abductor pollicis longus muscle
8 Opponens pollicis muscle
9 Adductor pollicis muscle
10 Tendon of flexor pollicis longus muscle
11 Triceps brachii muscle
12 Medial intermuscular septum
13 Medial epicondyle of humerus
14 Common flexor mass (divided)
15 Ulna
16 Interosseous membrane
17 Pronator quadratus muscle
18 Tendon of flexor carpi ulnaris muscle
19 Pisiform bone
20 Abductor digiti minimi muscle
21 Flexor digiti minimi brevis muscle
22 Tendons of flexor digitorum profundus muscle
23 Tendons of flexor digitorum superficialis muscle
24 Flexor retinaculum
25 Hypothenar muscles
26 Thenar muscles
27 Common synovial sheath of flexor tendons
28 Synovial sheath of tendon of flexor pollicis longus muscle
29 Digital synovial sheaths of flexor tendons

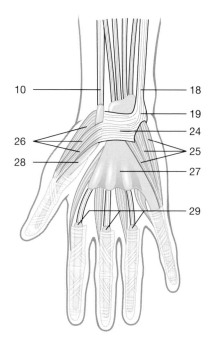

10

26
28

18

19

24

25

27

29

**Flexor muscles of forearm and hand,** deep layer (right side, anterior aspect). All flexors have been removed to display the pronator quadratus and pronator teres muscles together with the interosseous membrane. Forearm in supination.

**Synovial sheaths of flexor tendons,** indicated in blue (palmar aspect of right hand).

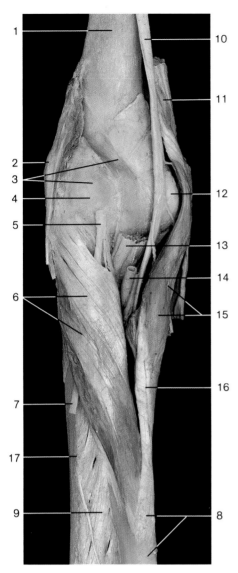

1 Humerus
2 Lateral epicondyle of humerus
3 Articular capsule
4 Position of capitulum of humerus
5 Deep branch of radial nerve
6 Supinator muscle
7 Entrance of deep branch of radial nerve to extensor muscles
8 Radius and insertion of pronator teres muscle
9 Interosseous membrane
10 Median nerve
11 Triceps brachii muscle
12 Trochlea of humerus
13 Tendon of biceps brachii muscle
14 Brachial artery
15 Pronator teres muscle
16 Tendon of pronator teres muscle
17 Ulna
18 Pronator quadratus muscle
19 Tendon of flexor carpi radialis muscle
20 Thenar muscles
21 Synovial sheath of tendon of flexor pollicis longus muscle
22 Fibrous sheath of flexor tendons
23 Digital synovial sheath of flexor tendons
24 Flexor digitorum superficialis muscle
25 Tendon of flexor carpi ulnaris muscle
26 Common synovial sheath of flexor tendons
27 Position of pisiform bone
28 Flexor retinaculum
29 Hypothenar muscles

**Right supinator muscle and elbow joint**
(anterior aspect). Forearm in pronation.

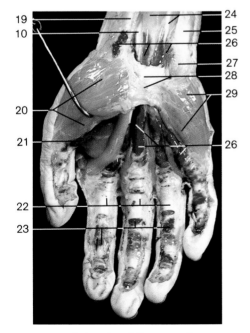

**Synovial sheaths of flexor tendons**
(palmar aspect of right hand). The sheaths
have been injected with blue gelatin.

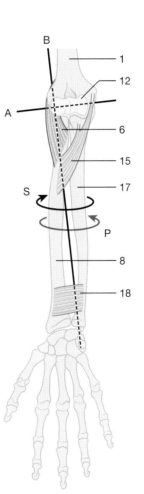

A = Axis of flexion and extension
B = Axis of rotation

Arrows:
S = Supination
P = Pronation

**Diagram illustrating the two axes of the elbow joint.**

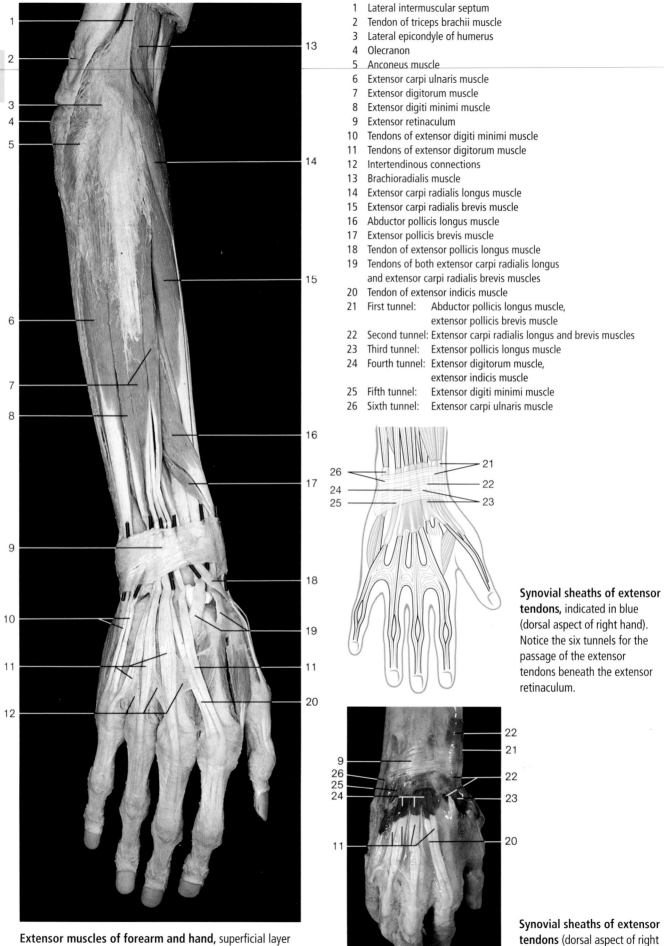

1   Lateral intermuscular septum
2   Tendon of triceps brachii muscle
3   Lateral epicondyle of humerus
4   Olecranon
5   Anconeus muscle
6   Extensor carpi ulnaris muscle
7   Extensor digitorum muscle
8   Extensor digiti minimi muscle
9   Extensor retinaculum
10  Tendons of extensor digiti minimi muscle
11  Tendons of extensor digitorum muscle
12  Intertendinous connections
13  Brachioradialis muscle
14  Extensor carpi radialis longus muscle
15  Extensor carpi radialis brevis muscle
16  Abductor pollicis longus muscle
17  Extensor pollicis brevis muscle
18  Tendon of extensor pollicis longus muscle
19  Tendons of both extensor carpi radialis longus
    and extensor carpi radialis brevis muscles
20  Tendon of extensor indicis muscle
21  First tunnel:    Abductor pollicis longus muscle,
                     extensor pollicis brevis muscle
22  Second tunnel: Extensor carpi radialis longus and brevis muscles
23  Third tunnel:    Extensor pollicis longus muscle
24  Fourth tunnel:  Extensor digitorum muscle,
                     extensor indicis muscle
25  Fifth tunnel:    Extensor digiti minimi muscle
26  Sixth tunnel:    Extensor carpi ulnaris muscle

**Synovial sheaths of extensor tendons,** indicated in blue (dorsal aspect of right hand). Notice the six tunnels for the passage of the extensor tendons beneath the extensor retinaculum.

**Extensor muscles of forearm and hand,** superficial layer (right side, posterior aspect). Tunnels for extensor tendons indicated by probes.

**Synovial sheaths of extensor tendons** (dorsal aspect of right hand). The sheaths have been injected with blue gelatin.

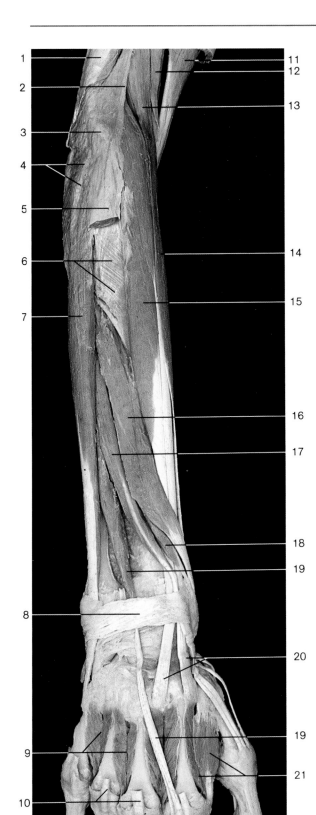

1 Triceps brachii muscle
2 Lateral intermuscular septum
3 Lateral epicondyle of humerus
4 Anconeus muscle
5 Extensor digitorum and extensor digiti minimi muscles (cut)
6 Supinator muscle
7 Extensor carpi ulnaris muscle
8 Extensor retinaculum
9 Third and fourth dorsal interossei muscles
10 Tendons of extensor digitorum muscle (cut)
11 Biceps brachii muscle
12 Brachialis muscle
13 Brachioradialis muscle
14 Extensor carpi radialis longus muscle
15 Extensor carpi radialis brevis muscle
16 Abductor pollicis longus muscle
17 Extensor pollicis longus muscle
18 Extensor pollicis brevis muscle
19 Extensor indicis muscle
20 Tendons of extensor carpi radialis longus and extensor carpi radialis brevis muscles
21 First dorsal interosseous muscle

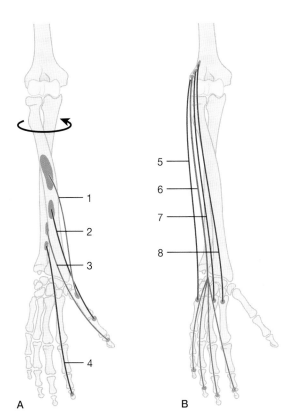

**Position and course of extensors of forearm and hand** (posterior aspect).

**A Extensors of thumb**

1 Abductor pollicis longus muscle (red)
2 Extensor pollicis brevis muscle (blue)
3 Extensor pollicis longus muscle (red)
4 Extensor indicis muscle (blue)

**B Extensors of fingers and hand**

5 Extensor carpi ulnaris muscle (blue)
6 Extensor digitorum muscle (red)
7 Extensor carpi radialis brevis muscle (blue)
8 Extensor carpi radialis longus muscle (blue)

**Extensor muscles of forearm and hand,** deep layer (right side, posterior aspect).

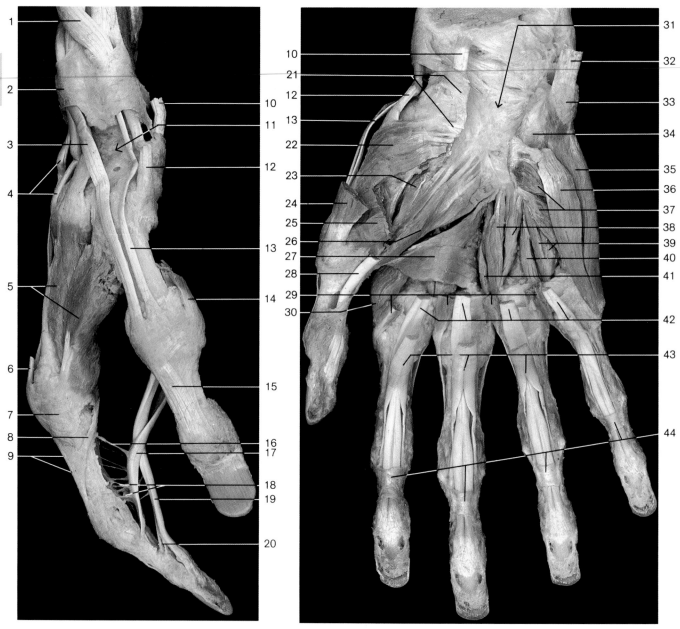

**Muscles of thumb and index finger** (medial aspect). The tendons of the extensor muscles of the thumb and the insertion of the flexor tendons of the index finger are displayed.

**Muscles of the hand** (right side, palmar aspect). The tendons of the flexor muscles and parts of the thumb muscles have been removed. The carpal tunnel has been opened.

1 Tendons of extensor pollicis brevis and abductor pollicis longus muscles
2 Extensor retinaculum
3 Tendon of extensor pollicis longus muscle
4 Tendons of extensor carpi radialis longus and brevis muscles
5 First dorsal interosseous muscle
6 Tendon of extensor digitorum muscle for index finger
7 Location of metacarpophalangeal joint
8 Tendon of lumbrical muscle
9 Extensor expansion of index finger
10 Tendon of flexor carpi radialis muscle (cut)
11 Anatomical snuffbox
12 Tendon of abductor pollicis longus muscle
13 Tendon of extensor pollicis brevis muscle
14 Tendon of abductor pollicis brevis muscle

15 Extensor expansion of extensor of thumb
16 Vinculum longum
17 Tendons of flexor digitorum superficialis muscle dividing to allow passage of deep tendons
18 Vincula of flexor tendons
19 Tendon of flexor digitorum profundus muscle
20 Vinculum breve
21 Radial carpal eminence (cut edge of flexor retinaculum)
22 Opponens pollicis muscle
23 Deep head of flexor pollicis brevis muscle
24 Abductor pollicis brevis muscle (cut)
25 Superficial head of flexor pollicis brevis muscle (cut)
26 Oblique head of adductor pollicis muscle
27 Transverse head of adductor pollicis muscle
28 Tendon of flexor pollicis longus muscle (cut)
29 Lumbrical muscles (cut)

30 First dorsal interosseous muscle
31 Position of carpal tunnel
32 Tendon of flexor carpi ulnaris muscle
33 Location of pisiform bone
34 Hook of hamate bone
35 Abductor digiti minimi muscle
36 Flexor digiti minimi brevis muscle
37 Opponens digiti minimi muscle
38 Second palmar interosseous muscle
39 Third palmar interosseous muscle
40 Fourth dorsal interosseous muscle
41 Third dorsal interosseous muscle
42 Tendon of flexor digitorum profundus muscle (cut)
43 Tendons of flexor digitorum superficialis muscle (cut)
44 Fibrous flexor sheaths

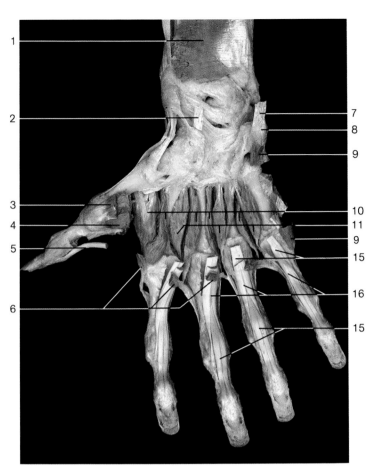

**Muscles of the hand,** deep layer (right side, palmar aspect). The thenar and hypothenar muscles have been removed to display the interossei muscles.

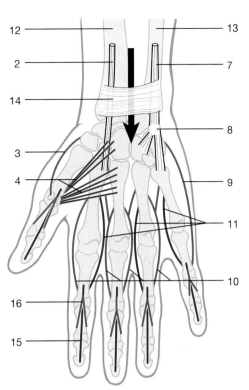

**Actions of interossei muscles** in abduction and adduction of fingers (palmar aspect of right hand).
Arrow: carpal tunnel.
Red = abduction (dorsal interossei, abductor digiti minimi, and abductor pollicis brevis muscles)
Blue = adduction (palmar interossei muscles, adductor pollicis muscle)

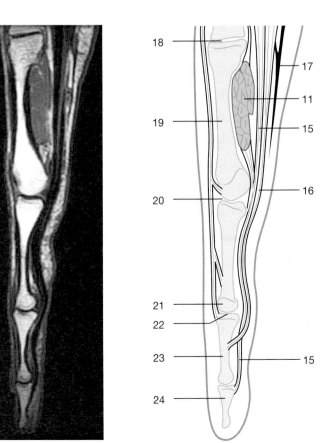

**Longitudinal section through the third finger** (MRI scan).
(Prof. Heuck, Munich, Germany.) Compare with the correspondent drawing.

1  Pronator quadratus muscle
2  Tendon of flexor carpi radialis muscle
3  Abductor pollicis brevis muscle (divided)
4  Adductor pollicis muscle (divided)
5  Tendon of flexor pollicis longus muscle
6  Lumbrical muscles (cut)
7  Tendon of flexor carpi ulnaris muscle
8  Pisiform bone
9  Abductor digiti minimi muscle (divided)
10  Dorsal interossei muscles
11  Palmar interossei muscles
12  Radius
13  Ulna
14  Flexor retinaculum
15  Tendons of flexor digitorum profundus muscle
16  Tendons of flexor digitorum superficialis muscle
17  Palmar aponeurosis
18  Carpometacarpal joint
19  Third metacarpal bone
20  Metacarpophalangeal joint
21  Head of third proximal phalanx
22  Proximal interphalangeal joint
23  Middle phalanx
24  Distal phalanx

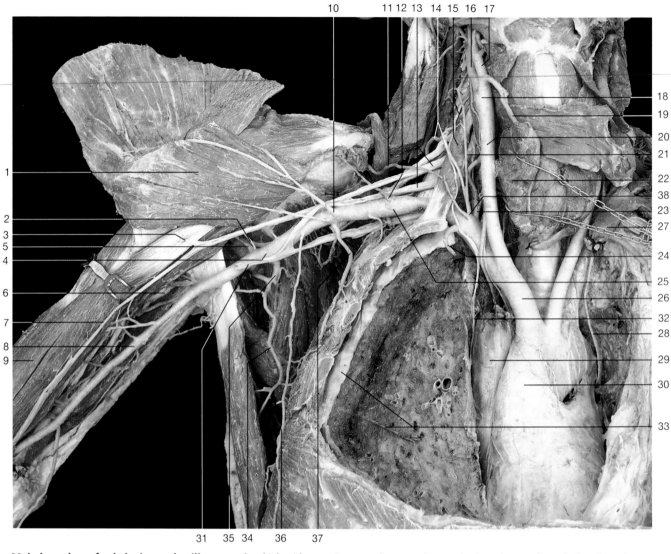

**Main branches of subclavian and axillary arteries** (right side, anterior aspect). Pectoralis muscles have been reflected, clavicle and anterior wall of thorax removed, and right lung divided. Left lung with pleura and thyroid gland have been reflected laterally to display aortic arch and common carotid artery with their branches.

| | | |
|---|---|---|
| 1　Pectoralis minor muscle (reflected) | 22　Thyroid gland | 43　Radial collateral artery |
| 2　Anterior circumflex humeral artery | 23　Inferior thyroid artery | 44　Radial recurrent artery |
| 3　Musculocutaneous nerve (divided) | 24　Internal thoracic artery | 45　Radial artery |
| 4　Axillary artery | 25　Right subclavian artery | 46　Anterior and posterior interosseous arteries |
| 5　Posterior circumflex humeral artery | 26　Brachiocephalic trunk | 47　Princeps pollicis artery |
| 6　Profunda brachii artery | 27　Left brachiocephalic vein (divided) | 48　Deep palmar arch |
| 7　Median nerve (var.) | 28　Left vagus nerve | 49　Common palmar digital arteries |
| 8　Brachial artery | 29　Superior vena cava (divided) | 50　Ulnar recurrent artery |
| 9　Biceps brachii muscle | 30　Ascending aorta | 51　Recurrent interosseous artery |
| 10　Thoraco-acromial artery | 31　Median nerve (divided) | 52　Common interosseous artery |
| 11　Suprascapular artery | 32　Phrenic nerve | 53　Ulnar artery |
| 12　Descending scapular artery | 33　Right lung (divided) and pulmonary pleura | 54　Superficial palmar arch |
| 13　Brachial plexus (middle trunk) | 34　Thoracodorsal artery | 55　Median nerve and brachial artery |
| 14　Transverse cervical artery | 35　Subscapular artery | 56　Biceps brachii muscle |
| 15　Anterior scalene muscle and phrenic nerve | 36　Lateral mammary branches (var.) | 57　Ulnar nerve |
| 16　Right internal carotid artery | 37　Lateral thoracic artery | 58　Flexor pollicis longus muscle |
| 17　Right external carotid artery | 38　Thyrocervical trunk | 59　Proper palmar digital arteries |
| 18　Carotid sinus | 39　Supreme intercostal artery | 60　Anterior interosseous artery |
| 19　Superior thyroid artery | 40　Superior ulnar collateral artery | 61　Flexor carpi ulnaris muscle |
| 20　Right common carotid artery | 41　Inferior ulnar collateral artery | 62　Superficial palmar branch of radial artery |
| 21　Ascending cervical artery | 42　Middle collateral artery | |

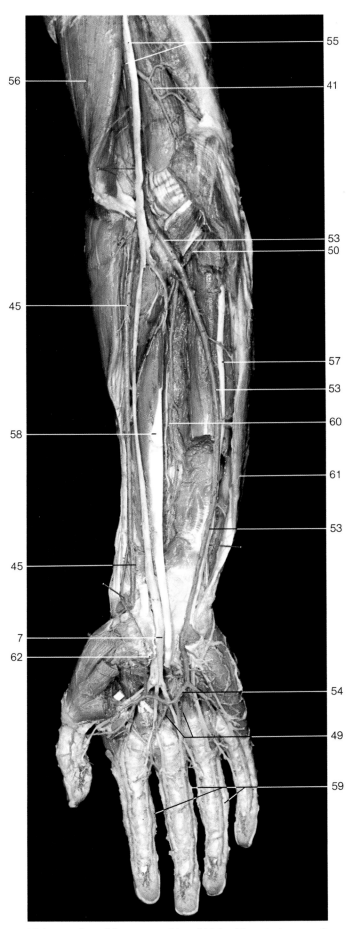

| | |
|---|---|
| 56 | 55 |
| | 41 |
| 45 | 53 |
| 58 | 50 |
| 45 | 57 |
| 7 | 53 |
| 62 | 60 |
| | 61 |
| | 53 |
| | 54 |
| | 49 |
| | 59 |

**Main arteries of forearm and hand** (right side, anterior aspect). The superficial flexor muscles have been removed, the carpal tunnel opened, and the flexor retinaculum cut. The arteries have been filled with colored resin.

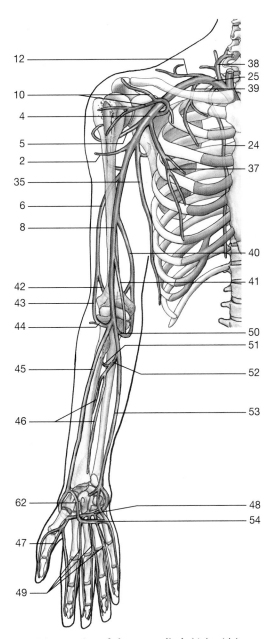

**Main arteries of the upper limb** (right side).

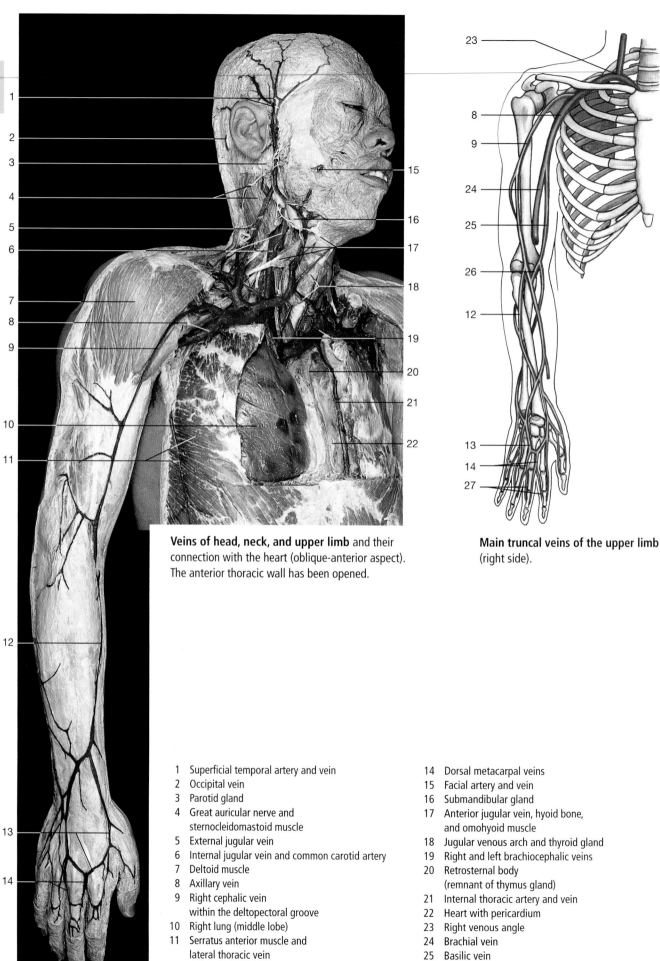

**Veins of head, neck, and upper limb** and their connection with the heart (oblique-anterior aspect). The anterior thoracic wall has been opened.

**Main truncal veins of the upper limb** (right side).

1   Superficial temporal artery and vein
2   Occipital vein
3   Parotid gland
4   Great auricular nerve and sternocleidomastoid muscle
5   External jugular vein
6   Internal jugular vein and common carotid artery
7   Deltoid muscle
8   Axillary vein
9   Right cephalic vein within the deltopectoral groove
10  Right lung (middle lobe)
11  Serratus anterior muscle and lateral thoracic vein
12  Cephalic vein on forearm
13  Venous network on dorsum of hand

14  Dorsal metacarpal veins
15  Facial artery and vein
16  Submandibular gland
17  Anterior jugular vein, hyoid bone, and omohyoid muscle
18  Jugular venous arch and thyroid gland
19  Right and left brachiocephalic veins
20  Retrosternal body (remnant of thymus gland)
21  Internal thoracic artery and vein
22  Heart with pericardium
23  Right venous angle
24  Brachial vein
25  Basilic vein
26  Median cubital vein
27  Digital veins

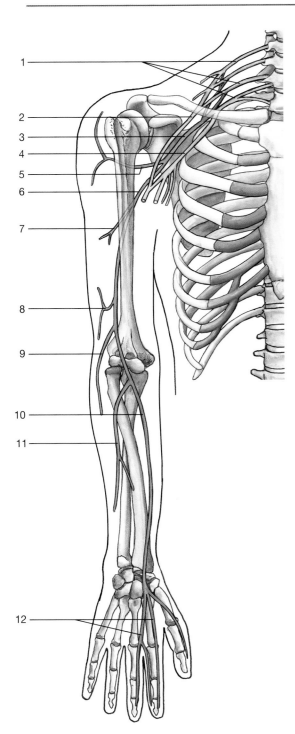

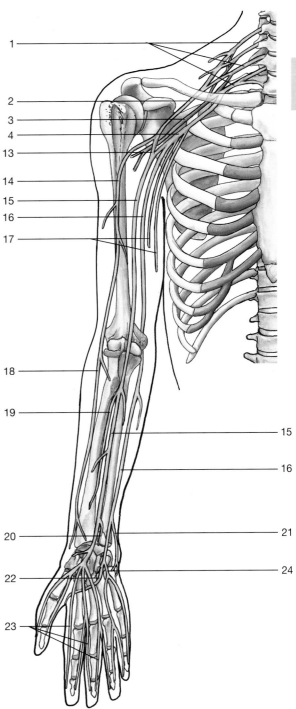

**Main branches of radial and axillary nerves**
(right side). The posterior trunk of brachial plexus is
indicated in orange.

**Main branches of musculocutaneous, median, and
ulnar nerves** (right side). The posterior trunk of brachial
plexus is indicated in orange.

| | |
|---|---|
| 1 | Brachial plexus |
| 2 | Lateral cord of brachial plexus |
| 3 | Posterior cord of brachial plexus |
| 4 | Medial cord of brachial plexus |
| 5 | Axillary nerve |
| 6 | Radial nerve |
| 7 | Posterior cutaneous nerve of arm |
| 8 | Lower lateral cutaneous nerve of arm |
| 9 | Posterior cutaneous nerve of forearm |
| 10 | Superficial branch of radial nerve |
| 11 | Deep branch of radial nerve |
| 12 | Dorsal digital nerves |

| | |
|---|---|
| 13 | Roots of median nerve |
| 14 | Musculocutaneous nerve |
| 15 | Median nerve |
| 16 | Ulnar nerve |
| 17 | Medial cutaneous nerves of arm and forearm |
| 18 | Lateral cutaneous nerve of forearm |
| 19 | Anterior interosseous nerve |
| 20 | Palmar branch of median nerve |
| 21 | Dorsal branch of ulnar nerve |
| 22 | Deep branch of ulnar nerve |
| 23 | Common palmar digital nerves of median nerve |
| 24 | Superficial branch of ulnar nerve |

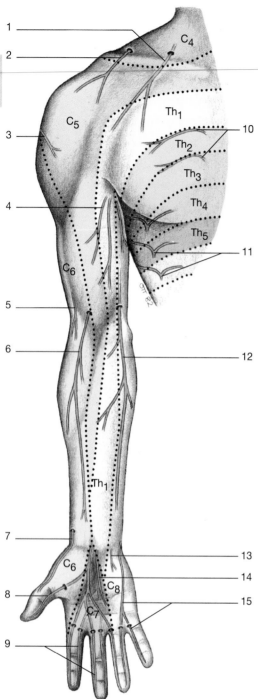

**Cutaneous nerves of the upper limb**
(right side, anterior aspect).

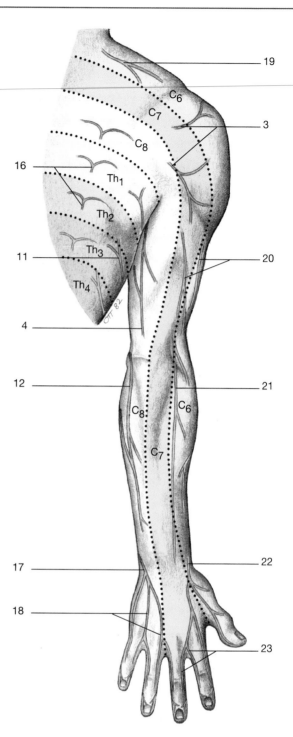

**Cutaneous nerves of the upper limb**
(right side, posterior aspect).

1   Medial supraclavicular nerve
2   Intermediate supraclavicular nerve
3   Upper lateral cutaneous nerve of arm
4   Terminal branches of intercostobrachial nerves
5   Lower lateral cutaneous nerve of arm
6   Lateral cutaneous nerve of forearm
7   Terminal branch of superficial branch of radial nerve
8   Palmar digital nerve of thumb (branch of median nerve)
9   Palmar digital branches of median nerve
10  Anterior cutaneous branches of intercostal nerves
11  Lateral cutaneous branches of intercostal nerves
12  Medial cutaneous nerve of forearm

13  Palmar cutaneous branch of ulnar nerve
14  Palmar branch of median nerve
15  Palmar digital branches of ulnar nerve
16  Cutaneous branches of dorsal rami of spinal nerves
17  Dorsal branch of ulnar nerve
18  Dorsal digital nerves
19  Posterior supraclavicular nerve
20  Posterior cutaneous nerve of arm
21  Posterior cutaneous nerve of forearm    } from radial nerve
22  Superficial branch
23  Dorsal digital branches

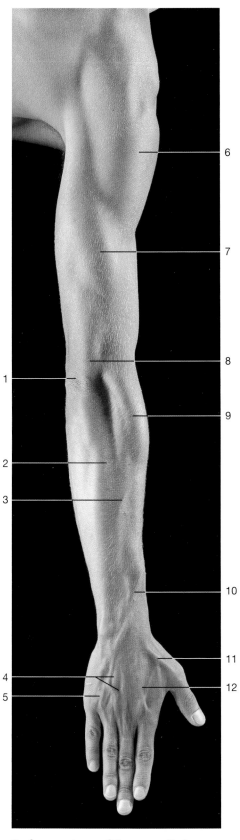

**Surface anatomy of the upper limb**
(right side, posterior aspect).

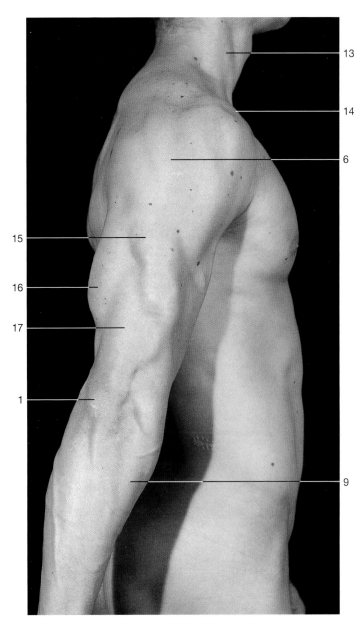

**Surface anatomy of the arm** (right side, lateral aspect).
The triceps brachii muscle is strongly contracted.

1   Olecranon
2   Extensor muscles of forearm
3   Accessory cephalic vein
4   Tendons of extensor digitorum
    muscle
5   Dorsal venous network
    of hand
6   Deltoid muscle
7   Triceps brachii muscle
8   Lateral epicondyle of humerus
9   Brachioradialis muscle
10  Cephalic vein

11  Tendon of abductor pollicis
    longus muscle
12  Tendon of extensor indicis
    muscle
13  Sternocleidomastoid muscle
14  Clavicle
15  Lateral head
    of triceps brachii muscle
16  Medial head
    of triceps brachii muscle
17  Tendon of triceps brachii muscle

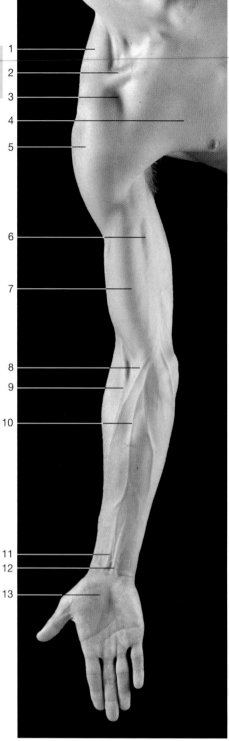

**Surface anatomy of the upper limb**
(right side, anterior aspect).

**Superficial veins of the arm** (right side, anterior aspect). The veins have been injected with blue gelatin.

| | |
|---|---|
| 1 Trapezius muscle | 8 Median cubital vein |
| 2 Clavicle | 9 Cephalic vein |
| 3 Deltopectoral triangle | 10 Median vein of forearm |
| 4 Pectoralis major muscle | 11 Tendon of flexor carpi radialis |
| 5 Deltoid muscle | 12 Tendon of palmaris longus muscle |
| 6 Brachial vein | 13 Location of adductor pollicis muscle |
| 7 Biceps brachii muscle | 14 Accessory cephalic vein |
| | 15 Basilic vein |

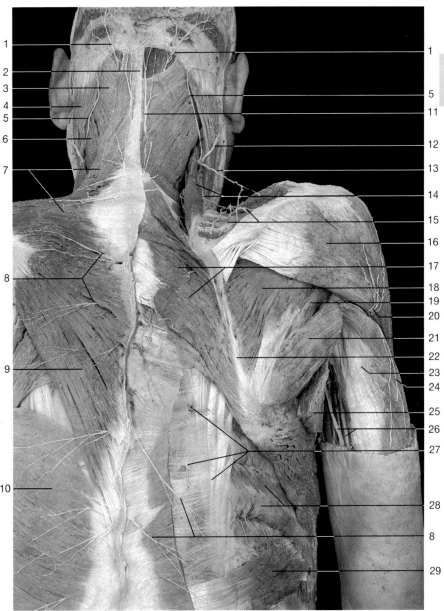

**Posterior regions of neck and shoulder** (left side: superficial layer; right side: trapezius and latissimus dorsi muscles have been removed). Dissection of dorsal branches of spinal nerves.

1   Greater occipital nerve
2   Ligamentum nuchae
3   Splenius capitis muscle
4   Sternocleidomastoid muscle
5   Lesser occipital nerve
6   Splenius cervicis muscle
7   Descending and transverse fibers of trapezius muscle
8   Medial cutaneous branches of dorsal rami of spinal nerves
9   Ascending fibers of trapezius muscle
10   Latissimus dorsi muscle
11   Cutaneous branch of third occipital nerve
12   Great auricular nerve
13   Accessory nerve (n. XI)
14   Posterior supraclavicular nerve and levator scapulae muscle
15   Branches of suprascapular artery

16   Deltoid muscle
17   Rhomboid major muscle
18   Infraspinatus muscle
19   Teres minor muscle
20   Upper lateral cutaneous nerve of arm (branch of axillary nerve)
21   Teres major muscle
22   Medial margin of scapula
23   Long head of triceps muscle
24   Posterior cutaneous nerve of arm (branch of radial nerve)
25   Latissimus dorsi muscle (divided)
26   Ulnar nerve and brachial artery
27   Lateral cutaneous branches of dorsal rami of spinal nerves and iliocostalis thoracis muscle
28   External intercostal muscle and seventh rib
29   Serratus posterior inferior muscle

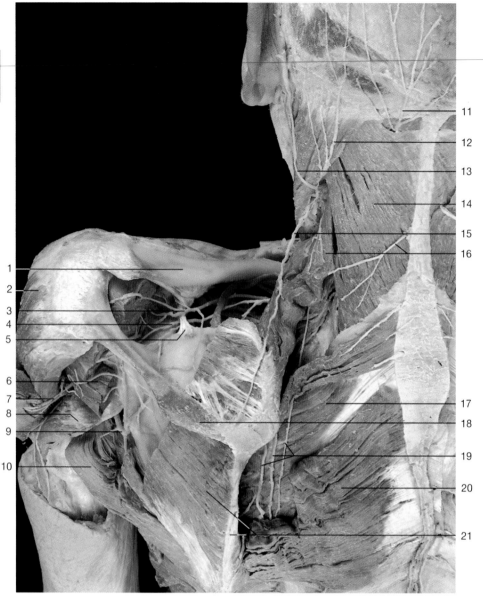

1   Clavicle
2   Deltoid muscle
3   Suprascapular artery
4   Suprascapular nerve
5   Superior transverse scapular
    ligament
6   Teres minor muscle
7   Axillary nerve and posterior
    circumflex humeral artery
8   Long head of triceps muscle
9   Circumflex scapular artery
10  Teres major muscle
11  Greater occipital nerve
12  Lesser occipital nerve
13  Great auricular nerve
14  Splenius capitis muscle
15  Accessory nerve (n. XI)
16  Third occipital nerve and
    levator scapulae muscle
17  Serratus posterior superior
    muscle
18  Spine of scapula
19  Descending scapular artery
    and dorsal scapular nerve
20  Rhomboid major muscle
21  Infraspinatus muscle and
    medial margin of scapula
22  Axillary artery
23  Radial nerve and brachial artery
24  Thoracodorsal artery
25  Thyrocervical trunk
26  Brachial plexus

**Posterior region of the shoulder,** deepest layer. Rhomboid and scapular muscles have been
fenestrated, the posterior part of deltoid muscle has been reflected.

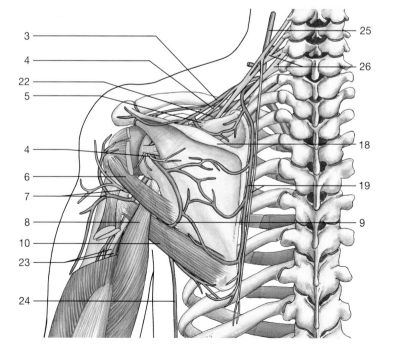

**Collateral circulation of the shoulder** (posterior
aspect). Anastomosis of suprascapular and circumflex
scapular arteries.

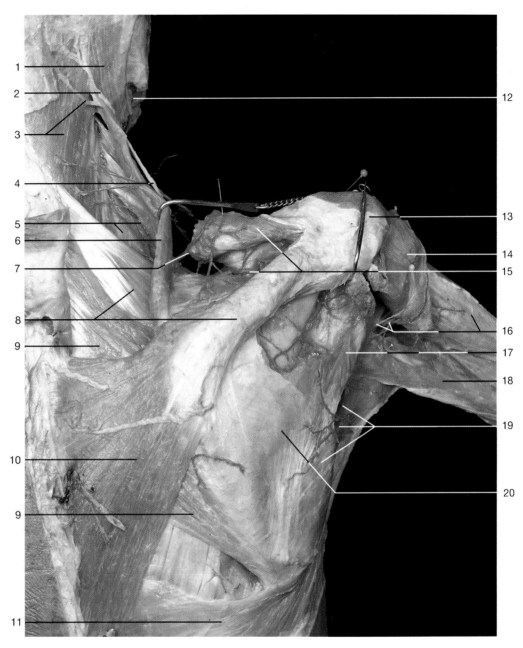

**Posterior region of the shoulder,** deep layer. The arteries of the scapular region have been injected with red gelatin. Trapezius, deltoid, and infraspinatus muscles have been partially removed or reflected.

| | | | |
|---|---|---|---|
| 1 | Sternocleidomastoid muscle | 10 | Trapezius muscle |
| 2 | Lesser occipital nerve | 11 | Latissimus dorsi muscle |
| 3 | Splenius capitis muscle and | 12 | Facial artery |
| | third occipital nerve | 13 | Acromion |
| 4 | Accessory nerve (n. XI) | 14 | Deltoid muscle |
| 5 | Splenius cervicis muscle and | 15 | Suprascapular artery and supraspinatus muscle |
| | transverse cervical artery (deep branch) | | (reflected) |
| 6 | Levator scapulae muscle | 16 | Axillary nerve, posterior circumflex humeral artery, |
| 7 | Transverse cervical artery | | and lateral head of triceps brachii muscle |
| | (superficial branch) | 17 | Teres minor muscle |
| 8 | Spine of scapula and | 18 | Long head of triceps brachii muscle |
| | serratus posterior superior muscle | 19 | Circumflex scapular artery and teres major muscle |
| 9 | Rhomboid major muscle | 20 | Infraspinatus muscle |

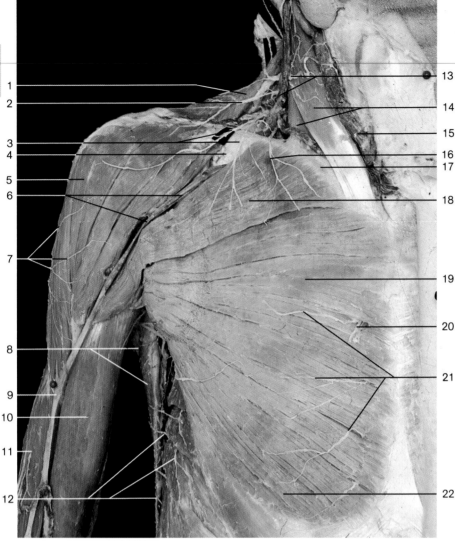

1 Trapezius muscle
2 Posterior supraclavicular nerve
3 Middle supraclavicular nerve
4 Deltopectoral triangle
5 Deltoid muscle
6 Cephalic vein
   within the deltopectoral groove
7 Upper lateral cutaneous nerve of arm
   (branch of axillary nerve)
8 Latissimus dorsi muscle
9 Cephalic vein
10 Biceps brachii muscle
11 Triceps brachii muscle
12 Lateral cutaneous branches
   of intercostal nerves
13 Transverse cervical nerve and
   external jugular vein
14 Sternocleidomastoid muscle
15 Anterior jugular vein
16 Anterior supraclavicular nerve
17 Clavicle
18 Clavicular part of pectoralis major muscle
19 Sternocostal part of pectoralis major
   muscle
20 Perforating branch of internal thoracic
   artery
21 Anterior cutaneous branches
   of intercostal nerves
22 Abdominal part of pectoralis major muscle
23 Sternocleidomastoid muscle,
   cervical branch of facial nerve, and
   anterior jugular vein
24 External jugular vein and
   transverse cervical nerve (inferior branch)
25 Sternoclavicular joint (opened)
   with articular disc
26 Pectoralis major muscle
27 Omohyoid muscle and
   external jugular vein
28 Jugular venous arch and sternohyoid muscle
29 Sternoclavicular joint (not opened)

**Anterior regions of shoulder and thoracic wall,** superficial layer. Dissection of the cutaneous nerves and veins.

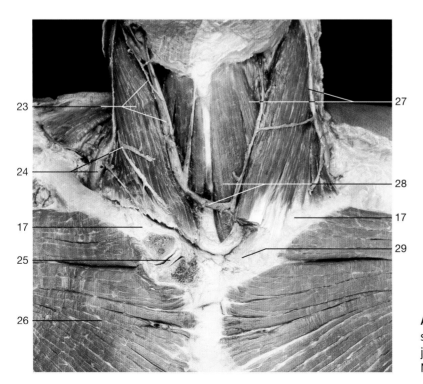

**Anterior regions of thoracic wall and neck.** The sternoclavicular joint is depicted. On the right side the joint has been opened by a coronal section. Note the articular disc.

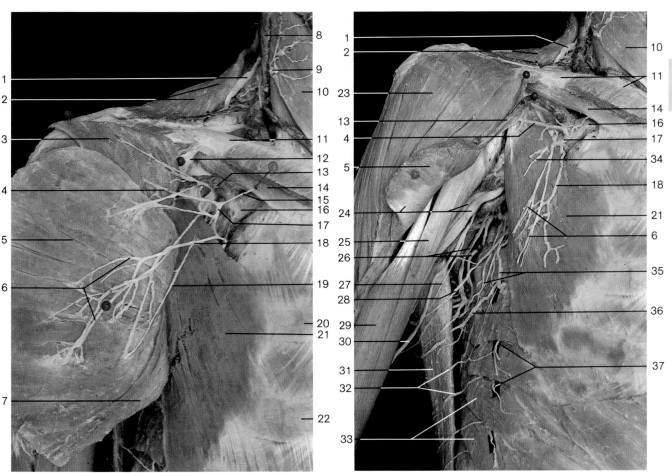

**Deltopectoral triangle and infraclavicular region** (anterior aspect). The pectoralis major muscle has been cut and reflected.

**Anterior regions of shoulder and thoracic wall** with axillary region, deep layer. The pectoralis major muscle has been cut and partly removed.

1   Accessory nerve
2   Trapezius muscle
3   Pectoralis major muscle (clavicular part)
4   Acromial branch of thoraco-acromial artery
5   Pectoralis major muscle
6   Lateral pectoral nerves
7   Abdominal part of pectoralis major muscle
8   External jugular vein
9   Cutaneous branches of cervical plexus
10  Sternocleidomastoid muscle
11  Clavicle
12  Clavipectoral fascia
13  Cephalic vein
14  Subclavius muscle
15  Clavicular branch of thoraco-acromial artery
16  Subclavian vein
17  Thoraco-acromial artery
18  Pectoral branch of thoraco-acromial artery
19  Medial pectoral nerve
20  Second rib

21  Pectoralis minor muscle
22  Third rib
23  Deltoid muscle
24  Pectoralis major muscle (reflected), brachial artery, and median nerve
25  Short head of biceps brachii muscle
26  Thoracodorsal artery and nerve
27  Medial cutaneous nerve of arm
28  Intercostobrachial nerve (Th$_2$)
29  Long head of biceps brachii muscle
30  Medial cutaneous nerve of forearm
31  Latissimus dorsi muscle
32  Lateral cutaneous branches of intercostal nerves (posterior branches)
33  Serratus anterior muscle
34  Medial pectoral nerve
35  Long thoracic nerve and lateral thoracic artery
36  Intercostobrachial nerve (Th$_3$)
37  Lateral cutaneous branches of intercostal nerves (anterior branches)

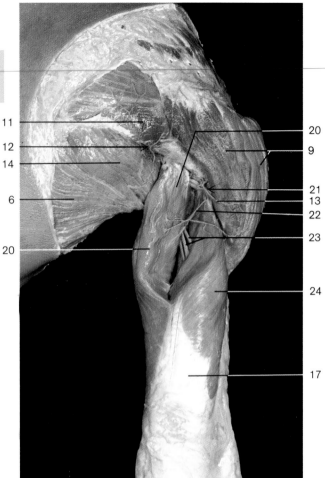

**Shoulder and arm** (posterior aspect). Dissection of the quadrangular and triangular spaces of the axillary region.

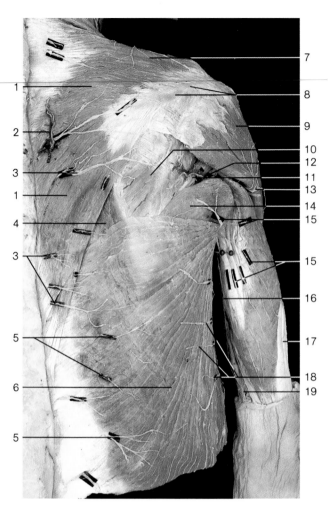

**Shoulder region and arm,** superficial layer (posterior aspect). Note the segmental arrangement of the cutaneous nerves of the back.

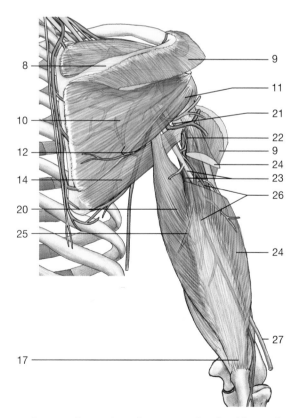

**Course of vessels and nerves at the shoulder region and arm** (posterior aspect).

1   Trapezius muscle
2   Dorsal branches of posterior intercostal artery and vein (medial cutaneous branches)
3   Medial branches of dorsal rami of spinal nerves
4   Rhomboid major muscle
5   Lateral branches of dorsal rami of spinal nerves
6   Latissimus dorsi muscle
7   Posterior supraclavicular nerves
8   Spine of scapula
9   Deltoid muscle
10  Infraspinatus muscle
11  Teres minor muscle
12  Triangular space with circumflex scapular artery and vein
13  Upper lateral cutaneous nerve of arm with artery
14  Teres major muscle
15  Terminal branches of intercostobrachial nerve
16  Medial cutaneous nerve of arm
17  Tendon of triceps brachii muscle
18  Lateral cutaneous branches of intercostal nerves
19  Medial cutaneous nerve of forearm
20  Long head of triceps brachii muscle
21  Quadrangular space with axillary nerve and posterior humeral circumflex artery
22  Anastomosis between profunda brachii artery and posterior humeral circumflex artery
23  Course of radial nerve and profunda brachii artery
24  Lateral head of triceps brachii muscle
25  Medial collateral artery
26  Radial collateral artery
27  Radial nerve

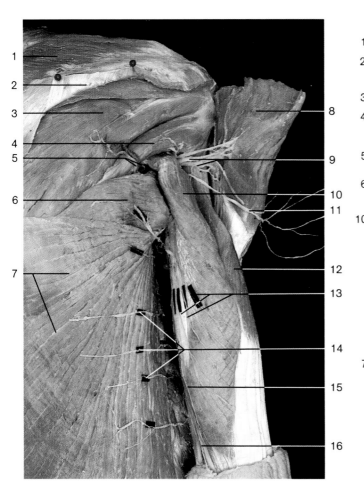

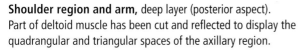

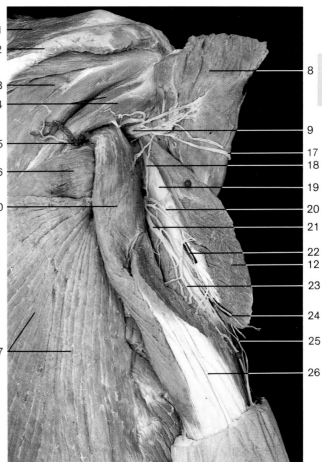

**Shoulder region and arm,** deep layer (posterior aspect). Part of deltoid muscle has been cut and reflected to display the quadrangular and triangular spaces of the axillary region.

**Shoulder region and arm,** deep layer (posterior aspect). The lateral head of the triceps brachii muscle has been cut to display the radial nerve and accompanying vessels.

1  Trapezius muscle
2  Spine of scapula
3  Infraspinatus muscle
4  Teres minor muscle
5  Triangular space containing circumflex scapular artery and vein
6  Teres major muscle
7  Latissimus dorsi muscle
8  Deltoid muscle (cut and reflected)
9  Quadrangular space containing axillary nerve and posterior circumflex humeral artery and vein
10  Long head of triceps brachii muscle
11  Cutaneous branch of axillary nerve
12  Lateral head of triceps brachii muscle
13  Terminal branches of intercostobrachial nerve

14  Lateral cutaneous branches of intercostal nerves
15  Medial cutaneous nerve of arm
16  Medial cutaneous nerve of forearm
17  Upper lateral cutaneous nerve of arm
18  Anastomosis between profunda brachii artery and posterior humeral circumflex artery
19  Humerus
20  Profunda brachii artery
21  Radial nerve
22  Radial collateral artery
23  Middle collateral artery
24  Lower lateral cutaneous nerve of arm
25  Posterior cutaneous nerve of forearm
26  Tendon of triceps brachii muscle

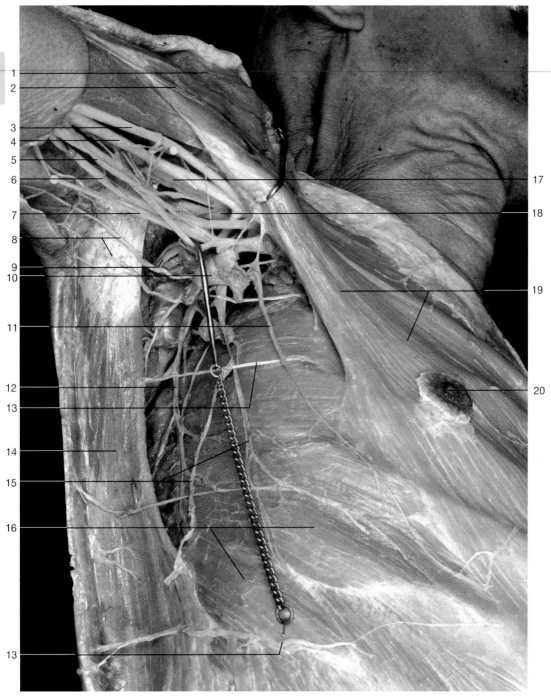

**Axillary region** (right side, inferior aspect). Dissection of superficial axillary lymph nodes and lymphatic vessels. The pectoralis major muscle has been slightly elevated.

| | | | |
|---|---|---|---|
| 1 | Deltoid muscle | 11 | Lateral thoracic artery |
| 2 | Cephalic vein | 12 | Thoracodorsal artery |
| 3 | Median nerve | 13 | Lateral cutaneous branch of intercostal nerve |
| 4 | Brachial artery | 14 | Latissimus dorsi muscle |
| 5 | Medial cutaneous nerves of arm and forearm | 15 | Thoraco-epigastric vein |
| 6 | Ulnar nerve | 16 | Serratus anterior muscle |
| 7 | Basilic vein | 17 | Musculocutaneous nerve |
| 8 | Intercostobrachial nerves | 18 | Radial nerve |
| 9 | Circumflex scapular artery | 19 | Pectoralis major muscle |
| 10 | Superficial axillary lymph nodes | 20 | Nipple |

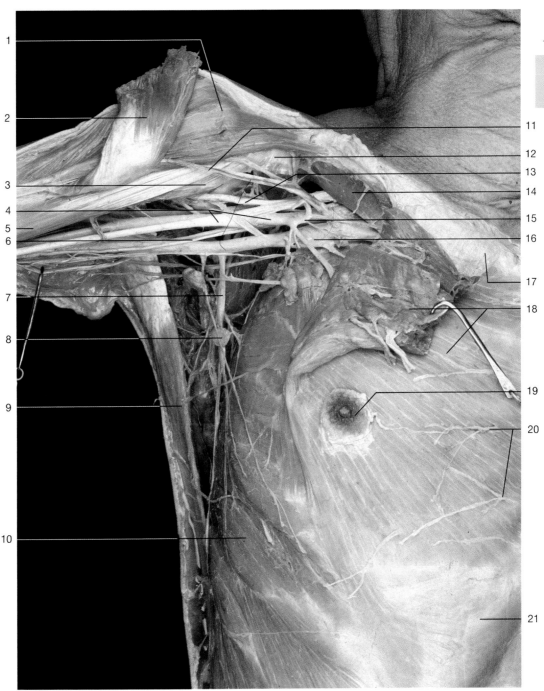

**Axillary region** (right side, anterior aspect). Dissection of deep axillary lymph nodes. Pectoralis major and minor muscles have been divided and reflected. Shoulder girdle and arm have been elevated and reflected.

| | | | |
|---|---|---|---|
| 1 | Deltoid muscle | 11 | Cephalic vein |
| 2 | Insertion of pectoralis major muscle | 12 | Insertion of pectoralis minor muscle (coracoid process) |
| 3 | Coracobrachialis muscle | 13 | Musculocutaneous nerve |
| 4 | Roots of median nerve and axillary artery | 14 | Subclavius muscle |
| 5 | Short head of biceps brachii muscle | 15 | Thoraco-acromial artery |
| 6 | Ulnar nerve and | 16 | Axillary vein |
| | medial cutaneous nerve of forearm | 17 | Clavicle |
| 7 | Thoraco-epigastric vein | 18 | Pectoralis major and minor muscles (reflected) |
| 8 | Deep axillary lymph nodes | 19 | Nipple |
| 9 | Latissimus dorsi muscle | 20 | Anterior cutaneous branches of intercostal nerves |
| 10 | Serratus anterior muscle | 21 | Anterior layer of rectus sheath |

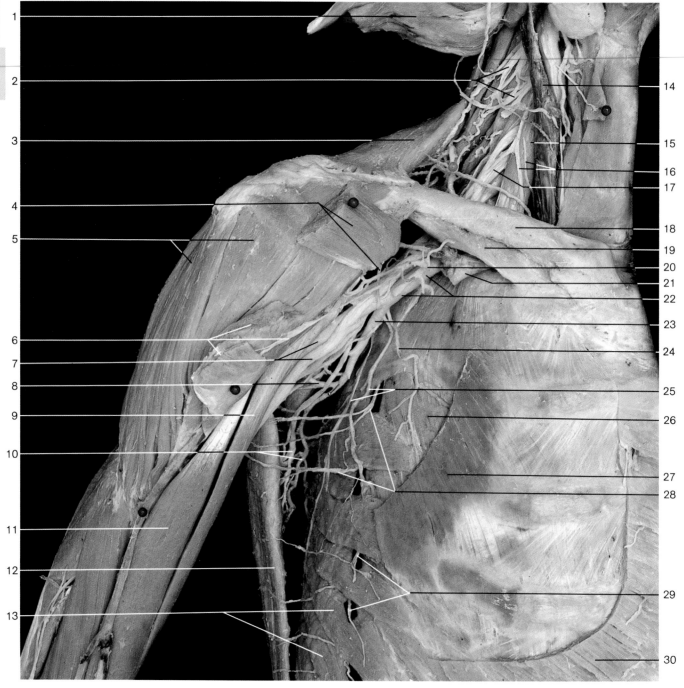

**Axillary region** (right side, anterior aspect). Pectoralis major and minor muscles have been cut and reflected to display the vessels and nerves of the axilla.

1  Sternocleidomastoid muscle (cut and reflected)
2  Cervical plexus
3  Trapezius muscle
4  Pectoralis minor muscle and medial pectoral nerve
5  Deltoid muscle
6  Pectoralis major muscle and lateral pectoral nerve
7  Median nerve and brachial artery
8  Circumflex scapular artery
9  Short head of biceps brachii muscle
10  Thoracodorsal artery and nerve
11  Long head of biceps brachii muscle
12  Latissimus dorsi muscle
13  Serratus anterior muscle
14  Internal jugular vein
15  Anterior scalene muscle

16  Phrenic nerve and ascending cervical artery
17  Brachial plexus (at the levels of the trunks)
18  Clavicle
19  Subclavius muscle
20  Thoraco-acromial artery
21  Subclavian vein (cut)
22  Axillary artery
23  Subscapular artery
24  Superior thoracic artery
25  Lateral thoracic artery and long thoracic nerve
26  External intercostal muscle
27  Insertion of pectoralis minor muscle
28  Intercostobrachial nerves
29  Lateral cutaneous branches of intercostal nerves
30  Insertion of pectoralis major muscle

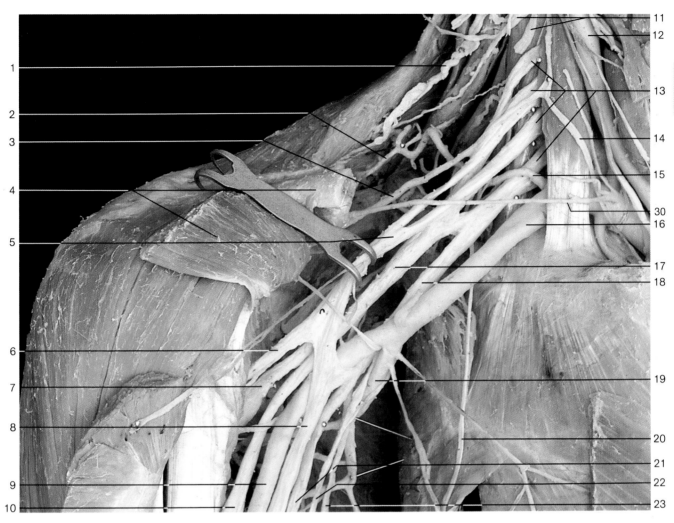

**Brachial plexus** (anterior aspect). The clavicle and the two pectoralis muscles have been partly removed.

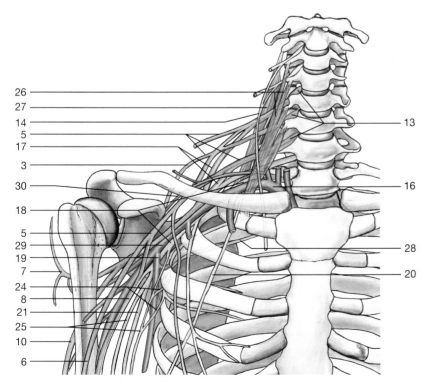

**Main branches of brachial plexus.** Posterior cord in orange, lateral cord in ocher, and medial cord in light yellow.

1 Accessory nerve
2 Dorsal scapular artery
3 Suprascapular nerve
4 Clavicle and pectoralis minor muscle
5 Lateral cord of brachial plexus
6 Musculocutaneous nerve
7 Axillary nerve
8 Median nerve
9 Brachial artery
10 Radial nerve
11 Cervical plexus
12 Common carotid artery
13 Roots of brachial plexus ($C_5$–$Th_1$)
14 Phrenic nerve
15 Transverse cervical artery
16 Subclavian artery
17 Posterior cord of brachial plexus
18 Medial cord of brachial plexus
19 Subscapular artery
20 Long thoracic nerve
21 Ulnar nerve
22 Medial cutaneous nerve of forearm
23 Thoracodorsal nerve
24 Intercostobrachial nerves
25 Medial cutaneous nerves
   of arm and forearm
26 Anterior scalene muscle
27 Middle scalene muscle
28 Intercostal nerve ($Th_3$)
29 Axillary artery
30 Suprascapular artery

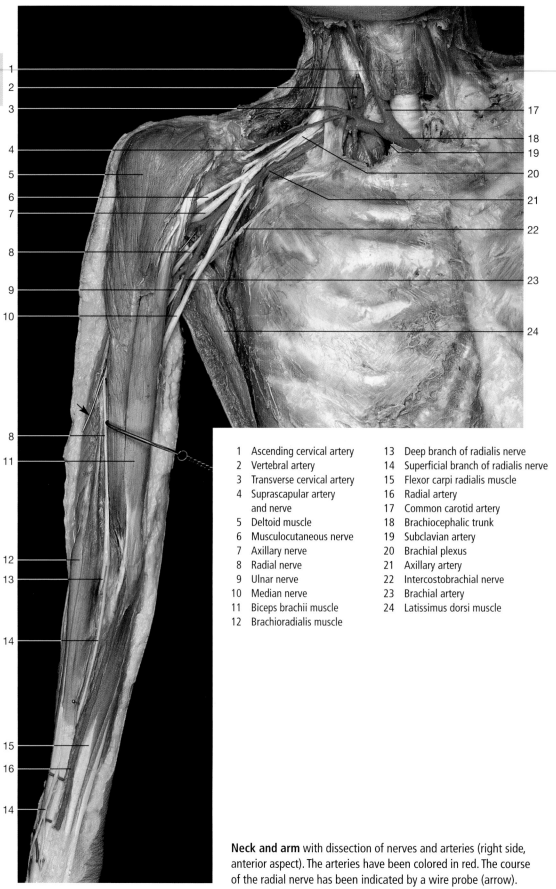

| | |
|---|---|
| 1 Ascending cervical artery | 13 Deep branch of radialis nerve |
| 2 Vertebral artery | 14 Superficial branch of radialis nerve |
| 3 Transverse cervical artery | 15 Flexor carpi radialis muscle |
| 4 Suprascapular artery | 16 Radial artery |
| and nerve | 17 Common carotid artery |
| 5 Deltoid muscle | 18 Brachiocephalic trunk |
| 6 Musculocutaneous nerve | 19 Subclavian artery |
| 7 Axillary nerve | 20 Brachial plexus |
| 8 Radial nerve | 21 Axillary artery |
| 9 Ulnar nerve | 22 Intercostobrachial nerve |
| 10 Median nerve | 23 Brachial artery |
| 11 Biceps brachii muscle | 24 Latissimus dorsi muscle |
| 12 Brachioradialis muscle | |

**Neck and arm** with dissection of nerves and arteries (right side, anterior aspect). The arteries have been colored in red. The course of the radial nerve has been indicated by a wire probe (arrow).

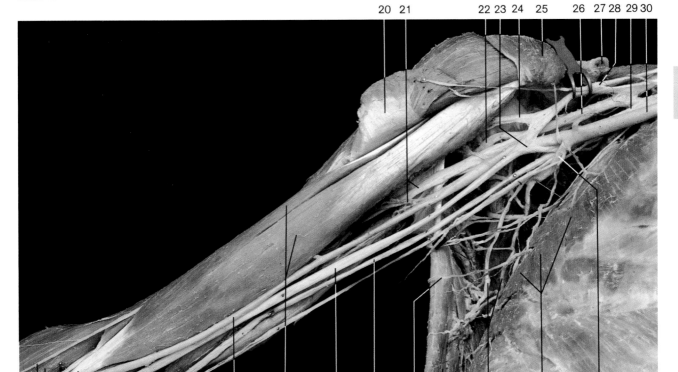

20  21        22 23 24  25      26  27 28 29 30

1  23 4   5 6 7  8 9 10  11    12    13      14      8    11   15  16    17      18      19

6          14        24        21        20    24

Arm with dissection of nerves and
vessels (right side, anterior aspect).
The shoulder girdle has been reflected
slightly.

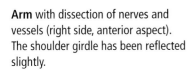

Arm with dissection of nerves and
vessels, deeper layer (right side, antero-
inferior aspect). The biceps brachii
muscle has been reflected.

8    31    11    13        16

| | | | |
|---|---|---|---|
| 1 | Radial artery and superficial branch of radial nerve | 8 | Median nerve |
| | | 9 | Medial epicondyle of humerus |
| 2 | Lateral cutaneous nerve of forearm | 10 | Inferior ulnar collateral artery |
| 3 | Brachioradialis muscle | 11 | Ulnar nerve |
| 4 | Ulnar artery | 12 | Medial cutaneous nerve of forearm |
| 5 | Tendon of biceps brachii muscle | 13 | Brachial artery |
| 6 | Brachialis muscle | 14 | Biceps brachii muscle |
| 7 | Pronator teres muscle | 15 | Intercostobrachial nerve (Th₃) |
| | | 16 | Latissimus dorsi muscle |

17  Thoracodorsal nerve and artery
18  Serratus anterior muscle
19  Subscapular artery
20  Pectoralis major muscle (reflected) and lateral pectoral nerve
21  Radial nerve and profunda brachii artery
22  Axillary nerve
23  Roots of the median nerve with axillary artery

24  Musculocutaneous nerve
25  Pectoralis minor muscle (reflected) and medial pectoral nerve
26  Posterior cord of brachial plexus
27  Clavicle (cut)
28  Lateral cord of brachial plexus
29  Medial cord of brachial plexus
30  Subclavian artery
31  Brachial vein

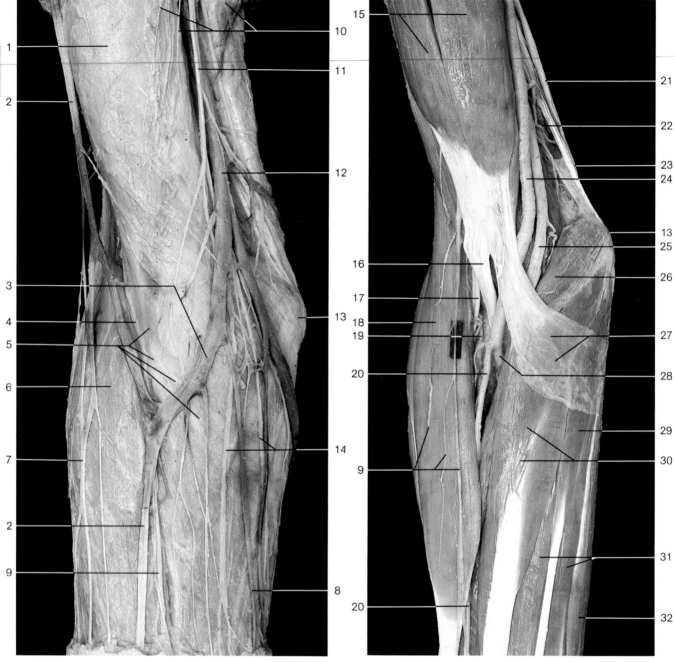

**Cubital region** (anterior aspect). Dissection of cutaneous nerves and veins.

**Cubital region,** superficial layer (anterior aspect). The fasciae of the muscles have been removed.

1   Biceps brachii muscle with fascia
2   Cephalic vein
3   Median cubital vein
4   Lateral cutaneous nerve of forearm
5   Tendon and aponeurosis of biceps brachii muscle (covered by the antebrachial fascia)
6   Brachioradialis muscle with fascia
7   Accessory cephalic vein
8   Median vein of forearm
9   Branches of lateral cutaneous nerve of forearm
10  Terminal branches of medial cutaneous nerve of arm
11  Medial cutaneous nerve of forearm
12  Basilic vein
13  Medial epicondyle of humerus
14  Terminal branches of medial cutaneous nerve of forearm
15  Biceps brachii muscle

16  Tendon of biceps brachii muscle
17  Radial nerve
18  Brachioradialis muscle
19  Radial recurrent artery
20  Radial artery
21  Ulnar nerve
22  Superior ulnar collateral artery
23  Medial intermuscular septum
24  Brachial artery
25  Median nerve
26  Pronator teres muscle
27  Bicipital aponeurosis
28  Ulnar artery
29  Palmaris longus muscle
30  Flexor carpi radialis muscle
31  Flexor digitorum superficialis muscle
32  Flexor carpi ulnaris muscle

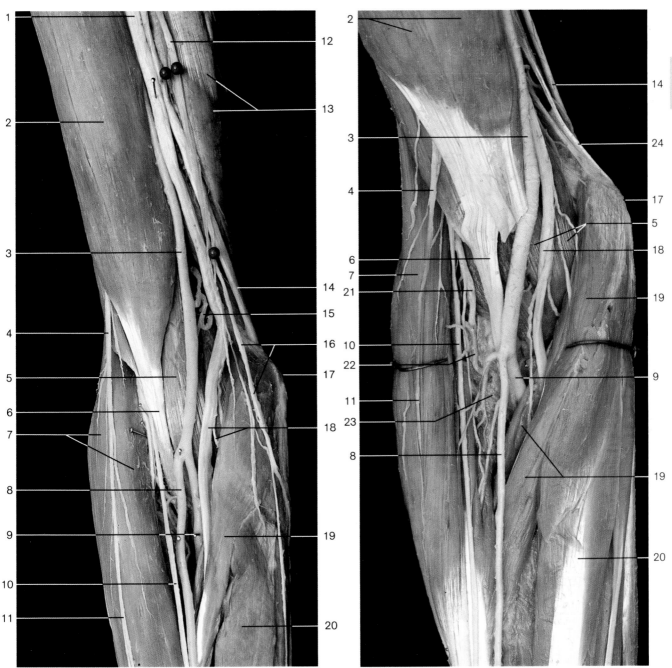

**Cubital region,** middle layer (anterior aspect). The bicipital aponeurosis has been removed.

**Cubital region,** middle layer (anterior aspect). Pronator teres and brachioradialis muscles have been slightly reflected.

| | |
|---|---|
| 1 Median nerve | 13 Triceps brachii muscle |
| 2 Biceps brachii muscle | 14 Ulnar nerve |
| 3 Brachial artery | 15 Inferior ulnar collateral artery |
| 4 Lateral cutaneous nerve of forearm (terminal branch of musculocutaneous nerve) | 16 Anterior branch of medial cutaneous nerve of forearm |
| 5 Brachialis muscle | 17 Medial epicondyle of humerus |
| 6 Tendon of biceps brachii muscle | 18 Median nerve with branches to pronator teres muscle |
| 7 Brachioradialis muscle | 19 Pronator teres muscle |
| 8 Radial artery | 20 Flexor carpi radialis muscle |
| 9 Ulnar artery | 21 Deep branch of radial nerve |
| 10 Superficial branch of radial nerve | 22 Radial recurrent artery |
| 11 Lateral cutaneous nerve of forearm | 23 Supinator muscle |
| 12 Medial cutaneous nerve of forearm | 24 Medial intermuscular septum of arm |

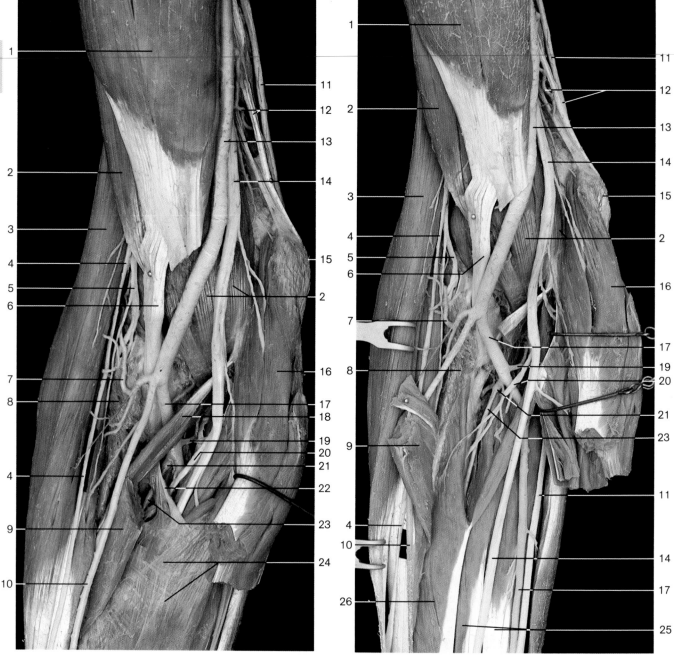

**Cubital region,** deep layer (anterior aspect). Pronator teres and flexor carpi ulnaris muscles have been cut and reflected.

**Cubital region,** deepest layer (anterior aspect). Flexor digitorum superficialis muscle and the ulnar head of the pronator teres muscle have been cut and reflected.

| | |
|---|---|
| 1 Biceps brachii muscle | 14 Median nerve |
| 2 Brachialis muscle | 15 Medial epicondyle of humerus |
| 3 Brachioradialis muscle | 16 Humeral head of pronator teres muscle |
| 4 Superficial branch of radial nerve | 17 Ulnar artery |
| 5 Deep branch of radial nerve | 18 Ulnar head of pronator teres muscle |
| 6 Tendon of biceps brachii muscle | 19 Ulnar recurrent artery |
| 7 Radial recurrent artery | 20 Anterior interosseous nerve |
| 8 Supinator muscle | 21 Common interosseous artery |
| 9 Insertion of pronator teres muscle | 22 Tendinous arch of flexor digitorum superficialis muscle |
| 10 Radial artery | 23 Anterior interosseous artery |
| 11 Ulnar nerve | 24 Flexor digitorum superficialis muscle |
| 12 Medial intermuscular septum of arm and superior ulnar collateral artery | 25 Flexor digitorum profundus muscle |
| 13 Brachial artery | 26 Flexor pollicis longus muscle |

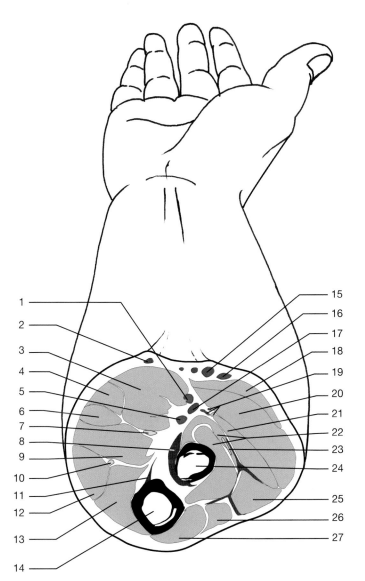

1   Radial artery
2   Basilic vein
3   Pronator teres muscle
4   Flexor carpi radialis muscle
5   Ulnar artery
6   Palmaris longus muscle
7   Median nerve
8   Tendon of biceps brachii muscle
9   Flexor digitorum superficialis muscle
10  Ulnar nerve
11  Tendon of brachialis muscle
12  Flexor carpi ulnaris muscle
13  Flexor digitorum profundus muscle
14  Ulna
15  Median cubital vein
16  Cephalic antebrachii vein
17  Radial vein
18  Brachioradialis muscle
19  Superficial branch of radial nerve,
    radial artery and vein
20  Extensor carpi radialis longus muscle
21  Extensor carpi radialis brevis muscle
22  Supinator muscle
23  Deep branch of radial nerve
24  Radius
25  Extensor digitorum muscle
26  Extensor carpi ulnaris muscle
27  Anconeus muscle

**Axial section through the forearm** distally of the elbow joint revealing the arrangement of muscles, nerves, and vessels (compare with the MRI scan below).

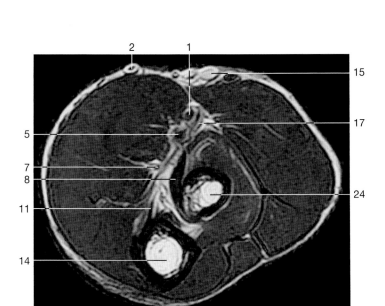

**Axial section through the forearm** distally of the elbow joint (MRI scan). (From Heuck et al., MRT-Atlas, 2009.) For details see schematic drawing above.

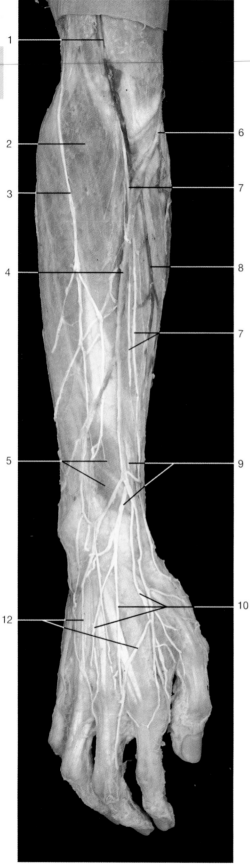

**Posterior regions of forearm and hand** with superficial veins and cutaneous nerves (right side).

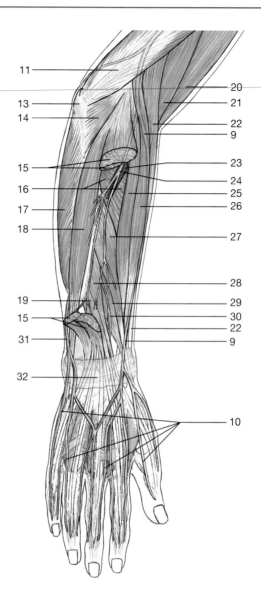

**Course of the nerves to forearm and hand**
(posterior aspect). Yellow = radial and ulnar nerves.

1   Cephalic vein
2   Brachioradialis muscle
    covered by its fascia
3   Posterior cutaneous nerve
    of forearm (branch of radial nerve)
4   Cephalic vein of forearm
5   Extensor pollicis longus and brevis
    muscles covered by their fascia
6   Median cubital vein
7   Lateral cutaneous nerves
    of forearm (branch of
    musculocutaneous nerve)
8   Intermedian vein of forearm
9   Superficial branch of radial nerve
10  Dorsal digital branches
    of radial nerve
11  Triceps brachii muscle
12  Dorsal venous network of hand
13  Olecranon
14  Anconeus muscle

15  Extensor digitorum and
    extensor digiti minimi muscles
16  Supinator muscle
17  Flexor carpi ulnaris muscle
18  Extensor carpi ulnaris muscle
19  Extensor indicis muscle
20  Biceps brachii muscle
21  Brachialis muscle
22  Brachioradialis muscle
23  Supinator channel
24  Deep branch of radial nerve
25  Extensor carpi radialis brevis muscle
26  Extensor carpi radialis longus muscle
27  Abductor pollicis longus muscle
28  Extensor pollicis longus muscle
29  Extensor pollicis brevis muscle
30  Posterior interosseus nerve
31  Ulnar nerve
32  Extensor retinaculum

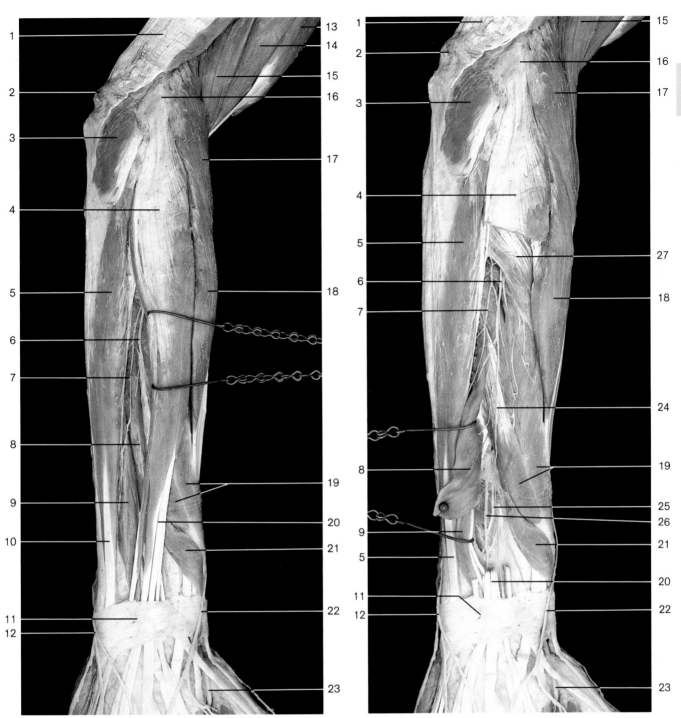

**Posterior region of the forearm** with vessels and nerves, superficial layer (right side).

**Posterior region of the forearm** with vessels and nerves, deep layer (right side).

| | | |
|---|---|---|
| 1 | Tendon of triceps brachii muscle | |
| 2 | Olecranon | |
| 3 | Anconeus muscle | |
| 4 | Extensor digitorum muscle | |
| 5 | Extensor carpi ulnaris muscle | |
| 6 | Deep branch of radial nerve | |
| 7 | Posterior interosseous artery | |
| 8 | Extensor pollicis longus muscle | |
| 9 | Extensor indicis muscle | |
| 10 | Tendon of extensor carpi ulnaris muscle | |
| 11 | Extensor retinaculum | |
| 12 | Dorsal branch of ulnar nerve | |
| 13 | Biceps brachii muscle | |
| 14 | Brachialis muscle | |
| 15 | Brachioradialis muscle | |
| 16 | Lateral epicondyle of humerus | |
| 17 | Extensor carpi radialis longus muscle | |
| 18 | Extensor carpi radialis brevis muscle | |
| 19 | Abductor pollicis longus muscle | |
| 20 | Tendons of extensor digitorum muscle | |
| 21 | Extensor pollicis brevis muscle | |
| 22 | Superficial branch of radial nerve | |
| 23 | Radial artery | |
| 24 | Posterior interosseous nerve | |
| 25 | Posterior interosseous branch of radial nerve | |
| 26 | Posterior branch of anterior interosseous artery | |
| 27 | Supinator muscle | |

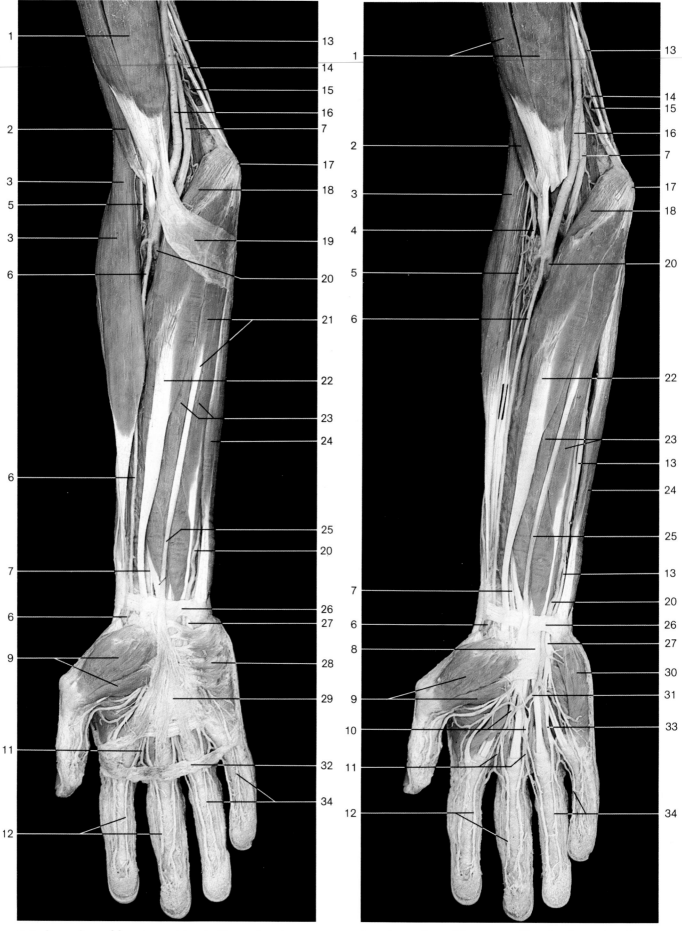

**Anterior regions of forearm and hand** with vessels and nerves, superficial layer (right side).

**Anterior regions of forearm and hand** with vessels and nerves, superficial layer (right side). The palmar aponeurosis of the hand and the bicipital aponeurosis have been removed.

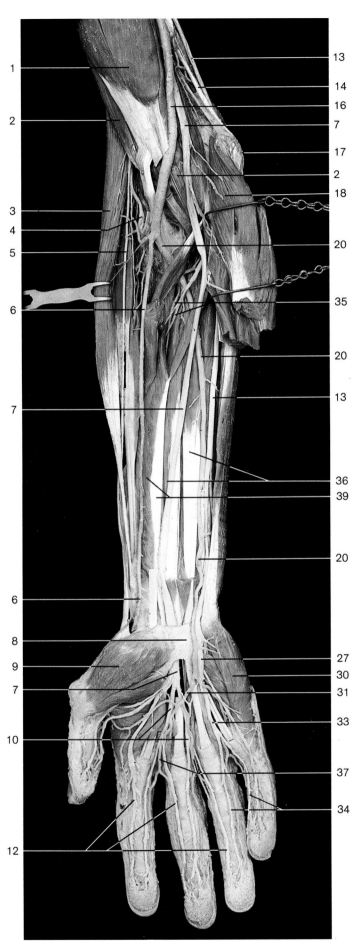

1   Biceps brachii muscle
2   Brachialis muscle
3   Brachioradialis muscle
4   Deep branch of radial nerve
5   Superficial branch of radial nerve
6   Radial artery
7   Median nerve
8   Flexor retinaculum
9   Thenar muscles
10  Common palmar digital nerves of median nerve
11  Common palmar digital arteries
12  Proper palmar digital nerves of median nerve
13  Ulnar nerve
14  Medial intermuscular septum of arm
15  Superior ulnar collateral artery
16  Brachial artery
17  Medial epicondyle of humerus
18  Pronator teres muscle
19  Bicipital aponeurosis
20  Ulnar artery
21  Palmaris longus muscle
22  Flexor carpi radialis muscle
23  Flexor digitorum superficialis muscle
24  Flexor carpi ulnaris muscle
25  Tendon of palmaris longus muscle
26  Remnant of antebrachial fascia
27  Superficial branch of ulnar nerve
28  Palmaris brevis muscle
29  Palmar aponeurosis
30  Hypothenar muscles
31  Superficial palmar arch
32  Superficial transverse metacarpal ligament
33  Common palmar digital branch of ulnar nerve
34  Proper palmar digital branches of ulnar nerve
35  Anterior interosseous artery and nerve
36  Flexor digitorum profundus muscle
37  Common palmar digital arteries
38  Palmar branch of median nerve
39  Flexor pollicis longus muscle
40  Palmar cutaneous branch of ulnar nerve

**Anterior regions of forearm and hand** with vessels and nerves, deep layer (right side). The superficial layer of the flexor muscles has been removed.

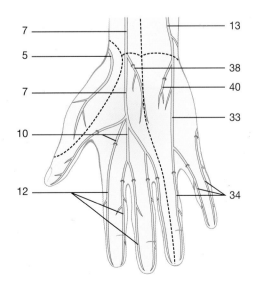

**Innervation pattern of the hand** (palmar aspect).
3½ digits by median nerve, 1½ digits by ulnar nerve.

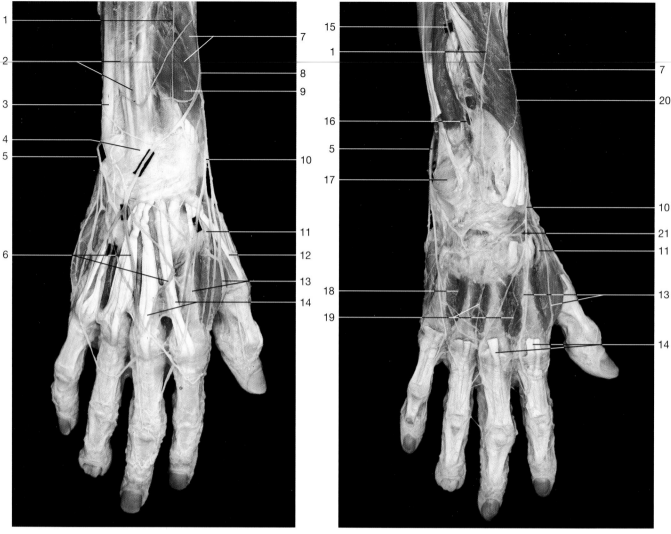

**Dorsum of the right hand,** superficial layer. Cutaneous nerves and veins are depicted.

**Dorsum of the right hand,** deeper layer. Extensor digitorum muscle has been partly removed.

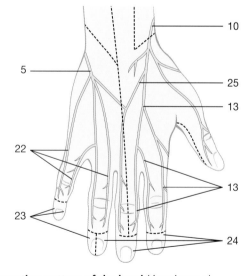

**Innervation pattern of the hand** (dorsal aspect).
2¹⁄₂ digits by radial nerve, 2¹⁄₂ digits by ulnar nerve.
Note that the terminal branches to the dorsal surfaces of the distal phalanges are derived from the palmar digital nerves. The cutaneous distribution varies; often 3¹⁄₂ digits are innervated by the radial and 1¹⁄₂ digits by the ulnar nerve.

1 Posterior cutaneous nerve of forearm (branch of radial nerve)
2 Extensor digitorum muscle
3 Tendon of extensor carpi ulnaris muscle
4 Extensor retinaculum
5 Ulnar nerve
6 Dorsal venous network of hand
7 Abductor pollicis brevis muscle
8 Cephalic vein
9 Extensor pollicis brevis muscle
10 Superficial branch of radial nerve
11 Radial artery
12 Tendon of extensor pollicis longus muscle
13 Dorsal digital branches of radial nerve
14 Tendons of extensor digitorum muscle with intertendinous connections
15 Posterior interosseus nerve (branch of the deep radial nerve)
16 Posterior interosseous artery
17 Styloid process of ulna
18 Dorsal interosseus muscle
19 Dorsal carpal branch of radial artery
20 Lateral cutaneous nerve of forearm
   (branch of musculocutaneous nerve)
21 Dorsal metacarpal artery
22 Dorsal digital branches of ulnar nerve
23 Regions supplied by palmar digital nerves (ulnar nerve)
24 Regions supplied by palmar digital nerves (median nerve)
25 Communicating branch with ulnar nerve

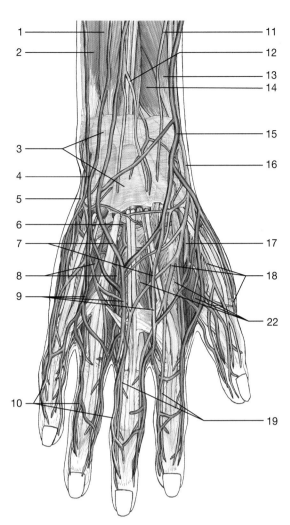

1  Extensor digiti minimi muscle
2  Extensor carpi ulnaris muscle
3  Extensor retinaculum
4  Basilic vein
5  Dorsal branch of ulnar nerve
6  Dorsal carpal branch of ulnar artery
7  Dorsal venous network of hand
8  Dorsal metacarpal arteries
9  Dorsal metacarpal veins
10  Dorsal digital veins
11  Lateral cutaneous nerve of forearm
12  Posterior cutaneous nerve of forearm
13  Abductor pollicis longus muscle
14  Abductor pollicis brevis muscle
15  Cephalic vein
16  Superficial branch of radial nerve
17  Radial artery
18  Dorsal digital branches of radial nerve
19  Dorsal digital nerves for the fingers
20  Hamate bone
21  Capitate bone
22  Dorsal interossei muscles
23  Collateral ligament
24  Proximal phalanges II–V
25  Middle phalanges II–V
26  Distal phalanges IV and V
27  Os trapezoideum
28  Metacarpal bones II–IV
29  Opponens pollicis muscle
30  Second metacarpophalangeal joint
31  Proper palmar digital artery

**Dorsum of the right hand,** superficial layer.
Cutaneous veins, nerves, and arteries are depicted.
The dorsal fascia of the hand has been removed.

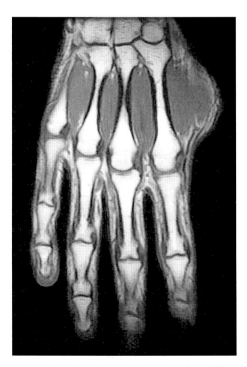

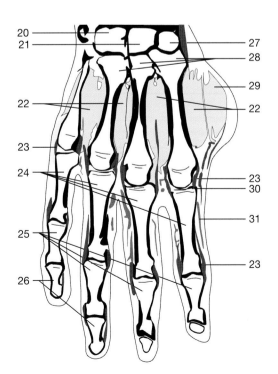

**Coronal section through the right hand** (dorsal aspect). (From Heuck et al., MRT-Atlas, 2009.)
For details see the schematic drawing alongside.

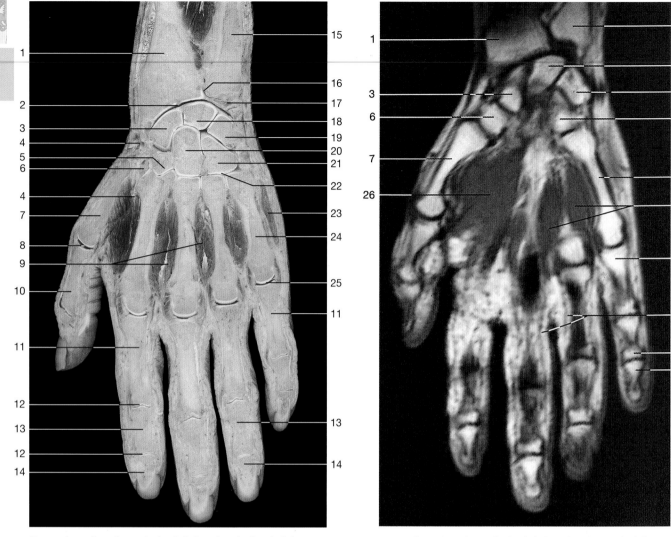

**Coronal section through the left hand** at the level of the interossei muscles (dorsal aspect).

**Coronal section through the left hand** at the level of the interossei muscles (dorsal aspect; MRI scan).
(Courtesy of Prof. Heuck, Munich, Germany.)

| | | | | | |
|---|---|---|---|---|---|
| 1 | Radius | 10 | Proximal phalanx of thumb | 19 | Triquetral bone |
| 2 | Radiocarpal joint | 11 | Proximal phalanx of fingers | 20 | Capitate bone |
| 3 | Scaphoid (navicular) bone | 12 | Interphalangeal joints | 21 | Hamate bone |
| 4 | Radial artery | 13 | Middle phalanx | 22 | Carpometacarpal joints |
| 5 | Trapezoid bone | 14 | Distal phalanx | 23 | Abductor digiti minimi muscle |
| 6 | Trapezium bone | 15 | Ulna | 24 | Fifth metacarpal bone |
| 7 | First metacarpal bone | 16 | Distal radio-ulnar joint | 25 | Metacarpophalangeal joint |
| 8 | Metacarpophalangeal joint of thumb | 17 | Articular disc | 26 | Adductor pollicis muscle |
| 9 | Interossei muscles | 18 | Lunate bone | 27 | Proper palmar digital arteries |

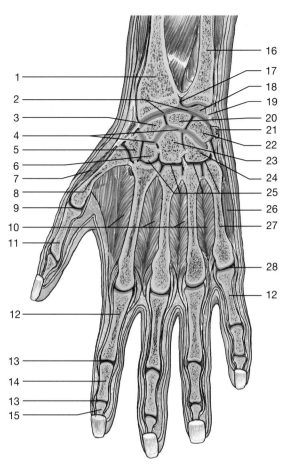

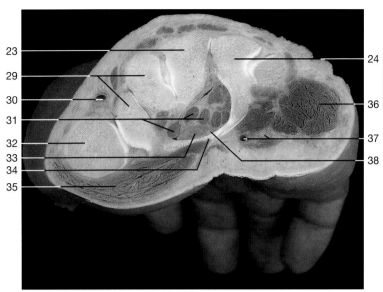

**Axial section through the right hand** at the level of the carpal tunnel (proximal aspect).

**Coronal section through the left hand** at the level of the interossei muscles (dorsal aspect).

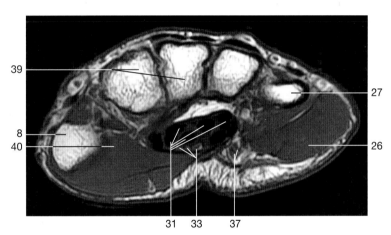

**Axial section through the right hand** at the level of the carpal tunnel (proximal aspect; MRI scan). (Courtesy of Prof. Heuck, Munich, Germany.)

| | |
|---|---|
| 1 | Radius |
| 2 | Radiocarpal joint |
| 3 | Scaphoid (navicular) bone |
| 4 | Metacarpal joint |
| 5 | Trapezium bone |
| 6 | Trapezoid bone |
| 7 | Opponens pollicis muscle |
| 8 | First metacarpal bone |
| 9 | First metacarpophalangeal joint |
| 10 | Interossei muscles |
| 11 | Proximal phalanx of thumb |
| 12 | Proximal phalanx of fingers |
| 13 | Interphalangeal joints |
| 14 | Middle phalanx |

| | |
|---|---|
| 15 | Distal phalanx |
| 16 | Ulna |
| 17 | Distal radio-ulnar joint |
| 18 | Articular disc |
| 19 | Ulnar collateral ligament |
| 20 | Lunate bone |
| 21 | Pisiforme bone |
| 22 | Triquetral bone |
| 23 | Capitate bone |
| 24 | Hamate bone |
| 25 | Carpometacarpal joints |
| 26 | Abductor digiti minimi muscle |
| 27 | Fifth metacarpal bone |
| 28 | Metacarpophalangeal joints |

| | |
|---|---|
| 29 | Trapezium and trapezoid bones |
| 30 | Radial artery |
| 31 | Tendons of flexor digitorum superficialis and profundus muscles |
| 32 | First metacarpal bone |
| 33 | Median nerve |
| 34 | Flexor retinaculum |
| 35 | Thenar muscles |
| 36 | Hypothenar muscles |
| 37 | Ulnar artery and nerve |
| 38 | Carpal tunnel |
| 39 | Second and third metacarpal bones |
| 40 | Adductor pollicis muscle |

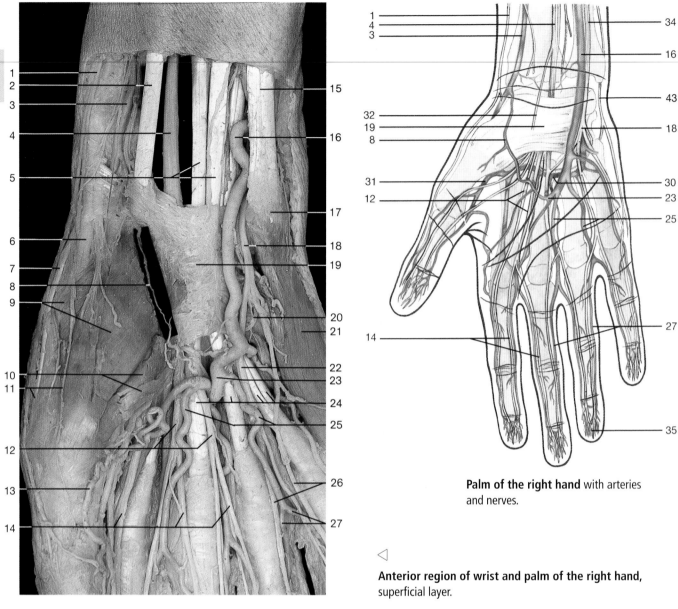

1
2
3
4
5
6
7
8
9
10
11
12
13
14

15
16
17
18
19
20
21
22
23
24
25
26
27

1
4
3

32
19
8

31
12

14

34
16

43
18

30
23
25

27

35

**Palm of the right hand** with arteries and nerves.

◁

**Anterior region of wrist and palm of the right hand,** superficial layer.

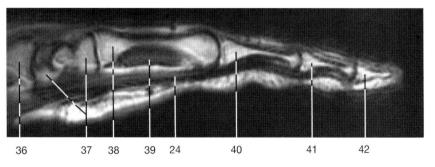

38    39    44    40    41    42

**Longitudinal section through the hand** at the level of the third finger.

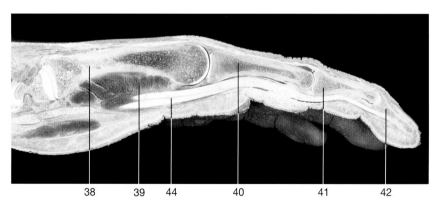

36    37    38    39    24    40    41    42

**Longitudinal section through the hand** at the level of the third finger (MRI scan). (Courtesy of Prof. Heuck, Munich, Germany.)

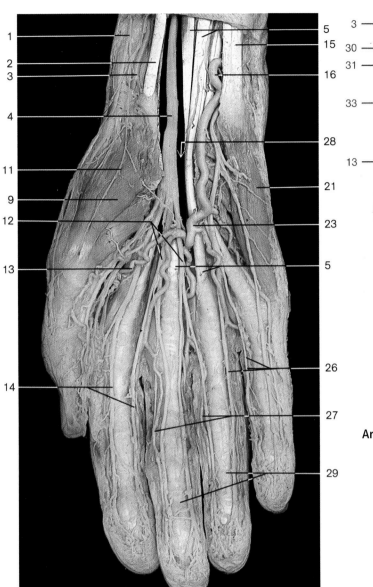

**Palm of the right hand,** middle layer. The flexor retinaculum has been removed.

**Arteriogram of the right hand** (palmar aspect).

1 Superficial branch of radial nerve
2 Tendon of flexor carpi radialis muscle
3 Radial artery
4 Median nerve
5 Tendon of flexor digitorum superficialis muscle
6 Tendon of abductor pollicis longus muscle
7 Tendon of extensor pollicis brevis muscle
8 Superficial palmar branch of radial artery
9 Abductor pollicis brevis muscle
10 Superficial head of flexor pollicis brevis muscle
11 Terminal branches of superficial branch of radial nerve
12 Common palmar digital nerves (median nerve)
13 Proper palmar digital arteries of thumb
14 Proper palmar digital nerves (median nerve)
15 Tendon of flexor carpi ulnaris muscle
16 Ulnar artery
17 Position of pisiform bone
18 Superficial branch of ulnar nerve
19 Flexor retinaculum
20 Deep branch of ulnar nerve
21 Abductor digiti minimi muscle
22 Common palmar digital nerve (ulnar nerve)

23 Superficial palmar arch
24 Tendons of flexor digitorum muscles
25 Common palmar digital arteries
26 Palmar digital nerves (ulnar nerve)
27 Proper palmar digital arteries
28 Carpal tunnel
29 Fibrous sheaths for the tendons of flexor digitorum muscles
30 Deep palmar arch
31 Princeps pollicis artery
32 Palmar branch of median nerve
33 Common digital palmar artery
34 Ulnar nerve
35 Capillary network of fingers
36 Radius
37 Carpal bones
38 Metacarpal bone
39 Interossei muscles
40 Proximal phalanx
41 Middle phalanx
42 Distal phalanx
43 Dorsal branch of ulnar nerve
44 Tendons of flexor digitorum profundus (upper) and superficialis (lower) muscles

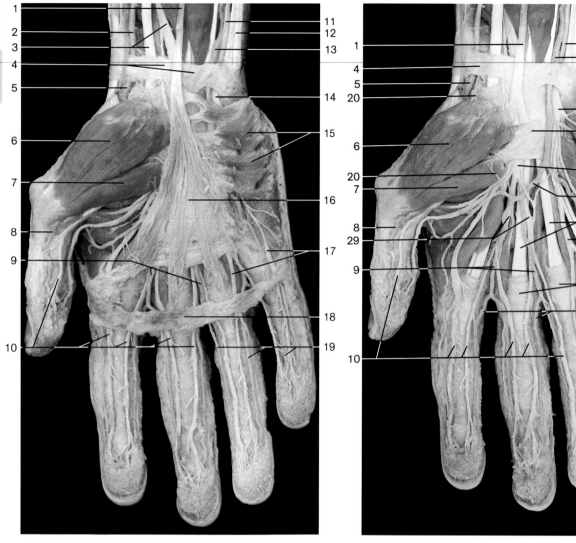

**Palm of the right hand,** superficial layer. Dissection of vessels and nerves.

**Palm of the right hand,** superficial layer. Dissection of vessels and nerves. The palmar aponeurosis has been removed to display the superficial palmar arch.

| | | | |
|---|---|---|---|
| 1 | Tendon of palmaris longus muscle | 17 | Palmar digital nerves (ulnar nerve) |
| 2 | Radial artery | 18 | Superficial transverse metacarpal ligament |
| 3 | Tendon of flexor carpi radialis muscle and median nerve | 19 | Proper palmar digital arteries |
| 4 | Distal part of antebrachial fascia | 20 | Superficial palmar branch of radial artery (contributing to the superficial palmar arch) |
| 5 | Radial artery passing into the anatomical snuffbox | 21 | Flexor retinaculum |
| 6 | Abductor pollicis brevis muscle | 22 | Median nerve |
| 7 | Superficial head of flexor pollicis brevis muscle | 23 | Abductor digiti minimi muscle |
| 8 | Palmar digital artery of thumb | 24 | Flexor digiti minimi brevis muscle |
| 9 | Common palmar digital arteries | 25 | Opponens digiti minimi muscle |
| 10 | Proper palmar digital nerves (median nerve) | 26 | Superficial palmar arch |
| 11 | Ulnar nerve | 27 | Tendons of flexor digitorum superficialis muscle |
| 12 | Tendon of flexor carpi ulnaris muscle | 28 | Common palmar digital branch of ulnar nerve |
| 13 | Ulnar artery | 29 | Common palmar digital branches of median nerve |
| 14 | Superficial branch of ulnar nerve | 30 | Fibrous sheaths of tendons of flexor muscles |
| 15 | Palmaris brevis muscle | | |
| 16 | Palmar aponeurosis | | |

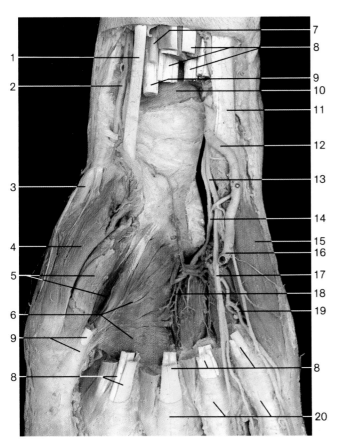

**Anterior region of wrist and palm of the right hand,** deep layer. The carpal tunnel has been opened, the tendons of the flexor muscles have been removed, and the superficial palmar arch has been cut.

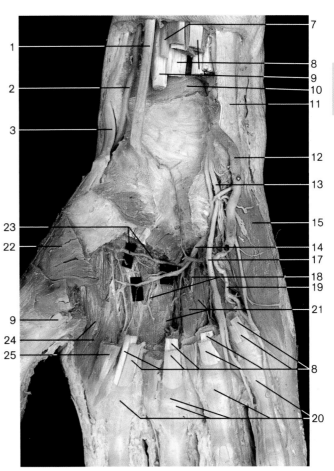

**Anterior region of wrist and palm of the right hand,** deep layer. Dissection of the deep palmar arch.

| | |
|---|---|
| 1 | Tendon of flexor carpi radialis muscle |
| 2 | Radial artery |
| 3 | Tendon of abductor pollicis longus muscle |
| 4 | Abductor pollicis brevis muscle |
| 5 | Superficial and deep heads of flexor pollicis brevis muscle |
| 6 | Oblique and transverse heads of adductor pollicis muscle |
| 7 | Median nerve |
| 8 | Tendons of flexor digitorum superficialis and profundus muscles |
| 9 | Tendon of flexor pollicis longus muscle |
| 10 | Pronator quadratus muscle |
| 11 | Tendon of flexor carpi ulnaris muscle |
| 12 | Ulnar artery |

| | |
|---|---|
| 13 | Superficial branch of ulnar nerve |
| 14 | Deep branch of ulnar nerve |
| 15 | Abductor digiti minimi muscle |
| 16 | Superficial palmar arch (cut end) |
| 17 | Common palmar digital nerve (ulnar nerve) |
| 18 | Palmar metacarpal arteries of deep palmar arch |
| 19 | Palmar digital artery of the fifth finger |
| 20 | Fibrous sheaths of tendons of flexor muscles |
| 21 | Palmar interossei muscles |
| 22 | Opponens pollicis muscle (cut) |
| 23 | Deep palmar arch |
| 24 | First dorsal interosseous muscle |
| 25 | First lumbrical muscle |

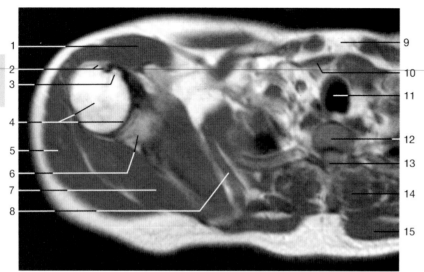

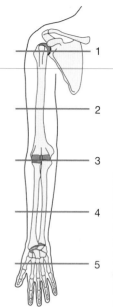

**Horizontal section through the right shoulder joint.** Section 1 (MRI scan, inferior aspect).

**Upper limb, location of sections 1–5** (MRI scans, p. 444: courtesy of Prof. Heuck, Munich, Germany; MRI scans, p. 445: courtesy of Prof. Bautz and Dr. Janka, Univ. Erlangen-Nuremberg, Germany).

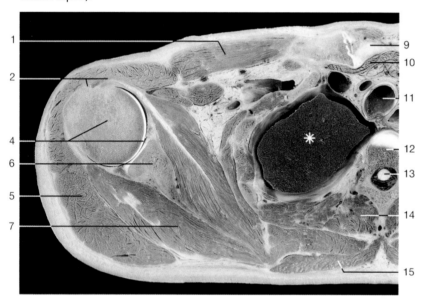

**Horizontal section through the right shoulder joint.** Section 1 (inferior aspect).
\* = Upper lobe of lung.

1　Pectoralis major muscle
2　Greater tubercle and tendon of biceps muscle
3　Lesser tubercle
4　Head of humerus and articular cavity of shoulder joint
5　Deltoid muscle
6　Scapula
7　Infraspinatus muscle
8　Serratus anterior muscle
9　Sternum
10　Infrahyoid muscles
11　Trachea
12　Body of thoracic vertebra
13　Vertebral canal and spinal cord
14　Deep muscles of the back
15　Trapezius muscle
16　Brachialis muscle
17　Radial nerve and profunda brachii artery

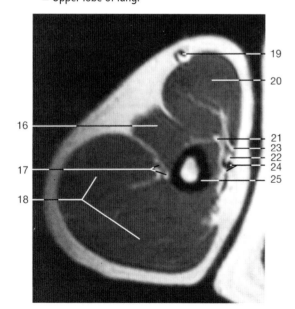

**Axial section through the middle of the right arm.** Section 2 (MRI scan, inferior aspect).

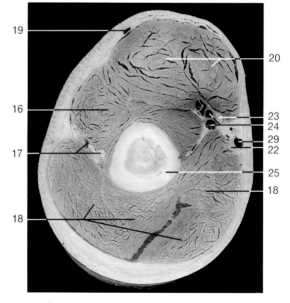

**Axial section through the middle of the right arm.** Section 2 (inferior aspect).

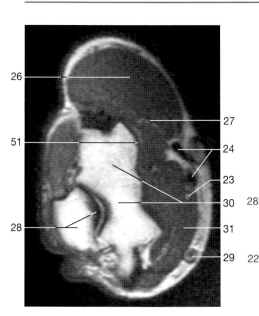

**Axial section through the right elbow joint.** Section 3 (MRI scan, inferior aspect).

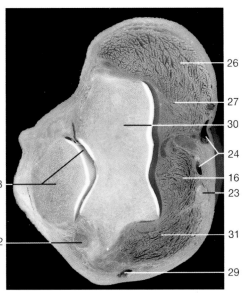

**Axial section through the right elbow joint.** Section 3 (inferior aspect).

18 Triceps brachii muscle
19 Cephalic vein
20 Biceps brachii muscle
21 Musculocutaneous nerve
22 Ulnar nerve
23 Median nerve
24 Brachial artery and vein
25 Shaft of humerus
26 Brachioradialis muscle
27 Radial nerve
28 Olecranon and
   articular cavity of elbow joint
29 Basilic vein
30 Humerus
31 Pronator teres muscle
32 Extensor muscles of forearm
33 Deep branch of radial nerve
34 Anterior interosseus artery
   and nerve
35 Interosseous membrane
36 Ulna
37 Radius
38 Superficial branch
   of radial artery
39 Flexor pollicis longus muscle
40 Flexor digitorum superficialis
   and profundus muscles
41 Ulnar nerve, artery, and vein
42 Flexor carpi ulnaris muscle
43 Radial artery
44 Third and fourth metacarpal
   bones
45 Carpal tunnel with tendons
   of flexor digitorum muscles
46 Hypothenar muscles
47 Median nerve
48 Interossei muscles
49 First metacarpal bone
50 Thenar muscles
51 Articular cavity
   of humeroradial joint

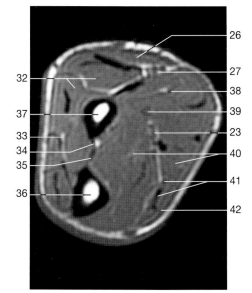

**Axial section through the middle of the right forearm.** Section 4 (MRI scan, inferior aspect).

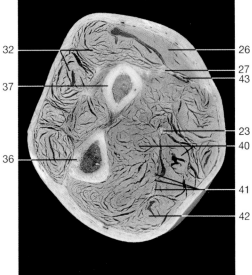

**Axial section through the middle of the right forearm.** Section 4 (inferior aspect).

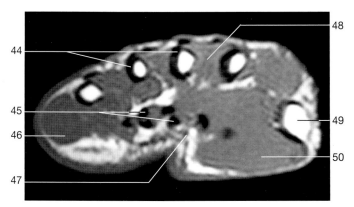

**Axial section through the right hand** at the level of the metacarpus. Section 5 (MRI scan, inferior aspect).

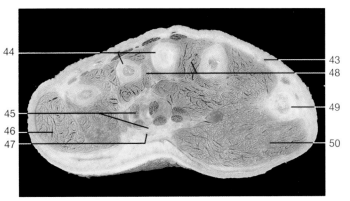

**Axial section through the right hand** at the level of the metacarpus. Section 5 (inferior aspect).

# 8 Lower Limb

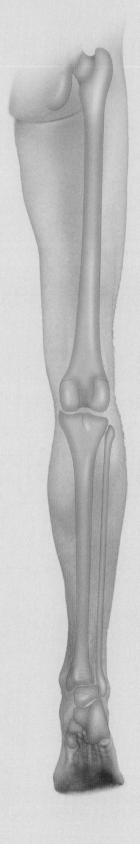

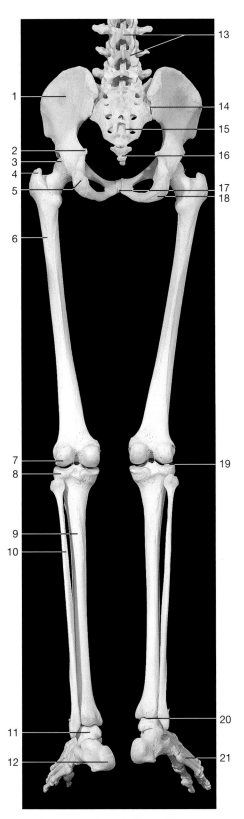

**Skeleton of pelvic girdle and lower limb** (posterior aspect).

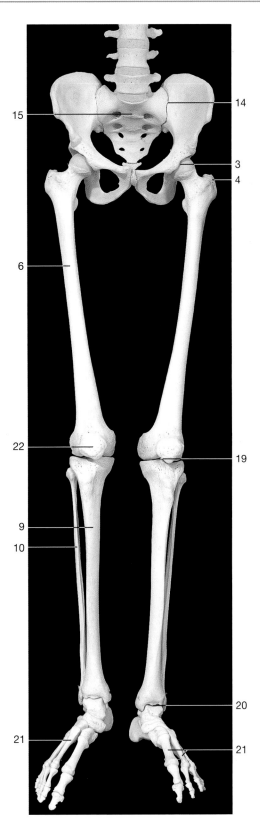

**Skeleton of pelvic girdle and lower limb** (anterior aspect).

| | | | | | |
|---|---|---|---|---|---|
| 1 | Ilium | 9 | Tibia | 17 | Pubic symphysis |
| 2 | Ischial spine | 10 | Fibula | 18 | Ischial tuberosity |
| 3 | Hip joint | 11 | Talus | 19 | Knee joint |
| 4 | Greater trochanter | 12 | Calcaneus | 20 | Ankle joint |
| 5 | Ischial tuberosity | 13 | Lumbar vertebrae | 21 | Metatarsal bones |
| 6 | Femur | 14 | Sacro-iliac joint | 22 | Patella |
| 7 | Lateral condyle of femur | 15 | Sacrum | | |
| 8 | Lateral condyle of tibia | 16 | Coccyx | | |

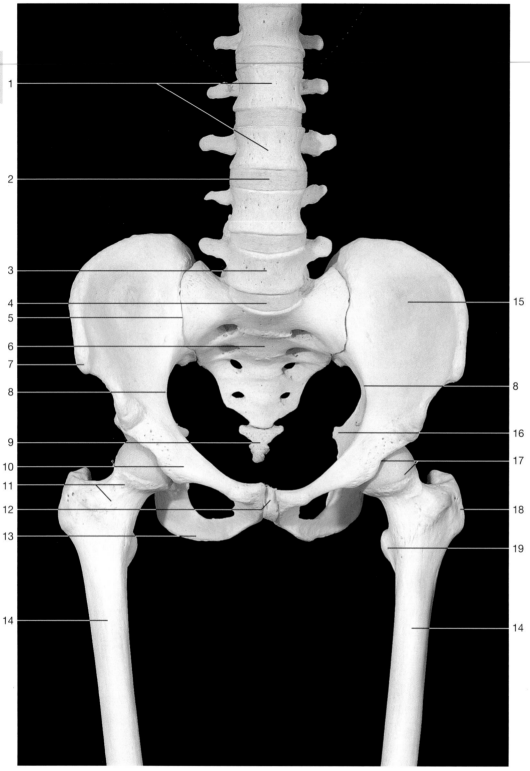

**Lumbar vertebrae and skeleton of pelvic girdle with both femurs** (anterior aspect).

1  Second and third lumbar vertebrae
2  Intervertebral disc
3  Fifth lumbar vertebra
4  Intervertebral disc between fifth lumbar vertebra and sacrum
5  Sacro-iliac joint
6  Sacrum
7  Anterior superior iliac spine
8  Linea terminalis
9  Coccyx
10  Pubis

11  Neck of femur
12  Pubic symphysis
13  Ischial tuberosity
14  Femur
15  Iliac fossa
16  Ischial spine
17  Head of femur (and localization of hip joint)
18  Greater trochanter
19  Lesser trochanter

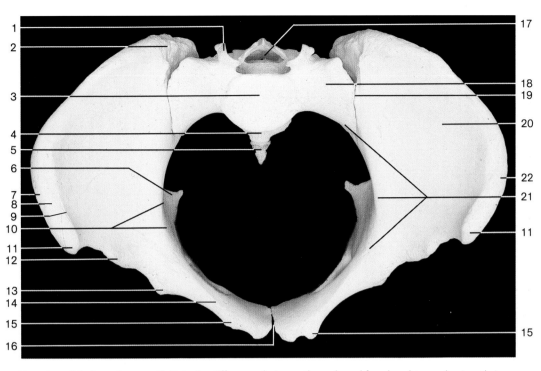

**Female pelvis** (superior aspect). Note the differences between the male and female pelvis, predominantly in the form and dimensions of the sacrum, the superior and inferior apertures, and the alae of the ilium.

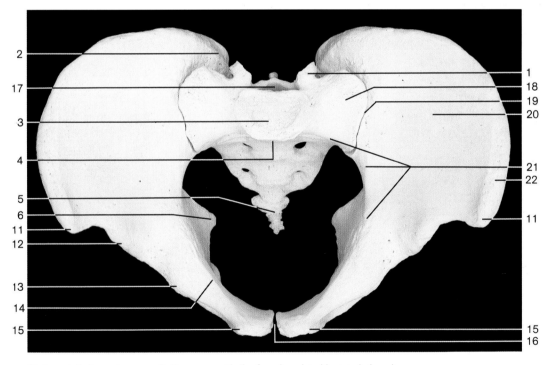

**Male pelvis** (superior aspect). Compare with the female pelvis (depicted above).

| | | | |
|---|---|---|---|
| 1 | Superior articular process of sacrum | 12 | Anterior inferior iliac spine |
| 2 | Posterior superior iliac spine | 13 | Iliopubic eminence |
| 3 | Base of sacrum | 14 | Pecten pubis |
| 4 | Sacral promontory | 15 | Pubic tubercle |
| 5 | Coccyx | 16 | Pubic symphysis |
| 6 | Ischial spine | 17 | Sacral canal |
| 7 | External lip ⎤ of iliac | 18 | Ala of sacrum |
| 8 | Intermediate line ⎬ crest | 19 | Position of sacro-iliac joint |
| 9 | Internal lip ⎦ | 20 | Iliac fossa |
| 10 | Arcuate line | 21 | Linea terminalis |
| 11 | Anterior superior iliac spine | 22 | Iliac crest |

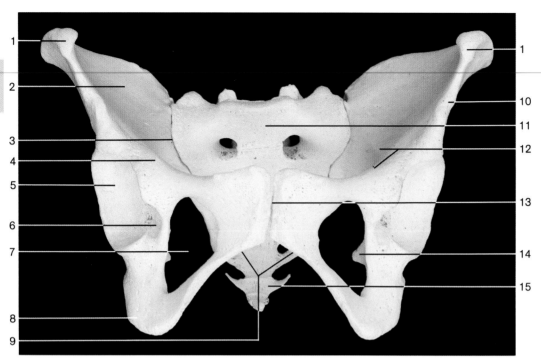

**Female pelvis** (anterior aspect). Note the differences between the form and dimensions of the male and female pelvis. The female pubic arch is wider than the male. The obturator foramen in the female pelvis is triangular, while that in the male pelvis is ovoid.

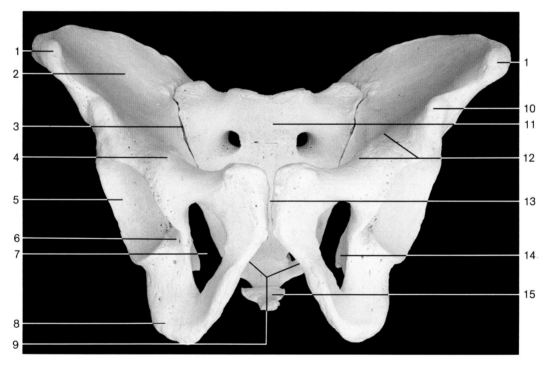

**Male pelvis** (anterior aspect). Compare with the female pelvis (depicted above).

| | | | |
|---|---|---|---|
| 1 | Anterior superior iliac spine | 9 | Pubic arch |
| 2 | Iliac fossa | 10 | Anterior inferior iliac spine |
| 3 | Position of sacro-iliac joint | 11 | Sacrum |
| 4 | Iliopubic eminence | 12 | Linea terminalis (at margin of superior aperture) |
| 5 | Lunate surface of acetabulum | 13 | Pubic symphysis |
| 6 | Acetabular notch | 14 | Ischial spine |
| 7 | Obturator foramen | 15 | Coccyx |
| 8 | Ischial tuberosity | | |

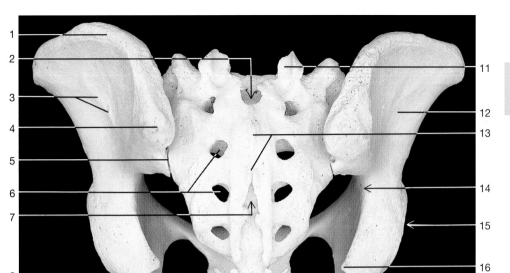

**Female pelvis** (posterior aspect). Note the differences between the female and male pelvis, especially with respect to the inferior aperture, the shape of the sacrum, the two sciatic notches, and the pubic arch.

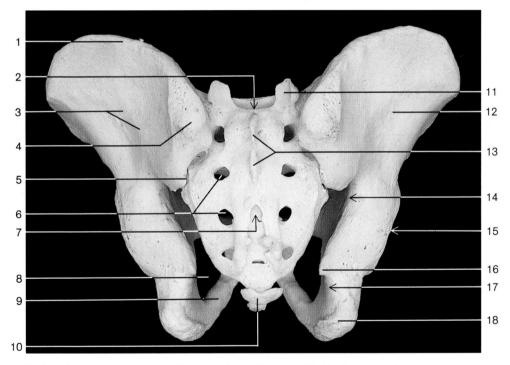

**Male pelvis** (posterior aspect). Compare with the female pelvis (depicted above).

| | | | |
|---|---|---|---|
| 1 | Iliac crest | 10 | Coccyx |
| 2 | Sacral canal | 11 | Superior articular process of sacrum |
| 3 | Posterior gluteal line | 12 | Gluteal surface of ilium |
| 4 | Posterior superior iliac spine | 13 | Median sacral crest |
| 5 | Position of sacro-iliac joint | 14 | Greater sciatic notch |
| 6 | Dorsal sacral foramina | 15 | Position of acetabulum |
| 7 | Sacral hiatus | 16 | Ischial spine |
| 8 | Obturator foramen | 17 | Lesser sciatic notch |
| 9 | Ramus of ischium | 18 | Ischial tuberosity |

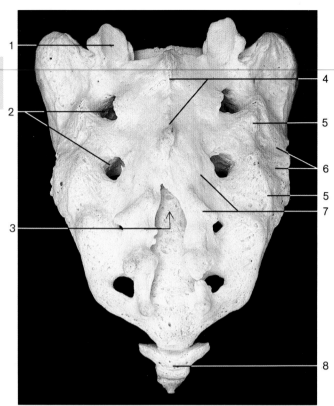

**Sacrum** (posterior aspect).

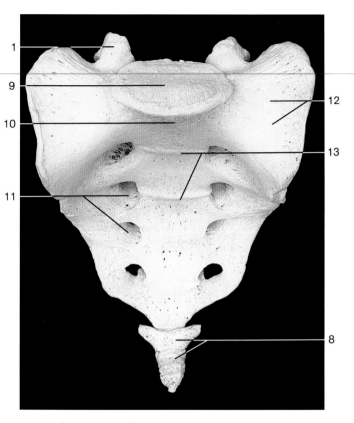

**Sacrum** (anterior aspect).

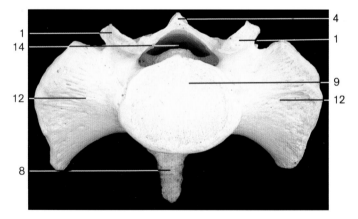

**Sacrum** (superior aspect).

1  Superior articular process of sacrum
2  Posterior sacral foramina
3  Sacral hiatus
4  Median sacral crest
5  Lateral sacral crest
6  Sacral tuberosity
7  Intermediate sacral crest
8  Coccyx
9  Base of sacrum
10  Sacral promontory
11  Anterior sacral foramina
12  Lateral part of sacrum (ala)
13  Transverse line of sacrum
14  Sacral canal
15  Linea terminalis
16  True conjugate
17  Diagonal conjugate
18  Transverse diameter
19  Oblique diameter
20  Inferior pelvic aperture or outlet

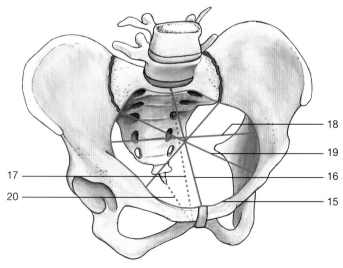

**Diameters of pelvis** (oblique-superior aspect).

The pelvic girdle is firmly connected to the vertebral column at the sacro-iliac joint. Therefore, the body can be kept upright more easily even if only one limb is used for support (as in walking). The mobility of the lower limb is more limited than that of the upper limb.

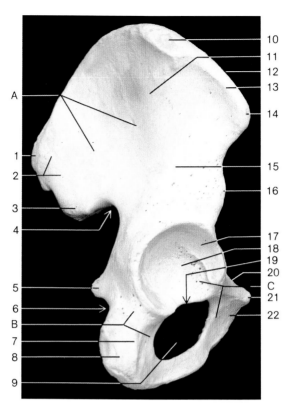

**Right hip bone** (lateral aspect).

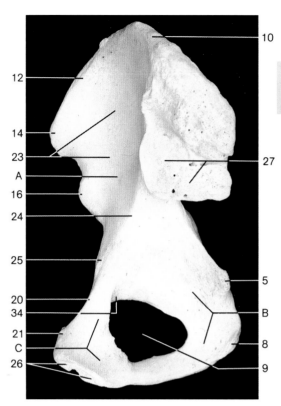

**Right hip bone** (medial aspect).

A = Ilium
B = Ischium
C = Pubis

1   Posterior superior iliac spine
2   Posterior gluteal line
3   Posterior inferior iliac spine
4   Greater sciatic notch
5   Ischial spine
6   Lesser sciatic notch
7   Body of ischium
8   Ischial tuberosity
9   Obturator foramen
10  Iliac crest
11  Anterior gluteal line
12  Internal lip of iliac crest
13  External lip of iliac crest
14  Anterior superior iliac spine
15  Inferior gluteal line
16  Anterior inferior iliac spine
17  Lunate surface of acetabulum
18  Acetabular fossa
19  Acetabular notch
20  Pecten pubis
21  Pubic tubercle
22  Body of pubis
23  Iliac fossa
24  Arcuate line
25  Iliopubic eminence
26  Symphysial surface of pubis
27  Auricular surface
28  Pelvic surface of sacrum
29  Superior articular process of sacrum
30  Dorsal sacral foramina
31  Sacral tuberosity
32  Lateral sacral crest
33  Median sacral crest
34  Obturator groove
35  Coccyx

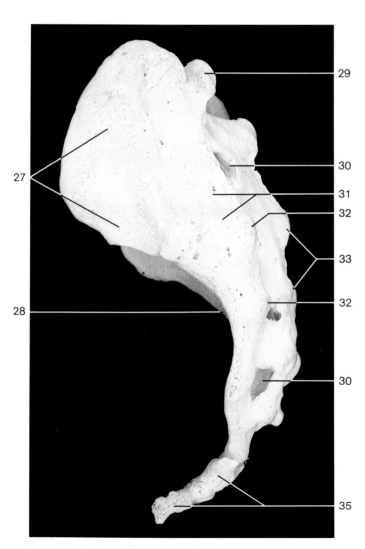

**Sacrum and coccyx** (lateral aspect).

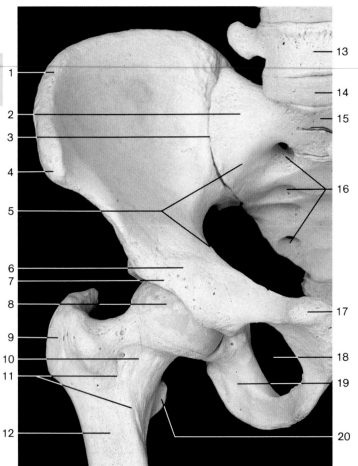

**Bones of the right hip joint** (anterior aspect).

1   Iliac crest
2   Lateral part of sacrum (ala)
3   Position of sacro-iliac joint
4   Anterior superior iliac spine
5   Linea terminalis
6   Iliopubic eminence
7   Bony margin of acetabulum
8   Head of femur
9   Greater trochanter
10  Neck of femur
11  Intertrochanteric line
12  Shaft of femur
13  Fifth lumbar vertebra
14  Intervertebral disc
    between fifth lumbar vertebra and sacrum (imitation)
15  Sacral promontory
16  Anterior sacral foramina
17  Pubic tubercle
18  Obturator foramen
19  Ramus of ischium
20  Lesser trochanter
21  Posterior sacral foramina
22  Greater sciatic notch
23  Ischial spine
24  Pubic symphysis
25  Pubis
26  Ischial tuberosity
27  Intertrochanteric crest
28  Symphysial surface

**Diameters of the pelvis**

A  =  True conjugate (11–11.5 cm) (conjugata vera)
B  =  Diagonal conjugate (12.5–13 cm)
C  =  Largest diameter of pelvis
D  =  Inferior pelvic aperture
E  =  Pelvic inclination (60°)

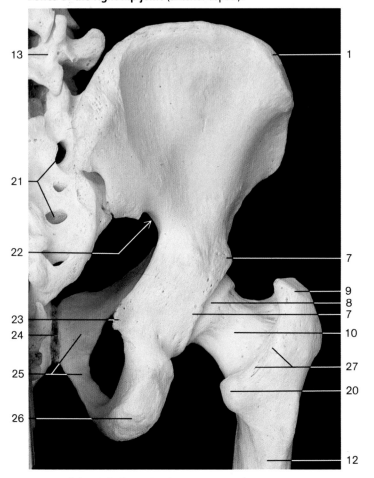

**Bones of the right hip joint** (posterior aspect).

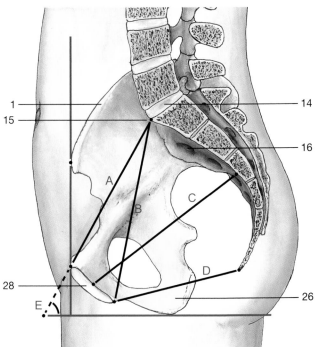

**Inclination and diameters of the female pelvis,**
right half (medial aspect).

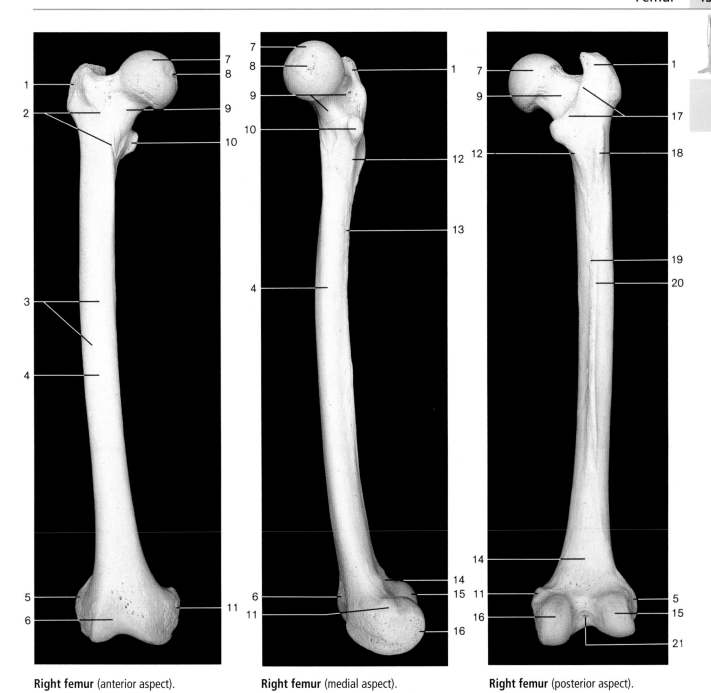

**Right femur** (anterior aspect).

**Right femur** (medial aspect).

**Right femur** (posterior aspect).

| | | | | | | | |
|---|---|---|---|---|---|---|---|
| 1 | Greater trochanter | 8 | Fovea of head | 15 | Lateral condyle |
| 2 | Intertrochanteric line | 9 | Neck | 16 | Medial condyle |
| 3 | Nutrient foramina | 10 | Lesser trochanter | 17 | Intertrochanteric crest |
| 4 | Shaft of femur (diaphysis) | 11 | Medial epicondyle | 18 | Third trochanter |
| 5 | Lateral epicondyle | 12 | Pectineal line | 19 | Medial lip of linea aspera |
| 6 | Patellar surface | 13 | Linea aspera | 20 | Lateral lip of linea aspera |
| 7 | Head | 14 | Popliteal surface | 21 | Intercondylar fossa |

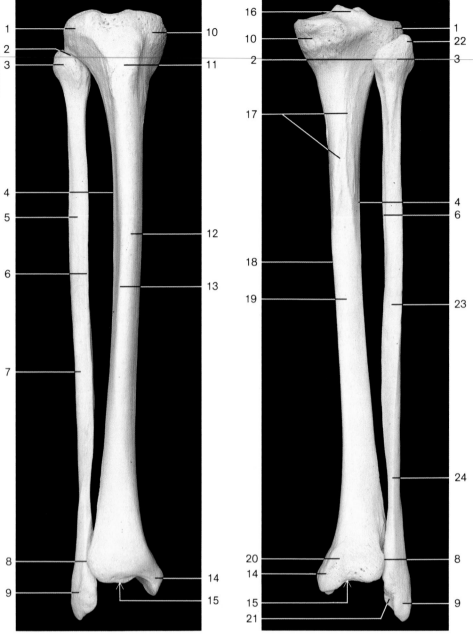

1   Lateral condyle of tibia
2   Position of tibiofibular joint
3   Head of fibula
4   Interosseous border of tibia
5   Shaft of fibula
6   Interosseous border of fibula
7   Lateral surface of fibula
8   Position of tibiofibular syndesmosis
9   Lateral malleolus
10  Medial condyle of tibia
11  Tuberosity of tibia
12  Shaft of tibia (diaphysis)
13  Anterior margin of tibia
14  Medial malleolus
15  Inferior articular surface
    of tibia
16  Intercondylar eminence
17  Soleal line
18  Medial border of tibia
19  Posterior surface of tibia
20  Malleolar sulcus of tibia
21  Malleolar articular surface
    of fibula
22  Apex of head of fibula
23  Posterior surface of fibula
24  Posterior border of fibula
25  Medial intercondylar tubercle
26  Posterior intercondylar area
27  Anterior intercondylar area
28  Lateral intercondylar tubercle

**Bones of the leg. Right tibia and fibula** (anterior aspect).

**Bones of the leg. Right tibia and fibula** (posterior aspect).

**Upper end of the right tibia with fibula** (from above), anterior margin of tibia above. Superior articular surface of tibia.

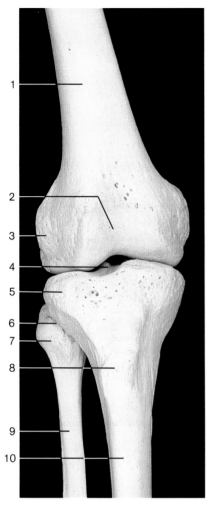

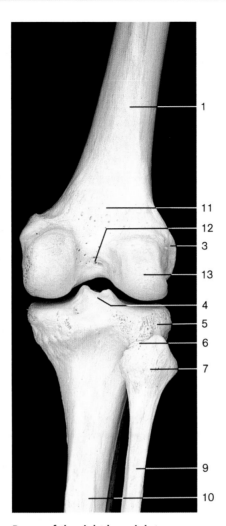

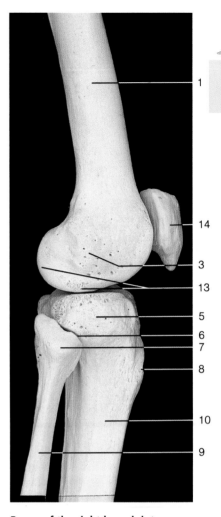

**Bones of the right knee joint** (anterior aspect).

**Bones of the right knee joint** (posterior aspect).

**Bones of the right knee joint** (lateral aspect).

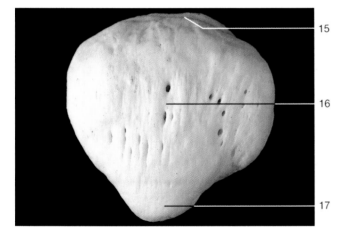

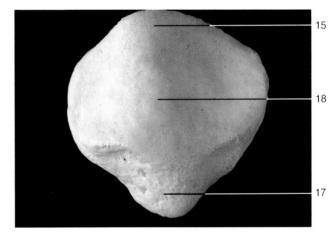

**Right patella** (anterior aspect).

**Right patella** (posterior aspect).

| | |
|---|---|
| 1 Femur | 10 Shaft of tibia |
| 2 Patellar surface of femur | 11 Popliteal surface of femur |
| 3 Lateral epicondyle of femur | 12 Intercondylar fossa of femur |
| 4 Intercondylar eminence of tibia | 13 Lateral condyle of femur |
| 5 Lateral condyle of tibia | 14 Patella |
| 6 Position of tibiofibular joint | 15 Base of patella |
| 7 Head of fibula | 16 Anterior surface of patella |
| 8 Tuberosity of tibia | 17 Apex of patella |
| 9 Fibula | 18 Articular surface of patella |

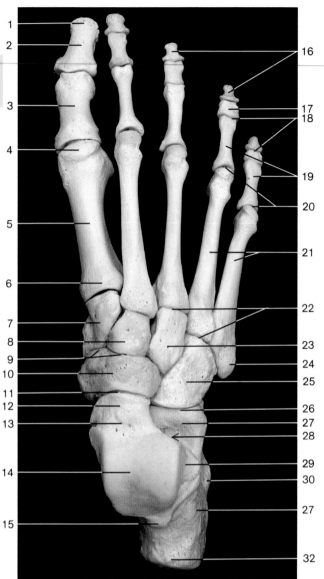

**Bones of the right foot** (dorsal aspect).

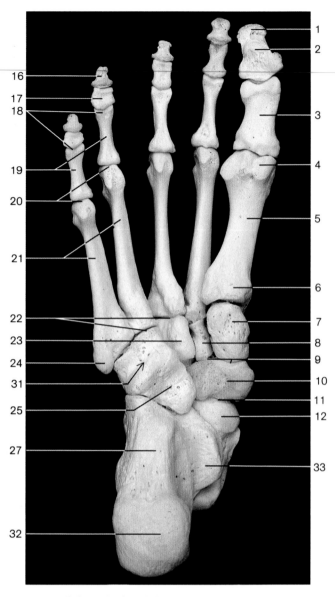

**Bones of the right foot** (plantar aspect).

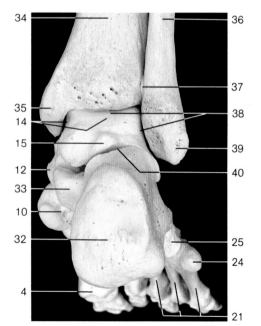

**Bones of the right foot** together with tibia and fibula (posterior aspect).

1   Tuberosity of distal phalanx of great toe
2   Distal phalanx of great toe
3   Proximal phalanx of great toe
4   Head of first metatarsal bone
5   First metatarsal bone
6   Base of first metatarsal bone
7   Medial cuneiform bone
8   Intermediate cuneiform bone
9   Position of cuneonavicular joint
10  Navicular bone

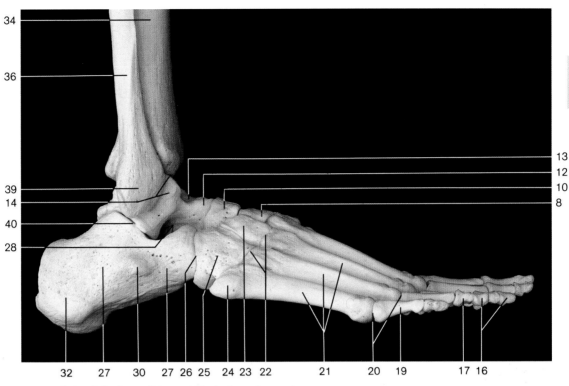

**Bones of the right foot, tibia, and fibula** (lateral aspect).

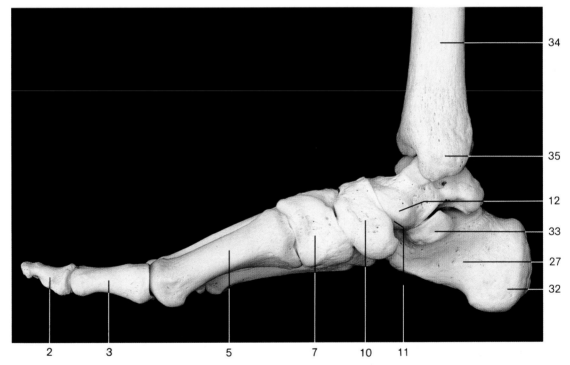

**Bones of the right foot, tibia, and fibula** (medial aspect).

| | | | | | |
|---|---|---|---|---|---|
| 11 | Position of talocalcaneonavicular joint | 21 | Metatarsal bones | 31 | Groove for the tendon of peroneus longus muscle |
| 12 | Head of talus | 22 | Position of tarsometatarsal joints | 32 | Calcaneal tuberosity |
| 13 | Neck of talus | 23 | Lateral cuneiform bone | 33 | Sustentaculum tali |
| 14 | Trochlea of talus | 24 | Tuberosity of fifth metatarsal bone | 34 | Tibia |
| 15 | Posterior talar process | 25 | Cuboid bone | 35 | Medial malleolus |
| 16 | Distal phalanges | 26 | Position of calcaneocuboid joint | 36 | Fibula |
| 17 | Middle phalanx | 27 | Calcaneus | 37 | Position of tibiofibular syndesmosis |
| 18 | Position of interphalangeal joints | 28 | Tarsal sinus | 38 | Position of ankle joint |
| 19 | Proximal phalanges | 29 | Lateral malleolar surface of talus | 39 | Lateral malleolus |
| 20 | Position of metatarsophalangeal joints | 30 | Peroneal trochlea of calcaneus | 40 | Position of subtalar joint |

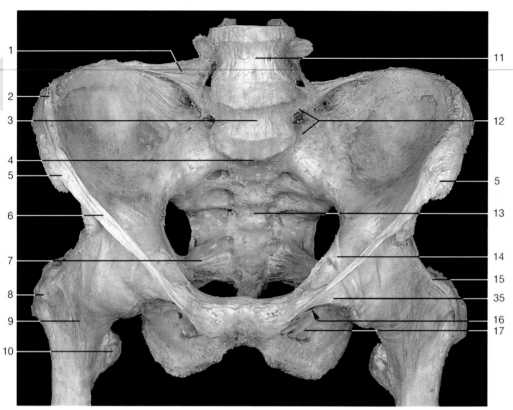

**Ligaments of pelvis and hip joint** (anterior aspect).

| | | | | | |
|---|---|---|---|---|---|
| 1 | Iliolumbar ligament | 13 | Sacrum | 26 | Articular capsule of hip joint |
| 2 | Iliac crest | 14 | Iliopectineal arch | 27 | Dorsal sacro-iliac ligaments |
| 3 | Fifth lumbar vertebra | 15 | Iliofemoral ligament (horizontal band) | 28 | Coccyx |
| 4 | Sacral promontory | 16 | Obturator canal | | with superficial dorsal |
| 5 | Anterior superior iliac spine | 17 | Obturator membrane | | sacrococcygeal ligament |
| 6 | Inguinal ligament | 18 | Greater sciatic foramen | 29 | Head of femur |
| 7 | Sacrospinous ligament | 19 | Sacrospinous ligament | 30 | Articular cartilage of head of femur |
| 8 | Greater trochanter | 20 | Sacrotuberous ligament | 31 | Articular cavity of hip joint |
| 9 | Iliofemoral ligament (vertical band) | 21 | Lesser sciatic foramen | 32 | Acetabular lip |
| 10 | Lesser trochanter | 22 | Ischial tuberosity | 33 | Spongy bone |
| 11 | Fourth lumbar vertebra | 23 | Ischiofemoral ligament | 34 | Ligament of head of femur |
| 12 | Iliolumbar and ventral sacro-iliac | 24 | Intertrochanteric crest | 35 | Pubofemoral ligament |
| | ligaments | 25 | Femur | 36 | Zona orbicularis |

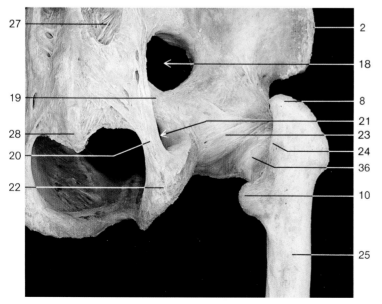

**Ligaments of pelvis and hip joint** (right posterior aspect).

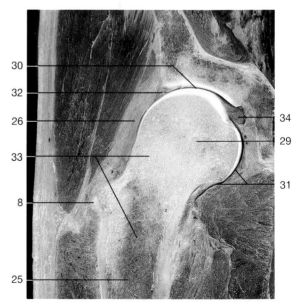

**Coronal section through the right hip joint** (anterior aspect).

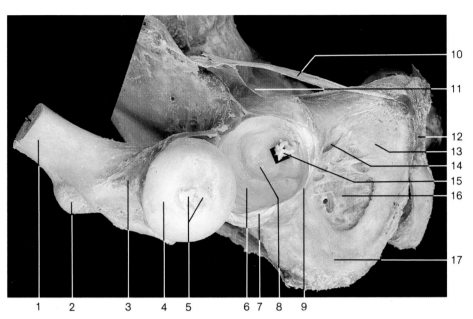

1   Femur
2   Lesser trochanter
3   Neck of femur
4   Head of femur
5   Fovea of head
     with cut edge of ligament of head
6   Lunate surface of acetabulum
7   Acetabular lip
8   Acetabular fossa
9   Transverse acetabular ligament
10  Inguinal ligament
11  Iliopectineal arch
12  Pubic symphysis
13  Pubis
14  Obturator canal
15  Ligament of head of femur
16  Obturator membrane
17  Ischium
18  Anterior longitudinal ligament
     (level of fifth lumbar vertebra)
19  Sacral promontory
20  Iliolumbar ligament
21  Iliac crest
22  Anterior superior iliac spine
23  Iliofemoral ligament
     (horizontal band)
24  Iliofemoral ligament
     (vertical band)
25  Greater trochanter
26  Pubofemoral ligament
27  Anterior inferior iliac spine
28  Ventral sacro-iliac ligaments
29  Sacrospinous ligament
30  Sacrotuberous ligament
31  Intertrochanteric line
32  Ischiofemoral ligament
33  Zona orbicularis

**Right hip joint,** opened (latero-anterior aspect). The ligament of the head of the femur has been divided, and the femur has been posteriorly reflected.

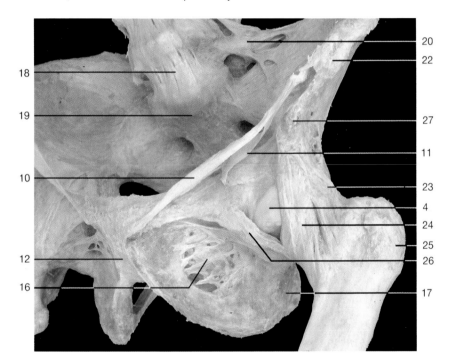

◁ **Ligaments of pelvis and hip joint** (antero-lateral aspect).

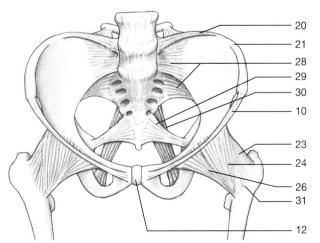

**Ligaments of pelvis and hip joint** (anterior aspect).

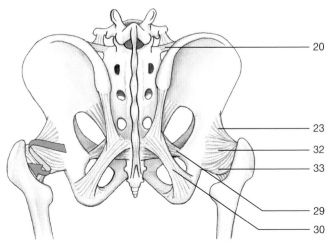

**Ligaments of pelvis and hip joint** (posterior aspect).

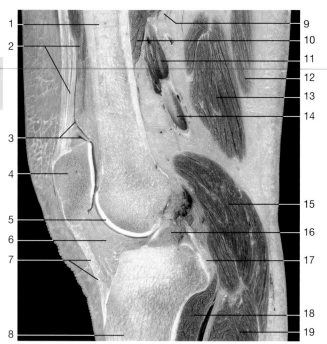

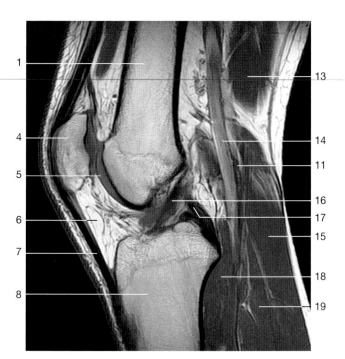

**Sagittal section through the knee joint** (lateral aspect). Anterior surface to the left.

**Sagittal section through the knee joint** (MRI scan). (From Heuck et al., MRT-Atlas, 2009.)

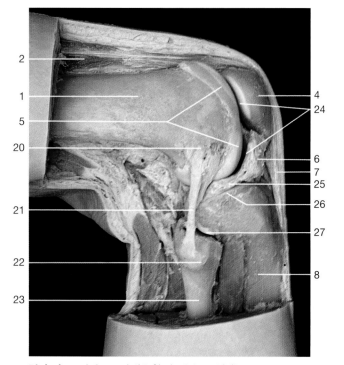

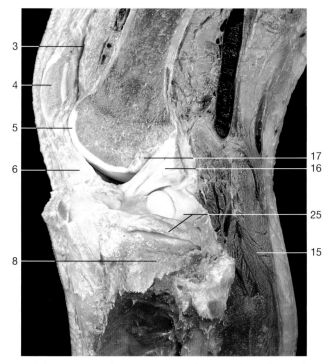

**Right knee joint** and tibiofibular joint with ligaments (lateral aspect). Note the position of the lateral meniscus.

**Left knee joint** with anterior cruciate ligament (lateral aspect).

| | | | | | |
|---|---|---|---|---|---|
| 1 | Femur | 10 | Adductor magnus muscle | 19 | Soleus muscle |
| 2 | Quadriceps femoris muscle | 11 | Popliteal vein | 20 | Lateral epicondyle of femur |
| 3 | Suprapatellar bursa and articular cavity | 12 | Semitendinosus muscle | 21 | Fibular collateral ligament |
| 4 | Patella | 13 | Semimembranosus muscle | 22 | Head of fibula |
| 5 | Articular cartilage of femur | 14 | Popliteal artery | 23 | Fibula |
| 6 | Infrapatellar fat pad | 15 | Gastrocnemius muscle | 24 | Articular cavity of knee joint |
| 7 | Patellar ligament | 16 | Anterior cruciate ligament | 25 | Lateral meniscus of knee joint |
| 8 | Tibia | 17 | Posterior cruciate ligament | 26 | Lateral condyle of tibia |
| 9 | Tibial nerve | 18 | Popliteus muscle | 27 | Tibiofibular joint |

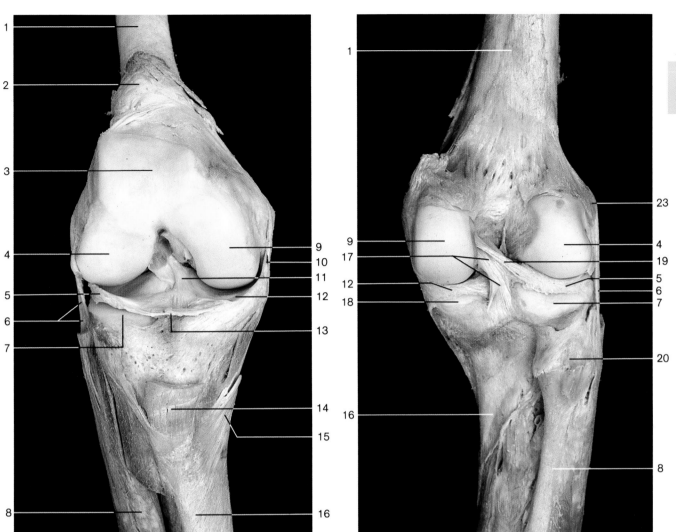

**Right knee joint with ligaments** (anterior aspect). The patella and articular capsule have been removed and the femur slightly flexed.

**Right knee joint with ligaments** (posterior aspect). The joint is extended and the articular capsule has been removed.

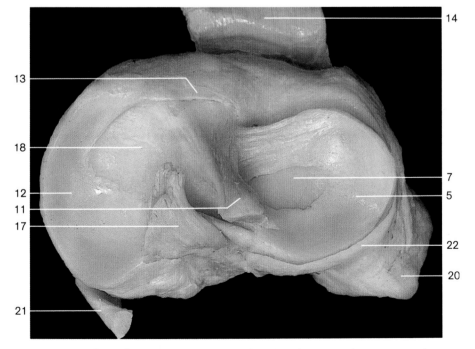

**Articular surface of right tibia, menisci, and cruciate ligaments** (superior aspect). Anterior margin of tibia above.

1   Femur
2   Articular capsule
    with suprapatellar bursa
3   Patellar surface
4   Lateral condyle of femur
5   Lateral meniscus of knee joint
6   Fibular collateral ligament
7   Lateral condyle of tibia
    (superior articular surface)
8   Fibula
9   Medial condyle of femur
10  Tibial collateral ligament
11  Anterior cruciate ligament
12  Medial meniscus of knee joint
13  Transverse ligament of knee
14  Patellar ligament
15  Common tendon of sartorius,
    semitendinosus, and gracilis muscles
16  Tibia
17  Posterior cruciate ligament
18  Medial condyle of tibia
    (superior articular surface)
19  Posterior meniscofemoral ligament
20  Head of fibula
21  Tendon of semimembranosus muscle
22  Posterior attachment
    of articular capsule of knee joint
23  Lateral epicondyle of femur

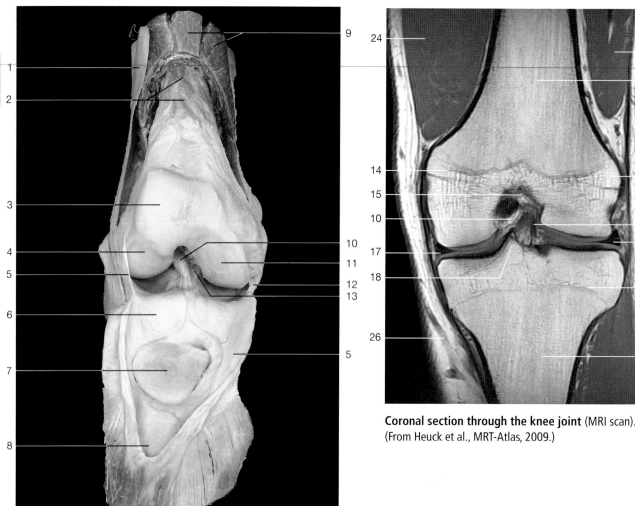

**Right knee joint,** opened (anterior aspect). The patellar ligament with the patella have been reflected.

**Coronal section through the knee joint** (MRI scan). (From Heuck et al., MRT-Atlas, 2009.)

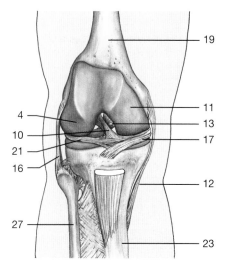

**Ligaments of the right knee joint** (anterior aspect).

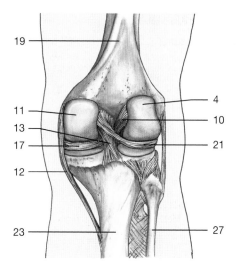

**Ligaments of the right knee joint** (posterior aspect).

1   Iliotibial tract
2   Articular muscle of knee
3   Patellar surface
4   Lateral condyle of femur
5   Articular capsule
6   Infrapatellar fat pad
7   Patella (articular surface)
8   Suprapatellar bursa
9   Quadriceps femoris muscle
10  Anterior cruciate ligament
11  Medial condyle of femur
12  Tibial collateral ligament
13  Posterior cruciate ligament
14  Medial epicondyle of femur
15  Intercondylar fossa of femur
16  Fibular collateral ligament
17  Medial meniscus of knee joint
18  Medial intercondylar tubercle
19  Femur
20  Lateral epicondyle of femur
21  Lateral meniscus of knee joint
22  Epiphysial line of tibia
23  Tibia
24  Vastus medialis muscle
25  Vastus lateralis muscle
26  Great saphenous vein
27  Fibula

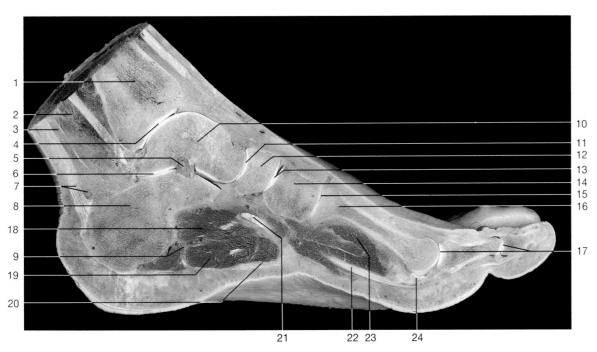

**Sagittal section through the foot** at the level of the first phalanx.

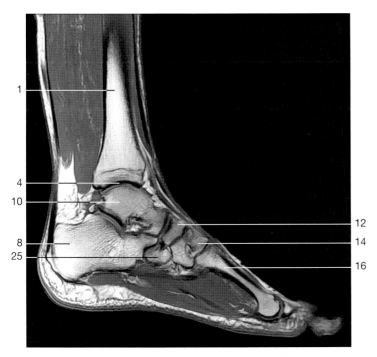

**Sagittal section through the foot and leg** (MRI scan).
(From Heuck et al., MRT-Atlas, 2009.)

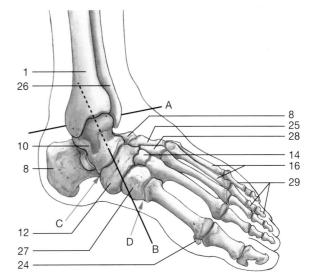

**Skeleton of the left foot.** Joints are indicated in blue.
Red lines = axis of joints.

A = Talocrural joint
B = Talocalcaneonavicular joint
C = Transverse tarsal joint (Chopart joint line)
D = Tarsometatarsal joints (Lisfranc joint line)

1 Tibia
2 Deep flexor muscles of leg
3 Superficial flexor muscles of leg
4 Ankle joint
5 Interosseous talocalcaneal ligament
6 Subtalar joint
7 Calcaneal or Achilles tendon and bursa
8 Calcaneus
9 Vessels and nerves of foot
10 Talus
11 Talocalcaneonavicular joint
12 Navicular bone
13 Cuneonavicular joint
14 Intermediate cuneiform bone
15 First tarsometatarsal joint
16 Metatarsal bones
17 Metatarsophalangeal and interphalangeal joints
18 Quadratus plantae muscle with flexor tendons
19 Flexor digitorum brevis muscle
20 Plantar aponeurosis
21 Tendon of tibialis posterior muscle
22 Tendon of flexor hallucis longus muscle
23 Flexor hallucis brevis muscle
24 Sesamoid bone
25 Cuboid bone
26 Fibula
27 Medial cuneiform bone
28 Lateral cuneiforme bone
29 Phalanges

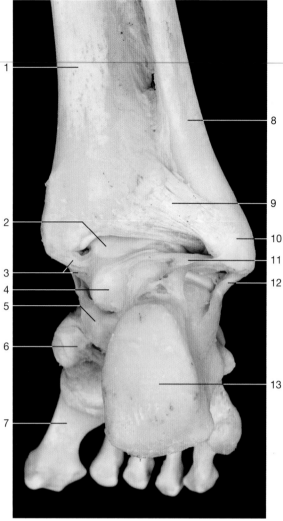

**Ligaments of the ankle joint of the right foot** (dorsal aspect).

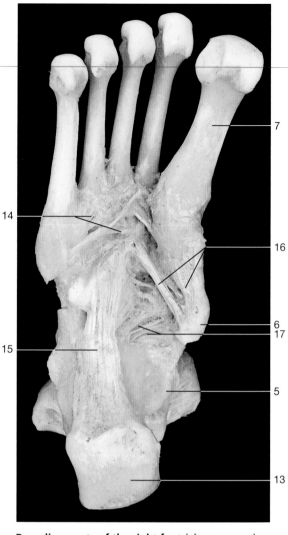

**Deep ligaments of the right foot** (plantar aspect). The toes have been removed.

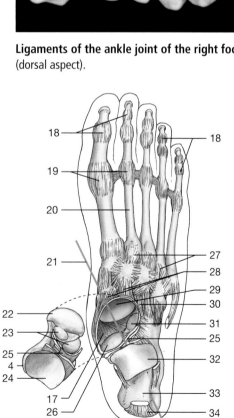

**Ligaments of the foot.** Top view of the talocal-caneonavicular joint. The talus has been rotated to show the articular surfaces of the joint.

| | | | |
|---|---|---|---|
| 1 | Tibia | 20 | Second metatarsal bone |
| 2 | Trochlea of talus | 21 | Axis for inversion and eversion of foot |
| 3 | Medial or deltoid ligament of ankle (posterior tibiotalar part) | 22 | Navicular articular surface of talus |
| 4 | Talus | 23 | Anterior and middle calcaneal surfaces of talus |
| 5 | Sustentaculum tali | 24 | Posterior calcaneal surface of talus |
| 6 | Navicular bone | 25 | Talocalcaneal interosseous ligament |
| 7 | First metatarsal bone | 26 | Middle talar articular surface of calcaneus |
| 8 | Fibula | 27 | Dorsal tarsometatarsal ligaments |
| 9 | Posterior tibiofibular ligament | 28 | Talonavicular ligament |
| 10 | Lateral malleolus | 29 | Articular surface of navicular bone |
| 11 | Posterior talofibular ligament | 30 | Bifurcate ligament |
| 12 | Calcaneofibular ligament | 31 | Anterior talar articular surface of calcaneus |
| 13 | Calcaneal tuberosity | 32 | Posterior talar articular surface of calcaneus |
| 14 | Plantar tarsometatarsal ligaments | 33 | Calcaneus |
| 15 | Long plantar ligament | 34 | Calcaneal or Achilles tendon and bursa |
| 16 | Plantar cuneonavicular ligaments | | |
| 17 | Plantar calcaneonavicular ligament | | |
| 18 | Articular capsules of interphalangeal joints | | |
| 19 | Articular capsules of metatarsophalangeal joints | | |

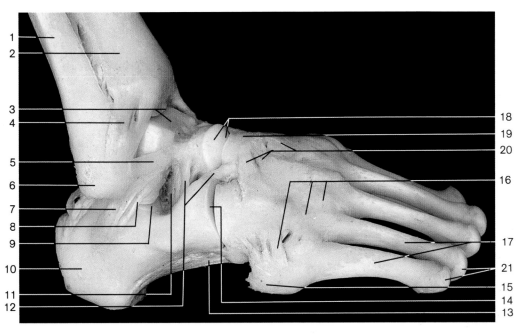

**Ligaments of the right foot** (lateral aspect).

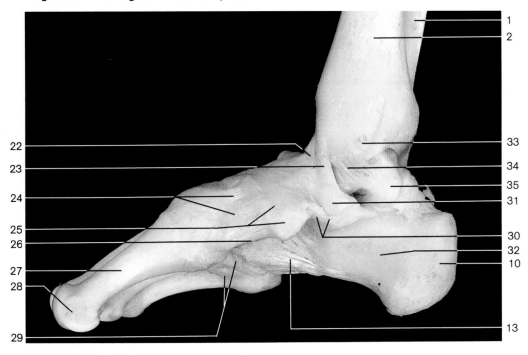

**Ligaments of the right foot** (medial aspect).

| | |
|---|---|
| 1 Fibula | 19 Navicular bone |
| 2 Tibia | 20 Dorsal cuneonavicular ligaments |
| 3 Trochlea of talus and ankle joint | 21 Heads of metatarsal bones |
| 4 Anterior tibiofibular ligament | 22 Medial or deltoid ligament of ankle (tibionavicular part) |
| 5 Anterior talofibular ligament | 23 Medial or deltoid ligament of ankle (tibiocalcaneal part) |
| 6 Lateral malleolus | 24 Dorsal cuneonavicular ligaments |
| 7 Calcaneofibular ligament | 25 Navicular bone |
| 8 Lateral talocalcaneal ligament | 26 Plantar cuneonavicular ligament |
| 9 Subtalar joint | 27 First metatarsal bone |
| 10 Calcaneal tuberosity | 28 Head of first metatarsal bone |
| 11 Interosseous talocalcaneal ligament | 29 Plantar tarsometatarsal ligaments |
| 12 Bifurcate ligament | 30 Plantar calcaneonavicular ligament |
| 13 Long plantar ligament | 31 Sustentaculum tali |
| 14 Calcaneocuboid joint | 32 Calcaneus |
| 15 Tuberosity of fifth metatarsal bone | 33 Medial malleolus |
| 16 Dorsal tarsometatarsal ligaments | 34 Medial or deltoid ligament of ankle |
| 17 Metatarsal bones | (posterior tibiotalar part) |
| 18 Head of talus and talocalcaneonavicular joint | 35 Talus |

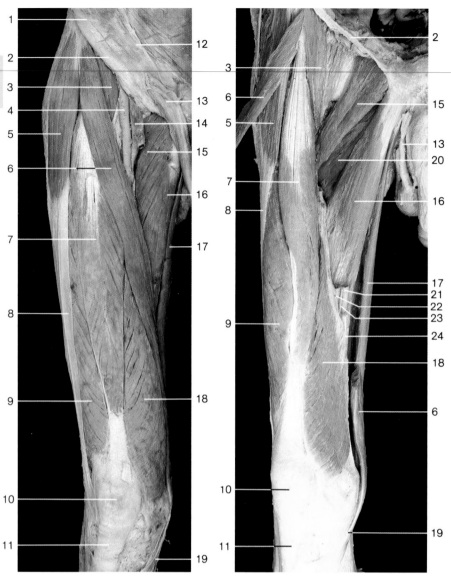

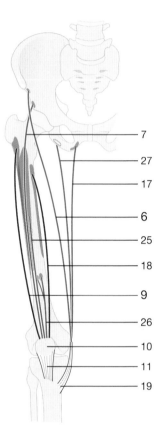

**Extensor and adductor muscles of the thigh** (right side, anterior aspect).

**Quadriceps muscle and superficial layer of adductor muscles of the thigh** (right side, anterior aspect). The sartorius muscle has been divided.

**Course of the extensor muscles of the thigh** and muscles inserting with common tendon on the tibia (anterior aspect).

| | |
|---|---|
| 1　Anterior superior iliac spine | |
| 2　Inguinal ligament | |
| 3　Iliopsoas muscle | |
| 4　Femoral artery | |
| 5　Tensor fasciae latae muscle | |
| 6　Sartorius muscle | |
| 7　Rectus femoris muscle | |
| 8　Iliotibial tract | |
| 9　Vastus lateralis muscle | |
| 10　Patella | |
| 11　Patellar ligament | |

12　Aponeurosis
　　of external abdominal oblique muscle
13　Spermatic cord
14　Femoral vein
15　Pectineus muscle
16　Adductor longus muscle
17　Gracilis muscle
18　Vastus medialis muscle
19　Common tendon of sartorius, gracilis, and semitendinosus muscles (pes anserinus)

20　Adductor brevis muscle
21　Femoral artery ⎫ entering the
22　Femoral vein　 ⎬ adductor canal
23　Saphenous nerve ⎭
24　Vasto-adductor membrane
25　Vastus intermedius muscle
26　Articularis genus muscle
27　Semitendinosus muscle

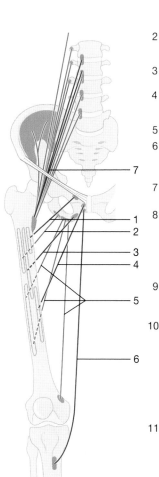

**Course of the adductor muscles of the thigh** (anterior aspect).

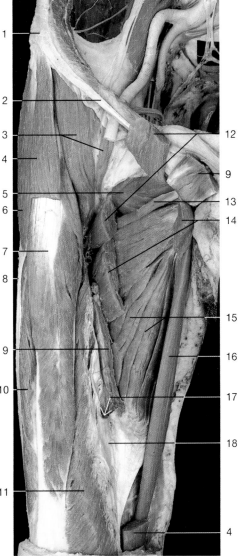

**Adductor magnus muscle and deep layer of adductor muscles of the thigh** (right side, anterior aspect). Pectineus, adductor longus, and brevis muscles have been divided.

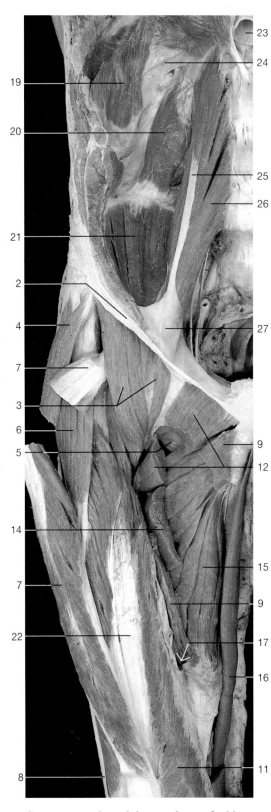

**Iliopsoas muscle and deepest layer of adductor muscles of the thigh** (right side, anterior aspect). Pectineus, adductor longus and brevis, and rectus femoris muscles have been divided.

1   Pectineus muscle (blue)
2   Adductor minimus muscle (red)
3   Adductor brevis muscle (blue)
4   Adductor longus muscle (blue)
5   Adductor magnus and minimus muscles (red)
6   Gracilis muscle (blue)
7   Iliopsoas muscle (blue and red)

1   Anterior superior iliac spine
2   Inguinal ligament
3   Iliopsoas muscle
4   Sartorius muscle
5   Obturator externus muscle
6   Tensor fasciae latae muscle
7   Rectus femoris muscle
8   Iliotibial tract
9   Adductor longus muscle (divided)
10  Vastus lateralis muscle
11  Vastus medialis muscle
12  Pectineus muscle (divided)
13  Adductor minimus muscle
14  Adductor brevis muscle (cut)
15  Adductor magnus muscle
16  Gracilis muscle
17  Adductor canal
18  Vasto-adductor membrane
19  Diaphragm
20  Quadratus lumborum muscle
21  Iliacus muscle
22  Vastus intermedius muscle

23  Aortic hiatus
24  Twelfth rib
25  Psoas minor muscle
26  Psoas major muscle
27  Iliopectineal arch

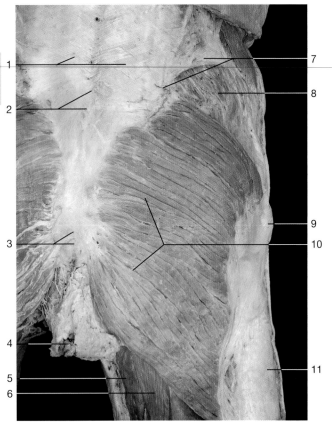

1
2
7
8
3
9
10
4
5
6
11

**Gluteal muscles,** superficial layer (right side, posterior aspect).

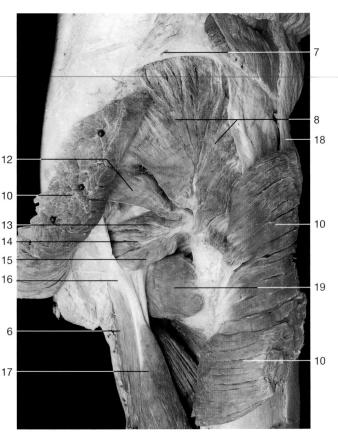

7
12
10
13
14
15
16
6
17
8
18
10
19
10

**Gluteal muscles,** deeper layer (right side, posterior aspect).

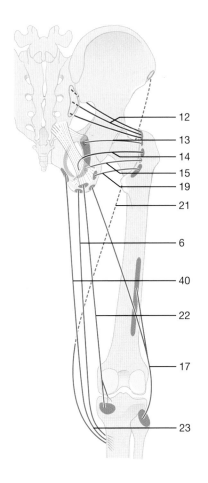

12
13
14
15
19
21
6
40
22
17
23

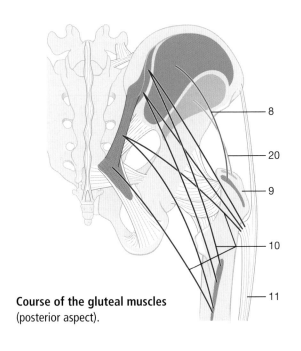

8
20
9
10
11

**Course of the gluteal muscles**
(posterior aspect).

◁

**Course of gluteal** (deeper layer) **and ischiocrural muscles**
(posterior aspect). The sartorius muscle is indicated by a dotted
line.

1   Thoracolumbar fascia
2   Spinous processes of lumbar vertebrae
3   Coccyx
4   Anus
5   Adductor magnus muscle
6   Semitendinosus muscle
7   Iliac crest
8   Gluteus medius muscle
9   Greater trochanter
10  Gluteus maximus muscle
11  Iliotibial tract
12  Piriformis muscle
13  Superior gemellus muscle
14  Obturator internus muscle
15  Inferior gemellus muscle
16  Ischial tuberosity
17  Biceps femoris muscle
18  Tensor fasciae latae muscle
19  Quadratus femoris muscle
20  Gluteus minimus muscle
21  Sartorius muscle
22  Semimembranosus muscle
23  Tendon of gracilis muscle
24  Tibial nerve
25  Medial head of gastrocnemius muscle
26  Common fibular nerve
27  Tendon of biceps femoris muscle
28  Lateral head of gastrocnemius muscle
29  Rectus femoris muscle
30  Vastus medialis muscle
31  Vastus intermedius muscle
32  Vastus lateralis muscle
33  Sciatic nerve
34  Gluteus maximus muscle (insertion)
35  Great saphenous vein
36  Femoral artery
37  Femoral vein
38  Adductor longus muscle
39  Femur
40  Gracilis muscle
41  Septum between semitendinosus
    and semimembranosus muscles

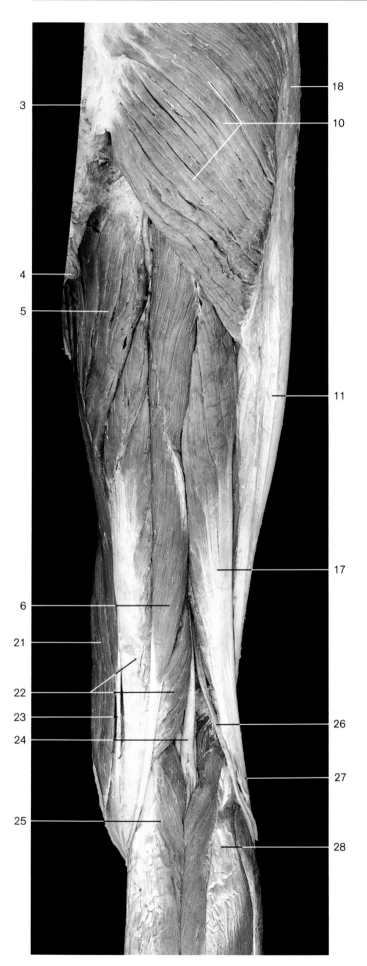

**Flexor muscles of the thigh,** superficial layer (right side, posterior aspect).

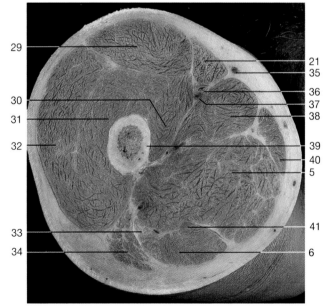

**Cross section through the right thigh** (inferior aspect). Anterior side on top.

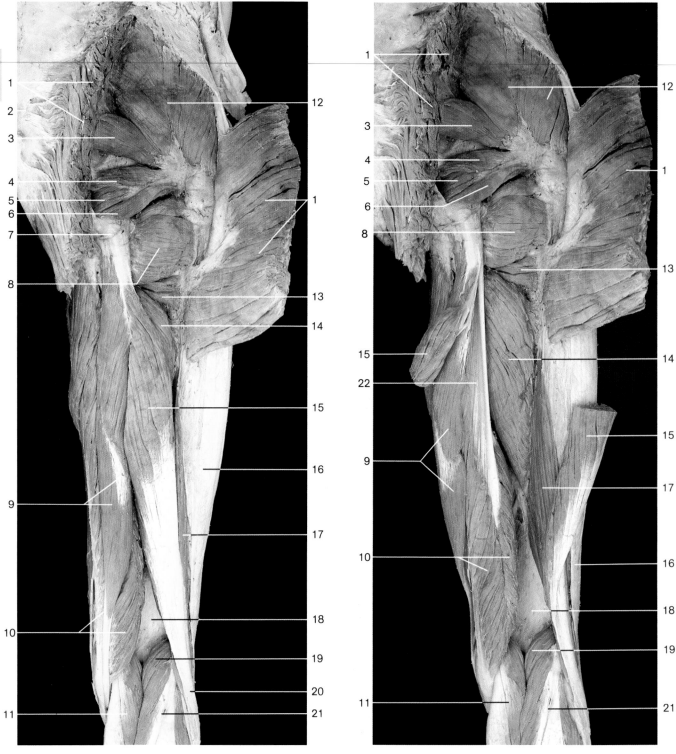

**Flexor muscles of the thigh** (right side, posterior aspect).
The gluteus maximus muscle has been cut and reflected.

**Flexor muscles of the thigh** (right side, posterior aspect).
The gluteus maximus muscle and the long head of biceps
femoris muscle have been divided and displaced.

| | | |
|---|---|---|
| 1  Gluteus maximus muscle (divided) | 9  Semitendinosus muscle with intermediate tendon | 17  Short head of biceps femoris muscle |
| 2  Position of coccyx | 10  Semimembranosus muscle | 18  Popliteal surface of femur |
| 3  Piriformis muscle | 11  Medial head of gastrocnemius muscle | 19  Plantaris muscle |
| 4  Superior gemellus muscle | 12  Gluteus medius muscle | 20  Tendon of biceps femoris muscle |
| 5  Obturator internus muscle | 13  Adductor minimus muscle | 21  Lateral head of gastrocnemius muscle |
| 6  Inferior gemellus muscle | 14  Adductor magnus muscle | 22  Tendon of semimembranosus muscle |
| 7  Ischial tuberosity | 15  Long head of biceps femoris muscle | |
| 8  Quadratus femoris muscle | 16  Iliotibial tract | |

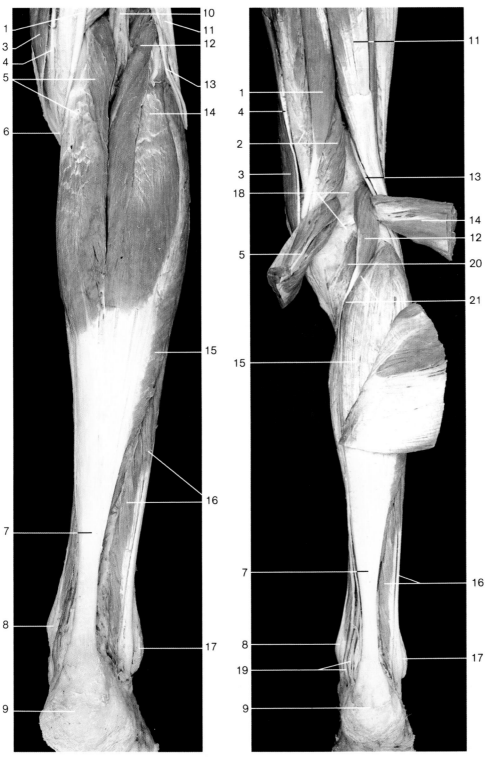

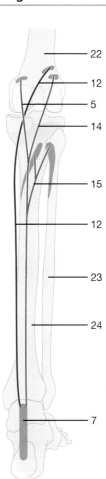

**Course of the flexor muscles of the leg** (posterior aspect).

**Flexor muscles of the leg** (right side, posterior aspect).

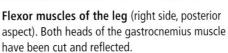

**Flexor muscles of the leg** (right side, posterior aspect). Both heads of the gastrocnemius muscle have been cut and reflected.

| | | |
|---|---|---|
| 1 Semitendinosus muscle | 9 Calcaneal tuberosity | 18 Popliteal fossa |
| 2 Semimembranosus muscle | 10 Tibial nerve | 19 Tibial nerve and |
| 3 Sartorius muscle | 11 Biceps femoris muscle | posterior tibial artery |
| 4 Tendon of gracilis muscle | 12 Plantaris muscle | 20 Popliteus muscle |
| 5 Medial head of gastrocnemius muscle | 13 Common fibular nerve | 21 Tendinous arch of soleus muscle |
| 6 Common tendon of gracilis, sartorius, and | 14 Lateral head of gastrocnemius muscle | 22 Femur |
| semitendinosus muscles (pes anserinus) | 15 Soleus muscle | 23 Fibula |
| 7 Calcaneal or Achilles tendon | 16 Peroneus longus and brevis muscles | 24 Tibia |
| 8 Medial malleolus | 17 Lateral malleolus | |

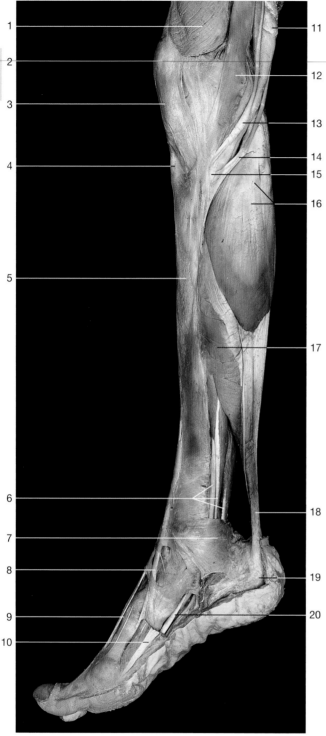

**Muscles of leg and foot** (right side, medial aspect).

**Popliteal region with plantaris and soleus muscles** (right side, posterior aspect). Notice the insertion of the tendon of semimembranosus muscle.

| | |
|---|---|
| 1 | Vastus medialis muscle |
| 2 | Patella |
| 3 | Patellar ligament |
| 4 | Tibial tuberosity |
| 5 | Tibia |
| 6 | Tendons of deep flexor muscles (from anterior to posterior: 1. tibialis posterior; 2. flexor digitorum longus; 3. flexor hallucis longus muscles) |
| 7 | Flexor retinaculum |
| 8 | Tendon of tibialis anterior muscle |
| 9 | Tendon of extensor hallucis longus muscle |
| 10 | Abductor hallucis muscle |
| 11 | Tendon of semimembranosus muscle |
| 12 | Sartorius muscle |
| 13 | Tendon of gracilis muscle |
| 14 | Tendon of semitendinosus muscle |
| 15 | Common tendon of gracilis, semitendinosus, and sartorius muscles (pes anserinus) |
| 16 | Medial head of gastrocnemius muscle |
| 17 | Soleus muscle |
| 18 | Calcaneal or Achilles tendon |
| 19 | Calcaneus muscle |
| 20 | Tendon of flexor hallucis longus muscle |
| 21 | Quadriceps femoris muscle (divided) |
| 22 | Tendon of adductor magnus muscle (divided) |
| 23 | Medial condyle of femur |
| 24 | Popliteal artery and vein, and tibial nerve |
| 25 | Tibia |
| 26 | Femur |
| 27 | Lateral epicondyle of femur |
| 28 | Oblique popliteal ligament |
| 29 | Lateral (fibular) collateral ligament |
| 30 | Plantaris muscle |
| 31 | Tendon of biceps femoris muscle (divided) |
| 32 | Tendinous arch of soleus muscle |

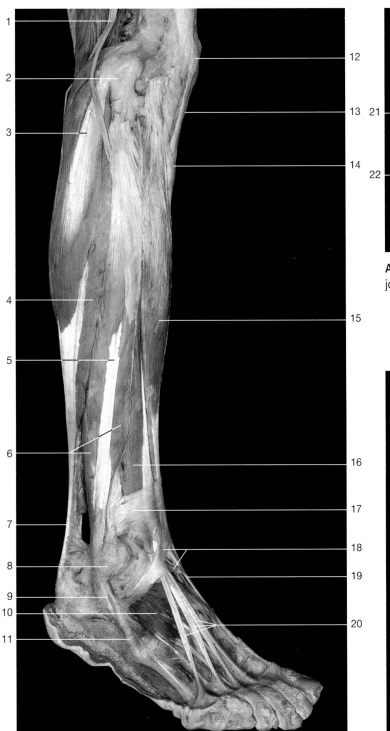

**Muscles of leg and foot** (right side, lateral aspect).

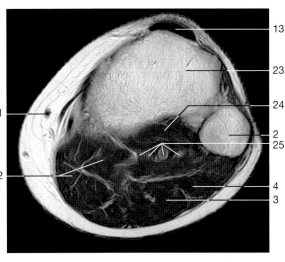

**Axial section through the right leg** distally of the knee joint (MRI scan). (From Heuck et al., MRT-Atlas, 2009.)

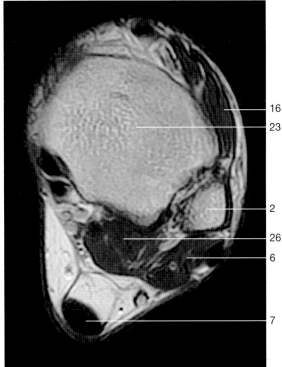

**Axial section through the right leg** cranially of the ankle joint (MRI scan). (From Heuck et al., MRT-Atlas, 2009.)

| | | |
|---|---|---|
| 1 Common fibular nerve | 10 Extensor digitorum brevis muscle | 19 Tendon of extensor hallucis longus muscle |
| 2 Head of fibula | 11 Tendon of peroneus brevis muscle | 20 Tendons of extensor digitorum longus muscle |
| 3 Lateral head of gastrocnemius muscle | 12 Patella | 21 Great saphenous vein |
| 4 Soleus muscle | 13 Patellar ligament | 22 Medial head of gastrocnemius muscle |
| 5 Peroneus longus muscle | 14 Tuberosity of tibia | 23 Tibia |
| 6 Peroneus brevis muscle | 15 Tibialis anterior muscle | 24 Popliteus muscle |
| 7 Calcaneal or Achilles tendon | 16 Extensor digitorum longus muscle | 25 Tibial nerve, popliteal artery, and veins |
| 8 Lateral malleolus muscle | 17 Superior extensor retinaculum | 26 Flexor hallucis longus muscle |
| 9 Tendon of peroneus longus muscle | 18 Inferior extensor retinaculum | |

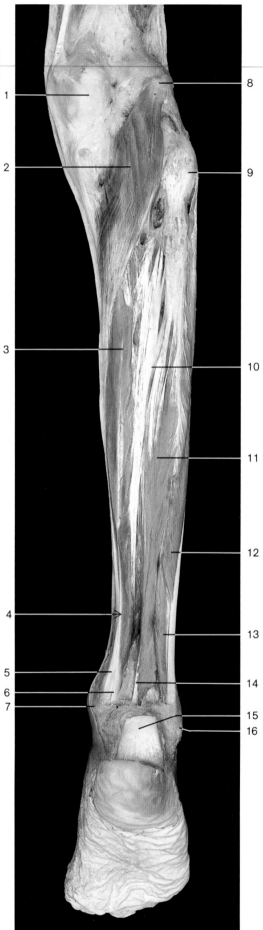

1　Medial condyle of femur
2　Popliteus muscle
3　Flexor digitorum longus muscle
4　Crossing of tendons in the leg
5　Tendon of tibialis posterior muscle
6　Tendon of flexor digitorum longus muscle
7　Medial malleolus
8　Lateral condyle of femur
9　Head of fibula
10　Tibialis posterior muscle
11　Flexor hallucis longus muscle
12　Peroneus longus muscle
13　Peroneus brevis muscle
14　Tendon of flexor hallucis longus muscle
15　Calcaneal or Achilles tendon (divided)
16　Lateral malleolus

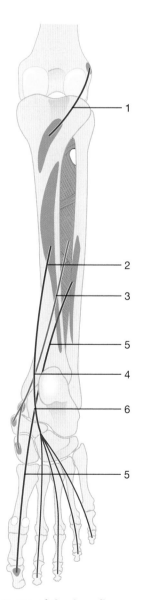

**Deep flexor muscles of leg and foot**
(right side, posterior aspect).

**Course of the deep flexor muscles of the leg** (posterior aspect).

1　Popliteus muscle (blue)
2　Flexor digitorum longus muscle (blue)
3　Tibialis posterior muscle (red)
4　Crossing of tendons in the leg
5　Flexor hallucis longus muscle (blue)
6　Crossing of tendons in the sole

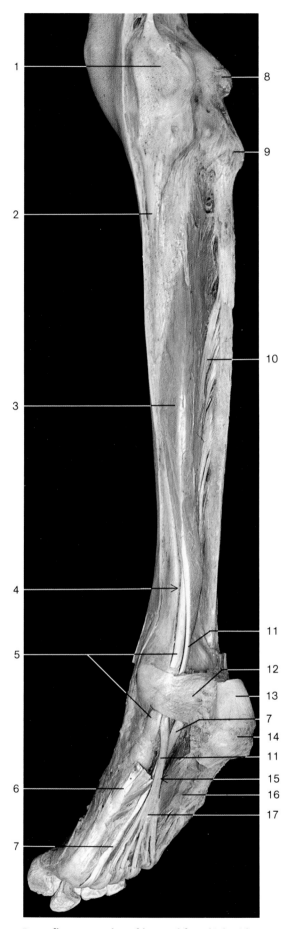

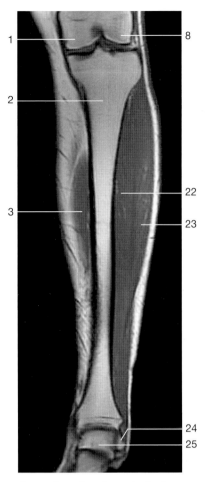

1  Medial condyle of femur
2  Tibia
3  Flexor digitorum longus muscle
4  Crossing of tendons in the leg
5  Tendon of tibialis posterior muscle
6  Abductor hallucis muscle
7  Tendon of flexor hallucis longus muscle
8  Lateral condyle of femur
9  Head of fibula
10  Tibialis posterior muscle
11  Tendon of flexor digitorum longus muscle
12  Flexor retinaculum
13  Calcaneal or Achilles tendon
14  Calcaneal tuberosity
15  Crossing of tendons in the sole
16  Quadratus plantae muscle
17  Tendons of flexor digitorum longus muscle
18  Tendon of tibialis anterior muscle
19  Area of insertion of tibialis posterior muscle
20  Lumbrical muscles
21  Flexor hallucis longus muscle
22  Tibialis anterior muscle
23  Extensor hallucis longus muscle
24  Lateral malleolus of fibula
25  Trochlea of talus

**Coronal section through the leg**
(MRI scan). (From Heuck et al., MRT-Atlas, 2009.)

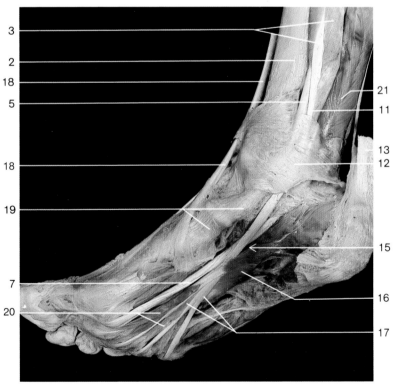

**Deep flexor muscles of leg and foot** (right side, posterior oblique-medial aspect). Flexor digitorum brevis and flexor hallucis longus muscles have been removed.

**Sole of the right foot with tendons of long flexor muscles** (oblique-medial and inferior aspect).

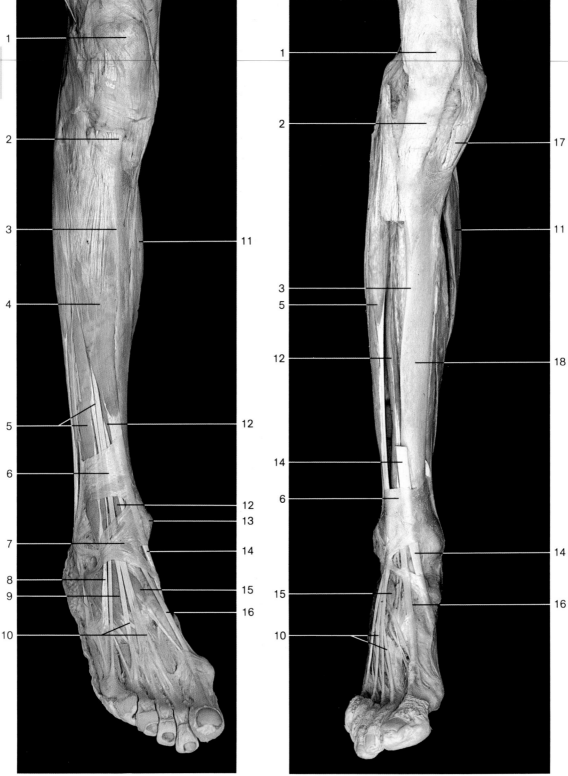

**Extensor muscles of leg and foot** (right side, oblique antero-lateral aspect).

**Extensor muscles of leg and foot** (right side, anterior aspect). Part of the tibialis anterior muscle has been removed.

| | | |
|---|---|---|
| 1 Patella | 8 Tendon of peroneus tertius muscle | 14 Tendon of tibialis anterior muscle |
| 2 Patellar ligament | 9 Extensor digitorum brevis muscle | 15 Extensor hallucis brevis muscle |
| 3 Anterior margin of tibia | 10 Tendons of extensor digitorum longus muscle | 16 Tendon of extensor hallucis longus muscle |
| 4 Tibialis anterior muscle | 11 Soleus muscle | 17 Common tendon of gracilis, semitendinosus, and sartorius muscles (pes anserinus) |
| 5 Extensor digitorum longus muscle | 12 Extensor hallucis longus muscle | 18 Tibia |
| 6 Superior extensor retinaculum | 13 Medial malleolus | |
| 7 Inferior extensor retinaculum | | |

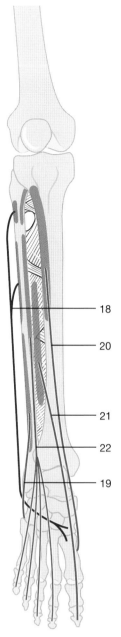

**Course of the extensor muscles of the leg** (anterior aspect).

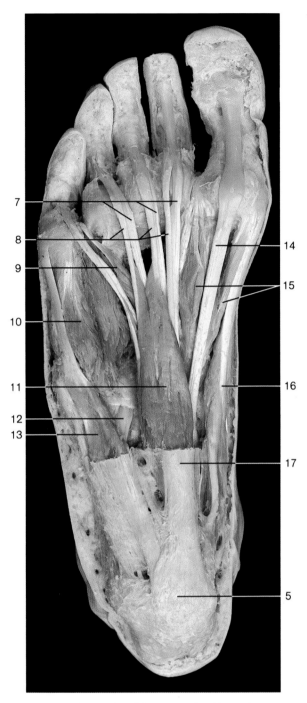

**Muscles of the sole of foot,** superficial layer. The plantar aponeurosis and the fasciae of the superficial muscles have been removed.

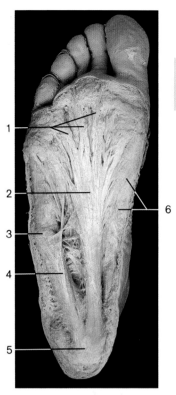

**Sole of the foot with the plantar aponeurosis.**

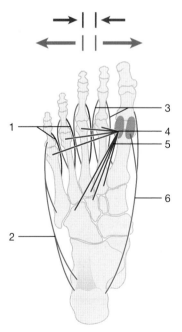

**Course of abductor and adductor muscles of the foot** (plantar aspect). Red arrows: abduction; blue arrows: adduction.

| | |
|---|---|
| 1 | Longitudinal bands of plantar aponeurosis |
| 2 | Plantar aponeurosis |
| 3 | Position of tuberosity of fifth metatarsal bone |
| 4 | Muscles of fifth toe with fascia |
| 5 | Calcaneal tuberosity |
| 6 | Muscles of great toe with fascia |
| 7 | Tendons of flexor digitorum longus muscle |
| 8 | Tendons of flexor digitorum brevis muscle |
| 9 | Lumbrical muscle |
| 10 | Flexor digiti minimi brevis muscle |
| 11 | Flexor digitorum brevis muscle |
| 12 | Tendon of peroneus longus muscle |
| 13 | Abductor digiti minimi muscle |
| 14 | Tendon of flexor hallucis longus muscle |
| 15 | Flexor hallucis brevis muscle |
| 16 | Abductor hallucis muscle |
| 17 | Plantar aponeurosis (cut) |
| 18 | Peroneus longus muscle |
| 19 | Peroneus brevis muscle |
| 20 | Tibialis anterior muscle |
| 21 | Extensor hallucis longus muscle |
| 22 | Extensor digitorum longus muscle |

1 Plantar interossei muscles (blue)
2 Abductor digiti minimi muscle (red)
3 Dorsal interossei muscles (red)
4 Transverse head of adductor hallucis muscle (blue)
5 Oblique head of adductor hallucis muscle (blue)
6 Abductor hallucis muscle (red)

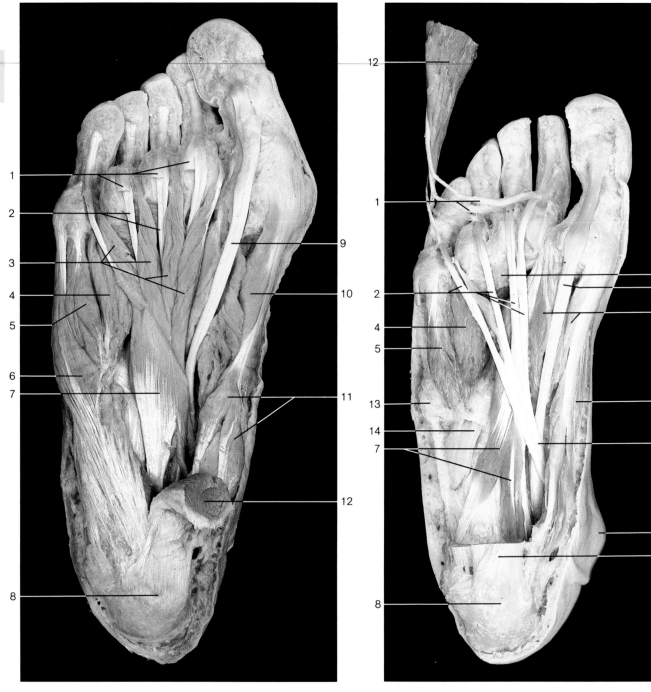

**Muscles of the sole of foot,** middle layer. The flexor digitorum brevis muscle has been divided.

**Muscles of the sole of foot,** middle layer. The tendons of the flexor muscles and the crossing of tendons are displayed. The flexor digitorum brevis muscle has been divided and reflected.

| | | |
|---|---|---|
| 1 Tendons of flexor digitorum brevis muscle | 8 Calcaneal tuberosity | 15 Transverse head of adductor hallucis muscle |
| 2 Tendons of flexor digitorum longus muscle | 9 Tendon of flexor hallucis longus muscle | 16 Crossing of tendons in the sole of foot |
| 3 Lumbrical muscles | 10 Flexor hallucis brevis muscle | 17 Medial malleolus |
| 4 Interossei muscles | 11 Abductor hallucis muscle | 18 Plantar aponeurosis (divided) |
| 5 Flexor digiti minimi brevis muscle | 12 Flexor digitorum brevis muscle (divided) | |
| 6 Abductor digiti minimi muscle | 13 Tuberosity of fifth metatarsal bone | |
| 7 Quadratus plantae muscle | 14 Tendon of peroneus longus muscle | |

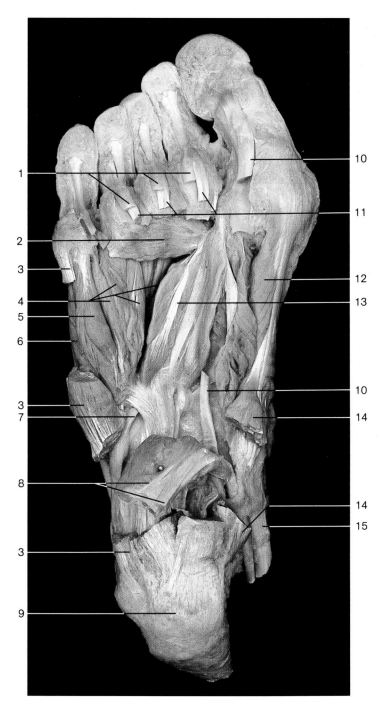

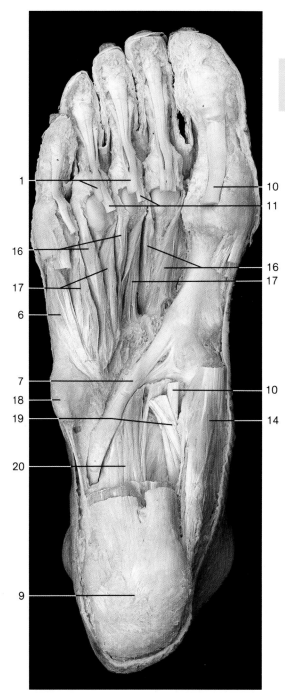

**Muscles of the sole of foot,** deep layer. The flexor digitorum brevis muscle has been removed, and the quadratus plantae, abductor hallucis, and digiti minimi muscles have been divided.

**Muscles of the sole of foot,** deepest layer. The interossei muscles and the canal for the tendon of peroneus longus muscle are shown.

| | | |
|---|---|---|
| 1 Tendons of flexor digitorum brevis muscle | 9 Calcaneal tuberosity | 17 Plantar interossei muscles |
| 2 Transverse head of adductor hallucis muscle | 10 Tendon of flexor hallucis longus muscle (divided) | 18 Tuberosity of fifth metatarsal bone |
| 3 Abductor digiti minimi muscle | 11 Tendons of flexor digitorum longus muscle | 19 Tendon of flexor digitorum longus muscle (crossing of plantar tendons) |
| 4 Interossei muscles | 12 Flexor hallucis brevis muscle | 20 Long plantar ligament |
| 5 Flexor digiti minimi brevis muscle | 13 Oblique head of adductor hallucis muscle | |
| 6 Opponens digiti minimi muscle | 14 Abductor hallucis muscle (cut) | |
| 7 Tendon of peroneus longus muscle | 15 Tendon of tibialis posterior muscle | |
| 8 Quadratus plantae muscle with tendon of flexor digitorum longus muscle | 16 Dorsal interossei muscles | |

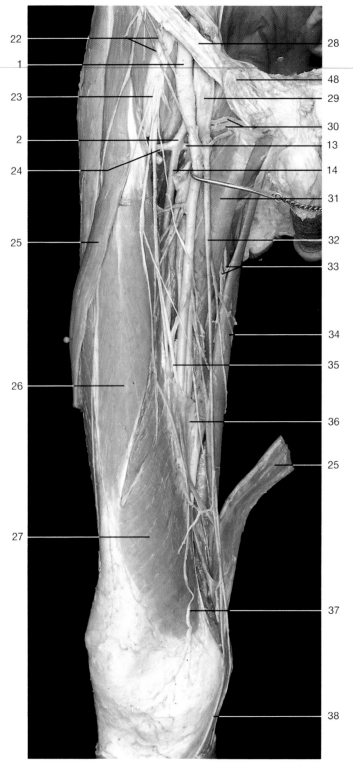

22
1
23
2
24
25
26
27

28
48
29
30
13
14
31
32
33
34
35
36
25
37
38

**Main arteries and nerves of the thigh** (right side, anterior aspect). The sartorius muscle has been divided and reflected. The femoral vein has been partly removed to show the deep femoral artery. Note that the vessels enter the adductor canal to reach the popliteal fossa.

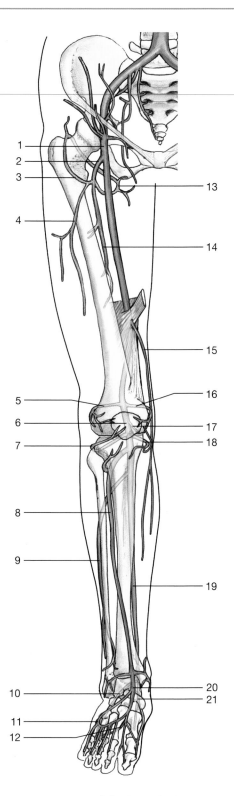

1
2
3
4
5
6
7
8
9
10
11
12

13
14
15
16
17
18
19
20
21

**Main arteries of the lower limb** (anterior aspect).

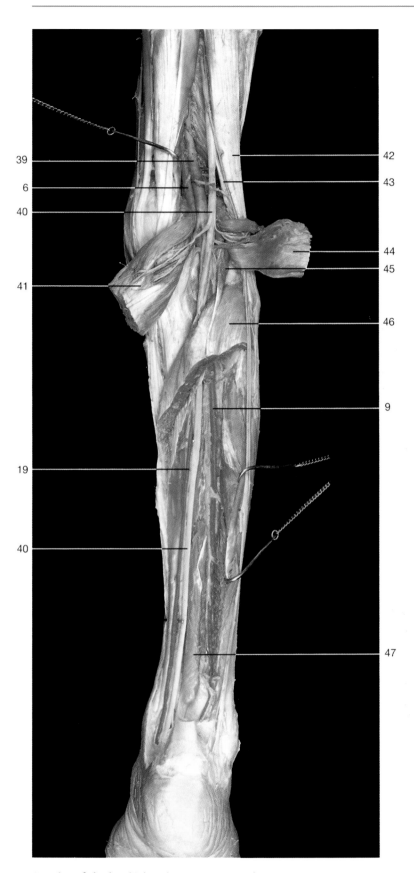

1 Femoral artery
2 Deep artery of thigh
3 Ascending branch
  of lateral circumflex femoral artery
4 Descending branch
  of lateral circumflex femoral artery
5 Lateral superior genicular artery
6 Popliteal artery
7 Lateral inferior genicular artery
8 Anterior tibial artery
9 Peroneal artery
10 Lateral plantar artery
11 Arcuate artery with dorsal metatarsal arteries
12 Plantar arch with plantar metatarsal arteries
13 Medial circumflex femoral artery
14 Deep artery of thigh with perforating arteries
15 Descending genicular artery
16 Medial superior genicular artery
17 Middle genicular artery
18 Medial inferior genicular artery
19 Posterior tibial artery
20 Dorsalis pedis artery
21 Medial plantar artery
22 Superficial and deep circumflex iliac arteries
23 Femoral nerve
24 Lateral circumflex femoral artery
25 Sartorius muscle (cut and reflected)
26 Rectus femoris muscle
27 Vastus medialis muscle
28 Inguinal ligament
29 Femoral vein (cut)
30 External pudendal artery and vein
31 Adductor longus muscle
32 Great saphenous vein
33 Obturator artery and nerve
34 Gracilis muscle
35 Saphenous nerve
36 Vasto-adductor membrane
37 Anterior cutaneous branch of femoral nerve
38 Infrapatellar branch of saphenous nerve
39 Popliteal vein
40 Tibial nerve
41 Medial head of gastrocnemius muscle
42 Biceps femoris muscle
43 Common fibular nerve
44 Lateral head of gastrocnemius muscle
45 Plantaris muscle
46 Soleus muscle
47 Flexor hallucis longus muscle
48 Spermatic cord

**Arteries of the leg** (right side, posterior aspect).

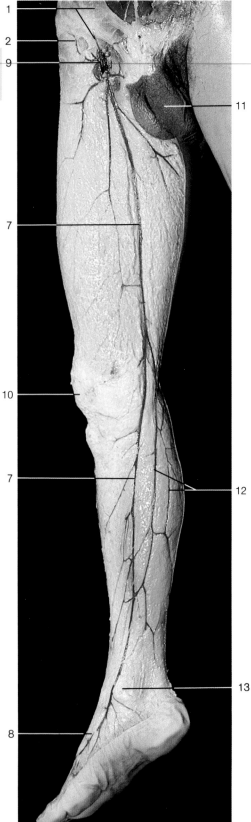

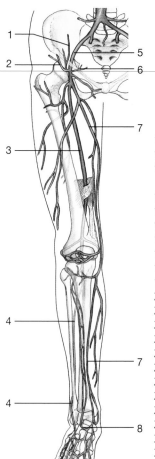

1   Superficial epigastric vein
2   Superficial circumflex iliac vein
3   Femoral vein
4   Small saphenous vein
5   External iliac vein
6   External pudendal vein
7   Great saphenous vein
8   Dorsal venous arch of foot
9   Saphenous opening with femoral vein
10  Patella
11  Penis
12  Anastomoses between great and
    small saphenous veins
13  Medial malleolus
14  Saphenous nerve
15  Posterior tibial artery and veins
16  Tibial nerve
17  Medial dorsal cutaneous nerve
18  Posterior tibial vein
19  Popliteal fossa
20  Perforating veins
21  Lateral malleolus
22  Superficial layer of crural fascia
23  Perforating veins I–III (of Cockett)
24  Tibia
25  Dorsal digital veins of foot
26  Dorsal venous arch of foot
27  Dorsal metatarsal veins
28  Anterior tibial artery and vein
29  Fibula
30  Peroneal artery and vein
31  Deep layer of crural fascia

**Main trunkal veins
of the lower limb**
(anterior aspect).

**Superficial veins of the lower limb** (right
side, medio-anterior aspect). The veins have
been injected with red solution.

**Medial malleolar region of the right foot.** ▷
Dissection of tibial nerve, posterior tibial
vessels, and great saphenous vein. The veins
have been injected with blue resin.

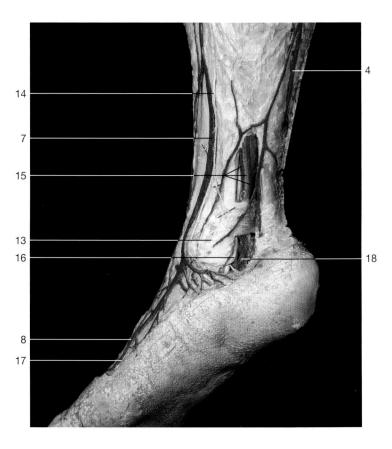

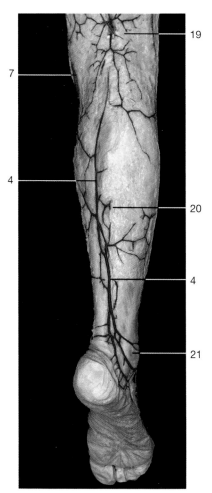

**Superficial veins of the leg** (right side, posterior aspect). The veins have been injected with blue resin.

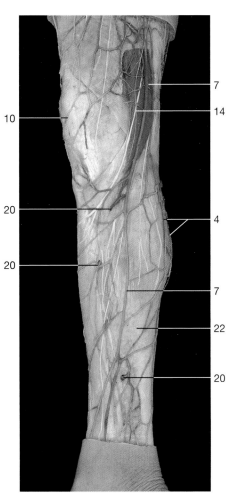

**Superficial veins of the leg** (left side, medial aspect). The perforating veins of Cockett have been dissected.

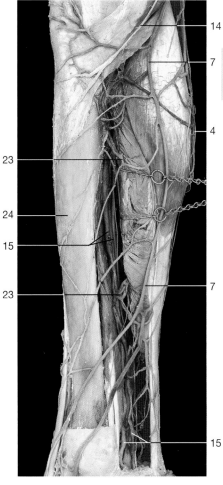

**Veins of the leg** (left side, medial aspect). The anastomoses between superficial and deeper veins are dissected.

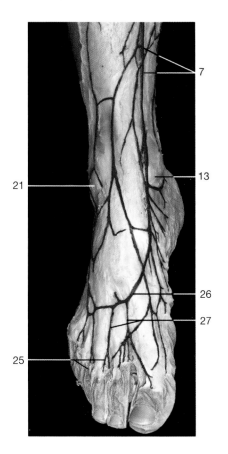

**Superficial veins of the dorsum of the right foot.** The veins have been injected with blue resin.

**Anastomoses between superficial ▷ and deep veins of the leg.** Arrows: directions of blood flow.

◁

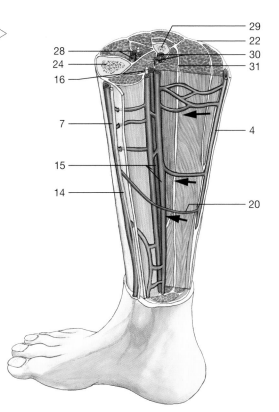

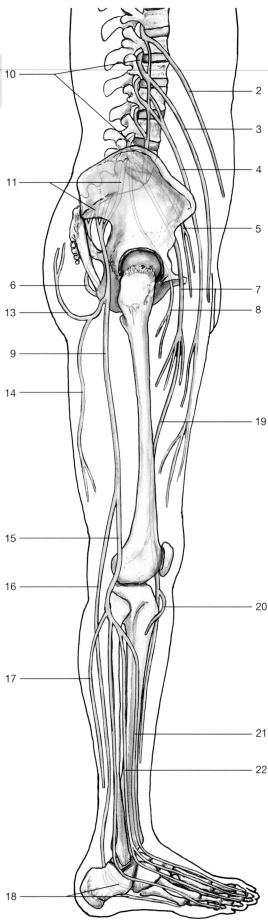

1   Subcostal nerve
2   Iliohypogastric nerve
3   Ilio-inguinal nerve
4   Lateral femoral cutaneous nerve
5   Genitofemoral nerve
6   Pudendal nerve
7   Femoral nerve
8   Obturator nerve
9   Sciatic nerve
10  Lumbar plexus (L$_1$–L$_4$)
11  Sacral plexus (L$_4$–S$_4$)
12  "Pudendal" plexus (S$_2$–S$_4$)
}  lumbosacral plexus
13  Inferior cluneal nerves
14  Posterior femoral cutaneous nerve
15  Common fibular nerve
16  Tibial nerve
17  Lateral sural cutaneous nerve
18  Medial and lateral plantar nerves
19  Saphenous nerve
20  Infrapatellar branch of saphenous nerve
21  Deep fibular nerve
22  Superficial fibular nerve
23  Anterior cutaneous branch of iliohypogastric nerve
24  Lateral cutaneous branch of iliohypogastric nerve
25  Femoral branch of genitofemoral nerve
26  Lateral cutaneous branches of intercostal nerves
27  Anterior cutaneous branches of intercostal nerves
28  Genital branch of genitofemoral nerve
29  Anterior scrotal nerves

**Nerves of the lower limb** (lateral aspect).

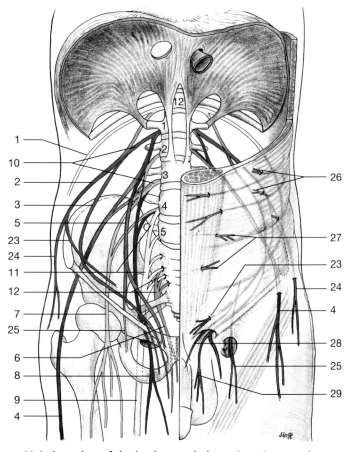

**Main branches of the lumbosacral plexus** (anterior aspect).

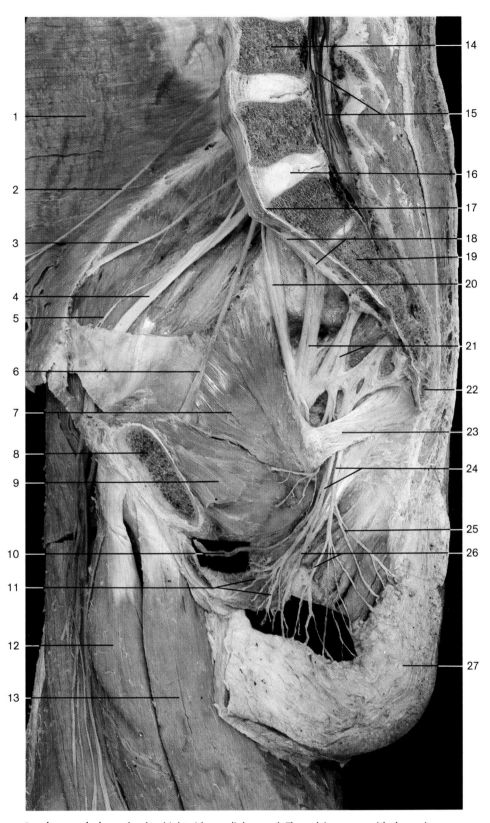

1   Transverse abdominal muscle
2   Iliohypogastric nerve
3   Ilio-inguinal nerve
4   Femoral nerve
5   Lateral femoral cutaneous nerve
6   Obturator nerve
7   Obturator internus muscle
8   Pubis (cut edge)
9   Levator ani muscle (remnant)
10  Dorsal nerve of penis
11  Posterior scrotal nerves
    of pudendal nerve
12  Adductor longus muscle
13  Gracilis muscle
14  Body of fourth lumbar vertebra
15  Cauda equina
16  Intervertebral disc
17  Sacral promontory
18  Sympathetic trunk
19  Sacrum
20  Lumbosacral trunk
21  Sacral plexus
22  Coccyx
23  Sacrospinous ligament
24  Pudendal nerve
25  Inferior rectal nerves
26  Perineal nerves of pudendal nerve
27  Subcutaneous fat tissue
    of gluteal region

**Lumbosacral plexus in situ** (right side, medial aspect). The pelvic organs with the peritoneum and part of the levator ani muscle have been removed.

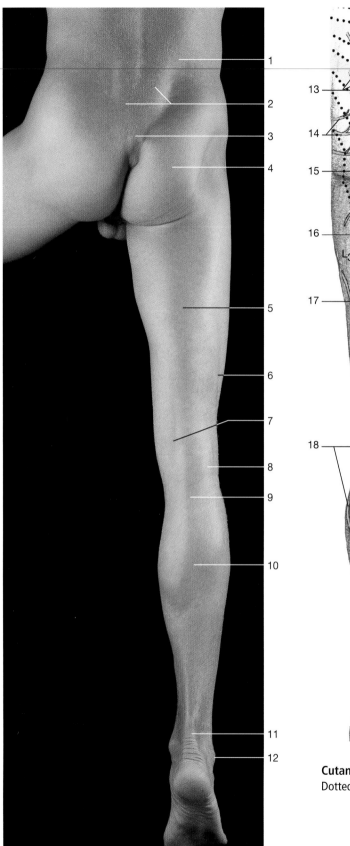

| | |
|---|---|
| 1 | Iliac crest |
| 2 | Sacrum |
| 3 | Coccyx |
| 4 | Gluteus maximus muscle |
| 5 | Ischiocrural muscles |
| 6 | Iliotibial tract |
| 7 | Tendon of semimembranosus muscle |
| 8 | Tendon of biceps femoris muscle |
| 9 | Popliteal fossa |
| 10 | Triceps surae muscle |
| 11 | Calcaneal or Achilles tendon |
| 12 | Lateral malleolus |
| 13 | Superior cluneal nerves |
| 14 | Middle cluneal nerves |
| 15 | Inferior cluneal nerves |
| 16 | Posterior femoral cutaneous nerve |
| 17 | Obturator nerve |
| 18 | Saphenous nerve |
| 19 | Iliohypogastric nerve |
| 20 | Lateral femoral cutaneous nerves |
| 21 | Common fibular nerve |
| 22 | Sural nerve |

**Cutaneous nerves of the lower limb** (posterior aspect). Dotted lines = border of segments.

**Surface anatomy of the lower limb** (right side, posterior aspect). The gluteal muscles are contracted.

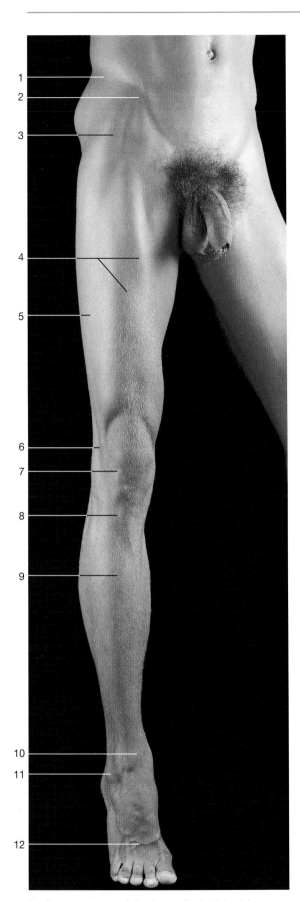

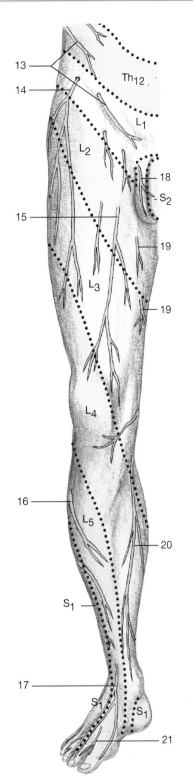

1   Iliac crest
2   Anterior superior iliac spine
3   Tensor fasciae latae muscle
4   Quadriceps femoris muscle
5   Iliotibial tract
6   Tendon of biceps femoris muscle
7   Patella
8   Patellar ligament
9   Tibia
10  Tendon of tibialis anterior muscle
11  Lateral malleolus
12  Dorsal venous arch of foot
13  Iliohypogastric nerve
14  Lateral femoral cutaneous nerve
15  Femoral nerve
16  Common fibular nerve
17  Superficial fibular nerve
18  Ilio-inguinal nerve
19  Obturator nerve
20  Saphenous nerve
21  Deep fibular nerve

**Cutaneous nerves of the lower limb** (anterior aspect).
Dotted lines = border of segments.

**Surface anatomy of the lower limb** (right side, anterior aspect).

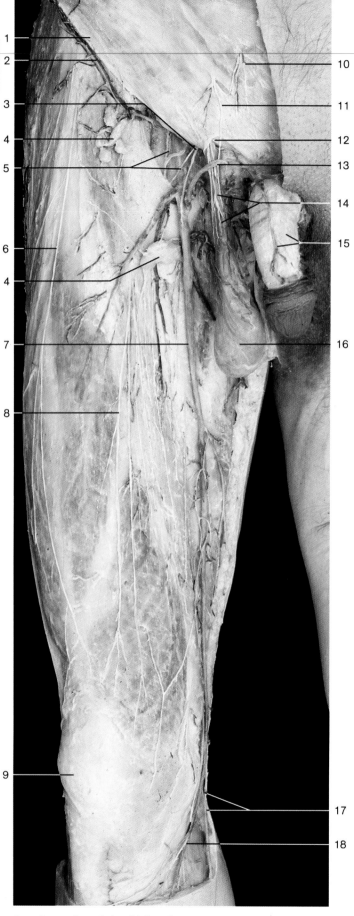

**Anterior region of the thigh** with cutaneous nerves and veins (right side).

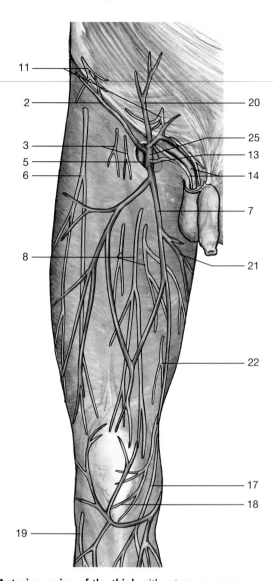

**Anterior region of the thigh** with cutaneous nerves and veins (right side; compare with the dissection alongside).

1  Inguinal ligament
2  Superficial circumflex iliac vein
3  Femoral branch of genitofemoral nerve
4  Superficial inguinal lymph nodes
5  Saphenous opening with femoral artery and vein
6  Lateral femoral cutaneous nerve
7  Great saphenous vein
8  Anterior cutaneous branches of femoral nerve
9  Patella
10 Terminal branches of subcostal nerve
11 Terminal branches of iliohypogastric nerve
12 Superficial inguinal ring
13 External pudendal vein
14 Spermatic cord
   with genital branch of genitofemoral nerve
15 Penis with superficial dorsal vein of penis
16 Testis and its coverings
17 Saphenous nerve
18 Infrapatellar branch of saphenous nerve
19 Lateral sural cutaneous nerve
20 Superficial epigastric vein
21 Accessory saphenous vein
22 Cutaneous branch of obturator nerve
23 Femoral nerve
24 Femoral artery
25 Femoral vein
26 Superficial and inferior inguinal lymph nodes (enlarged)
27 Lymphatic vessels
28 Sartorius muscle
29 Iliohypogastric nerve

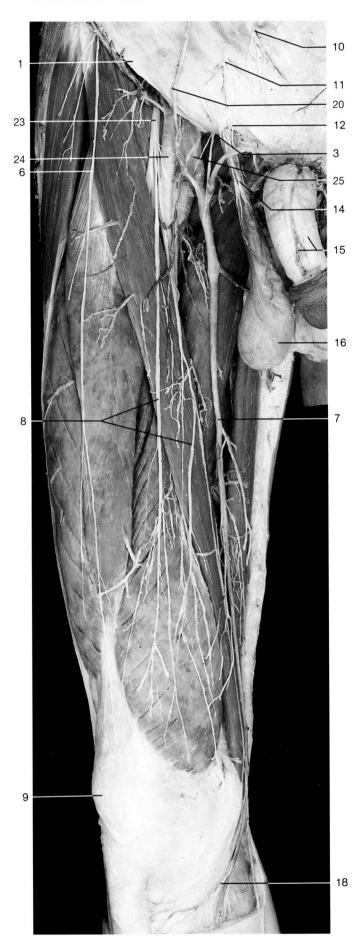

**Anterior region of the thigh** with cutaneous nerves and veins
(right side). The fascia lata and the fasciae of the thigh muscles
have been removed.

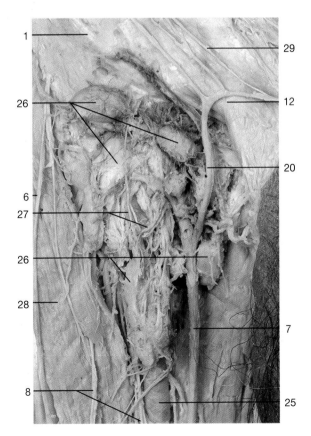

**Inguinal nodes with lymphatic vessels** (anterior
aspect).

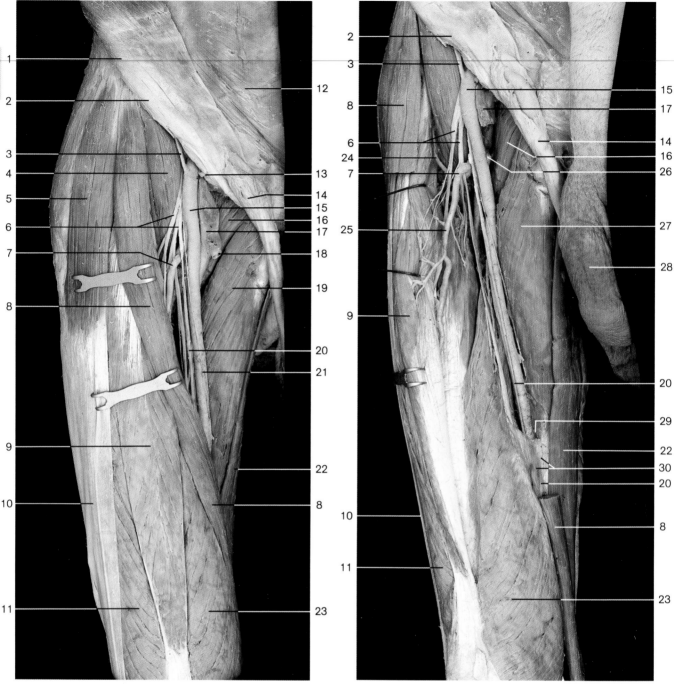

**Anterior region of the thigh** (right side, anterior aspect). The fascia lata has been removed and the sartorius muscle has been slightly reflected.

**Anterior region of the thigh** (right side, anterior aspect). The fascia lata has been removed and the sartorius muscle has been divided.

1 Anterior superior iliac spine
2 Inguinal ligament
3 Deep circumflex iliac artery
4 Iliopsoas muscle
5 Tensor fasciae latae muscle
6 Femoral nerve
7 Lateral circumflex femoral artery
8 Sartorius muscle
9 Rectus femoris muscle
10 Iliotibial tract
11 Vastus lateralis muscle
12 Anterior sheath of rectus abdominis muscle
13 Inferior epigastric artery
14 Spermatic cord
15 Femoral artery

16 Pectineus muscle
17 Femoral vein
18 Great saphenous vein (divided)
19 Adductor longus muscle
20 Saphenous nerve
21 Muscular branch of femoral nerve
22 Gracilis muscle
23 Vastus medialis muscle
24 Ascending branch of lateral circumflex femoral artery
25 Descending branch of lateral circumflex femoral artery
26 Medial circumflex femoral artery
27 Adductor longus muscle
28 Penis
29 Entrance to adductor canal
30 Vasto-adductor membrane of fascia beneath sartorius muscle

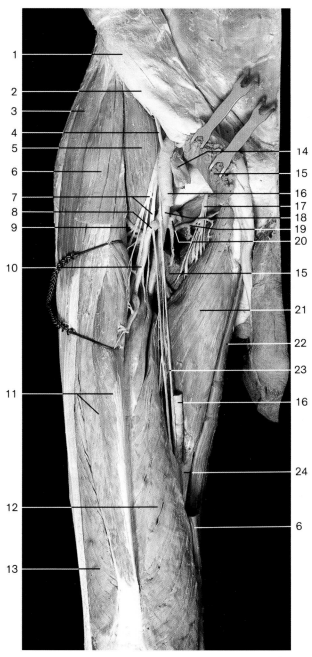

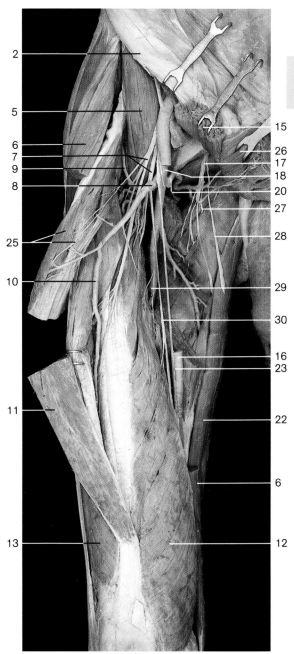

**Anterior region of the thigh** (right side, anterior aspect). The fascia lata has been removed. Sartorius and pectineus muscles, and the femoral artery have been cut to display the deep femoral artery with its branches. The rectus femoris muscle has been slightly reflected.

**Anterior region of the thigh** (right side, anterior aspect). The sartorius, pectineus, adductor longus, and rectus femoris muscles have been divided and reflected. The greater part of the femoral artery has been removed.

1 Anterior superior iliac spine
2 Inguinal ligament
3 Tensor fasciae latae muscle
4 Deep circumflex iliac artery
5 Iliopsoas muscle
6 Sartorius muscle (cut)
7 Femoral nerve
8 Lateral circumflex femoral artery
9 Ascending branch of lateral circumflex femoral artery
10 Descending branch of lateral circumflex femoral artery
11 Rectus femoris muscle
12 Vastus medialis muscle
13 Vastus lateralis muscle
14 Femoral vein
15 Pectineus muscle (cut)
16 Femoral artery (cut)

17 Obturator nerve
18 Deep artery of thigh
19 Ascending branch of medial circumflex femoral artery
20 Medial circumflex femoral artery
21 Adductor longus muscle
22 Gracilis muscle
23 Saphenous nerve
24 Distal part of vasto-adductor membrane
25 Rectus femoris muscle
   with muscular branches of femoral nerve
26 Adductor longus muscle (divided)
27 Posterior branch of obturator nerve
28 Anterior branch of obturator nerve
29 Point at which perforating artery branches off
   from deep artery of thigh
30 Muscular branch of femoral nerve to vastus medialis muscle

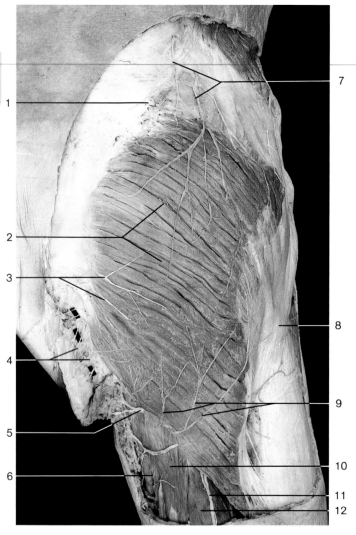

1  Iliac crest
2  Gluteus maximus muscle
3  Middle cluneal nerves
4  Anococcygeal nerves
5  Perineal branch of posterior femoral cutaneous nerve
6  Adductor magnus muscle
7  Superior cluneal nerves
8  Position of greater trochanter
9  Inferior cluneal nerves
10 Semitendinosus muscle
11 Posterior femoral cutaneous nerve
12 Long head of biceps femoris muscle

**Gluteal region** (right side). Dissection of the cutaneous nerves.

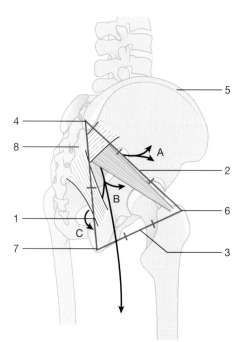

**Location of the sciatic foramina in relation to the bones at the gluteal region** (postero-lateral aspect).

**A  Suprapiriform foramen
(of greater sciatic foramen)**

Superior gluteal artery, vein, and nerve

**B  Infrapiriform foramen
(of greater sciatic foramen)**

Sciatic nerve
Inferior gluteal artery, vein, and nerve
Posterior femoral cutaneous nerve
Internal pudendal artery and vein
Pudendal nerve
Internal obturator nerve
Nerve to quadratus femoris muscle

**C  Lesser sciatic foramen**

Pudendal nerve
Internal pudendal artery and vein
Internal obturator nerve

**Red lines**

1  **Spine-tuber line**
   (the infrapiriform foramen is situated in the middle of this line)
2  **Spine-trochanter line**
   (the suprapiriform foramen is located in the upper third)
3  **Tuber-trochanter line**
   (the ischiadic nerve can be found between the middle and posterior third)

**Other structures**

4  Posterior superior iliac spine
5  Iliac crest
6  Greater trochanter
7  Ischial tuberosity
8  Sacrum

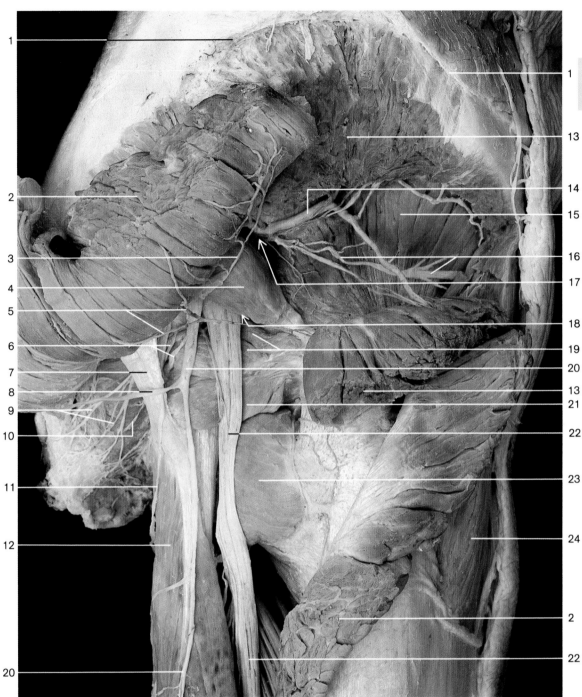

**Gluteal region** (right side). Gluteus maximus and gluteus medius muscles have been divided and reflected. Notice the position of the foramina above and below the piriformis muscle and the lesser sciatic foramen.

1  Iliac crest
2  Gluteus maximus muscle (cut)
3  Inferior gluteal nerve
4  Piriformis muscle
5  Muscular branches of inferior gluteal artery
6  Pudendal nerve and internal pudendal artery within the lesser sciatic foramen (entrance to the pudendal canal)
7  Sacrotuberous ligament
8  Inferior cluneal nerve
9  Inferior rectal nerves
10  Inferior rectal arteries
11  Perforating cutaneous nerve of posterior femoral cutaneous nerve

12  Long head of biceps femoris muscle
13  Gluteus medius muscle (cut)
14  Deep branch of superior gluteal artery
15  Gluteus minimus muscle
16  Superior gluteal nerve
17  Suprapiriform foramen ⎫ greater sciatic foramen
18  Infrapiriform foramen ⎭
19  Obturator internus and superior gemellus muscles
20  Posterior femoral cutaneous nerve
21  Inferior gemellus muscle
22  Sciatic nerve
23  Quadratus femoris muscle
24  Tensor fasciae latae muscle

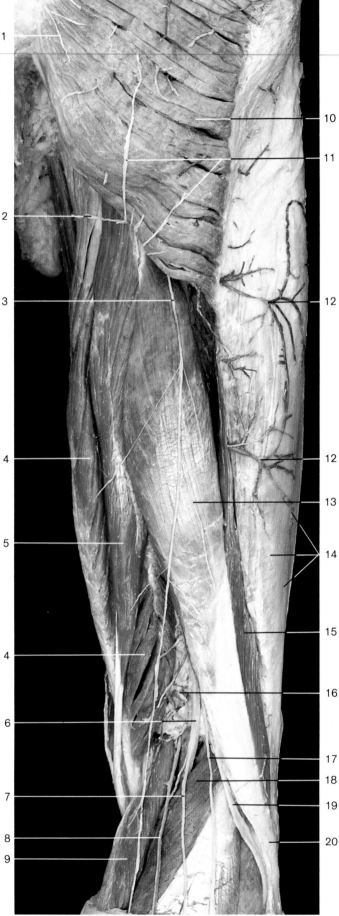

1 Middle cluneal nerves
2 Perineal branch of posterior femoral cutaneous nerve
3 Posterior femoral cutaneous nerve
4 Semimembranosus muscle
5 Semitendinosus muscle
6 Tibial nerve
7 Medial sural cutaneous nerve
8 Small saphenous vein
9 Medial head of gastrocnemius muscle
10 Gluteus maximus muscle
11 Inferior cluneal nerves
12 Cutaneous veins
13 Long head of biceps femoris muscle
14 Iliotibial tract
15 Short head of biceps femoris muscle
16 Popliteal fossa
17 Lateral sural cutaneous nerve
18 Lateral head of gastrocnemius muscle
19 Common fibular nerve
20 Tendon of biceps femoris muscle
21 Inferior gluteal nerve
22 Sacrotuberous ligament
23 Inferior rectal branches of pudendal nerve
24 Anus
25 Gluteus medius muscle
26 Piriformis muscle
27 Sciatic nerve
28 Inferior gluteal artery
29 Gluteus maximus muscle (cut)
30 Quadratus femoris muscle
31 Sciatic nerve dividing into its two branches
   (the common fibular nerve and the tibial nerve)
32 Muscular branches of sciatic nerve to the ischiocrural muscles
33 Popliteal artery
34 Popliteal vein
35 Small saphenous vein (cut)
36 Long head of biceps femoris muscle (cut)
37 Superficial fibular nerve

**Gluteal and posterior regions of the thigh** with cutaneous nerves (right side). The fascia lata and the fasciae of the muscles have been removed.

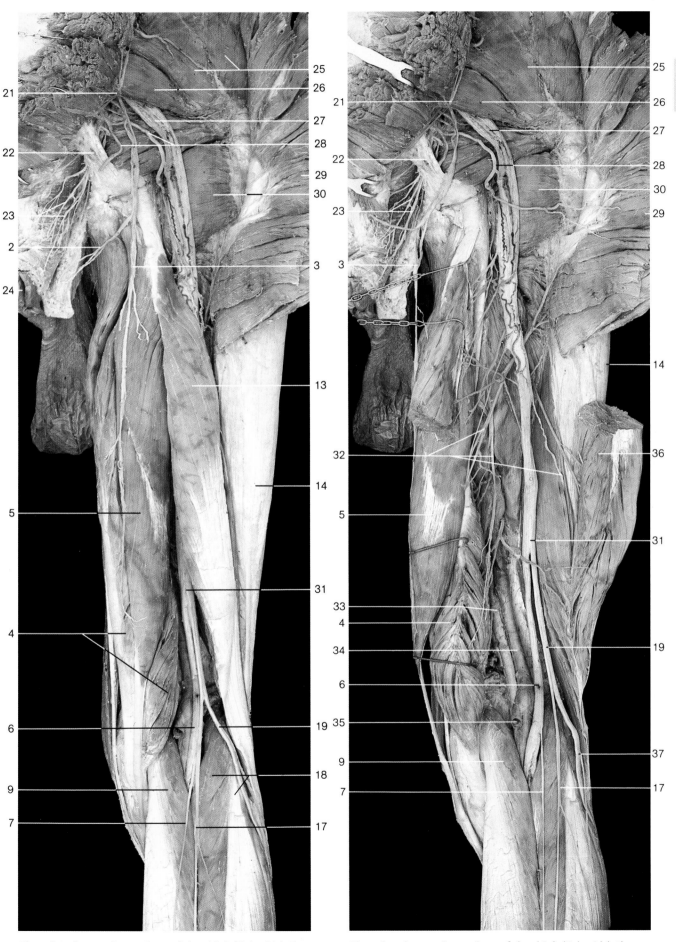

**Gluteal and posterior regions of the thigh** (right side). The gluteus maximus muscle has been divided and reflected.

**Gluteal and posterior regions of the thigh** (right side). The gluteus maximus muscle and the long head of the biceps femoris muscle have been divided and reflected.

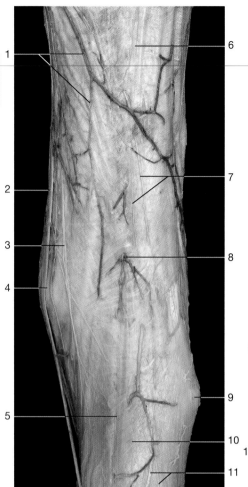

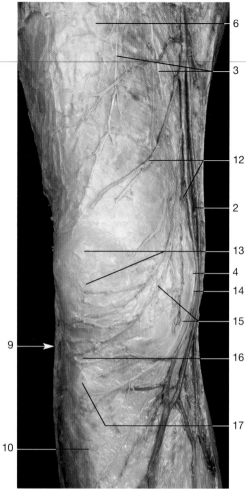

1   Cutaneous veins (tributaries of great saphenous vein)
2   Great saphenous vein
3   Cutaneous branches of femoral nerve
4   Position of medial condyle of femur
5   Position of small saphenous vein
6   Fascia lata
7   Terminal branches of posterior femoral cutaneous nerve
8   Cutaneous veins of popliteal fossa
9   Position of head of fibula
10  Superficial layer of fascia cruris
11  Lateral sural cutaneous nerve
12  Venous network around knee
13  Patella
14  Saphenous nerve
15  Infrapatellar branch of saphenous nerve
16  Patellar ligament
17  Position of tibial tuberosity
18  Sartorius muscle
19  Semimembranosus muscle
20  Gastrocnemius muscle
21  Popliteal vein
22  Tibial nerve
23  Biceps femoris muscle
24  Popliteal artery
25  Lateral inferior genicular artery
26  Fibula

**Posterior region of the knee** with cutaneous nerves and veins (right side).

**Anterior region of the knee** with cutaneous nerves and veins (right side).

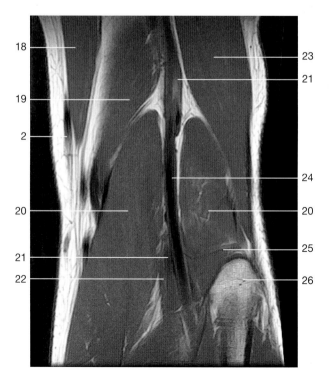

**Coronal section through the popliteal fossa** (MRI scan).
(From Heuck et al., MRT-Atlas, 2009.)

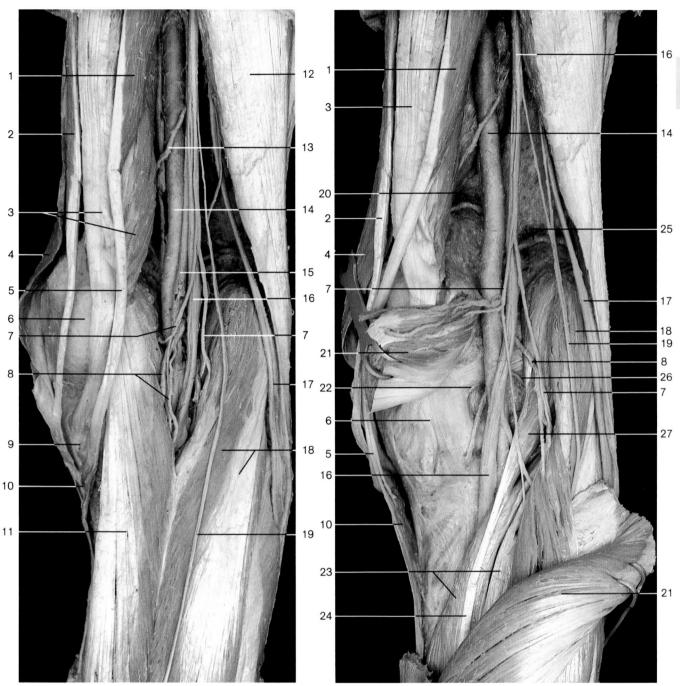

**Popliteal fossa,** middle layer (right side). The gastrocnemius muscle has been divided and reflected.

**Popliteal fossa,** deep layer (right side). Gastrocnemius and soleus muscles have been divided and reflected.

| | |
|---|---|
| 1 Semitendinosus muscle | 14 Popliteal artery |
| 2 Gracilis muscle | 15 Popliteal vein |
| 3 Semimembranosus muscle | 16 Tibial nerve |
| 4 Sartorius muscle | 17 Common fibular nerve |
| 5 Tendon of semitendinosus muscle | 18 Lateral head of gastrocnemius muscle |
| 6 Position of medial condyle of femur | 19 Medial sural cutaneous nerve |
| 7 Muscular branches of tibial nerve | 20 Medial superior genicular artery |
| 8 Sural arteries and veins | 21 Medial head of gastrocnemius muscle (cut and reflected) |
| 9 Tendon of semimembranosus muscle | 22 Medial inferior genicular artery |
| 10 Common tendon of gracilis, semitendinosus, and sartorius muscles (pes anserinus) | 23 Soleus muscle |
| 11 Medial head of gastrocnemius muscle | 24 Tendon of plantaris muscle |
| 12 Biceps femoris muscle | 25 Lateral superior genicular artery |
| 13 Muscular branch of popliteal artery | 26 Lateral inferior genicular artery |
| | 27 Plantaris muscle |

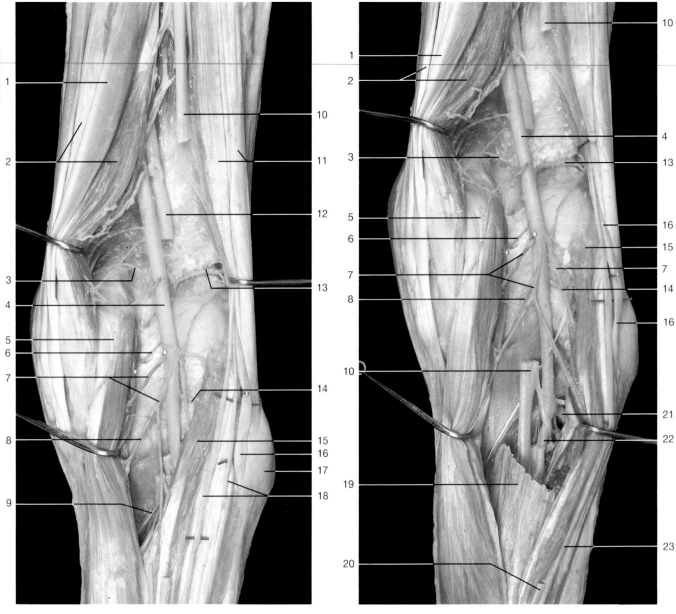

**Popliteal fossa,** deep layer (right side). The muscles have been reflected to display the genicular arteries.

**Popliteal fossa,** deepest layer (right side). Tibial nerve and popliteal vein have been partly removed and a portion of the soleus muscle was cut away to display the anterior tibial artery.

1  Semitendinosus muscle
2  Semimembranosus muscle
3  Medial superior genicular artery
4  Popliteal artery
5  Medial head of gastrocnemius muscle
6  Middle genicular artery
7  Muscular branches of popliteal artery
8  Medial inferior genicular artery
9  Tendon of plantaris muscle
10  Tibial nerve (cut)
11  Biceps femoris muscle
12  Popliteal vein (cut)

13  Lateral superior genicular artery
14  Lateral inferior genicular artery
15  Lateral head of gastrocnemius muscle
16  Common fibular nerve
17  Head of fibula
18  Lateral sural cutaneous nerves
19  Soleus muscle
20  Medial sural cutaneous nerve
21  Anterior tibial artery
22  Posterior tibial artery
23  Lateral sural cutaneous nerve

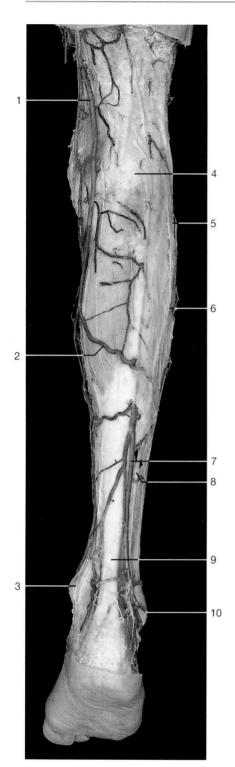

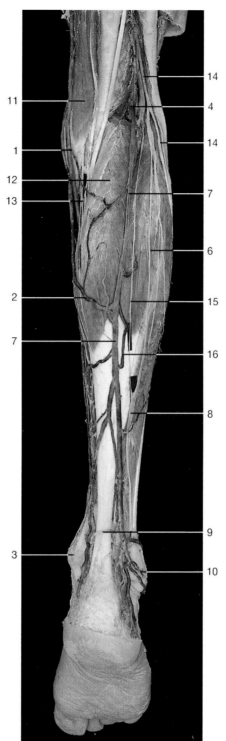

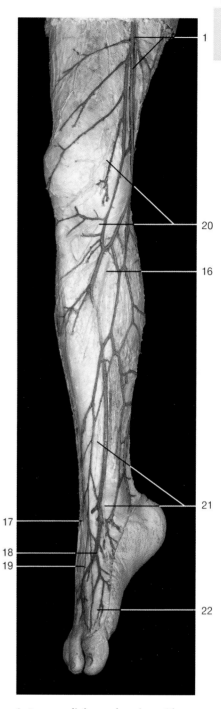

**Posterior crural region and popliteal fossa** with cutaneous veins and nerves (right side).

**Posterior crural region and popliteal fossa** with cutaneous veins and nerves (right side). The superficial layer of the crural fascia has been removed.

**Antero-medial crural region** with cutaneous veins and nerves (right side).

| | | | |
|---|---|---|---|
| 1 | Great saphenous vein | 8 | Sural nerve |
| 2 | Anastomosis between small and great saphenous veins | 9 | Calcaneal or Achilles tendon |
| | | 10 | Lateral malleolus |
| 3 | Medial malleolus | 11 | Semitendinosus muscle |
| 4 | Popliteal fossa | 12 | Medial head of gastrocnemius muscle |
| 5 | Position of head of fibula | 13 | Saphenous nerve |
| 6 | Lateral sural cutaneous nerve | 14 | Common fibular nerve |
| 7 | Small saphenous vein | 15 | Medial sural cutaneous nerve |

| | |
|---|---|
| 16 | Perforating veins |
| 17 | Superficial fibular nerve |
| 18 | Dorsal venous arch of foot |
| 19 | Intermediate dorsal cutaneous nerve |
| 20 | Infrapatellar branches of saphenous nerve |
| 21 | Terminal branches of saphenous nerve |
| 22 | Medial dorsal cutaneous nerve |

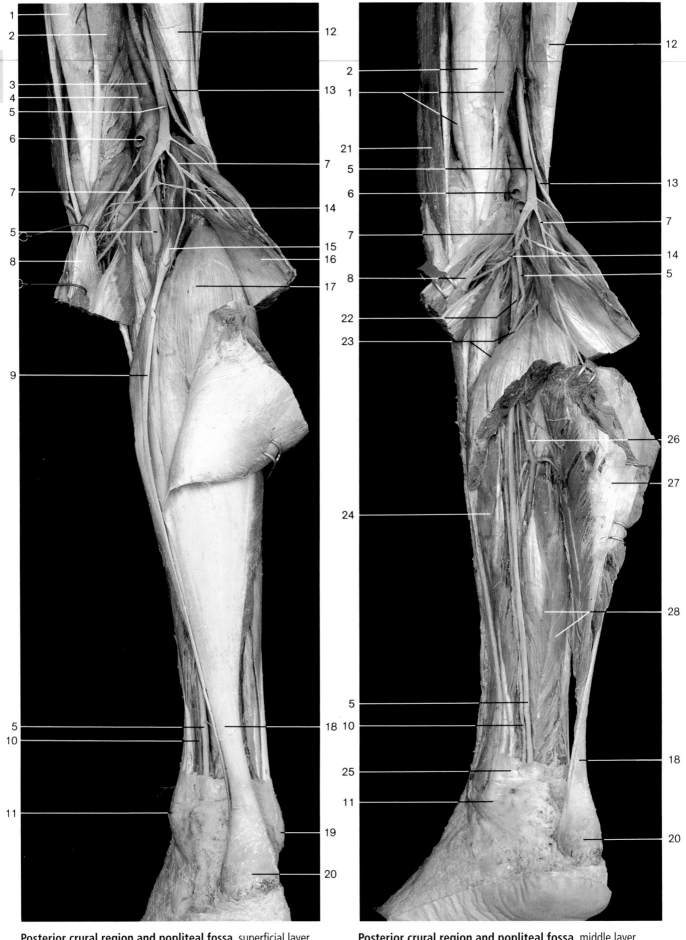

**Posterior crural region and popliteal fossa,** superficial layer (right side). The cutaneous veins and nerves have been removed.

**Posterior crural region and popliteal fossa,** middle layer (right side). The medial head of gastrocnemius muscle has been divided and reflected.

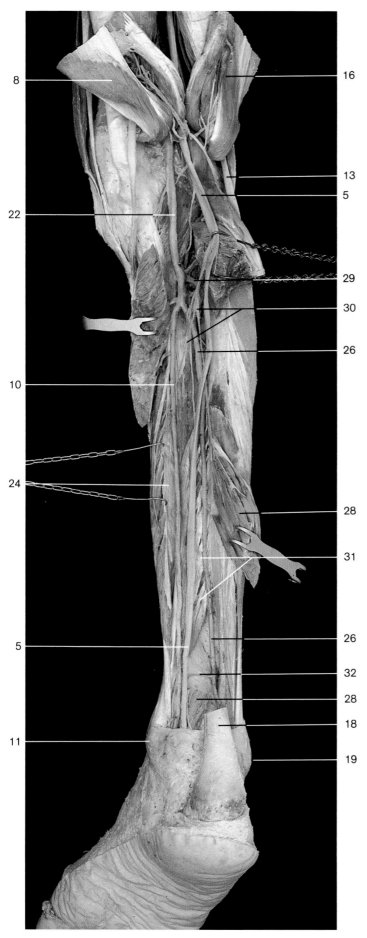

1  Semimembranosus muscle
2  Semitendinosus muscle
3  Popliteal vein
4  Popliteal artery
5  Tibial nerve
6  Small saphenous vein (cut)
7  Muscular branch of tibial nerve
8  Medial head of gastrocnemius muscle
9  Tendon of plantaris muscle
10  Posterior tibial artery
11  Medial malleolus
12  Biceps femoris muscle
13  Common fibular nerve
14  Sural arteries
15  Plantaris muscle
16  Lateral head of gastrocnemius muscle
17  Soleus muscle
18  Calcaneal or Achilles tendon
19  Lateral malleolus
20  Calcaneal tuberosity
21  Sartorius muscle
22  Popliteal artery
23  Tendinous arch of soleus muscle
24  Flexor digitorum longus muscle
25  Flexor retinaculum
26  Peroneal artery
27  Triceps surae muscle (cut)
28  Flexor hallucis longus muscle
29  Anterior tibial artery
30  Muscular branches of tibial nerve
31  Tibialis posterior muscle
32  Communicating branch of peroneal artery
33  Tendon of tibialis anterior muscle
34  Tibia
35  Tendon of extensor hallucis longus muscle
36  Tendons of extensor digitorum longus muscle
37  Anterior tibial artery
38  Fibula
39  Tendons of peroneus longus and brevis muscles

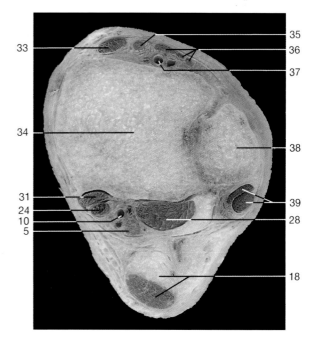

**Posterior crural region and popliteal fossa,** deep layer (right side). Triceps surae (gastrocnemius and soleus) and flexor hallucis longus muscles have been cut and reflected.

**Cross section through the leg,** superior to the malleoli (inferior aspect).

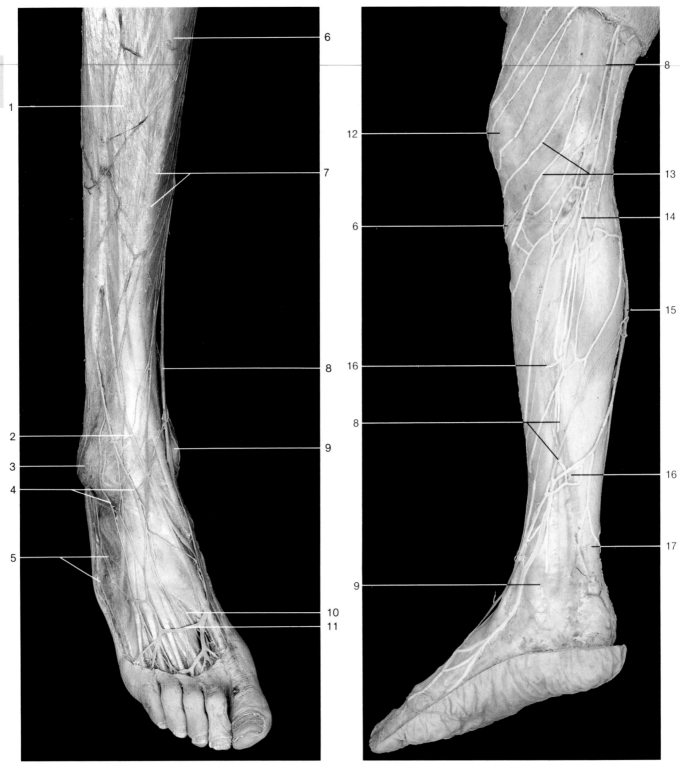

**Anterior crural region and dorsum of the foot** with cutaneous nerves and veins (right side).

**Medial crural region and foot** with cutaneous nerves and veins (right side).

1  Superficial crural fascia
2  Medial dorsal cutaneous branch of superficial fibular nerve
3  Lateral malleolus
4  Intermediate dorsal cutaneous branch of superficial fibular nerve
5  Lateral dorsal cutaneous branch of sural nerve
6  Position of tibial tuberosity
7  Anterior margin of tibia
8  Great saphenous vein
9  Medial malleolus

10  Deep fibular nerve
11  Dorsal venous arch of foot
12  Position of patella
13  Infrapatellar branches of saphenous nerve
14  Saphenous nerve
15  Small saphenous vein
16  Perforating vein
17  Calcaneal or Achilles tendon

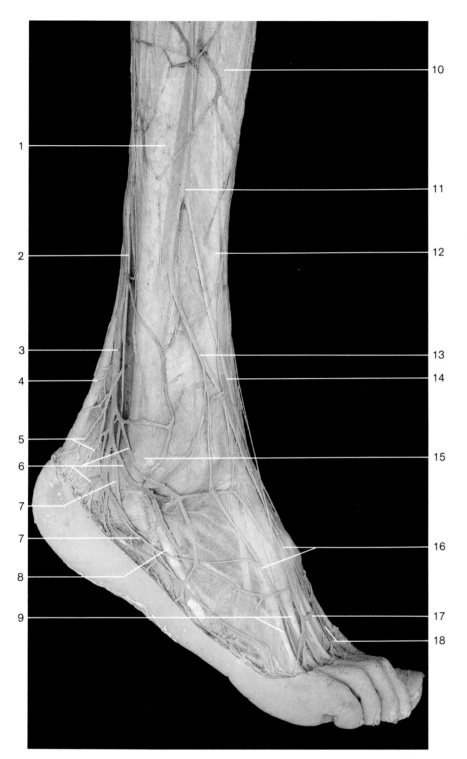

**Lateral crural region and foot** with cutaneous nerves and veins (right side).

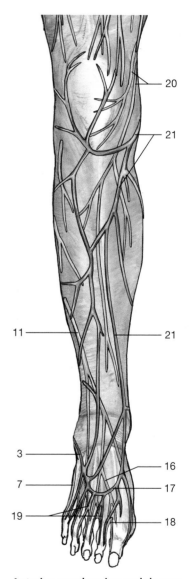

**Anterior crural region and dorsum of the foot** with cutaneous nerves and veins.

1   Position of fibula
2   Sural nerve
3   Small saphenous vein
4   Calcaneal or Achilles tendon
5   Lateral calcaneal branches
    of sural nerve
6   Venous plexus of lateral malleolus
7   Lateral dorsal cutaneous branch
    of sural nerve
8   Tendon of peroneus brevis muscle
9   Tendons of extensor digitorum
    longus muscle
10  Crural fascia

11  Superficial fibular nerve
12  Position of tibia
13  Intermediate dorsal cutaneous branch
    of superficial fibular nerve
14  Medial dorsal cutaneous branch
    of superficial fibular nerve
15  Lateral malleolus
16  Dorsal digital nerves
17  Dorsal venous arch of foot
18  Deep fibular nerve
19  Dorsal metatarsal veins
20  Saphenous nerve
21  Great saphenous vein

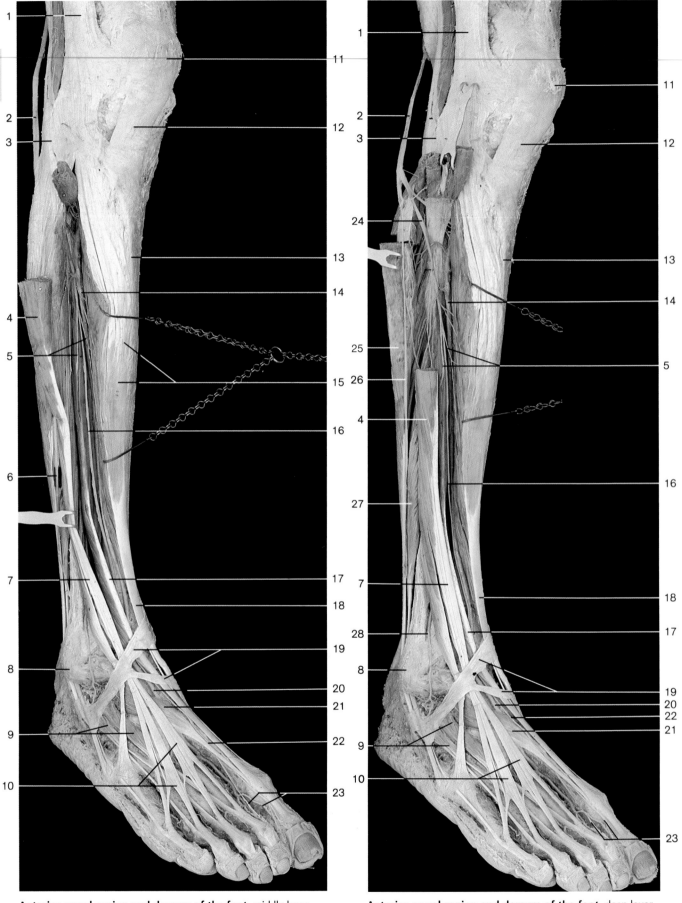

**Anterior crural region and dorsum of the foot,** middle layer
(right side, antero-lateral aspect). The extensor digitorum longus
muscle has been divided and reflected laterally.

**Anterior crural region and dorsum of the foot,** deep layer
(right side, antero-lateral aspect). Extensor digitorum longus
and peroneus longus muscles have been divided or removed.
The common fibular nerve has been elevated to show its course
around the head of fibula.

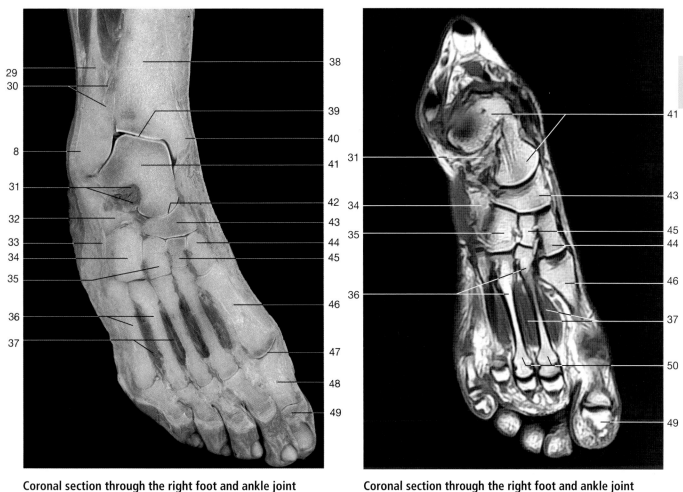

**Coronal section through the right foot and ankle joint** (dorsal aspect).

**Coronal section through the right foot and ankle joint** (MRI scan). (From Heuck et al., MRT-Atlas, 2009.)

**Synovial sheaths of extensor tendons** (dorsal aspect). The sheaths have been injected with blue gelatin.

| | |
|---|---|
| 1 Iliotibial tract | 29 Fibula |
| 2 Common fibular nerve | 30 Distal tibiofibular joint (syndesmosis) |
| 3 Position of head of fibula | 31 Talocalcaneal interosseous ligament |
| 4 Extensor digitorum longus muscle | 32 Calcaneus |
| 5 Muscular branches of deep fibular nerve | 33 Tendon of peroneus brevis muscle |
| 6 Superficial fibular nerve | 34 Cuboid bone |
| 7 Tendon of extensor digitorum longus muscle | 35 Lateral cuneiform bone |
| 8 Lateral malleolus | 36 Metatarsal bones |
| 9 Extensor digitorum brevis muscle with tendons | 37 Dorsal interossei muscles |
| 10 Tendons of extensor digitorum longus muscle | 38 Tibia |
| 11 Patella | 39 Ankle joint |
| 12 Patellar ligament | 40 Medial malleolus |
| 13 Anterior margin of tibia | 41 Talus |
| 14 Anterior tibial artery | 42 Talocalcaneonavicular joint |
| 15 Tibialis anterior muscle | 43 Navicular bone |
| 16 Deep fibular nerve | 44 Medial cuneiform bone |
| 17 Extensor hallucis longus muscle | 45 Intermediate cuneiform bone |
| 18 Tendon of tibialis anterior muscle | 46 First metatarsal bone |
| 19 Inferior extensor retinaculum | 47 Metatarsophalangeal joint of great toe |
| 20 Dorsalis pedis artery | 48 Proximal phalanx of great toe |
| 21 Extensor hallucis brevis muscle | 49 Distal phalanx of great toe |
| 22 Deep fibular nerve (on dorsum of foot) | 50 Heads of the second and third metatarsal bones |
| 23 Terminal branches of deep fibular nerve | 51 Synovial sheath of tendons of extensor digitorum longus muscle |
| 24 Deep fibular nerve | |
| 25 Peroneus longus muscle (cut) | 52 Synovial sheath of tendon of tibialis anterior muscle |
| 26 Superficial fibular nerve (with peroneal muscles laterally reflected) | |
| 27 Peroneus brevis muscle | 53 Synovial sheath of tendon of extensor hallucis longus muscle |
| 28 Lateral anterior malleolar artery | |

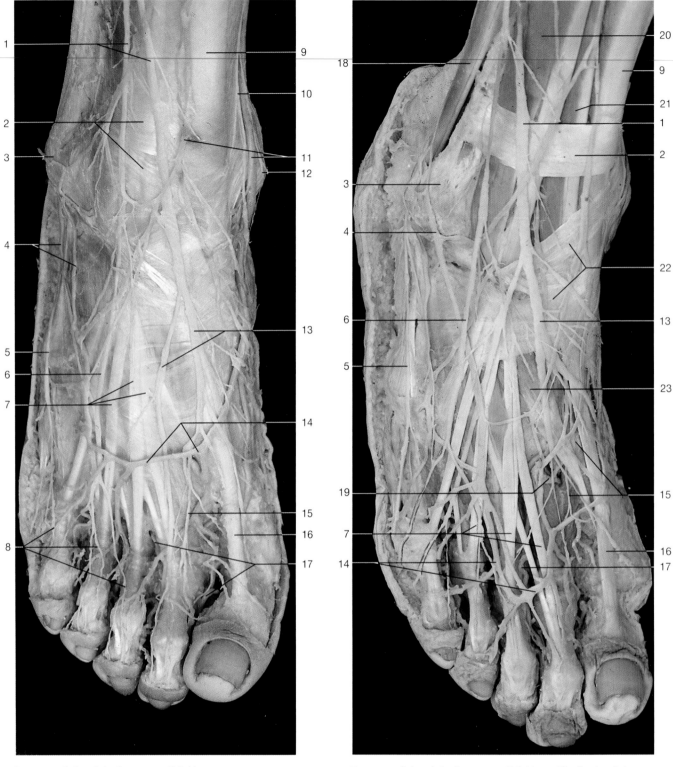

**Dorsum of the right foot,** superficial layer.

**Dorsum of the right foot,** superficial layer. The fascia of the dorsum has been removed.

| | | |
|---|---|---|
| 1 | Superficial fibular nerve | 9 | Tendon of tibialis anterior muscle | 17 | Dorsal digital arteries |
| 2 | Superior extensor retinaculum | 10 | Saphenous nerve | 18 | Peroneal muscles |
| 3 | Lateral malleolus | 11 | Venous network of medial malleolus and | 19 | Deep plantar branch |
| 4 | Venous network of lateral malleolus and | | tributaries of great saphenous vein | | of dorsalis pedis artery |
| | tributaries of small saphenous vein | 12 | Medial malleolus | | anastomosing with plantar arch |
| 5 | Lateral dorsal cutaneous branch | 13 | Medial dorsal cutaneous nerves | 20 | Extensor digitorum longus muscle |
| | of sural nerve | 14 | Dorsal venous arch of foot | 21 | Extensor hallucis longus muscle |
| 6 | Intermediate dorsal cutaneous nerve | 15 | Dorsal digital nerve | 22 | Inferior extensor retinaculum |
| 7 | Tendons of extensor digitorum longus muscle | | (of deep fibular nerve) | 23 | Extensor hallucis brevis muscle |
| 8 | Dorsal digital nerves | 16 | Tendon of extensor hallucis longus muscle | | |

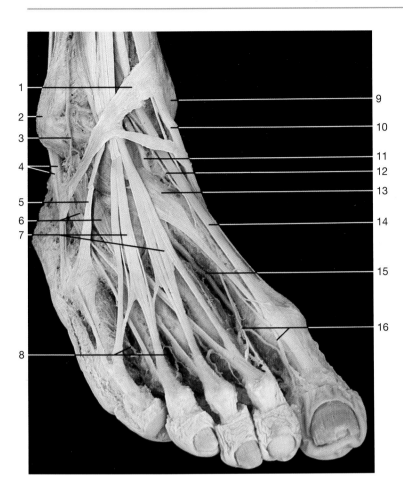

1   Inferior extensor retinaculum
2   Lateral malleolus
3   Lateral anterior malleolar artery
4   Tendons of peroneal muscles
5   Tendon of peroneus tertius muscle
6   Extensor digitorum brevis muscle
7   Tendons of extensor digitorum longus muscle
8   Dorsal metatarsal arteries
9   Medial malleolus
10  Tendon of tibialis anterior muscle
11  Dorsalis pedis artery
12  Deep fibular nerve (on dorsum of foot)
13  Extensor hallucis brevis muscle
14  Tendon of extensor hallucis longus muscle
15  Dorsalis pedis artery
    with deep plantar branch to the plantar arch
16  Terminal branches of deep fibular nerve
17  Lateral tarsal artery
18  Extensor digitorum brevis muscle (divided)
19  Arcuate artery
20  Dorsal interossei muscles
21  Deep fibular nerve

**Dorsum of the right foot,** middle layer. The cutaneous nerves have been removed.

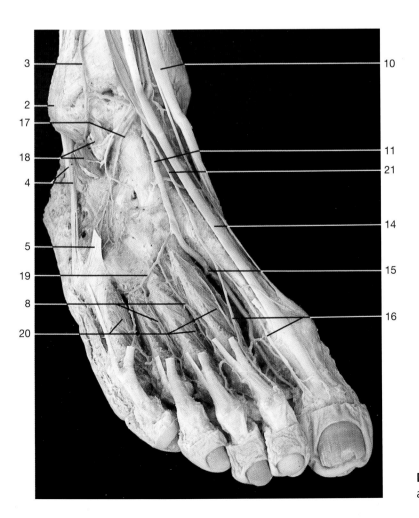

**Dorsum of the right foot,** deep layer. Extensor digitorum and hallucis brevis muscles have been removed.

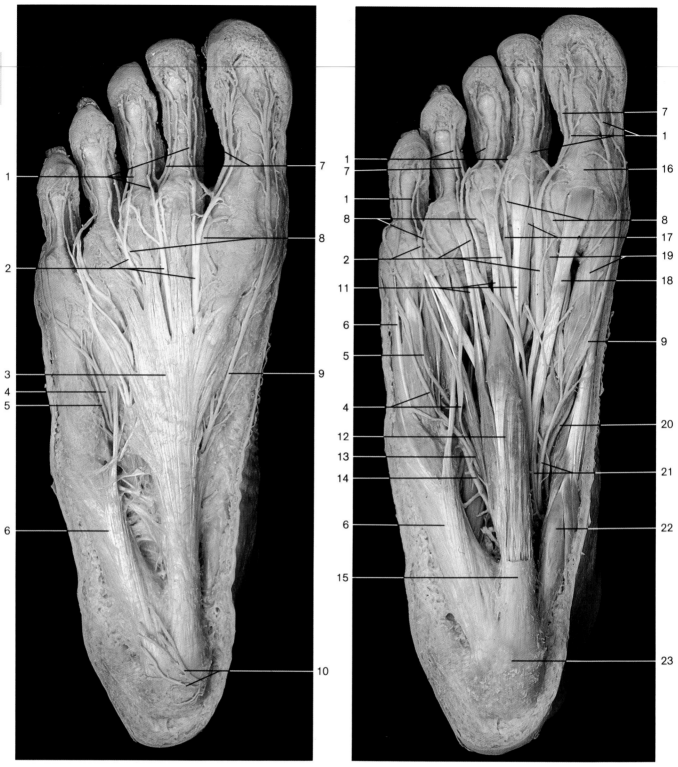

**Sole of the right foot,** superficial layer. Dissection of cutaneous nerves and vessels.

**Sole of the right foot,** middle layer. The plantar aponeurosis has been removed.

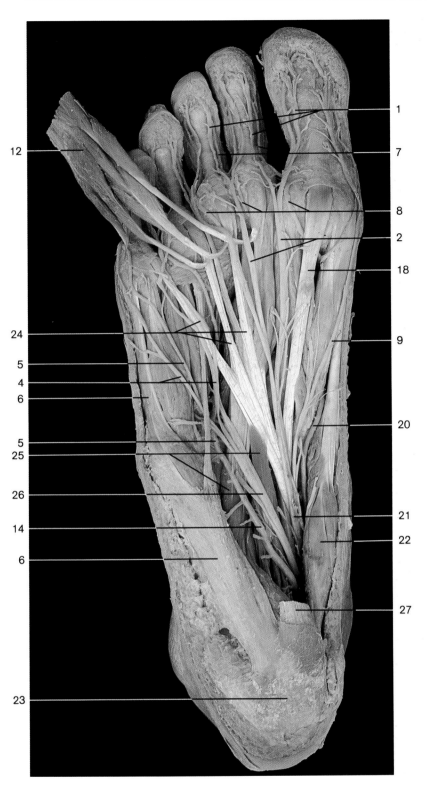

1   Proper plantar digital nerves
2   Common plantar digital nerves
3   Plantar aponeurosis
4   Superficial branch of lateral plantar nerve
5   Superficial branch of lateral plantar artery
6   Abductor digiti minimi muscle
7   Proper plantar digital arteries
8   Common plantar digital arteries
9   Digital branch of medial plantar nerve
    to great toe
10  Medial calcaneal branches
11  Tendons of flexor digitorum brevis muscle
12  Flexor digitorum brevis muscle
13  Superficial branch of lateral plantar nerve
14  Lateral plantar artery
15  Plantar aponeurosis (remnant)
16  Fibrous sheath of toe
17  Lumbrical muscles
18  Tendon of flexor hallucis longus muscle
19  Flexor hallucis brevis muscle
20  Medial plantar artery
21  Medial plantar nerve
22  Abductor hallucis muscle
23  Calcaneal tuberosity
24  Tendons of flexor digitorum longus muscle
25  Quadratus plantae muscle
26  Lateral plantar nerve
27  Flexor digitorum brevis muscle (cut)
28  Synovial sheaths of tendons
    of flexor digitorum longus and brevis muscles
29  Plantar arch
30  Deep branch of lateral plantar nerve

**Sole of the right foot,** middle layer. Dissection of vessels and nerves. The flexor digitorum brevis muscle has been divided and anteriorly reflected.

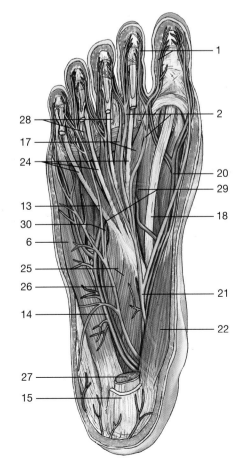

**Sole of the right foot** with vessels and nerves. The flexor digitorum brevis muscle has been removed. Light blue = synovial sheaths of flexor tendons.

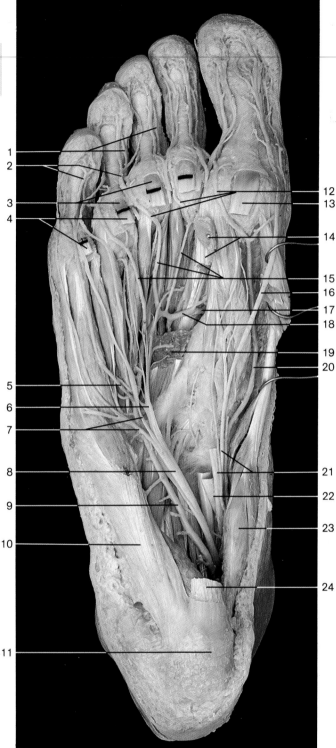

1   Proper plantar digital arteries
2   Proper plantar digital nerves
3   Tendons of flexor digitorum brevis muscle
4   Tendons of flexor digitorum longus muscle
5   Superficial branch of lateral plantar artery
6   Deep branch of lateral plantar nerve
7   Superficial branch of lateral plantar nerve
8   Lateral plantar nerve
9   Lateral plantar artery
10  Abductor digiti minimi muscle
11  Calcaneal tuberosity
12  Common plantar digital arteries
13  Tendon of flexor hallucis longus muscle
14  Insertion of both heads of adductor hallucis muscle
15  Plantar metatarsal arteries
16  Medial proper plantar digital nerve
17  Deep plantar branch of dorsal metatarsal artery
    (perforating branch)
18  Plantar arch
19  Oblique head of adductor hallucis muscle (cut)
20  Medial plantar artery
21  Medial plantar nerve
22  Crossing of tendons in the sole of foot
    (flexor hallucis longus and flexor digitorum longus muscles)
23  Abductor hallucis muscle
24  Origin of flexor hallucis brevis muscle
25  Medial cuneiform and first metatarsal bones
26  Tendon of peroneus longus muscle
27  Abductor hallucis and flexor hallucis brevis muscles
28  Medial plantar artery, vein, and nerve
29  Fourth and fifth metatarsal bones
30  Lateral plantar artery, vein, and nerve
31  Flexor digitorum brevis muscle
32  Plantar aponeurosis

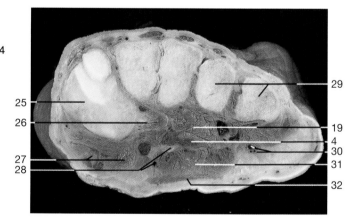

**Sole of the right foot,** deep layer. Dissection of vessels and nerves. The flexor digitorum brevis muscle, the quadratus plantae muscle with the tendons of the flexor digitorum longus muscle, and some branches of the medial plantar nerve have been removed. The flexor hallucis brevis and adductor hallucis muscles have been cut and portions removed to show the somewhat atypical course of the medial plantar artery and deep muscles of the foot.

**Cross section through the right foot** at the level of the metatarsal bones (posterior aspect).

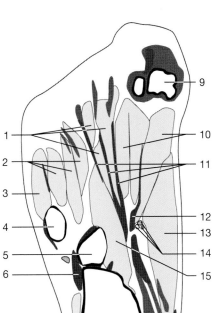

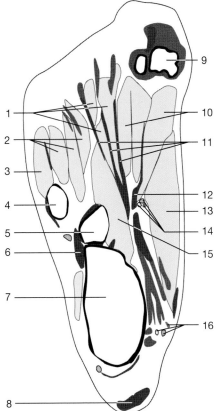

**Sole of the right foot** (MRI scan). (From Heuck et al., MRT-Atlas, 2009.) For details see schematic drawing alongside.

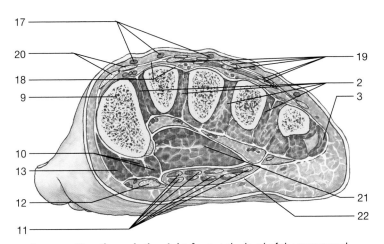

**Cross section through the right foot** at the level of the metatarsal bones (posterior aspect; compare with the dissection on the previous page).

1 Lumbrical muscles
2 Plantar interossei muscles
3 Abductor digiti minimi muscle
4 Tuberosity of fifth metatarsal bone
5 Cuboid bone
6 Tendon of peroneus longus muscle
7 Calcaneus
8 Calcaneal or Achilles tendon
9 First metatarsal bone
10 Flexor hallucis brevis muscle
11 Tendons of flexor digitorum longus and brevis muscles
12 Tendon of flexor hallucis longus muscle
13 Abductor hallucis muscle
14 Medial plantar artery, vein, and nerve
15 Quadratus plantae muscle
16 Lateral plantar artery, vein, and nerve
17 Dorsal venous network of foot
18 Superficial and deep dorsal fascia of foot
19 Tendons of extensor digitorum longus and brevis muscles
20 Tendons of extensor hallucis longus and brevis muscles
21 Adductor hallucis muscle
22 Plantar aponeurosis

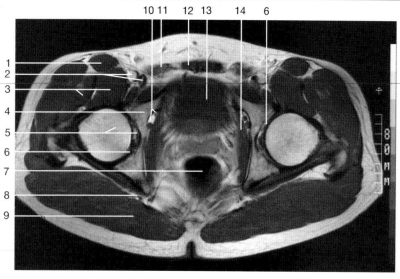

Axial section through the pelvis at the level of the hip joints. Section 1 (MRI scan, inferior aspect).

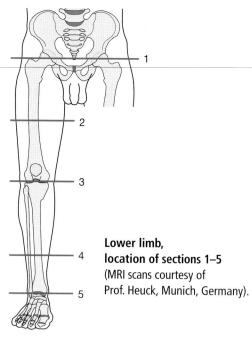

**Lower limb,
location of sections 1–5**
(MRI scans courtesy of
Prof. Heuck, Munich, Germany).

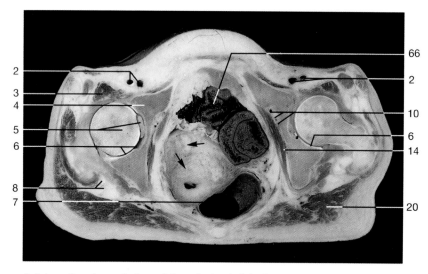

Axial section through the pelvis at the level of the hip joints in a female. Section 1 (inferior aspect). Arrows: uterus (myometrium with myoma).

1   Sartorius muscle
2   Femoral artery and vein
3   Iliopsoas muscle
4   Pubis
5   Head of femur with ligament of head of femur
6   Articular cavity
7   Rectum
8   Sciatic nerve and accompanying artery
9   Gluteus maximus muscle
10  Obturator artery, vein, and nerve
11  Rectus abdominis muscle
12  Pyramidalis muscle
13  Urinary bladder
14  Obturator internus muscle
15  Rectus femoris muscle
16  Vastus intermedius and vastus lateralis muscles
    of quadriceps femoris muscle

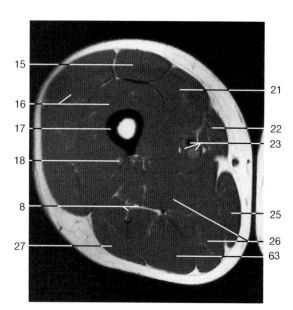

Axial section through the middle of the right thigh. Section 2 (MRI scan, inferior aspect).

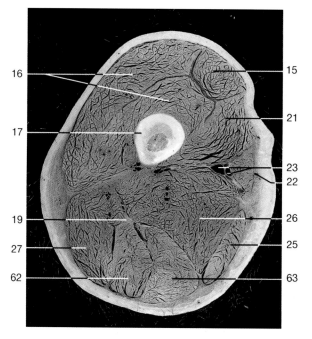

Axial section through the middle of the right thigh. Section 2 (inferior aspect).

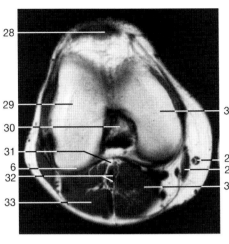

**Axial section through the right knee joint.** Section 3 (MRI scan, inferior aspect).

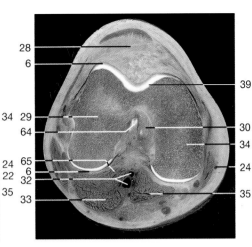

**Axial section through the right knee joint.** Section 3 (inferior aspect).

17  Femur
18  Perforating artery
19  Sciatic nerve
20  Gluteus maximus muscle (insertion)
21  Vastus medialis muscle
22  Sartorius muscle
23  Femoral artery and vein
24  Great saphenous vein
25  Gracilis muscle
26  Adductor muscles
27  Biceps femoris muscle
28  Patellar ligament
29  Lateral condyle of femur
30  Posterior cruciate ligament
31  Tibial nerve
32  Popliteal artery and vein
33  Lateral head
    of gastrocnemius muscle
34  Medial condyle of femur
35  Medial head
    of gastrocnemius muscle
36  Tibialis anterior muscle
37  Tibia
38  Deep fibular nerve,
    anterior tibial artery, and vein
39  Patellar surface
40  Peroneus longus and brevis muscles
41  Fibula
42  Soleus muscle
43  Flexor digitorum longus muscle
44  Tibialis posterior muscle
45  Posterior tibial artery and vein,
    and tibial nerve
46  Peroneal artery
47  Small saphenous vein and
    sural nerve
48  Extensor hallucis longus muscle
49  Extensor digitorum longus muscle
50  Tendon of peroneus longus muscle
51  Lateral malleolus of fibula
52  Peroneus brevis muscle
53  Tendon of tibialis anterior muscle
54  Dorsalis pedis artery
55  Medial malleolus of tibia
56  Tendon of tibialis posterior muscle
57  Tendon of flexor digitorum longus
    muscle with synovial sheath
58  Flexor hallucis longus muscle
59  Posterior tibial artery and vein
60  Lateral and medial plantar nerves
61  Calcaneal or Achilles tendon
62  Semitendinosus muscle
63  Semimembranosus muscle
64  Anterior cruciate ligament
65  Plantaris muscle
66  Small intestine

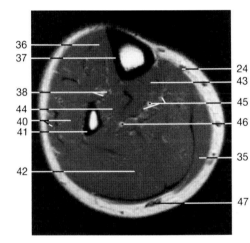

**Axial section through the middle of the right leg.** Section 4 (MRI scan, inferior aspect).

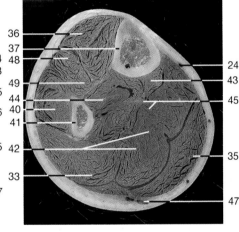

**Axial section through the middle of the right leg.** Section 4 (inferior aspect).

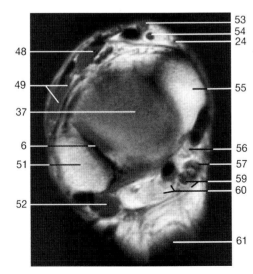

**Axial section through the end of the right leg.** Section 5 (MRI scan, inferior aspect).

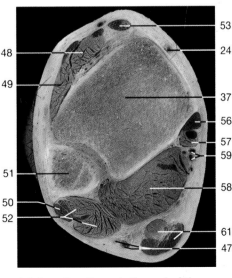

**Axial section through the end of the right leg.** Section 5 (inferior aspect).

# Index

Page numbers in **bold** indicate main discussions.

Page numbers in **bold** indicate main discussions.

Page numbers in **bold** indicate main discussions.

Page numbers in **bold** indicate main discussions.

Page numbers in **bold** indicate main discussions.

Page numbers in **bold** indicate main discussions.

Page numbers in **bold** indicate main discussions.

Page numbers in **bold** indicate main discussions.

Page numbers in **bold** indicate main discussions.

Page numbers in **bold** indicate main discussions.

Page numbers in **bold** indicate main discussions.

Page numbers in **bold** indicate main discussions.

Page numbers in **bold** indicate main discussions.

Page numbers in **bold** indicate main discussions.

Page numbers in **bold** indicate main discussions.

Page numbers in **bold** indicate main discussions.

Page numbers in **bold** indicate main discussions.

Page numbers in **bold** indicate main discussions.

Page numbers in **bold** indicate main discussions.

Page numbers in **bold** indicate main discussions.

Page numbers in **bold** indicate main discussions.

Page numbers in **bold** indicate main discussions.

Page numbers in **bold** indicate main discussions.

Page numbers in **bold** indicate main discussions.

Page numbers in **bold** indicate main discussions.

Page numbers in **bold** indicate main discussions.

Page numbers in **bold** indicate main discussions.

Page numbers in **bold** indicate main discussions.

Page numbers in **bold** indicate main discussions.

Page numbers in **bold** indicate main discussions.

Page numbers in **bold** indicate main discussions.